Handbook of Hematology and Oncology

Handbook of Hematology and Oncology

Editor: Dylan Hill

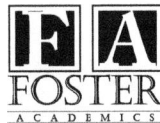

FA
FOSTER
ACADEMICS

www.fosteracademics.com

www.fosteracademics.com

FA
FOSTER
ACADEMICS

Cataloging-in-Publication Data

Handbook of hematology and oncology / edited by Dylan Hill.
      p. cm.
Includes bibliographical references and index.
ISBN 978-1-63242-940-7
1. Hematology. 2. Oncology. 3. Blood--Diseases. 4. Cancer. 5. Leukemia. I. Hill, Dylan.
RC636 .H36 2020
616.15--dc23

Foster Academics,
118-35 Queens Blvd., Suite 400,
Forest Hills, NY 11375, USA

ISBN 978-1-63242-940-7 (Hardback)

Contents

Preface

Hematology is the branch of medicine that delves on the study of the cause, prognosis, treatment, and prevention of diseases related to blood. Such diseases include hemophilia, blood clots, other bleeding disorders and blood cancers such as lymphoma, leukemia and multiple myeloma. These diseases affect the production of blood and its components such as hemoglobin, platelets, bone marrow, blood vessels, blood cells, etc. Oncology is a branch of medicine that involves the prevention, diagnosis, and treatment of cancer. Blood cancer is caused when tumors of the hematopoietic and lymphoid tissues or lymphoid malignancies affect the blood, lymph, lymphatic system and bone marrow. Bleeding manifestations such as blood vomiting, bleeding gums, bloodstained urine, etc. are some common symptoms of blood cancer. This book is a valuable compilation of topics, ranging from the basic to the most complex advancements in the fields of hematology and oncology. From theories to research to practical applications, case studies related to all contemporary topics of relevance have been included in it. Students, researchers, experts and all associated with these fields of study will benefit alike from this book.

The information contained in this book is the result of intensive hard work done by researchers in this field. All due efforts have been made to make this book serve as a complete guiding source for students and researchers. The topics in this book have been comprehensively explained to help readers understand the growing trends in the field.

I would like to thank the entire group of writers who made sincere efforts in this book and my family who supported me in my efforts of working on this book. I take this opportunity to thank all those who have been a guiding force throughout my life.

Editor

miR-519a enhances chemosensitivity and promotes autophagy in glioblastoma by targeting STAT3/Bcl2 signaling pathway

Hong Li[1†], Lei Chen[2†], Jun-jie Li[2], Qiang Zhou[2], Annie Huang[5], Wei-wen Liu[6], Ke Wang[1], Liang Gao[1], Song-tao Qi[2,3,4] and Yun-tao Lu[2,3,4*]

Abstract

Background: Chemoresistance to temozolomide (TMZ) is a major challenge in the treatment of glioblastoma (GBM). We previously found that *miR-519a* functions as a tumor suppressor in glioma by targeting the signal transducer and activator of transcription 3 (STAT3)-mediated autophagy oncogenic pathway. Here, we investigated the effects of *miR-519a* on TMZ chemosensitivity and autophagy in GBM cells. Furthermore, the underlying molecular mechanisms and signaling pathways were explored.

Methods: In the present study, two stable TMZ-resistant GBM cell lines were successfully generated by exposure of parental cells to a gradually increasing TMZ concentration. After transfecting U87-MG/TMZ and U87-MG cells with *miR-519a* mimic or inhibitor, a series of biochemical assays such as MTT, apoptosis, and colony formation were performed to determine the chemosensitive response to TMZ. The autophagy levels in GBM cells were detected by transmission electron microscopy, LC3B protein immunofluorescence, and Western blotting analysis. Stable knockdown and overexpression of *miR-519a* in GBM cells were established using lentivirus. A xenograft nude mouse model and in situ brain model were used to examine the in vivo effects of *miR-519a*. Tumor tissue samples were collected from 48 patients with GBM and were used to assess the relationship between *miR-519a* and STAT3 expression.

Results: TMZ treatment significantly upregulated *miR-519a* in U87-MG cells but not in U87-MG/TMZ cells. Moreover, the expression of *miR-519a* and baseline autophagy levels was lower in U87-MG/TMZ cells as compared to U87-MG cells. *miR-519a* dramatically enhanced TMZ-induced autophagy and apoptotic cell death in U87-MG/TMZ cells, while inhibition of *miR-519a* promoted TMZ resistance and reduced TMZ-induced autophagy in U87-MG cells. Furthermore, *miR-519a* induced autophagy through modification of STAT3 expression. The in vivo results showed that *miR-519a* can enhance apoptosis and sensitized GBM to TMZ treatment by promoting autophagy and targeting the STAT3/Bcl-2/Beclin-1 pathway. In human GBM tissues, we found an inverse correlation between *miR-519a* and STAT3 expression.

Conclusions: Our results suggested that *miR-519a* increased the sensitivity of GBM cells to TMZ therapy. The positive effects of *miR-519a* may be mediated through autophagy. In addition, *miR-519a* overexpression can induce autophagy by inhibiting STAT3/Bcl-2 pathway. Therefore, a combination of *miR-519a* and TMZ may represent an effective therapeutic strategy in GBM.

Keywords: *miR-519a*, Signal transducer and activator of transcription 3, Glioblastoma, Autophagy, Chemoresistance

* Correspondence: lllu2000yun@gmail.com
†Hong Li and Lei Chen contributed equally to this work.
[2]Department of Neurosurgery, Nanfang Hospital, Southern Medical University, Guangzhou 510515, Guangdong Province, People's Republic of China
[3]Nanfang Neurology Research Institution, Nanfang Hospital, Guangzhou 510515, Guangdong Province, People's Republic of China
Full list of author information is available at the end of the article

Background

Glioblastoma (GBM) is the most common primary malignant brain tumor in adults [1]. Multimodality treatment such as cytoreductive surgery followed by radiotherapy with concomitant and adjuvant temozolomide (TMZ) chemotherapy has been widely accepted as the new standard of care for patients with newly diagnosed GBM. However, the prognosis of TMZ-treated patients remains dismal, with a median survival of 12.1–14.6 months [2–4]. Intrinsic or acquired chemoresistance to TMZ is a major clinical obstacle for the treatment of GBM patients. Therefore, a better understanding of the molecular mechanisms underlying TMZ chemoresistance may lead to improved clinical outcomes in GBM patients.

Recently, several studies have shown that anticancer therapies can induce autophagy, which constitutes a novel mechanism of chemoresistance in cancer [5–8]. Autophagy is a highly evolutionarily conserved process that occurs in virtually all eukaryotic cells and has been implicated in various physiological and pathological conditions [9]. In some cases, autophagy induces apoptotic death in GBM cells upon TMZ treatment, and treatment with autophagy inducer rapamycin can further enhance chemotherapy-induced apoptosis [10–14]. In other cases, TMZ-induced autophagy may delay cell death [15–17]. Therefore, modulation of autophagy in response to TMZ treatment may hold great promise for circumventing chemotherapeutic resistance and improving anticancer efficacy in GBM patients. However, the roles of autophagy in regulating GBM cell death and survival remain controversial.

MicroRNAs (miRs) are small, non-coding RNA molecules (20–22 nucleotides in length) that negatively regulate gene expression by binding to the 3′-untranslated region (3′UTR) of target mRNAs [18]. miRs have been shown to be key players in a wide range of biological processes, including proliferation, apoptosis, and migration [19]. Recent evidence has indicated that miRs can regulate the chemosensitivity of glioma cells to TMZ by modulating autophagy signaling [20]. Previously, we demonstrated that miR-519a is closely related to improved prognosis of GBM patients [21]. However, the molecular mechanisms underlying the role of miR-519a in the chemoresistance of GBM remain unclear.

Signal transducer and activator of transcription 3 (STAT3) functions as a signal messenger and transcription factor, which regulates the transcription of downstream target genes during malignant transformation and tumor development. Several studies have demonstrated that STAT3 overexpression in glioma cells can promote tumor progression [22–24]. A growing body of evidence has implicated STAT3 in the regulation of autophagy, from the assembly of autophagosomes to their maturation [25]. In addition, differential localization of STAT3 may regulate autophagy in distinct ways [25]. For instance, nuclear STAT3 may upregulate BCL2 expression and lead to autophagy inhibition [26]. Therefore, a better understanding of the role of STAT3 signaling in regulating autophagy may provide new insights into the mechanisms of chemoresistance and the potential strategies to overcome TMZ chemoresistance in GBM.

In the present study, we evaluated whether miR-519a can affect the chemosensitivity of TMZ in GBM. Furthermore, the roles of miR-519a in the modulation of autophagy via STAT3/Bcl-2/Beclin-1 signaling pathway were investigated.

Methods

Cell lines and reagents

U87-MG cells were obtained from the Cell Bank of the Chinese Academy of Sciences (Shanghai, China) and were cultured in Dulbecco's modified Eagle's medium (DMEM) with 10% fetal bovine serum (FBS; Gibco, Carlsbad, CA, USA), 100 U/mL penicillin, and 100 mg/mL streptomycin (Gibco) at 37 °C in a humidified incubator with 5% CO_2. The methods for culturing patient-derived GBM cell line G131212 were described previously [21]. TMZ-resistant cell lines were generated by iterative pulse exposure of U87-MG and G131212 GBM cells to TMZ. The derived resistant cell lines were designated as U87-MG/TMZ and G131212/TMZ, respectively. Meanwhile, a stock solution of TMZ (100 mM; cat. no. T2577; Sigma-Aldrich, St. Louis, MO, USA) was dissolved in dimethylsulfoxide (DMSO; cat. no. D2650; Sigma-Aldrich) and stored at − 20 °C. 3-Methyladenine (3-MA; cat. no. M9281; Sigma-Aldrich) was prepared freshly in DMEM at 60 °C and then diluted to 5 mM before use.

Oligonucleotides and siRNA transfection

The miRNA mimic, miRNA inhibitor, STAT3 siRNA, and scrambled siRNA were synthesized by RiBoBio (China). The oligonucleotide sequences were listed in Table S1 (Additional file 1: Table S1). The miRNA overexpression vector pCMV-MIR519A (MI0003182) and the empty vector control were obtained from OriGene (Rockville, MD, USA). The miR-519a sponge and empty vector control were purchased from GeneChem (China). Transfections were performed using Lipofectamine 2000 reagent (cat. no. 11668-019; Invitrogen, Carlsbad, CA, USA) according to the manufacturer's instructions.

Cell viability assay

Cell viability was assessed by using MTT assays. First, cells were seeded in 96-well plates at a density of 8000 cells per well. After an overnight incubation, the cells were treated under the indicated conditions. At the end of the treatment, 0.5 mg/mL MTT was added to each well and incubated for 4 h. Then, the supernatants were aspirated carefully, and formazan crystals were dissolved in DMSO. Finally, the absorbance was measured at 550 nm using Thermo Varioskan Flash reader (Thermo Fisher Scientific, Waltham, MA, USA).

Colony forming cell assay

Cells (200 cells/well) were seeded onto 6-well culture plates and cultured in DMEM supplemented with 10% FBS. The cells were treated with the indicated agents and incubated for 10–14 days at 37 °C and 5% CO_2. Colonies were then stained with 0.1% crystal violet (Sigma-Aldrich) and counted. In some experiments, cells were pre-treated for 1 h with 3-MA (Sigma-Aldrich) or rapamycin (Abcam, San Francisco, CA, USA), followed by an incubation period of 24 h. For each set of clones, three independent assays were carried out.

Cell apoptosis assay

GBM cells were transfected with miRNAs (or anti-miRNAs) and/or incubated with 400 μM TMZ for 36 h. Subsequently, cells were harvested and stained with propidium iodide (PI) and annexin V-fluorescein isothiocyanate (FITC) for apoptotic analysis. The percentage of apoptotic cells was calculated as the sum of early and late apoptotic cells located in the lower and upper right quadrants, respectively.

Green fluorescent protein-LC3 puncta assay

GBM green fluorescent protein (GFP)-LC3 stable cells were transfected with miRNAs or anti-miRNAs. Two days after the transfection, cells were fixed with 4% paraformaldehyde. GFP-LC3 dot formation was observed under a confocal laser scanning microscope (FLUOVIEW FV10i; Olympus, Japan). The average number of GFP-LC3 dots/cell was counted in at least 200 cells.

Transmission electron microscopy (TEM)

GBM cells were subjected to different treatments. The freshly harvested tumors from mice were fixed overnight with 2.5% glutaraldehyde at 4 °C and post-fixed in 1% osmic acid. The fixed samples were then dehydrated using a graded series of ethanol (70–100%) and embedded in EPON resin. Ultrathin sections were cut with an ultramicrotome and double-stained with uranyl acetate and lead citrate. The stained sections were then examined using a TEM (H-7650; Hitachi, Tokyo, Japan).

Construction of stable lentiviral clones

Lentiviral expressing GFP empty vector (NC-LV), GFP vector overexpressing *miR-519a* (LV-*miR-519a*), or GFP vector inhibiting *miR-519a* expression (LV-anti-*miR-519a*) was constructed by Systems Biosciences Inc. (Mountain View, CA, USA). Virus production and cell transduction in GBM cells were performed as previously described [21],

and cells were selected in puromycin (1 μg/mL). The selected cells were sorted by flow cytometry to maintain a GFP-positive rate for at least 95%.

Western blotting

Western blotting was performed as described previously [27]. The antibodies including anti-LC3B (cat. no. 4445), anti-BECN1/Beclin (cat. no. 3495), anti-STAT3 (cat. no. 12640), anti-phospho-STAT3 (Tyr705; cat. no. 9145), and anti-CASP3/caspase-3 (cat. no. 9915) were purchased from Cell Signaling Technology, while anti-Bax (cat. no. sc-7480) and anti-Bcl-2 (cat. no. sc-509) were obtained from Santa Cruz Biotechnology, Santa Cruz, CA, USA.

RNA isolation and quantitative reverse transcription polymerase chain reaction

Total miRNA from cultured cells was extracted using TRIzol reagent (cat. no. 15596-026; Invitrogen), and the RNA purity was evaluated by A260/A280 ratio of 1.9–2.0. cDNA was synthesized from 1 μg of total RNA using PrimeScript RT reagent kit (cat. no. RR047A; Takara, Shiga, Japan). The primers used for PCR amplification were listed in Table S2 (Additional file 2: Table S2). The expression levels of target genes were quantified on a Stratagene Mx-3005p instrument (Agilent Technologies Inc., USA) by using Maxima SYBR Green/ROX qPCR Master Mix (cat. no. K0222; Thermo Scientific). Triplicate samples were examined.

Tumor xenograft assays in nude mice

BALB/c nude mice (4–5 weeks old) were provided by the Experimental Animal Center of Southern Medical University. U87-MG cells with stable expression of lentivirus *miR-519a* or U87-MG/TMZ cells with stable expression of *miR-519a* shRNA were injected into the left flank of the mice, while control cells were injected into the right flank of the mice. Mice were injected intraperitoneally (i.p.) with phosphate-buffered saline alone (control) or TMZ (Merck Co., NJ, USA; 20 mg/kg/mouse) once every other day for 3 weeks, starting on day 3. Tumor volume and animal weight were assessed every 4 days. Tumor volume was calculated using the following formula: volume $(mm^3) = 4/3 \times 3.14 \times$ radius $(mm)^3$. Mice were humanely sacrificed on day 24. Tissue blocks were subjected to immunohistochemical staining and TEM analysis.

For survival analysis in the orthotopic xenograft model, nude mice were randomly divided into four groups: LV-anti-*miR-519a* group, LV-anti-NC group, LV-anti-NC+TMZ group, and LV-anti-*miR-519a*+TMZ group. In this model, 3×10^5 cells were stereotactically implanted into the right striatum of the mice. Twenty four days after injection, tumor burden of mice was assessed using magnetic resonance imaging (MRI) scanner (Bruker Medical Inc., Billerica, MA, USA). The

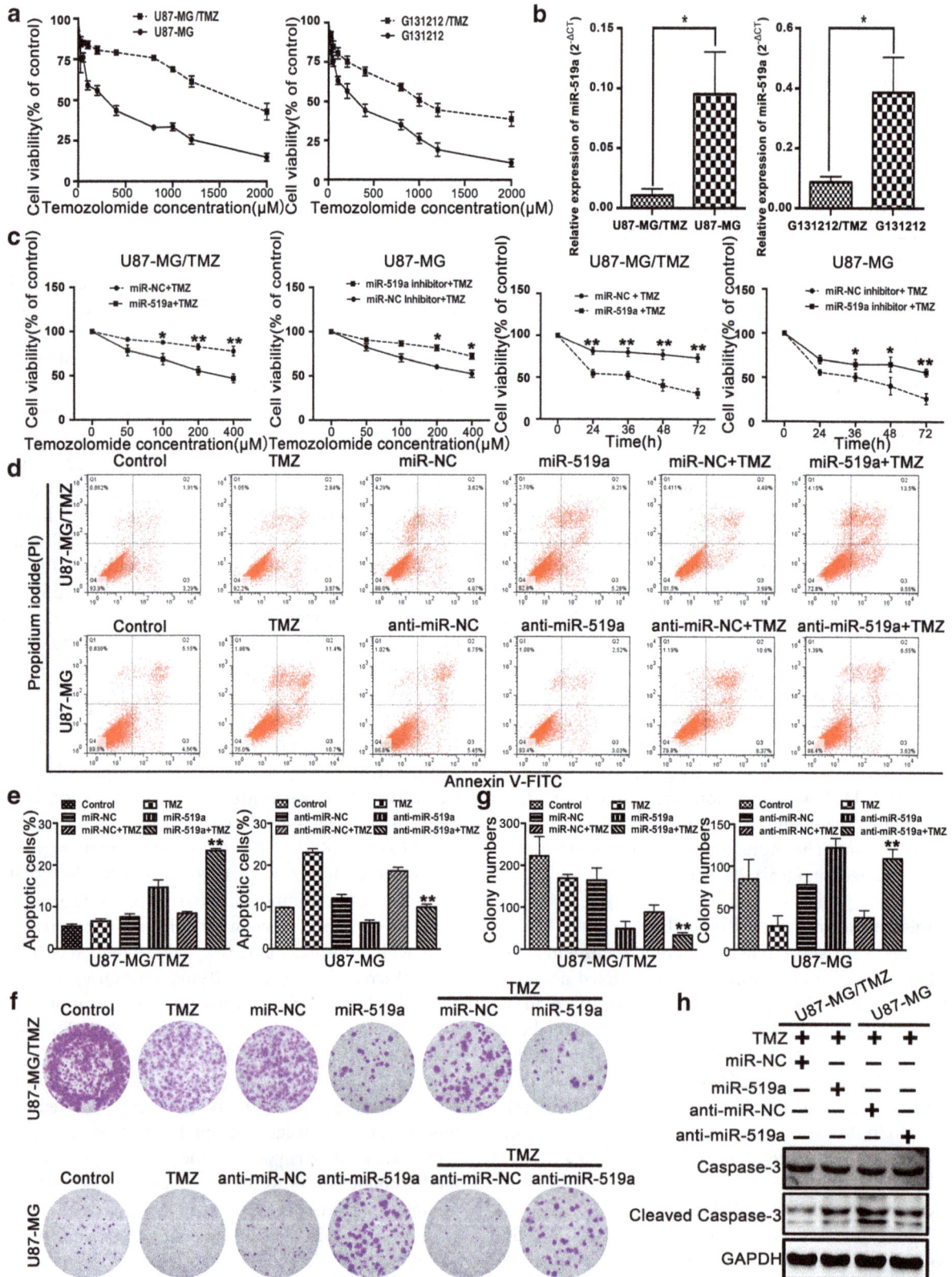

Fig. 1 (See legend on next page.)

number of surviving nude mice was recorded, and survival analysis was performed by Kaplan-Meier survival curves.

Patient samples

In this study, 24 patients with recurrent GBM treated with TMZ before second surgery and 24 patients with primary GBM without TMZ treatment were recruited from Nanfang Hospital (Guangzhou, China). Tissue samples were retrieved from the Department of Pathology and subjected to sectioning process. Subsequently, the tissue sections were fixed and immunohistochemically stained with anti-LC3B anti-STAT3, and anti-CASP3/caspase-3 antibodies (cat. no. 4445, 12649, and 9915, respectively; Cell Signaling Technology, Danvers, MA, USA).

Statistical analysis

All experiments were performed in triplicate and repeated at least once. All data were expressed as means ± standard deviation. If the homogeneity of variance assumption was met, one-way analysis of variance (ANOVA) was performed to determine the differences between groups, while least significant difference (LSD) test was used to compare the means of two groups. If the variance was heterogeneous, Welch test was applied to compare the differences between groups, while Dunnett's T3 test was used for pairwise comparisons. p values of less than 0.05 were considered statistically significant.

Results

miR-519a sensitized GBM cells to TMZ treatment

A stable TMZ-resistant phenotype of parental U87-MG cells (a GBM cell line) and G131212 cells (patient-derived GBM cells) was established by repetitive pulse exposure to increasing concentrations of TMZ for 6 months [28]. Both TMZ-resistant U87-MG/TMZ and G131212/TMZ cells exhibited lower sensitivity to TMZ and lower proliferation doubling times than the respective parental cells (Fig. 1a and Additional file 3: Figure S1).

To determine the effect of *miR-519a* on the chemosensitivity of TMZ, we first examined the expression levels of *miR-519a* in resistant sublines. As shown in Fig. 1b, the expression of *miR-519a* was lower in the resistant U87-MG/TMZ and G131212/TMZ cells compared to their

respective parental sensitive cells. Moreover, TMZ may induce the expression of *miR-519a* in U87-MG cells but not in U87-MG/TMZ cells (Additional file 4: Figure S2).

To further confirm the role of *miR-519a* in TMZ chemoresistance of GBM cells, we transiently transfected U87-MG (or U87-MG/TMZ) cells with *miR-519a* inhibitor (or *miR-519a* mimic) and evaluated the effects of miR by using MTT and clonogenic assays. We found that *miR-519a* sensitized the U87-MG/TMZ cells to TMZ and confirmed that anti-*miR-519a* induced TMZ resistance in U87-MG cells (Fig. 1c). The results of flow cytometry analysis revealed that *miR-519a* overexpression significantly increased GBM cell apoptosis caused by TMZ treatment, whereas downregulation of *miR-519a* inhibited TMZ-induced apoptosis in U87-MG cells (Fig. 1d, e). Colony formation in U87-MG/TMZ cells was markedly lower than that in the control group, while higher colony formation was found in U87-MG cells (Fig. 1f). These results were validated by using the overexpressing vector pCMV-MIR-519a or the inhibition vector *miR-519a* sponge (Additional file 5: Figure S3).

Furthermore, Western blot analysis showed that TMZ-induced cellular apoptosis was greatly enhanced by *miR-519a* compared to NC, while knockdown of endogenous *miR-519a* decreased TMZ-induced cell apoptosis (Fig. 1h). Moreover, *miR-519a* can effectively sensitize GBM cells to irradiation treatment (Additional file 6: Figure S4). Collectively, these data supported that *miR-519a* may enhance TMZ chemosensitivity in GBM cells.

miR-519a promoted TMZ-induced autophagy in GBM cells

The results of both immunofluorescence (Fig. 2a) and Western blotting (Fig. 2b) showed that U87-MG/TMZ cells had lower autophagic activity than U87-MG cells. Meanwhile, the sensitivity of both TMZ-sensitive and TMZ-resistant cells was tested, with regard to autophagy inducers, including low glucose (LG), chloroquine (CQ), and rapamycin (Rapa) at different concentrations. These results indicated that U87-MG cells were sensitive to all the tested concentrations of rapamycin, whereas the growth of U87MG/TMZ cells was not affected by rapamycin (Additional file 7: Figure S5). It is thereby proposed that the lack of autophagy is a possible mechanism for TMZ resistance.

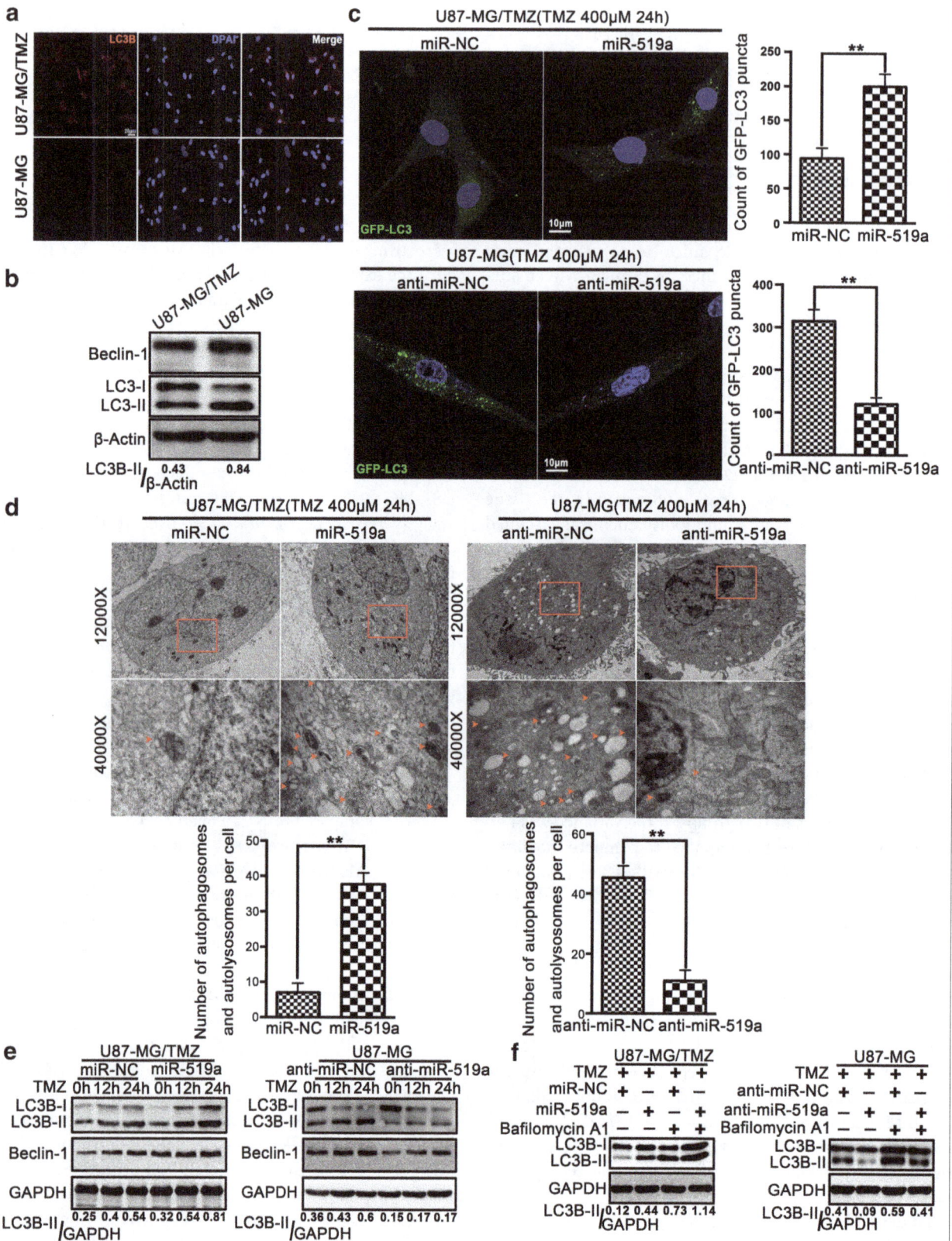

Fig. 2 (See legend on next page.)

(See figure on previous page.)
Fig. 2 *miR-519a* enhanced TMZ-induced autophagy in GBM cells. The expression levels of LC3-II in U87-MG/TMZ and U87-MG cells were evaluated by immunofluorescence assays (**a**) and Western blotting (**b**). Red indicates LC3B and blue indicates nuclei. **c** Both U87-MG/TMZ and U87-MG cells were transfected with GFP-LC3 construct expressing either *miR-519a* or anti-*miR-519a*, followed by treatment with 400 μM TMZ. The numbers of GFP-LC3 puncta were quantified using confocal laser scanning microscopy. **d** Both U87-MG/TMZ and U87-MG cells were transfected with either *miR-519a* or anti-*miR-519a* for 24 h, followed by treatment with 400 μM TMZ. Cell samples were prepared for transmission electron microscopy analysis. The arrows indicate autophagic vacuoles. **e** U87-MG/TMZ cells transfected with *miR-519a* and parental U87-MG cells transfected with anti-*miR-519a* were exposed to 400 μM TMZ at different time points (0–24 h). Whole cell lysates were analyzed by Western blotting. **f** U87-MG/TMZ cells transfected with or without *miR-519a* and treated with or without 400 μM TMZ after incubation with 20 nM bafilomycin A1 for 2 h. U87-MG cells transfected with or without anti-*miR-519a* were treated with 20 nM bafilomycin A1 for 2 h. Cell lysates were analyzed by Western blotting. *p < 0.05, **p < 0.01

In order to determine the effects of *miR-519a* on autophagy induction following TMZ treatment, U87-MG/TMZ cells were transfected with *miR-519a* and U87-MG cells were transfected with anti-*miR-519a* prior to TMZ treatment. In addition, GFP-LC3 was stably expressed in U87-MG and U87-MG/TMZ cells to facilitate the visualization of autophagy. As compared with control cells, overexpression of *miR-519a* enhanced TMZ-induced GFP-LC3 puncta formation in U87-MG/TMZ cells, whereas knockdown of *miR-519a* in U87MG cells inhibited the formation of TMZ-induced GFP-LC3 puncta (Fig. 2c). Besides, TEM was used to count the number of autophagic vacuoles per cell. The results revealed that the number of autophagic vacuoles per cell was markedly increased in *miR-519a*-overexpressing U87-MG/TMZ cells and decreased in *miR-519a*-knockdown U87-MG cells after TMZ treatment (Fig. 2d).

In order to detect the occurrence of autophagy after TMZ treatment in the presence or absence of *miR-519a*, we conducted Western blot analysis to examine the levels of two autophagy-related proteins: LC3B and Beclin-1. As shown in Fig. 2e, the expression levels of LC3-II and Beclin-1 proteins were increased in *miR-519-a*-overexpressing U87-MG/TMZ cells. On the other hand, knockdown of *miR-519a* inhibited the expression of LC3-II and Beclin-1 in U87-MG cells. Since the increased LC3-II may be due to either autophagy induction or inhibition of autophagic flux [29], BafA1, an inhibitor of fusion between autophagosomes and lysosomes, was used in this study. Twenty-four hours after TMZ treatment, the BafA1-treated negative control cells displayed markedly increased accumulation of LC3II, and the ectopic expression of miR-519a may enhance these effects (Fig. 2f). Taken together, our data indicated that the inductive effects of miR-519a on autophagy can be resulted from the induction of early stages of autophagy, rather than from the suppression of autophagosome degradation.

miR-519a sensitized GBM cells to TMZ treatment by promoting autophagy

Both 3-MA and rapamycin were not able to affect the viability of U87MG and U87MG/TMZ cells, respectively,

without TMZ treatment. Indeed, pre-treatment of U87-MG cells with 3-MA (an inhibitor of autophagy) significantly attenuated TMZ-induced cytotoxicity, while rapamycin enhanced TMZ cytotoxicity in U87-MG/TMZ cells (Additional file 8: Figure S6). These results further suggested that autophagy may contribute to the chemosensitivity of TMZ in GBM cells. To confirm whether autophagy is responsible for the cellular sensitization during TMZ chemotherapy enhanced by *miR-519a*, we assessed the cell apoptosis rate after the inhibition and induction of autophagic activity in both U87-MG/TMZ and U87-MG cells, respectively. Treatment with 3-MA significantly attenuated the anti-proliferative effects of *miR-519a* in miR-519a-overexpressing U87-MG/TMZ cells, whereas rapamycin treatment reversed the chemoresistance of TMZ in U87-MG cells transfected with anti-*miR-519a*, as indicated by MTT and colony formation assays, respectively (Fig. 3a, b, e).

The results of flow cytometry assays clearly showed that 3-MA significantly attenuated TMZ-induced apoptosis in *miR-519a*-overexpressing U87-MG/TMZ cells, whereas rapamycin enhanced TMZ-induced apoptosis in *miR-519a*-knockdown U87-MG cells (Fig. 3c, dc, d). In particular, 3-MA strongly inhibited the transformation of LC3-I into LC3-II and decreased the TMZ-induced activation of caspase-3 in *miR-519a*-overexpressing U87-MG/TMZ cells (Fig. 3f). Meanwhile, rapamycin significantly promoted the LC3-II accumulation and increased the TMZ-induced activation of caspase-3 in *miR-519a*-knockdown U87-MG cells (Fig. 3f). These findings strongly suggested that the enhanced apoptosis of GBM cells induced by the combination of *miR-519a* and TMZ is dependent on autophagy.

miR-519a induced autophagy through modification of STAT3 expression

We have previously demonstrated that *miR-519a* can target STAT3 in GBM [21] and speculated that STAT3 may be involved in *miR-519a*-enhanced autophagy after TMZ treatment. Thus, qRT-PCR and Western blotting analysis were performed to determine the expression levels of STAT3 in both U87-MG and U87-MG/TMZ

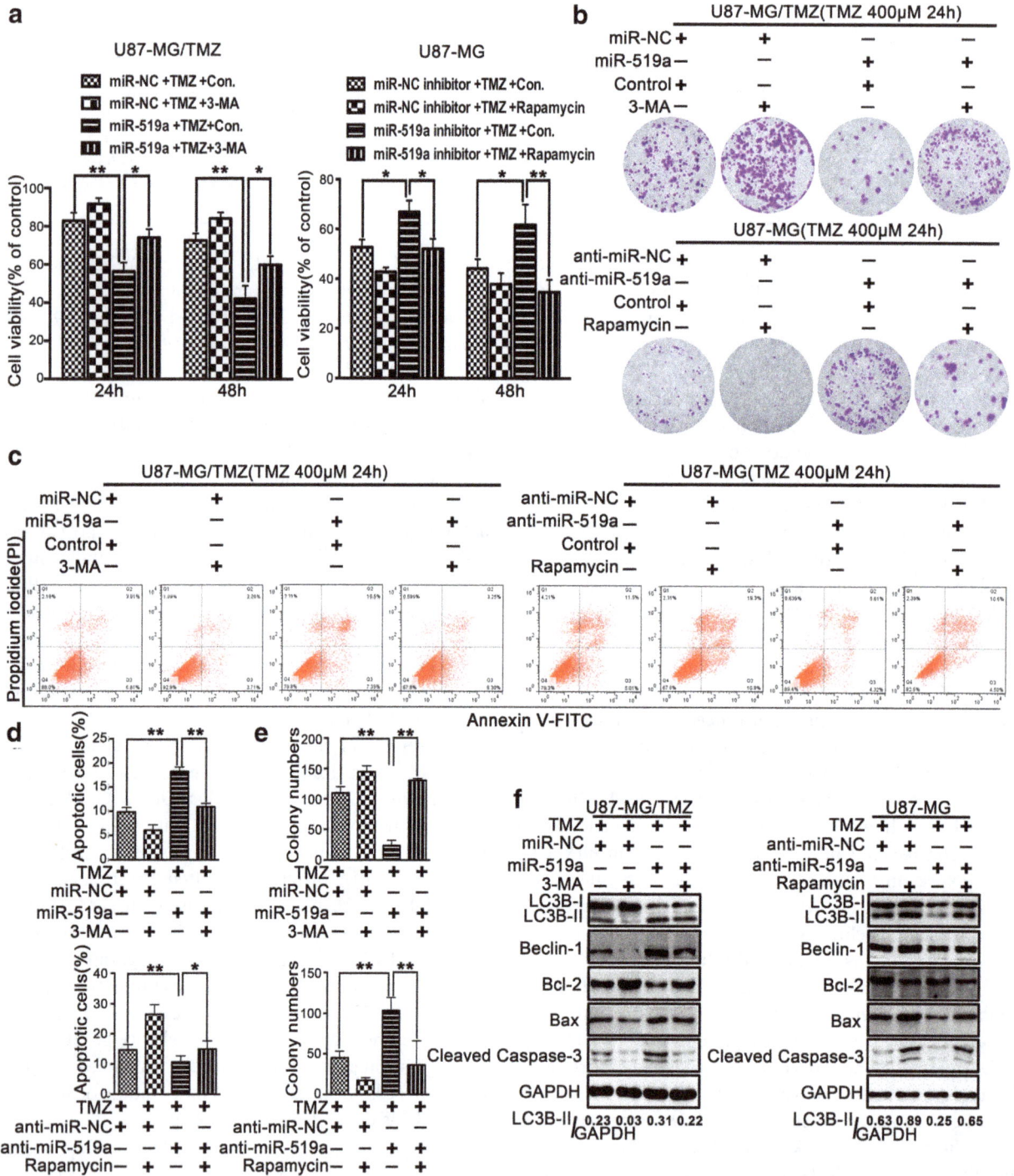

Fig. 3 *miR-519a* sensitized GBM cells to TMZ treatment partly regulated by autophagy. U87-MG/TMZ cells transfected with *miR-519a* were treated with or without 400 µM TMZ after incubation with 3-MA (an inhibitor of autophagy) for 2 h. U87-MG cells transfected with anti-*miR-519a* were treated with or without 200 nM rapamycin for 2 h. The cells were then analyzed for the following: **a** assessment of proliferation by MTT assay; **b**, **e** assessment of colony formation; **c**, **d** assessment of apoptosis by FACS analysis of PI-stained cells; and **f** assessment of caspase-3 activity. *p < 0.05, **p < 0.01

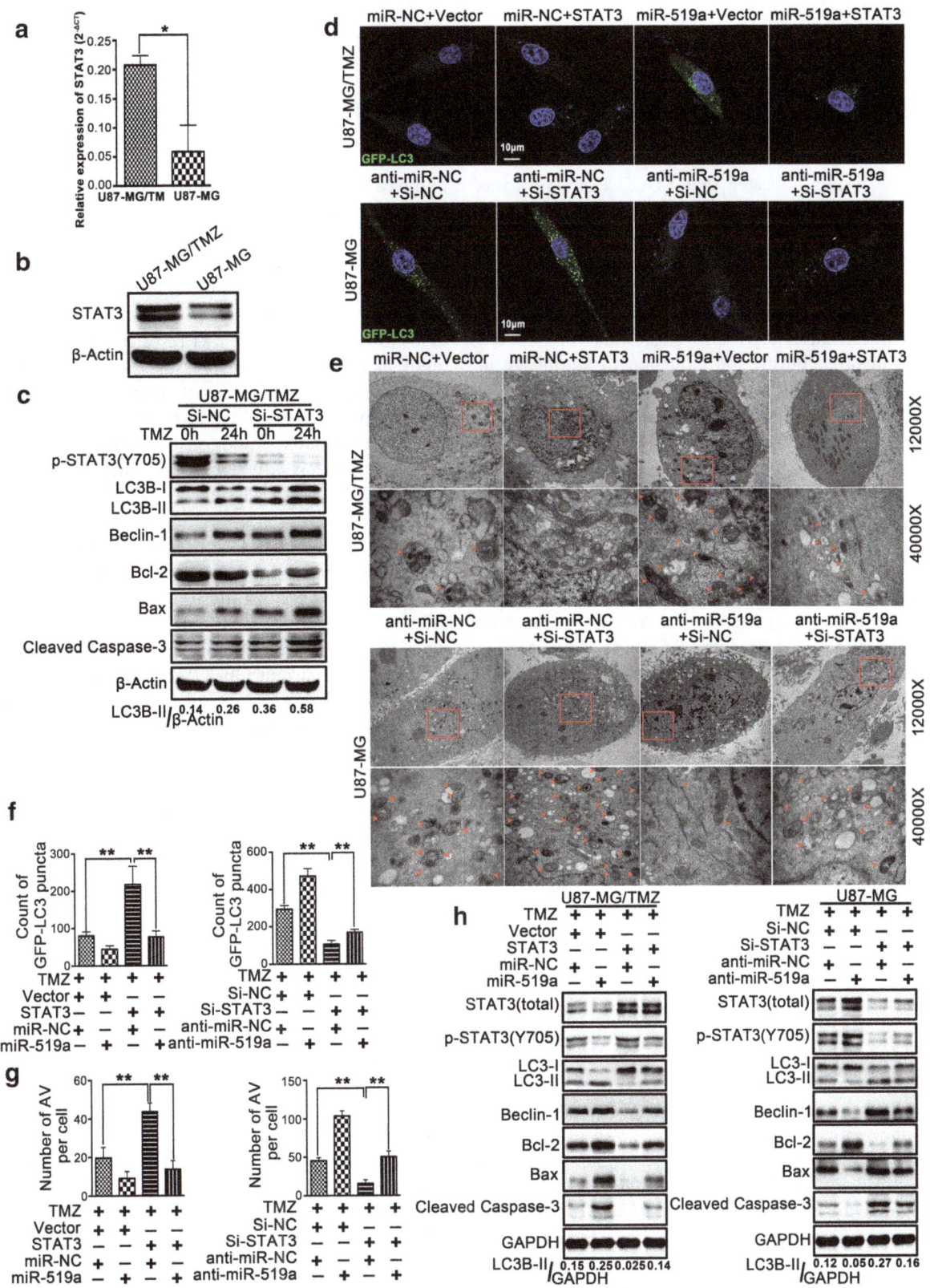

Fig. 4 (See legend on next page.)

cells. The results indicated that STAT3 expression was increased in U87-MG/TMZ cells (Fig. 4a, b).

A total of three siRNAs were constructed, and the one with the most efficient knockdown of STAT3 was chosen (Additional file 9: Figure S7). Transfection with STAT3 siRNA inhibited both basal autophagy and TMZ-induced autophagy, thus suggesting that STAT3 may be involved during the induction of autophagy in GBM cells (Fig. 4c). Furthermore, we constructed STAT3-expressing plasmids and siRNA to evaluate whether co-transfection with *miR-519a* mimic or inhibitor can counteract the effect of STAT3-expressing plasmids or STAT3 siRNA in GBM cells.

Ectopic expression of STAT3 significantly attenuated the effects of *miR-519a* on autophagy induction in U87-MG/TMZ cells, while suppression of STAT3 can stimulate anti-*miR-519a*-dependent autophagy in U87-MG cells. Moreover, ectopic expression of STAT3 may decrease the number of GFP-LC3 dots (Fig. 4d, f) and autophagic vacuoles (Fig. 4e, g) induced by *miR-519a*. The results of Western blotting analysis also revealed that STAT3 significantly attenuated the *miR-519a*-enhanced autophagy and apoptosis in GBM cells (Fig. 4h). Collectively, these findings suggested that STAT3 was critical for *miR-519a*-enhanced autophagy after TMZ treatment in GBM cells.

miR-519a sensitized GBM cells to TMZ treatment in vivo

To investigate the effects of *miR-519a* in vivo, we established U87-MG/TMZ cells with stable overexpression of *miR-519a* and U87-MG cells with stable knockdown of *miR-519a*. Both U87-MG/TMZ and U87-MG cells were infected with LV-miR-519a and LV-anti-miR-519a before they were applied to a subcutaneous xenograft model. After treatment with TMZ, tumors derived from *miR-519-a*-overexpressing U87-MG/TMZ cells grew more slowly and had lower tumor weight than those derived from cells harboring empty vector. Meanwhile, downregulation of *miR-519a* expression by LV-anti-miR-519a suppressed the chemosensitivity of U87-MG cells to TMZ (Fig. 5a–c).

Immunohistochemical analysis revealed that *miR-519a* increased the levels of LC3B, Bax, and cleaved caspase-3 and decreased the levels of phospho-STAT3 and Bcl-2, or vice versa in xenograft tumors (Fig. 5d). TEM results demonstrated that forced expression of *miR-519a* increased the numbers of autophagic vacuoles in GBM tissues, whereas knockdown of *miR-519a* decreased the

numbers of autophagic vacuoles after TMZ treatment (Fig. 5f, g). These in vivo findings suggested that the chemosensitizing effect of *miR-519a* may be contributed to autophagy induction.

Additionally, the antitumor efficacy of *miR-519a* was examined in an orthotopic G131212/TMZ xenograft model. MRI results on day 24 revealed lower tumor volumes in *miR-519a*-overexpressing tumor cells than in control (Fig. 5h). Further results from Kaplan-Meier survival analysis showed that *miR-519a* can improve the survival time after tumor cell implantation (Fig. 5i). These in vivo results supported that *miR-519a* can sensitize GBM cells to TMZ.

miR-519a was associated with chemoresistance of GBM

To further evaluate the clinical role of *miR-519a* in clinical samples (Additional file 10: Table S3), we performed qRT-PCR assays to detect the expression levels of *miR-519a* and STAT3 in brain tissues from patients with primary and recurrent GBM. We identified downregulation of *miR-519a* and upregulation of STAT3 in recurrent GBM tissues compared to primary GBM tissues (Fig. 6a). A significant inverse correlation was found between *miR-519a* and STAT3 expression levels (Fig. 6b). Similarly, the results from immunohistochemical staining showed the increased STAT3 expression and reduced LC3B and cleaved caspase-3 levels in recurrent GBM tissues compared to primary GBM tissues (Fig. 6c). Therefore, these differences strongly suggested an apparent association between *miR-519a*, STAT3, and LC3B in GBM patients.

Discussion

GBM is the most common type of malignant brain tumor [30]. Even after multimodality treatment including radical surgery, radiation, and chemotherapy, the median survival time of GBM is approximately 1 year from diagnosis. De novo and acquired resistance to TMZ in GBM cells have emerged as a challenging problem in clinical practice [31]. Therefore, identifying the mechanisms underlying TMZ chemoresistance shed light on a novel combination therapy strategy to circumvent acquired resistance in GBM patients. Numerous studies have reported that miRNA dysfunction may be involved in tumor progression and therapeutic resistance [20, 32, 33]. Moreover, the therapeutic potential of miR-NAs in cancer, either alone or in combination with

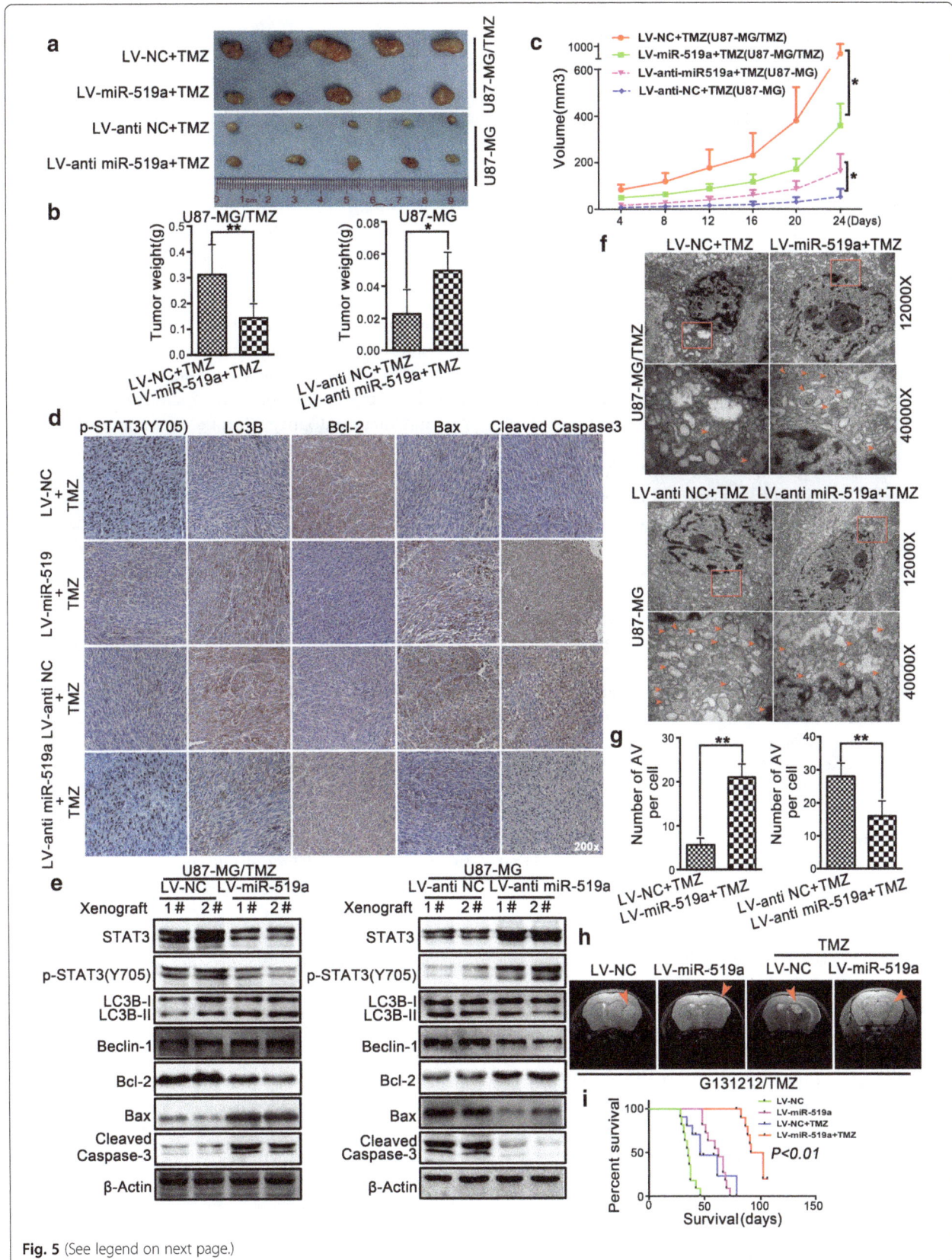

Fig. 5 (See legend on next page.)

(See figure on previous page.)
Fig. 5 *miR-519a* enhanced the antitumor efficacy of TMZ in vivo. The dissected tumors were collected at the end of drug administration (**a**), and tumor weight was measured (**b**). The tumor volume was calculated as $4/3 \times 3.14 \times$ radius (mm)^3 (**c**). Immunohistochemical analysis (**d**) and Western blot analysis (**e**) of phospho-STAT3, LC3B, Bcl-2, Bax, and cleaved caspase-3 levels in xenograft tumors. Xenograft tumors were subjected to TEM. AV (autophagic vacuoles) = autophagosomes and lysosomes (**f, g**). Coronal T2-weighted MRI of tumors acquired from patient-derived GBM cells (G131212/TMZ) from one animal in each treatment group (red arrow) in the brain samples on day 24 after treatment (**h**). The survival of mice with orthotopic tumors was measured by Kaplan-Meier survival curves (**i**). *$p < 0.05$, **$p < 0.01$

conventional drugs, has been demonstrated in several published studies (reviewed in [34]). Previously, we reported that *miR-519a* is downregulated in GBM cells, and overexpression of *miR-519a* may suppress GBM cell proliferation [21]. However, the pivotal role of *miR-519a* in the modulation of TMZ sensitivity is still not fully understood. In this study, we demonstrated that the expression of *miR-519a* was reduced in chemoresistant GBM tissues and TMZ-resistant cells, thus suggesting that low levels of *miR-519a* were associated with TMZ resistance. In addition, our results showed that *miR-519a* enhanced chemosensitivity in GBM cells, mainly through TMZ-induced autophagy and apoptosis.

Both prosurvival and prodeath roles of autophagy have been proposed in GBM cells in response to metabolic and therapeutic stress and are dependent on the cellular context and duration or degree of stress stimuli. Moreover, accumulating evidence has revealed a correlative relationship between chemoresistance and reduced autophagic activity in GBM cells [35–37]. Consistent with previous studies, we found that the basal level of autophagy was lower in TMZ-resistant U87-MG/TMZ cells than in parental GBM cells, suggesting an inverse correlation between reduced autophagy and chemoresistance (Additional file 11). Therefore, restoration of autophagic activity in resistant GBM cells may be a promising strategy to overcome chemoresistance and improve the effectiveness of chemotherapy. In this study, we demonstrated that the enhanced autophagy by forced *miR-519a* expression can sensitize GBM cells to TMZ. Additionally, these effects were attenuated by co-treatment with autophagic blockers (3-MA), suggesting the involvement of autophagic pathway. These results are consistent with previous research demonstrating that autophagy induction can lead to the suppression of GBM cell growth [10–14]. Furthermore, the combination of *miR-519a* and TMZ induced prodeath autophagy, suggesting that the autophagic response of GBM cells to TMZ can be modified when administered in combination with other antitumor agents.

Because the autophagy-related signal pathway is complex, additional studies are needed to elucidate the mechanisms of cell autophagy regulation. Beclin-1 may bind to and be inhibited by Bcl-2 protein to prevent cell autophagy [38, 39]. Furthermore, STAT3/Bcl-2/Beclin-1 signaling is associated with the induction of autophagy. Previous reports have showed that STAT3 has the ability

to transcriptionally activate the apoptosis-inhibitory protein BCL2, which also inhibits the induction of autophagy by dissociating the Bcl-2/Beclin-1 complex. Upon activation, STAT3 upregulates BCL2 expression and consequently leads to autophagy inhibition [33, 40, 41]. In our study, transfection with STAT3 siRNA also inhibited both basal autophagy and TMZ-induced autophagy, suggesting that STAT3 was involved in the induction of autophagy in GBM. Moreover, dysfunction of miRNAs can modulate autophagy through a variety of mechanisms in GBM [20, 32, 33]. We previously demonstrated that *miR-519a* functions as a tumor suppressor in glioma by targeting STAT3 [21]; therefore, we hypothesized that *miR-519a*-mediated prodeath autophagy may occur via targeting of STAT3 to sensitize U87-MG/TMZ cells to TMZ. Indeed, in this study, we found that *miR-519a* promoted the autophagy of GBM cells by enhancing dissociation of the Bcl-2/Beclin-1 complex and enhanced therapeutic efficacy in vivo and in vitro. We further improved our understanding of the molecular basis of *miR-519a* in GBM. Advances in molecular biology have promoted our understanding of the molecular basis of GBM and provide tools with which to improve therapy. There are many tools, including decoy oligonucleotides/antisense oligonucleotide/RNA interference and guanine-rich oligonucleotides, that have been very promising in modulating STAT3 pathway and facilitating the development of new drugs for clinical applications [42]. miR-519a, as a small molecule, may be a favorable candidate for analysis in clinical trials.

More recently, several studies have suggested that autophagy plays a prodeath role in GBM cells treated with chemotherapeutic agents, by enhancing autophagy-mediated apoptosis instead of autophagic cell death [41–43]. Mu et al. [43] observed an induced autophagy and apoptosis in GBM cells treated with a combination treatment of β-elemene and gefitinib. Bak et al. [44] reported that enhanced autophagy contributes to the synergistic effects of vitamin D in TMZ-based GBM chemotherapy. Peng-Hsu et al. [45] found that *miR-128* promotes apoptotic death in glioma cells through non-protective autophagy formation. Our results, in agreement with previous findings [41–43], showed that autophagy inhibition by 3-MA may reduce apoptosis during combined treatment of *miR-519a* and TMZ, whereas rapamycin-induced autophagy can enhance

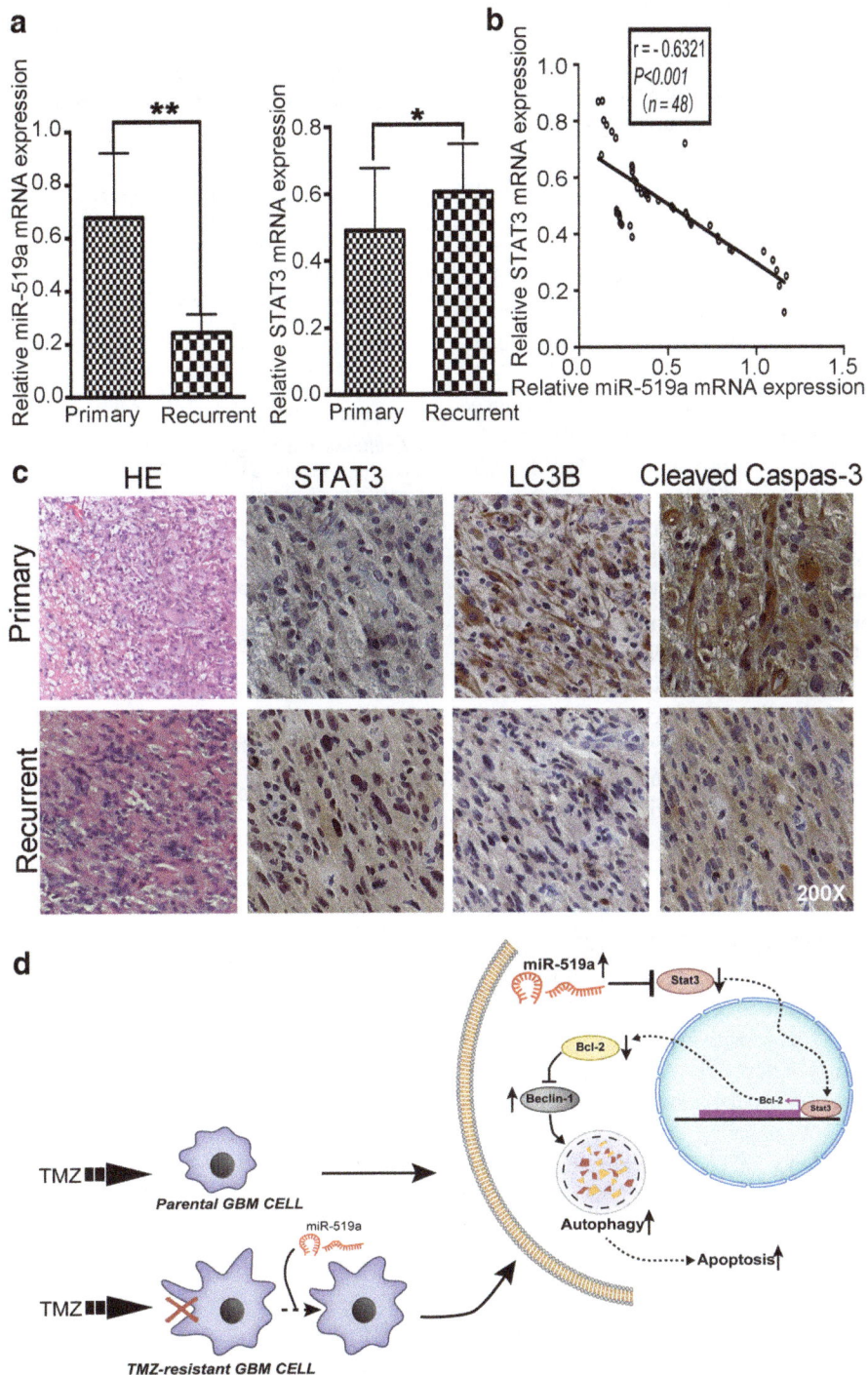

Fig. 6 *miR-519a* was associated with chemoresistance. **a** *miR-519a* expression was assessed in primary ($n = 24$) and recurrent GBM tissue samples ($n = 24$). **b** Expression levels of *miR-519a* were inversely correlated with *STAT3* mRNA in tissue samples, as measured by linear regression analysis. **c** Expression of STAT3, LC3B, and cleaved caspase-3 in primary and recurrent GBM tissue samples were determined by immunochemical staining (magnification × 200). **d** Schematic illustration of the mechanisms underlying *miR-519a* induced chemosensitivity to TMZ. Pointed arrows and blunted arrows indicate both activation and repression, respectively. *$p < 0.05$, **$p < 0.01$

apoptosis following combined treatment of anti-*miR-519a* and TMZ. Nevertheless, emerging evidence has suggested a crosstalk between autophagic and apoptotic pathways [46].

Since the autophagy-related pathway network can be complex, additional studies are required to elucidate the molecular mechanisms underlying cell autophagy. STAT3/Bcl-2/Beclin-1 signaling has been proposed to be associated with autophagy induction. Notably, Beclin-1 may be bound to or inhibited by Bcl-2 protein in order to prevent cell autophagy [38, 39]. STAT3 is able to induce BCL2 transcriptional activation, which inhibits the induction of autophagy by dissociating the Bcl-2/Beclin-1 complex [33, 40, 41]. In this study, transfection with STAT3 siRNA inhibited both basal autophagy and TMZ-induced autophagy, suggesting that STAT3 signaling pathway is involved in TMZ-induced autophagy in GBM cells. Additionally, dysfunction of miRNAs can modulate autophagy in GBM cells through various mechanisms [20, 32, 33]. We previously demonstrated that *miR-519a* functions as a tumor suppressor in glioma by targeting STAT3 [21]. In the present study, we confirmed that *miR-519a* sensitized U87-MG/TMZ cells to TMZ and triggered autophagy-mediated apoptosis via STAT3 pathway. Indeed, we found that *miR-519a* promoted the autophagy of GBM cells via dissociation of Bcl-2/Beclin-1 complex. These results significantly improved our understanding of the molecular basis of *miR-519a* in GBM cells with TMZ resistance.

Conclusions

The results of this study suggested that *miR-519a* may hold a great potential to overcome TMZ chemoresistance in GBM. In vivo and in vitro analysis clearly indicated that *miR-519a* increased TMZ sensitivity by promoting GBM cell apoptosis through autophagy. Additionally, overexpression of *miR-519a* can induce autophagy via the inhibition of STAT3/Bcl-2 signaling pathway. Therefore, *miR-519a* in combination with TMZ therapy could render a more effective therapeutic approach for GBM.

Additional files

Additional file 1: Table S1. Sequences of siRNAs and miRNA used in this study. (DOCX 58 kb)

Additional file 2: Table S2. List of primer sequences used in this study. (DOCX 48 kb)

Additional file 3: Figure S1. Determination of cell growth rates by using doubling time assay. U87-MG and U87-MG/TMZ cells displayed doubling times of 37.1 and 29.2 h, respectively. Each bar represents the mean ± s.d. of three independent experiments. (TIF 107 kb)

Additional file 4: Figure S2. TMZ enhanced the expression of *miR-519a* in U87-MG cells but showed no effect on U87-MG/TMZ cells. U87-MG cells and U87-MG/TMZ cells were treated with different concentrations of TMZ for 24 h or with 200 μM TMZ for the indicated times. The expression

of *miR-519a* was measured by qRT-PCR. a TMZ enhanced the levels of *miR-519a* in U87-MG cells in a concentration-dependent manner. b TMZ induced *miR-519a* upregulation in a time-dependent manner. Each bar represents the mean ± s.d. of three independent experiments. *p < 0.05, **p < 0.01, NS > 0.05 vs. control group. (TIF 1152 kb)

Additional file 5: Figure S3. *miR-519a* sensitized GBM cells to TMZ treatment. a Cell viability of U87-MG/TMZ and U87-MG cells transfected with pCMV-miR-519a or *miR-519a* sponge and then treated with or without TMZ at various concentrations (or times). b Colony formation in U87-MG/TMZ and U87-MG cells transfected with pCMV-miR-519a or *miR-519a* sponge and then treated with or without TMZ at various concentrations (or times). Each bar represents the mean ± s.d. of three independent experiments. NS > 0.05, *p < 0.05, **p < 0.01. (TIF 4190 kb)

Additional file 6: Figure S4. *miR-519a* enhanced radiosensitivity in GBM cells. a Cell viability of GBM cells after treatment. Each bar represents the mean ± standard deviation of three independent experiments. b Clonogenic survival of GBM cells transfected with *miR-519a* or anti-miR-519a. Each bar represents the mean ± s.d. of three independent experiments. *p < 0.05, **p < 0.01. (TIF 1670 kb)

Additional file 7: Figure S5. Cellular viability assay for TMZ-sensitive and -resistant cells. a U87-MG/TMZ and U87-MG cells were cultured in normal medium, with low glucose (LG), or in the presence of chloroquine (CQ). b The cell viability of U87-MG/TMZ and U87-MG treated with different concentrations of rapamycin for 72 h. The cell viability for a and b was evaluated by MTT assays. Data represent the mean (± standard deviation) of three independent experiments. *p < 0.05, **p < 0.01, NS > 0.05 vs. control group. (TIF 816 kb)

Additional file 8: Figure S6. Effects of 3-MA, rapamycin(Rapa), and/or their combination with TMZ on the viability of U87-MG/TMZ and U87-MG cells. a Rapamycin is not able to affect the viability of U87MG/TMZ cells. b 3-MA is not able to affect the viability of U87MG. Each bar represents the mean ± s.d. of three independent experiments. NS > 0.05,*p < 0.05. (TIF 538 kb)

Additional file 9: Figure S7. The knockdown efficiency of siSTAT3. Cells transfected with STAT3 siRNAs (NS, #1, #2, or #3) were treated with or without TMZ (400 μm) for 48 h. qRT-PCR (a) and Western blot analysis (b) for the respective target genes were carried out 48 h after transfection. Immunoblots (c) of the extracts for the indicated proteins in U87-MG cells. GAPDH was used as a loading control for Western blots. **p < 0.01 vs. Si-NC group. (TIF 599 kb)

Additional file 10: Table S3. Clinical information of patients with recurrent GBM. (DOCX 105 kb)

Additional file 11: Supplemental Material and Methods. (DOCX 104 kb)

Abbreviations
3'-UTR: 3'-Untranslated region; AV: Autophagic vacuole; GBM: Glioblastoma; GFP: Green fluorescent protein; miR-519a: MicroRNA-519a; miRNA: MicroRNA; PCR: Polymerase chain reaction; TEM: Transmission electron microscopy; TMZ: Temozolomide

Funding
This work was supported by the National Natural Science Foundation of China (grant no. 81772656), Natural Science Foundation of Guangdong Province (grant nos. 2014A030313298 and 2016A030313563), and the National Key Clinical Specialist Construction Program of China.

Authors' contributions
LYT, QST, and HAN conceived the study. LH, CL, LJJ, LWW, and ZQ carried out the experiments. LYT, QST, GL, and WK analyzed the data. LH and LYT wrote the manuscript. All authors have read and approved the final version of the manuscript.

Competing interests

The authors declare that they have no competing interests.

Author details

[1]Department of Neurosurgery, Shanghai Tenth People's Hospital, Tongji University School of Medicine, Shanghai 200072, People's Republic of China. [2]Department of Neurosurgery, Nanfang Hospital, Southern Medical University, Guangzhou 510515, Guangdong Province, People's Republic of China. [3]Nanfang Neurology Research Institution, Nanfang Hospital, Guangzhou 510515, Guangdong Province, People's Republic of China. [4]Nanfang Glioma Center, Guangzhou 510515, Guangdong Province, People's Republic of China. [5]Brain Tumor Research Center, The Hospital for Sick Children, Toronto, Canada. [6]Department of Plastic and Aesthetic Surgery, Nanfang Hospital, Southern Medical University, Guangzhou 510515, Guangdong Province, People's Republic of China.

References

1. Mostafa H, et al. Immune phenotypes predict survival in patients with glioblastoma multiforme. J Hematol Oncol. 2016;9(1):77.
2. Stupp R, et al. Radiotherapy plus concomitant and adjuvant temozolomide for glioblastoma. N Engl J Med. 2005;352(10):987–96.
3. Li B, et al. TMEM140 is associated with the prognosis of glioma by promoting cell viability and invasion. J Hematol Oncol. 2015;8:89.
4. Wang Z, et al. The D domain of LRRC4 anchors ERK1/2 in the cytoplasm and competitively inhibits MEK/ERK activation in glioma cells. J Hematol Oncol. 2016;9(1):130.
5. von Ahrens D, et al. The role of stromal cancer-associated fibroblasts in pancreatic cancer. J Hematol Oncol. 2017;10(1):76.
6. Lee SW, et al. The synergistic effect of combination temozolomide and chloroquine treatment is dependent on autophagy formation and p53 status in glioma cells. Cancer Lett. 2015;360(2):195–204.
7. Zanotto-Filho A, et al. Autophagy inhibition improves the efficacy of curcumin/temozolomide combination therapy in glioblastomas. Cancer Lett. 2015;358(2):220–31.
8. Yoshida GJ. Therapeutic strategies of drug repositioning targeting autophagy to induce cancer cell death: from pathophysiology to treatment. J Hematol Oncol. 2017;10(1):67.
9. He C, Klionsky DJ. Regulation mechanisms and signaling pathways of autophagy. Annu Rev Genet. 2009;43:67–93.
10. Franzetti E, et al. Autophagy precedes apoptosis during the remodeling of silkworm larval midgut. Apoptosis. 2012;17(3):305–24.
11. Zhang N, et al. PARP and RIP 1 are required for autophagy induced by 11'-deoxyverticillin A, which precedes caspase-dependent apoptosis. Autophagy. 2011;7(6):598–612.
12. Daido S, et al. Pivotal role of the cell death factor BNIP3 in ceramide-induced autophagic cell death in malignant glioma cells. Cancer Res. 2004; 64(12):4286–93.
13. Lorente M, et al. Stimulation of the midkine/ALK axis renders glioma cells resistant to cannabinoid antitumoral action. Cell Death Differ. 2011;18(6):959–73.
14. Bhoopathi P, et al. Cathepsin B facilitates autophagy-mediated apoptosis in SPARC overexpressed primitive neuroectodermal tumor cells. Cell Death Differ. 2010;17(10):1529–39.
15. Hu YL, et al. Hypoxia-induced autophagy promotes tumor cell survival and adaptation to antiangiogenic treatment in glioblastoma. Cancer Res. 2012; 72(7):1773–83.
16. Rosenfeld MR, et al. Pharmacokinetic analysis and pharmacodynamic evidence of autophagy inhibition in patients with newly diagnosed glioblastoma treated on a phase I trial of hydroxychloroquine in combination with adjuvant temozolomide and radiation (ABTC 0603). J Clin Oncol. 2010;28:15.
17. Lin CJ, et al. Inhibition of mitochondria- and endoplasmic reticulum stress-mediated autophagy augments temozolomide-induced apoptosis in glioma cells. PLoS One. 2012;7(6):e38706.
18. Braoudaki M, et al. Microrna expression signatures predict patient progression and disease outcome in pediatric embryonal central nervous system neoplasms. J Hematol Oncol. 2014;7:96.
19. Kasinski AL, Slack FJ. Epigenetics and genetics. MicroRNAs en route to the clinic: progress in validating and targeting microRNAs for cancer therapy. Nat Rev Cancer. 2011;11(12):849–64.
20. Chen G, et al. MicroRNA-181a sensitizes human malignant glioma U87MG cells to radiation by targeting Bcl-2. Oncol Rep. 2010;23(4):997–1003.
21. Hong L, et al. MiR-519a functions as a tumor suppressor in glioma by targeting the oncogenic STAT3 pathway. J Neuro-Oncol. 2016;128(1):35–45.
22. Brantley EC, Benveniste EN. Signal transducer and activator of transcription-3: a molecular hub for signaling pathways in gliomas. Mol Cancer Res. 2008; 6(5):675–84.
23. Lee K, et al. Proteome-wide discovery of mislocated proteins in cancer. Genome Res. 2013;23(8):1283–94.
24. Dasqupta A, et al. Stat3 activation is required for the growth of U87 cell-derived tumours in mice. Eur J Cancer. 2009;45(4):677–84.
25. You L, et al. The role of STAT3 in autophagy. Autophagy. 2015;11(5):729–39.
26. Feng Y, et al. Metformin promotes autophagy and apoptosis in esophageal squamous cell carcinoma by downregulating Stat3 signaling. Cell Death Dis. 2014;5:e1088.
27. Lu Y, et al. MIR517C inhibits autophagy and the epithelial-to-mesenchymal (-like) transition phenotype in human glioblastoma through KPNA2-dependent disruption of TP53 nuclear translocation. Autophagy. 2015; 11(12):2213–32.
28. Happold C, et al. Distinct molecular mechanisms of acquired resistance to temozolomide in glioblastoma cells. J Neurochem. 2012;122(2):444–55.
29. Hosokawa N, et al. Nutrient-dependent mTORC1 association with the ULK1-Atg13-FIP200 complex required for autophagy. Mol Biol Cell. 2009;20(7): 1981–91.
30. Gravina GL, et al. The brain-penetrating CXCR4 antagonist, PRX177561, increases the antitumor effects of bevacizumab and sunitinib in preclinical models of human glioblastoma. J Hematol Oncol. 2017;10(1):5.
31. Oermann E, et al. CyberKnife enhanced conventionally fractionated chemoradiation for high grade glioma in close proximity to critical structures. J Hematol Oncol. 2010;3:22.
32. Weidhaas JB, et al. MicroRNAs as potential agents to alter resistance to cytotoxic anticancer therapy. Cancer Res. 2007;67(23):11111–6.
33. Zou Z, et al. MicroRNA-30a sensitizes tumor cells to cis-platinum via suppressing beclin 1-mediated autophagy. J Biol Chem. 2012;287(6):4148–56.
34. Naidu S, et al. MiRNA-based therapeutic intervention of cancer. J Hematol Oncol. 2015;8:68.
35. Shi F, et al. The PI3K inhibitor GDC-0941 enhances radiosensitization and reduces chemoresistance to temozolomide in GBM cell lines. Neuroscience. 2017;346:298–308.
36. Liu YQ, et al. Identification of an annonaceous acetogenin mimetic, AA005, as an AMPK activator and autophagy inducer in colon cancer cells. PLoS One. 2012;7(10):e47049.
37. Fu J, et al. Glioblastoma stem cells resistant to temozolomide-induced autophagy. Chin Med J. 2009;122(11):1255–9.
38. Pattingre S, et al. Bcl-2 antiapoptotic proteins inhibit Beclin 1-dependent autophagy. Cell. 2005;122(6):927–39.
39. Akar U, et al. Silencing of Bcl-2 expression by small interfering RNA induces autophagic cell death in MCF-7 breast cancer cells. Autophagy. 2008;4(5): 669–79.
40. Seca H, et al. Targeting miR-21 induces autophagy and chemosensitivity of leukemia cells. Curr Drug Targets. 2013;14(10):1135–43.
41. Wang Z, et al. MicroRNA-25 regulates chemoresistance-associated autophagy in breast cancer cells, a process modulated by the natural autophagy inducer isoliquiritigenin. Oncotarget. 2014;5(16):7013–26.
42. Furqan M, et al. STAT inhibitors for cancer therapy. J Hematol Oncol. 2013;6:90
43. Mu L, et al. Beta-Elemene enhances the efficacy of gefitinib on glioblastoma multiforme cells through the inhibition of the EGFR signaling pathway. Int J Oncol. 2016;49(4):1427–36.
44. Bak D, et al. Autophagy enhancement contributes to the synergistic effect of vitamin D in temozolomide-based glioblastoma chemotherapy. Exp Ther Med. 2016;11(6):2153–62.
45. Chen PH, et al. The inhibition of microRNA-128 on IGF-1-activating mTOR signaling involves in temozolomide-induced glioma cell apoptotic death. PLoS One. 2016;11(11):e167096.
46. Eisenberg-Lerner A, et al. Life and death partners: apoptosis, autophagy and the cross-talk between them. Cell Death Differ. 2009;16(7):966–75.

2

The lncRNA NEAT1 activates Wnt/β-catenin signaling and promotes colorectal cancer progression via interacting with DDX5

Meng Zhang[1,2,3†], Weiwei Weng[1,3,4†], Qiongyan Zhang[1,3,4], Yong Wu[3,4], Shujuan Ni[1,3,4], Cong Tan[1,3,4], Midie Xu[1,3,4], Hui Sun[1,3,4], Chenchen Liu[4,6], Ping Wei[1,3,4,5,6*] and Xiang Du[1,2,3,4,5*]

Abstract

Background: The long noncoding RNA nuclear-enriched abundant transcript 1 (NEAT1) has been reported to be overexpressed in colorectal cancer (CRC). However, its underlying mechanisms in the progression of CRC have not been well studied.

Methods: To investigate the clinical significance of NEAT1, we analyzed its expression levels in a publicly available dataset and in 71 CRC samples from Fudan University Shanghai Cancer Center. Functional assays, including the CCK8, EdU, colony formation, wound healing, and Transwell assays, were used to determine the oncogenic role of NEAT1 in human CRC progression. Furthermore, RNA pull-down, mass spectrometry, RNA immunoprecipitation, and Dual-Luciferase Reporter Assays were used to determine the mechanism of NEAT1 in CRC progression. Animal experiments were used to determine the role of NEAT1 in CRC tumorigenicity and metastasis in vivo.

Results: NEAT1 expression was significantly upregulated in CRC tissues compared with its expression in normal tissues. Altered NEAT1 expression led to marked changes in proliferation, migration, and invasion of CRC cells both in vitro and in vivo. Mechanistically, we found that NEAT1 directly bound to the DDX5 protein, regulated its stability, and sequentially activated Wnt signaling. Our study showed that NEAT1 indirectly activated the Wnt/β-catenin signaling pathway via DDX5 and fulfilled its oncogenic functions in a DDX5-mediated manner. Clinically, concomitant NEAT1 and DDX5 protein levels negatively correlated with the overall survival and disease-free survival of CRC patients.

Conclusions: Our findings indicated that NEAT1 activated Wnt signaling to promote colorectal cancer progression and metastasis. The NEAT1/DDX5/Wnt/β-catenin axis could be a potential therapeutic target of pharmacological strategies.

Keywords: NEAT1, lncRNA, DDX5, β-Catenin, Colorectal cancer

Background

Colorectal cancer (CRC) is the third most common cancer and the third leading cause of cancer-related death in men and women in the USA, accounting for one-tenth of all cancer-related deaths in women and men [1]. Treatment regimens for advanced CRC involve combination chemotherapies, which are toxic and largely ineffective but have remained the backbone of treatment over the past decade [2]. Hence, genetic and epigenetic alterations and their underlying mechanisms in CRC should be explored more intensively to discover prognostic biomarkers and therapeutic targets for CRC.

Long noncoding RNAs (lncRNAs) are defined as RNA polymerase II transcripts longer than 200 nucleotides in length that lack a significant protein-coding capacity [3, 4]. Over the past two decades, the biogenesis and functional mechanisms of miRNAs have been extensively elucidated. Nevertheless, the roles of lncRNAs remain unclear. lncRNAs have a great biological significance in the occurrence and progression of cancers because they can interact with cancer stem cells and then affect cancer metastasis and recurrence [5]. lncRNAs potentially act through various mechanisms that may be related to a

* Correspondence: weiping@fudan.edu.cn; dx2008cn@163.com
†Meng Zhang and Weiwei Weng contributed equally to this work.
¹Department of Pathology, Fudan University Shanghai Cancer Center, Shanghai 200032, China
Full list of author information is available at the end of the article

wide range of subcellular localizations, expression levels, and stability in mammalian cells [6, 7]. As expected, increasing evidence suggests that many lncRNAs fulfill their functions through specific interactions with other cellular factors (proteins, DNA, and other RNA molecules). Hence, finding lncRNA interacting partners is considered a strategy to gain insights into their molecular mechanisms [6].

Many lncRNAs potentially act as scaffolds to bring together different proteins or bridge protein complexes via their protein interaction capabilities [8]. For example, NEAT1 and MALAT1 bind multiple proteins localized to paraspeckles and nuclear speckles, respectively [9–11]. The lncRNA NEAT1 is abnormally upregulated in somatic malignancies and has been found to promote tumor growth in CRC [12–14]. Nevertheless, elucidating the molecular mechanisms underlying the oncogenic functions of NEAT1 requires further effort. Identifying the upstream and downstream targets of NEAT1 will elucidate its critical role in tumor progression.

In most cases, inappropriate activation of the proto-oncoprotein β-catenin is thought to induce tumor formation. Mutations of the tumor suppressors APC and axin, which are found in many colorectal tumors, prevent β-catenin degradation, and phosphorylation [15, 16]. All of these mutations cause both nuclear accumulation of β-catenin, thereby contributing to its ability to bind T cell transcription factors, and upregulation of proto-oncogenes, such as c-myc, Axin2, and cyclin D1 [17–19]. Recently, decreased NEAT1 expression was reported to inhibit Wnt/β-catenin signaling pathway activity. However, the molecular mechanisms underlying this phenomenon are unknown.

In this study, we revealed the key functions of NEAT1 in the proliferation, migration, and invasion of CRC cells both in vitro and in vivo. Notably, we provided evidence that NEAT1 directly bound to DDX5 and enhanced its protein stability. NEAT1 activated the transcriptional activity of β-catenin to promote CRC tumor progression in a DDX5-mediated manner. Clinically, NEAT1 expression was elevated in CRC tissues and positively correlated with DDX5 expression. Taken together, these results suggest that NEAT1 and DDX5 in combination may be valuable prognostic predictors for CRC. Thus, the NEAT1/DDX5/β-catenin axis appears to be a promising target for CRC therapy.

Methods

Please find the complete Materials and Methods in Additional file 1.

CRC patient information

Fresh samples were obtained from 71 newly diagnosed CRC patients who underwent no preoperative therapy prior to surgical resection at Fudan University Shanghai Cancer Center (FDUSCC) between 2008 and 2009. This study was approved by the institutional review board of Shanghai Cancer Center. The median follow-up time was 80 months, and the longest follow-up was 87 months.

Transient and stable transfections

NEAT1 siRNAs (si1: sense 5′-GACCGUGGUUUGUU ACUAUdTdT-3′, antisense 5′-AUAGUAACAAACCA CGGUCdTdT-3′; si2: sense 5′-GUUGGUCAUUCCUA AAUCUTT-3′, antisense 5′-AGAUUUAGGAAUGACC AACTT-3′), si-DDX5 (sense: 5′-GCAAGUAGCUGCUG AAUAUUU-3′, antisense: 5′-pAUAUUCAGCAGCUA CUUGCUU-3′), and a scramble siRNA were purchased from GenePharma (Shanghai, China). ShNEAT1 lentiviruses (5′-GACCGUGGUUUGUUACUAU-3′) and shNC (representing the sh-negative control, 5′-UUCUCCGAACG UGUCACGU-3′) were generated by Sbo-Bio (Shanghai, China). Transient transfection of pc3.1-NEAT1, pc3.1 (control vector), or siRNA was performed using Lipofectamine 3000 (Invitrogen, CA, USA) according to the manufacturer's instructions. To establish stable cell lines, shNEAT1 lentiviruses were transduced into HCT116 and SW1116 cells with polybrene (5 μg/mL; Sigma-Aldrich, MO, USA). Then, the cells were selected with 0.5 μg/mL of puromycin for 14 days. The transfection efficiencies were verified by RT-qPCR and western blotting.

Animal experiments

This study complied with the Animal Care guidelines of FDUSCC. Male BALB/c nude mice (6 weeks old) were housed under specific pathogen-free conditions. HCT116-shNC and HCT116-shNEAT1 cells were injected either subcutaneously ($n = 4$, 5×10^6/mouse) or into the tail vein ($n = 4$, 2×10^6/mouse). The mice were sacrificed after 4–6 weeks. The tumors and lungs of the mice were removed, fixed in 10% formalin, and stored at − 80 °C for the subsequent analyses. Each animal experiment was performed in triplicate.

Western blotting

The standard western blotting assay was performed as previously described [20]. The specific primary antibodies are listed in Additional file 2: Table S1.

RNA pull-down, mass spectrometry, and RNA immunoprecipitation assays

RNA pull-down was performed using the Magnetic RNA-Protein Pull-Down kit (Pierce, MA, USA) in accordance with the manufacturer's instructions. The protein bands on the gel were silver-stained. Bands of interest were identified by mass spectrometry (MS) and confirmed by western blotting. RNA immunoprecipitation (RIP) was performed using the Magna RIP RNA-Binding Protein Immunoprecipitation Kit (Millipore, MA, USA) according to the manufacturer's protocol.

Promoter reporter and Dual-Luciferase Assay

The DDX5 promoter was cloned into the pGL3 basic luciferase reporter vectors (Promega, USA). In total, 5000 cells were seeded into each well of a 96-well plate and transfected with 100 ng of the TOP/FOP-flash reporter plasmids (Millipore, MA, USA), 100 ng of an expression vector (pGL3-DDX5 or pGL3-Basic) or 0.25 μl of siRNA. DDX5 promoter activity and TOP/FOP-flash were normalized by cotransfection with 10 ng of a Renilla luciferase reporter. After 24 h of incubation, the luciferase activity was detected using the Dual-Luciferase Reporter Assay System (Promega, USA).

Reproducibility

Each experiment was independently repeated at least three times, and the data were presented as the mean ± SD. For the western blotting, EdU, wound healing, RIP, and Transwell assays, the representative results of three independent experiments are shown.

Statistical analysis

Comparisons between groups were analyzed using Student's t tests for the mRNA levels, and clinicopathological parameters were compared using the χ^2 test. Correlations between the mRNA levels were calculated with Spearman's rank correlation coefficients. Survival curves were plotted using the Kaplan-Meier method and compared using the log-rank test. $p < 0.05$ was considered significant. All statistical analyses were conducted using the SPSS 19.0 statistical software (SPSS Inc., IL, USA).

Results

NEAT1 is upregulated in human CRC tissues and is associated with a poor prognosis in CRC patients

To investigate the clinical significance of NEAT1, we analyzed its expression levels in the publicly available TCGA dataset and in data from 71 CRC samples from FDUSCC. Both datasets showed that NEAT1 expression was significantly upregulated in the tumor tissues compared to the levels in the normal tissues (Fig. 1a, b). Correlations between the clinicopathological features of the CRC patients and the NEAT1 levels are summarized in Additional file 2: Table S3. NEAT1 was not related to age, gender, AJCC stage, T stage, N stage, and other features. The univariate Cox proportional hazards models for overall survival (OS) and disease-free survival (DFS) are summarized in Additional file 2: Table S4. Our results revealed that patients with high NEAT1 expression (divided by the mean value) showed obviously poorer

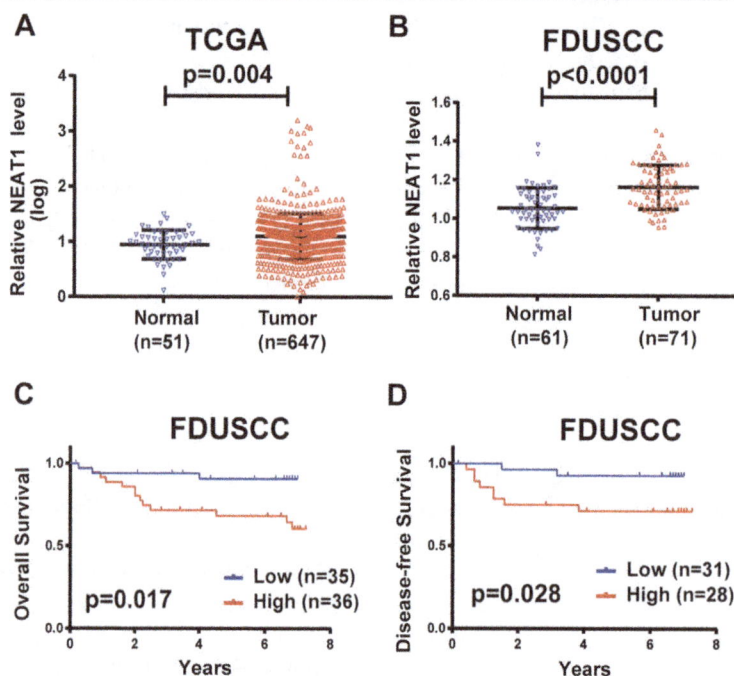

Fig. 1 NEAT1 is upregulated in human CRC patients and predicts a poor prognosis. **a** NEAT1 expression in TCGA CRC RNA-seq dataset (normal $n = 51$, tumor $n = 647$). **b** NEAT1 expression in the FDUSCC dataset (normal $n = 61$, tumor $n = 71$). **c–d** Kaplan-Meier analyses of the FDUSCC dataset. **c** High NEAT1 expression predicted shorter OS than that of patients with low NEAT1 expression. **d** High NEAT1 expression predicted shorter DFS than that of patients with low NEAT1 expression

OS than those with low NEAT1 expression [23/35 (65.7%) vs. 32/36 (88.9%), HR 4.457, 95% CI 1.267–15.685, $p = 0.017$, Fig. 1c]. In addition, 8 of the 28 (28.6%) patients with high NEAT1 expression experienced recurrence, whereas only 2 of the 31 (6.452%) patients with low NEAT1 relapsed. The Kaplan-Meier curves showed that patients with high NEAT1 expression has poorer DFS than those with relatively low NEAT1 expression ($p = 0.028$, Fig. 1d).

NEAT1 mediates cell proliferation in vitro and tumorigenicity in vivo

To assess the functional role of NEAT1 in colorectal cancer cells, first we examined the baseline NEAT1 RNA levels in eight CRC cell lines (RKO, CACO2, SW1116, LOVO, SW480, SW620, HT29, and HCT116) by RT-qPCR (Fig. 2a). NEAT1 was expressed at much higher levels in the HCT116 and SW1116 cells and relatively lower levels in the HT29 cells and was mainly located in the nucleus (Additional file 3: Figure S1A). Next, HCT116 and SW1116 cells were transfected with the NEAT1 siRNA and HT29 cells were transfected with the NEAT1 plasmid. The knockdown and overexpression efficiencies were verified by RT-PCR (Fig. 2b). The CCK8 assay showed that downregulation of NEAT1 significantly attenuated cell proliferation of the HCT116 and SW1116 cells, whereas forced NEAT1 expression had the opposite effect in the HT29 cells (Fig. 2c). This result was also confirmed by the EdU and colony formation assays (Fig. 2d, e, Additional file 3: Figure S1B-C).

Furthermore, our results showed that repression of NEAT1 induced late apoptosis (Additional file 4: Figure S2A-B) and G0/G1 phase arrest (Additional file 4: Figure S2D) in HCT116 and SW1116 cells. The western blotting analysis verified increased PARP1 and cleaved caspase 3 expression (Additional file 4: Figure S2C) and decreased cyclin D1 and p27 expression. In contrast, the G2/M transition-related markers cyclin B1 and CDC25B were not obviously altered (Additional file 4: Figure S2E). These results suggested that NEAT1 promoted CRC cell proliferation by reducing cell apoptosis and inducing the G1 to S phase cell cycle transition.

To further validate these effects in vivo, we injected HCT116-shNEAT1 and HCT116-shNC cells into the subcutis of nude mice. Consistent with our in vitro results, the volumes and weights of the tumors formed by the HCT116-shNEAT1 cells were significantly smaller than those formed by the control cells (Fig. 2f–h). The Ki-67 index was lower in the NEAT1 knockdown groups (Fig. 2i). These results suggested that NEAT1 promoted the tumorigenesis of CRC cells both in vitro and in vivo.

Altered NEAT1 affected CRC cell migration and invasion in vitro and in vivo

To determine the effect of altered NEAT1 expression on the migration and invasion of CRC cells, NEAT1-siRNA-transfected and NEAT1 plasmid-transfected CRC cells were wounded by scratching and maintained for 24 h. Knockdown of NEAT1 significantly inhibited the flattening and spreading abilities of the HCT116 and SW1116 cells (Fig. 3a, b, Additional file 5: Figure S3A), whereas overexpression of NEAT1 strongly promoted the flattening and spreading abilities of the HT29 cells (Fig. 3c, Additional file 5: Figure S3A). This result was also confirmed by the Transwell assay. We found that the invasive abilities of the NEAT1-siRNA-transfected HCT116 and SW1116 cells were significantly inhibited (Fig. 3d, Additional file 5: Figure S3B), whereas the invasive ability was higher in the NEAT1-transfected HT29 cells than in the control cells (Fig. 3e, Additional file 5: Figure S3B). Accordingly, the RT-qPCR and western blotting results showed that downregulation of NEAT1 resulted in higher E-cadherin expression and lower N-cadherin expression at both the mRNA and protein levels (Fig. 3f, Additional file 5: Figure S3C). The cell migration and invasion markers MMP2 and MMP9 were also decreased when NEAT1 was downregulated (Fig. 3f). However, overexpression of NEAT1 led to increased N-cadherin, MMP2, and MMP9 and decreased E-cadherin expression (Fig. 3f).

Next, we evaluated the functional role of NEAT1 in CRC cell metastasis in vivo. We injected HCT116-shNEAT1 and HCT116-shNC cells into the tail veins of mice in groups of four. The number of lung metastatic tumor nodules was decreased in the HCT116-shNEAT1 group compared with that of the HCT116-shNC group (Fig. 3g). Consistent with the effects of NEAT1 expression on migration and invasion in vitro, NEAT1 knockdown significantly abrogated metastasis both in vitro and in vivo.

NEAT1 interacted and enhanced with DDX5 stability

As described above, NEAT1 plays an important role in CRC progression, although the detailed mechanism remains unknown. Because lncRNAs can interact with proteins, a biotin RNA-protein pull-down assay was performed to identify potential proteins binding to NEAT1 (Fig. 4a). Interestingly, DDX5 was identified as an interacting target of NEAT1 by MS analysis (Additional file 6: Table S6), and an immunoprecipitation assay further confirmed that DDX5 directly bound to NEAT1 (Fig. 4b). Intriguingly, the RIP assay confirmed the interaction between DDX5 and NEAT1 in extracts from HCT116 cells. SNRNP70 was used as the positive control (Fig. 4c). Collectively, these results demonstrated a direct interaction between DDX5 and NEAT1.

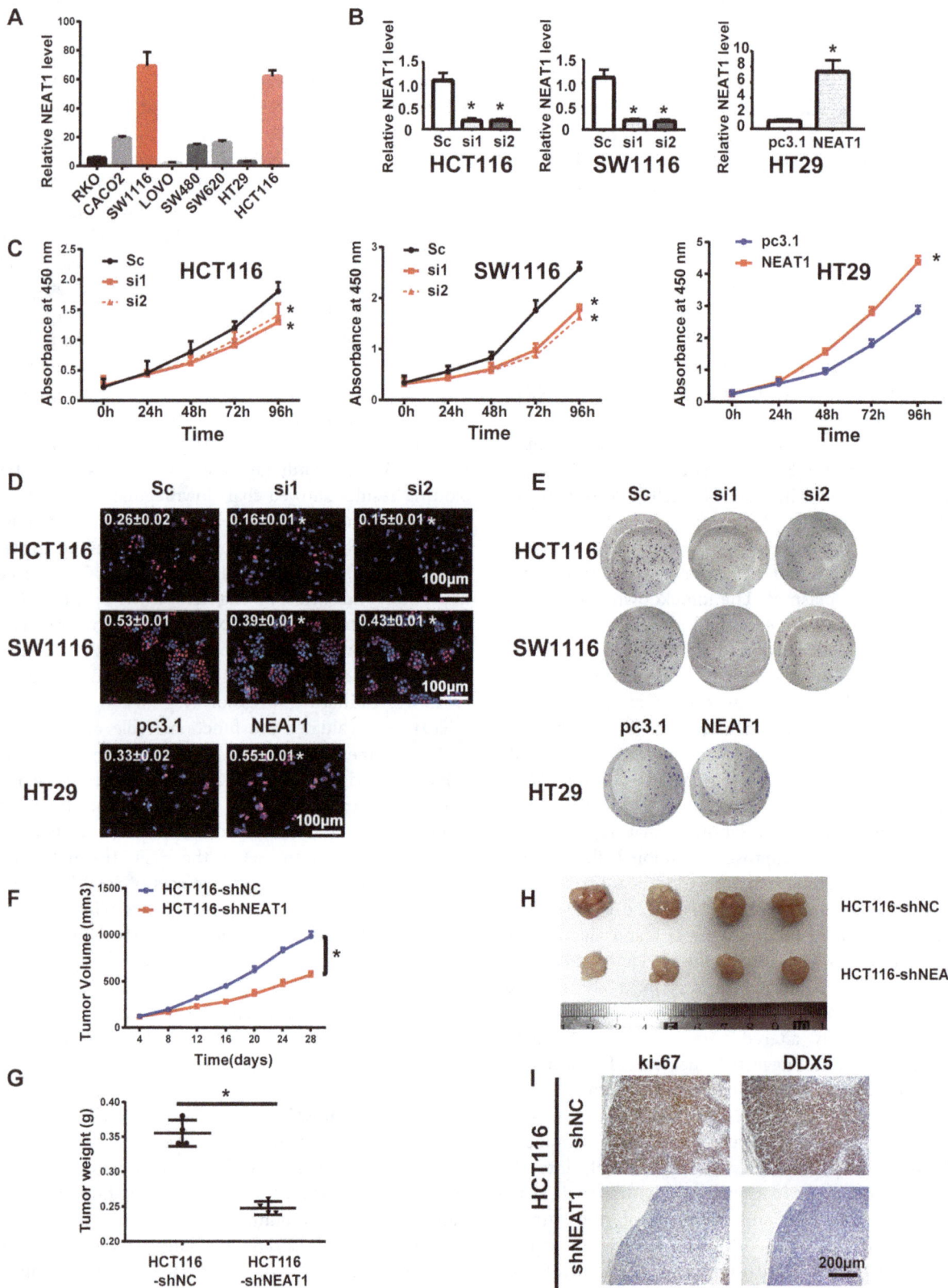

Fig. 2 (See legend on next page.)

(See figure on previous page.)

Fig. 2 NEAT1 promoted CRC cell proliferation in vitro and in vivo. **a** The baseline NEAT1 RNA levels in eight CRC cell lines detected by RT-qPCR. **b** The efficiency of NEAT1 knockdown or overexpression was detected by RT-qPCR in the indicated cells transfected with siRNAs or plasmids (*$p < 0.05$). **c** CCK8 and **d** EdU assays showing that knockdown of NEAT1 suppressed cell proliferation in the HCT116 and SW1116 cell lines (*$p < 0.05$) and that upregulation of NEAT1 promoted cell proliferation in the HT29 cell line (*$p < 0.05$). **e** Colony formation assays for the indicated cells after transfection with siRNAs or plasmids (*$p < 0.05$). The nude mouse xenograft model showed that knockdown of NEAT1 decreased tumor growth (**f**) and the tumor weights (**g**) compared with those of the HCT116-shNC cells (*$p < 0.05$). **h** Representative images of tumors in nude mice. **i** Representative images of IHC staining for ki-67 and DDX5 (**Sc** represents scramble)

Next, we analyzed the regulatory effects of NEAT1 on DDX5. We found that downregulation of NEAT1 effectively reduced the DDX5 protein level but not the mRNA level in the HCT116 and SW1116 cells (Fig. 4d, e). In addition, immunohistochemistry analysis of xenografts showed that nude mice in the NEAT1-knockdown group exhibited lower DDX5 expression (Fig. 2i). To further clarify the mechanism underlying the regulation of DDX5 expression by NEAT1, first we examined whether NEAT1 could

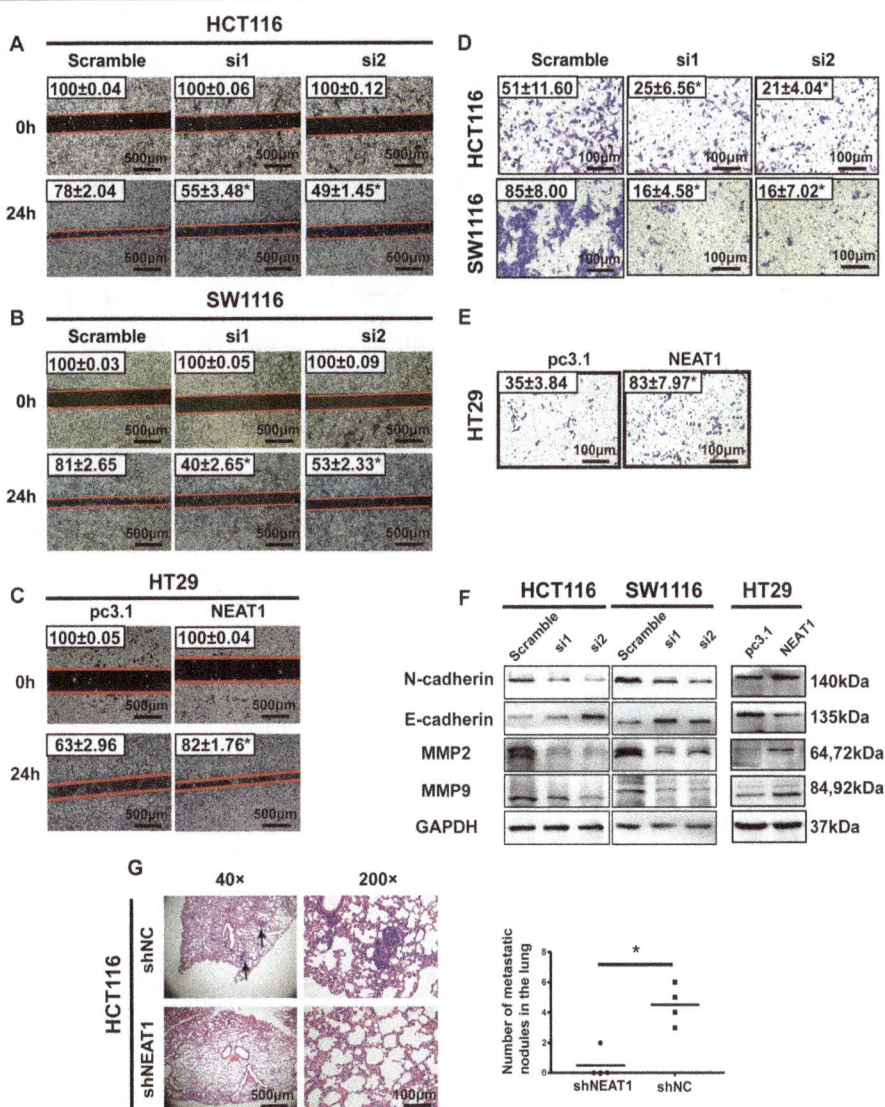

Fig. 3 Repression of NEAT1-inhibited cell invasion and migration in vitro and in vivo. Representative images (×40) of wound healing assays in HCT116 (**a**), SW1116 (**b**), and HT29 (**c**) cells (*$p < 0.05$). **d** Representative images (×200) of Transwell invasion assays for the indicated cells (*$p < 0.05$). **e** Representative images of Transwell invasion assays for HT29 cells. **f** Western blotting results for N-cadherin, E-cadherin, MMP2, and MMP9. **g** Representative images of lung metastasis in nude mice with HE staining

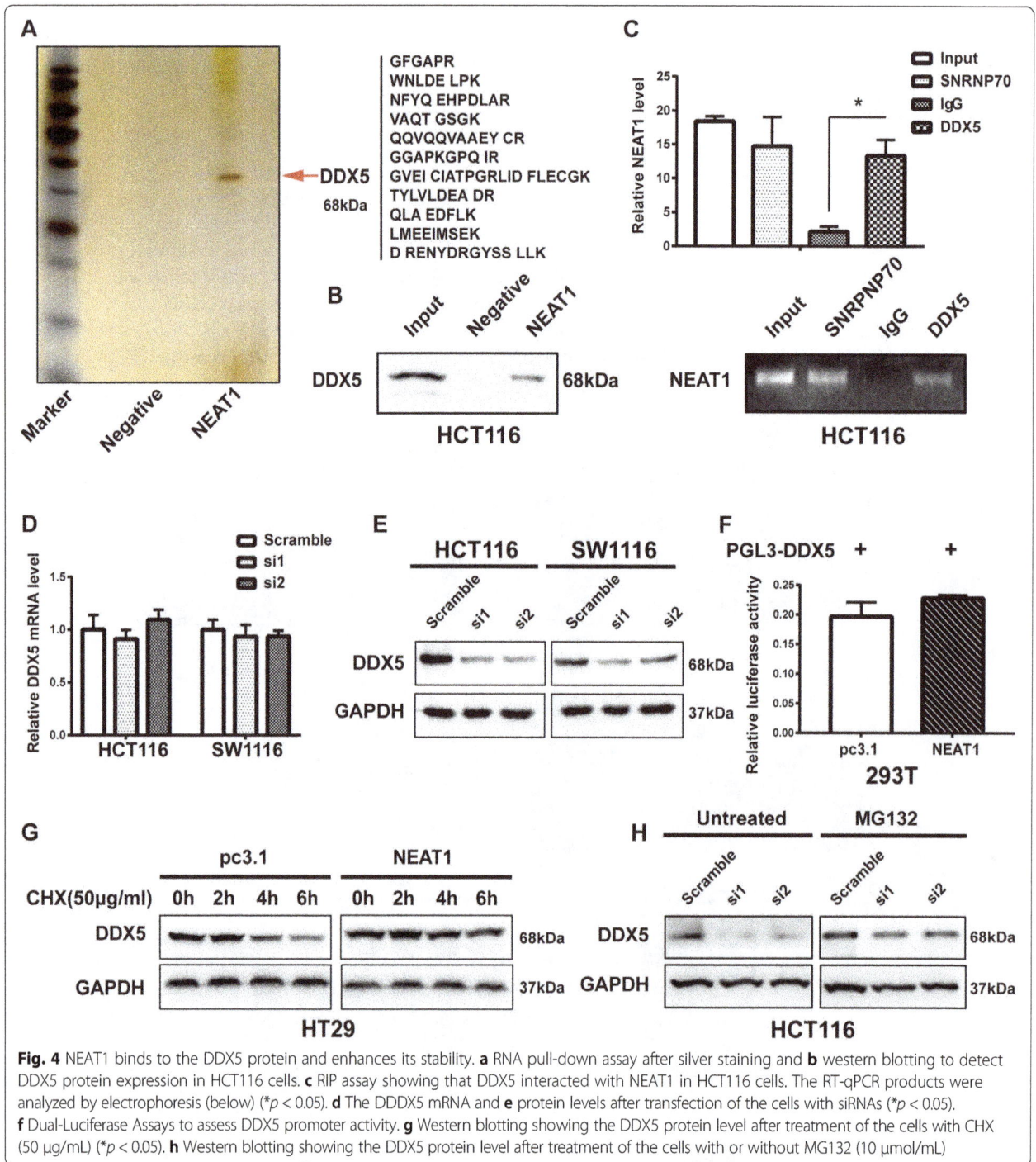

Fig. 4 NEAT1 binds to the DDX5 protein and enhances its stability. **a** RNA pull-down assay after silver staining and **b** western blotting to detect DDX5 protein expression in HCT116 cells. **c** RIP assay showing that DDX5 interacted with NEAT1 in HCT116 cells. The RT-qPCR products were analyzed by electrophoresis (below) (*$p < 0.05$). **d** The DDDX5 mRNA and **e** protein levels after transfection of the cells with siRNAs (*$p < 0.05$). **f** Dual-Luciferase Assays to assess DDX5 promoter activity. **g** Western blotting showing the DDX5 protein level after treatment of the cells with CHX (50 μg/mL) (*$p < 0.05$). **h** Western blotting showing the DDX5 protein level after treatment of the cells with or without MG132 (10 μmol/mL)

directly regulate the transcriptional activity of DDX5. Our results showed that DDX5 promoter activity was not increased in NEAT1-transfected HCT116 cells (Fig. 4f), suggesting that NEAT1 might participate in regulation of DDX5 at the posttranscriptional level. Therefore, we used the protein synthesis inhibitor cycloheximide (CHX) to observe the effect of NEAT1 on DDX5 degradation. The western blotting results showed that overexpression of

NEAT1 in HT29 cells enhanced DDX5 protein stability (Fig. 4g). Moreover, the 26S proteasome inhibitor MG132 rescued the reduction of DDX5 caused by repression of NEAT1 in HCT116 cells (Fig. 4h), suggesting that NEAT1 elevated DDX5 by reducing its degradation. Taken together, our data indicated that NEAT1 directly bound the DDX5 protein and enhanced its stability in CRC cells.

NEAT1 activated Wnt/β-catenin signaling by targeting DDX5

Recently, decreased NEAT1 expression was reported to inhibit Wnt/β-catenin signaling pathway activity in glioblastoma [21]. In our study, we performed a TOP/FOP-flash luciferase assay; the results revealed that Wnt/β-catenin signaling was inhibited by NEAT1 depletion (Fig. 5b). However, the Dual-Luciferase Reporter Assay showed that NEAT1 did not influence the activity of the β-catenin 3′-UTR (Fig. 5a), which indicated that NEAT1 did not regulate β-catenin directly. DDX5 reportedly forms a complex with β-catenin and promotes its transcriptional ability to activate gene transcription [22]. Co-IP assays detected an interaction between endogenous DDX5 and β-catenin (Fig. 5d) in HCT116 cells, and knockdown of DDX5 reduced the β-catenin level (Fig. 5e). We speculated that NEAT1 might activate Wnt/β-catenin signaling by targeting DDX5. To explore the effects of NEAT1 on Wnt/β-catenin signaling, we examined the levels of the Wnt/β-catenin signaling targets Axin2,

c-myc, and cyclin D1. The RT-qPCR and western blotting analyses showed that downregulation of NEAT1 reduced the mRNA (Additional file 5: Figure S3D) and protein (Fig. 5c) levels of Wnt/β-catenin signaling target genes. Furthermore, the increased TOP/FOP-flash luciferase activity resulting from NEAT1 overexpression was significantly suppressed by si-DDX5 (Fig. 5b), suggesting that NEAT1-induced activation of Wnt/β-catenin signaling was dependent on DDX5 expression. The RT-qPCR and western blotting analyses showed that downregulation of DDX5 did not reduce the NEAT1 RNA level but did abrogate the increase in the Axin2, c-myc, and cyclin D1 levels (Fig. 5f, Additional file 5: Figure S3E). Collectively, our results suggest that NEAT1 indirectly promotes β-catenin transcriptional activation by binding to DDX5.

NEAT1 facilitated tumor proliferation and metastasis in a DDX5-mediated manner

To elucidate whether NEAT1 functioned in CRC cells in a DDX5-mediated manner, we performed CCK-8 and

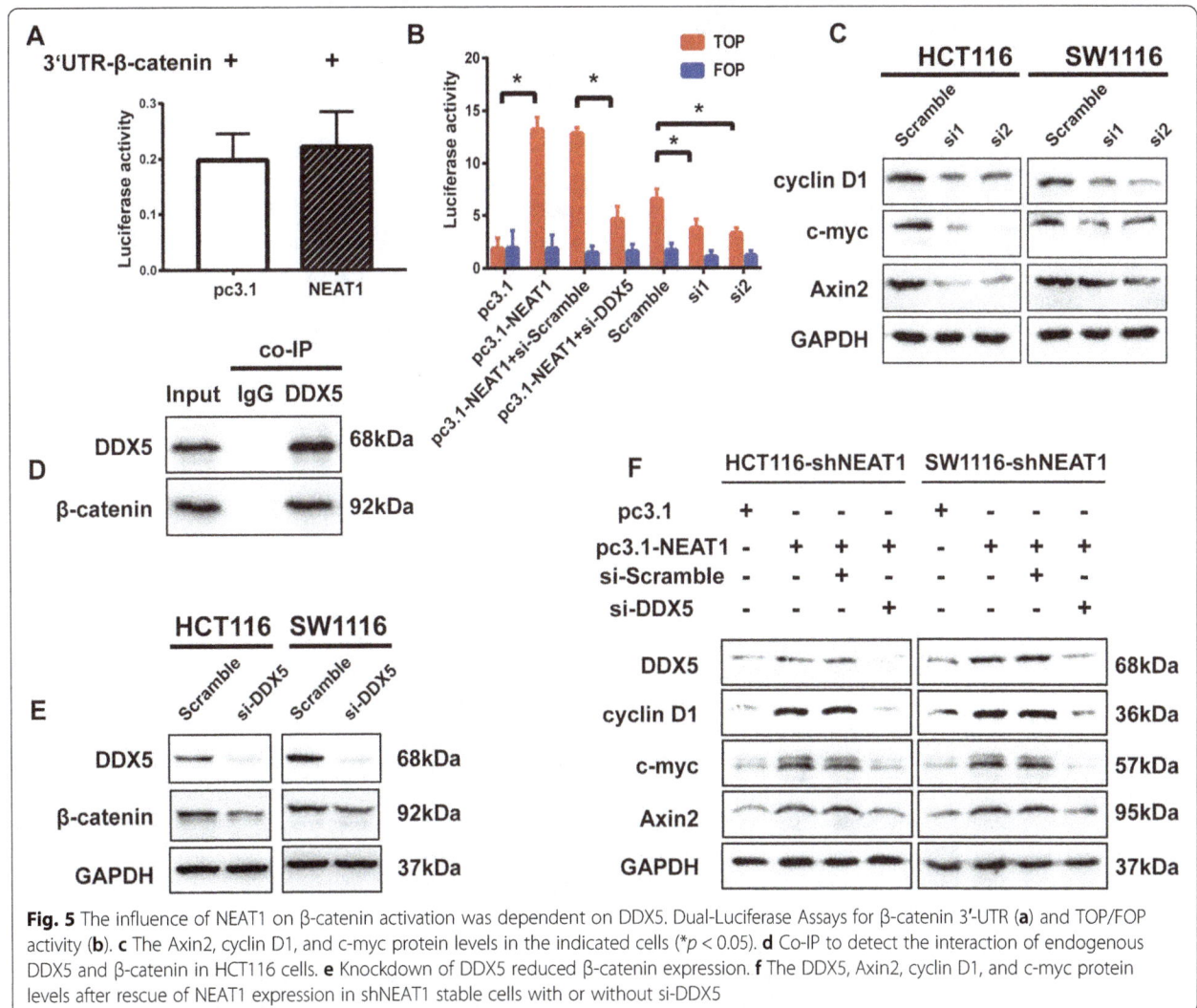

Fig. 5 The influence of NEAT1 on β-catenin activation was dependent on DDX5. Dual-Luciferase Assays for β-catenin 3′-UTR (a) and TOP/FOP activity (b). c The Axin2, cyclin D1, and c-myc protein levels in the indicated cells (*p < 0.05). d Co-IP to detect the interaction of endogenous DDX5 and β-catenin in HCT116 cells. e Knockdown of DDX5 reduced β-catenin expression. f The DDX5, Axin2, cyclin D1, and c-myc protein levels after rescue of NEAT1 expression in shNEAT1 stable cells with or without si-DDX5

EdU assays. The results showed that overexpression of NEAT1 recovered the proliferation potential of HCT116 and SW1116 NEAT1 stable knockdown cells, which nevertheless was impaired by the simultaneous downregulation of DDX5 (Fig. 6d, e). Similarly, the effect of NEAT1 on the invasion and migration of CRC cells was also partially attenuated by repression of DDX5 (Fig. 6c, d). Therefore, we hypothesized that NEAT1 facilitated tumor proliferation and metastasis in a DDX5-mediated manner.

Clinical associations between NEAT1 and DDX5 in human CRC samples

Finally, we tested the clinical association between NEAT1 and DDX5 in the FDUSCC dataset. Immunohistochemistry analysis of CRC samples showed that DDX5 was located in the cell nucleus and was overexpressed in cancerous tissues compared to normal tissues (Fig. 7a). In addition, DDX5 expression was correlated with NEAT1 expression in 71 CRC samples ($p < 0.01$, Fig. 7b). The survival analysis demonstrated that CRC patients with positive DDX5 expression (H score ≥ 50) had poorer OS and DFS than those with negative DDX5 expression (Fig. 7c, d). Next, the patients were divided into three groups based on their NEAT1 and DDX5 expression levels. Patients with positive NEAT1 and DDX5 expression had the poorest OS and DFS. In contrast, those with negative NEAT1 and DDX5 expression had the best OS ($p = 0.008$) and DFS ($p = 0.016$) (Fig. 7e, f). In addition, the multivariate COX analysis showed that the combination of NEAT1 and DDX5 was an independent prognostic indicator of OS ($p = 0.024$, HR = 6.916, 95% CI 1.291–37.051, Additional file 2: Table S5).

Discussion

Nuclear lncRNAs participate in many critical biological processes and are often dysregulated in a variety of cancers, including CRC. However, further investigations are required to elucidate how individual lncRNAs function [23]. Our study contributes to understanding the role of NEAT1 upregulation in CRC progression. Our results suggest that NEAT1 promotes CRC tumor growth and metastasis by stabilizing the DDX5 protein, thereby activating β-catenin gene transcription.

The role of NEAT1 in tumors seems to be controversial. Some studies have shown that NEAT1 is an oncogene in various cancers, such as lung cancer, breast cancer, prostate cancer, colorectal cancer, and pancreatic cancer [12, 24–26]. In prostate cancer, *Chakravarty D* et al. [24] demonstrated that NEAT1 was recruited to the promoters of well-characterized prostate cancer-related genes and contributed to an epigenetic "on" state. Other studies have shown that NEAT1 acts as a tumor suppressor and a target of p53. *Adriaens* et al. [27] showed that NEAT1 promoted ATR signaling in response to replication stress and was engaged in a negative feedback loop that attenuated oncogene-dependent activation of p53. *Blume CJ* et al. [28] indicated that NEAT1 and lincRNA-p21 were induced in response to DNA damage in the presence of functional p53 but not in chronic lymphocytic leukemia with a p53 mutation. *Masashi Idogawa* et al. [29] showed that p53 could induce NEAT1 expression in cells with wild-type p53, such as A549 and MCF7, but that NEAT1 was not increased at all in HCT116 (p53–/–) cells. Therefore, the role of NEAT1 in tumor cells may be cell-type dependent, although this possibility needs to be further studied.

NEAT1 is an essential component of nuclear paraspeckles [30], which contain ribonucleoprotein complexes formed around NEAT1 [9]. At present, NEAT1 is thought to be exclusive to the nucleus and mainly function as a transcriptional regulator. In our study, we found that NEAT1 was mainly located in the nucleus with a small amount in the cytoplasm, which was consistent with the report of Chiu et al. [31]. Furthermore, we found that NEAT1 interacted with DDX5 and enhanced its stability posttranslationally, which seemed to be inconsistent with its traditional function; however, a number of posttranscriptional functions for nuclear lncRNAs are also emerging (e.g., HOTAIR assists in assembling the chromatin modification complex in the nucleus). Yoon JH et al. [32] showed evidence that HOTAIR promoted the ubiquitination of Ataxin-1 by Dzip3 and Snurportin-1 by Mex3b and increased their degradation. Because Dzip3 was localized in the cytoplasm, the enhanced ubiquitination of Ataxin-1 might be linked to the cytoplasmic presence of HOTAIR. Mex3b and Snurportin-1 localized in both the nucleus and the cytoplasm, which suggested that HOTAIR-facilitated ubiquitination could occur in both cellular compartments [32].

Studies have reported that acetylation and sumoylation of DDX5 increase its stability. Thus, NEAT1 may form complexes with a histone acetyltransferase or SUMO-conjugating enzymes and interact with their substrate DDX5. By facilitating formation of the complexes, NEAT1 mediates the proteolysis of DDX5.

DDX5 is a prototypical member of the DEAD box family of RNA helicases and plays important roles in multiple biological processes, including cell proliferation, early organ development, and maturation [33–35]. DDX5 exhibited clear cell cycle-related localization in the nucleus, and its expression was related to tumor progression and transformation [36]. DDX5 was determined to be overexpressed in colon cancer, and the degree of its expression was associated with progression of the disease from polyp to adenoma to adenocarcinoma [22]. DDX5 may affect β-catenin in two ways: in the

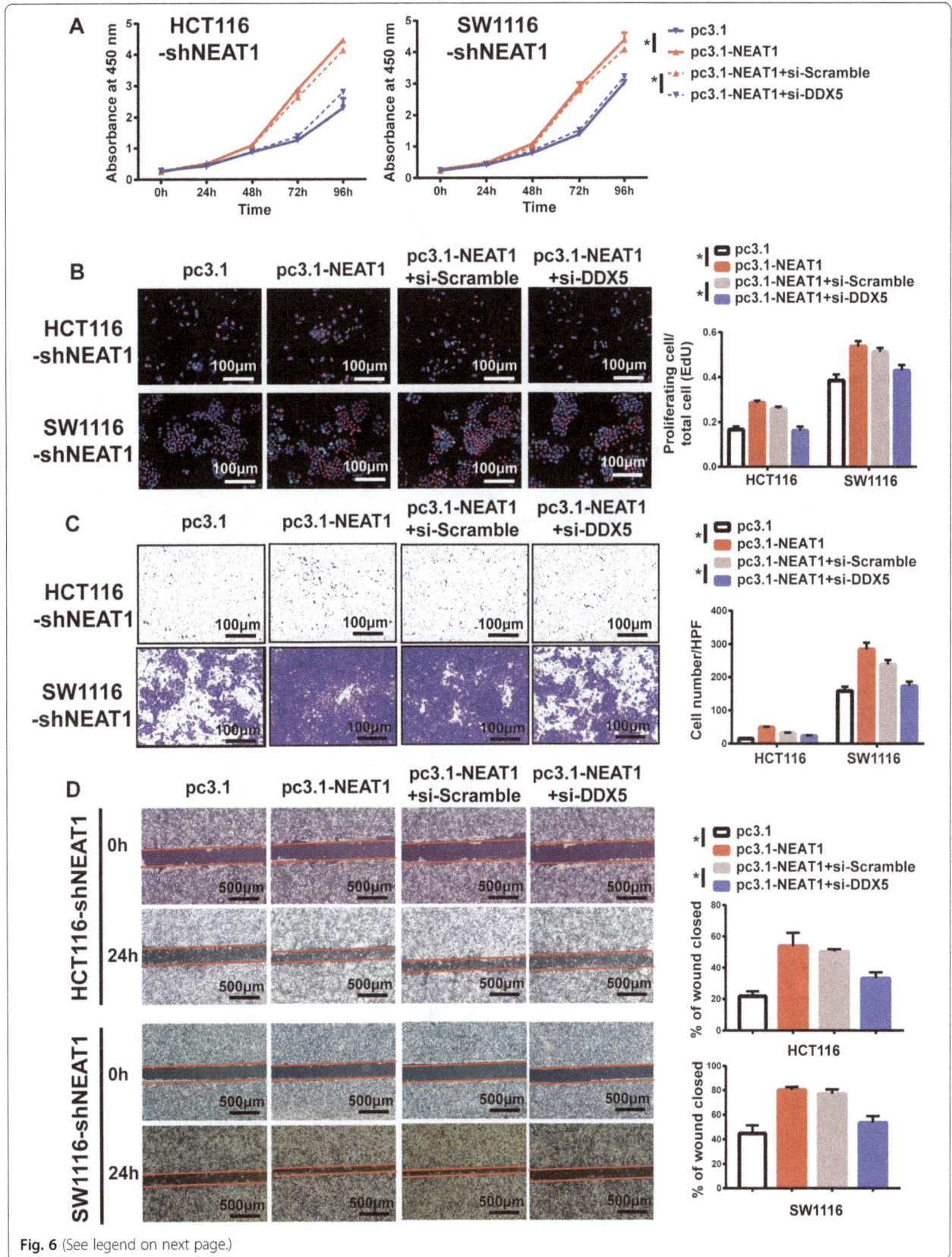

Fig. 6 (See legend on next page.)

(See figure on previous page.)
Fig. 6 NEAT1 facilitated CRC cell progression in a DDX5-mediated manner. **a** CCK-8 and **b** EdU assay results showing that knockdown of DDX5 partially attenuated the enhanced cell proliferation induced by overexpression of NEAT1 in HCT116-shNEAT1 and SW1116-shNEAT1 cells (*$p < 0.05$). Representative images of the **c** Transwell invasion assays and **d** wound healing assays showing that DDX5 repression rescued the enhanced invasion and migration abilities induced by NEAT1 overexpression (*$p < 0.05$)

cytoplasm by protecting β-catenin from degradation via dissociation from the cytoplasmic APC/axin/GSK-3β complex or in the nucleus by augmenting β-catenin transcriptional activity [22]. The IHC analyses of DDX5 expression in nude mice and the tissue microarrays in our study indicated that the latter possibility was more likely. DDX5 can directly bind β-catenin and TCF4 to activate β-catenin transcription [22, 37, 38]. To the best of our knowledge, β-catenin plays important roles in CRC progression. Thus, we investigated whether NEAT1 affected β-catenin in a manner that was dependent on or independent of DDX5. Because NEAT1 was located in the cell nucleus, we conceived that it might affect

β-catenin transcriptional activity. Our results confirmed that NEAT1 indirectly promoted β-catenin transcriptional activation in a manner that was dependent upon DDX5. Furthermore, NEAT1 regulated DDX5 expression by enhancing its protein stability.

Finally, our study investigated the clinical significance of NEAT1 and DDX5. NEAT1 was positively correlated with DDX5 expression in 71 CRC patients. Interestingly, although NEAT1 alone could not predict the DFS of CRC patients, patients with high NEAT1 expression together with positive DDX5 expression had the worst OS and DFS. These findings highlight that NEAT1 acts as an onco-lncRNA by regulating DDX5 in CRC.

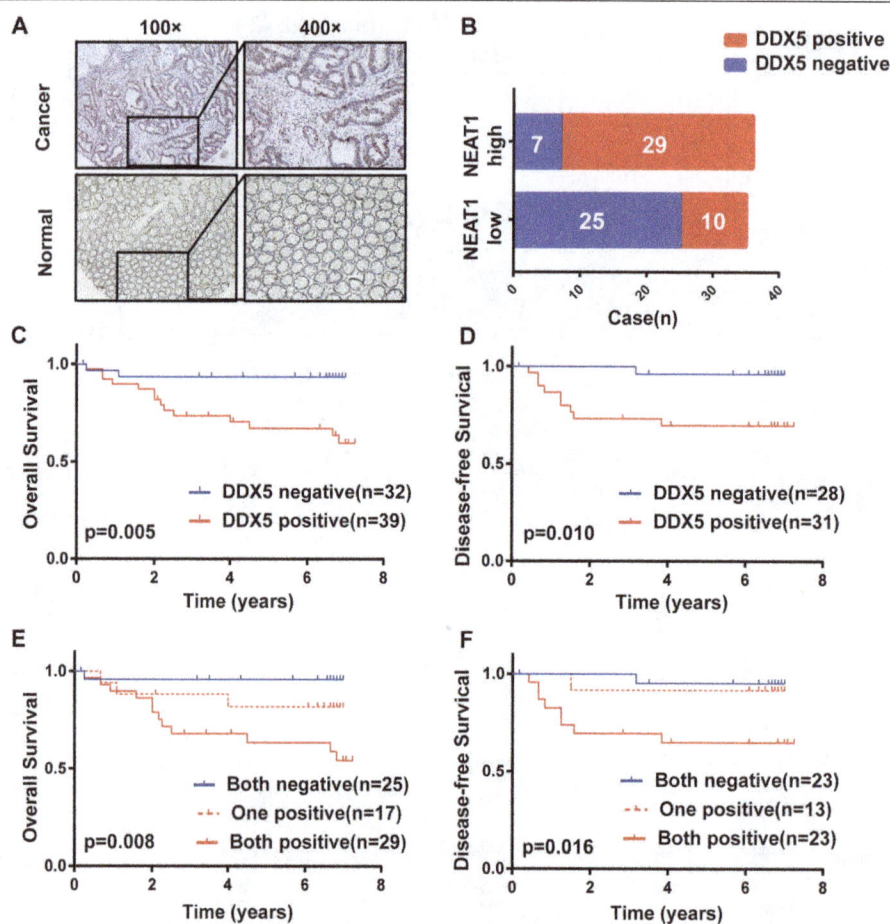

Fig. 7 NEAT1 and DDX5 expression in clinical CRC samples. **a** Representative images of DDX5 detected by IHC. **b** The chi-square test identified an association between DDX5 and NEAT1 in the CRC samples ($n = 71$, $p < 0.01$). **c–f** Kaplan-Meier analyses of the FDUSCC dataset. Patients with high DDX5 expression had poorer OS (**c**) and DFS (**d**) than those with negative expression. The patients were divided into three groups based on NEAT1 and DDX5 expression (negative or positive). Both positive groups had the poorest prognoses with the lowest OS (**e**) and DFS (**f**)

The lncRNA NEAT1 activates Wnt/β-catenin signaling and promotes colorectal cancer progression...

27

Conclusions

In summary, our study demonstrated important roles of NEAT1 in CRC progression and showed that NEAT1 activated β-catenin transcriptional activity by directly binding DDX5, which might reflect the underlying molecular mechanisms of their biological functions. These findings provide new insights into the roles of lncRNAs in CRC progression. Together with further research, these findings may prove to be clinically useful strategies for CRC treatment.

Additional files

Additional file 1: Supplemental materials and methods. (DOCX 20 kb)

Additional file 2: Table S1. Primary antibodies for western blot. **Table S2.** Primers for real-time PCR. **Table S3.** Association between clinicopathological features and NEAT1 expression. **Table S4.** Univariate Cox proportional hazards model for overall survival (OS) and disease-free survival (DFS). **Table S5.** Multivariate Cox proportional hazards model for OS and DFS. (DOCX 29 kb)

Additional file 3: Figure S1. (A) NEAT1 was mainly located in nuclear. (B) Column chart of EdU assay of indicated CRC cells (*$p < 0.05$). (C) Quantitative results for colony formation assay of indicated CRC cells (*$p < 0.05$). (TIF 16126 kb)

Additional file 4: Figure S2. (A–B). Knockdown of NEAT1 increased the proportion of late apoptotic cells (*$p < 0.05$). (C) Western blot showed that knockdown of NEAT1 enhanced PARP1 and caspase-3 cleavage. (D) Repression of NEAT1 inhibited the transition from the G0/G1 to the S phase of the cell cycle (*$p < 0.05$). (E) Western blot showed the reduction of cyclin D1 and p27 after NEAT1 repression. (c-PARP1 represents cleaved-PARP1; c-caspase3 represents cleaved-caspase3). (TIF 1695 kb)

Additional file 5: Figure S3. Quantitative results for wound healing assays (A) and Transwell assays (B) of indicated CRC cells. (C) The mRNA level of N-cadherin and E-cadherin (*$p < 0.05$). (D) The mRNA level of Axin2, cyclin D1, and c-myc for indicated cells (*$p < 0.05$). (E) The mRNA level changes of DDX5, Axin2, cyclin D1, and c-myc after NEAT1 expression rescued in shNEAT1 stable cells with or without si-DDX5 (*$p < 0.05$). (Sc represents scramble) (TIF 986 kb)

Additional file 6: Table S6. Mass spectrometry analysis for RNA pull-down. (XLSX 78 kb)

Abbreviations

CHX: Cycloheximide; CRC: Colorectal cancer; DFS: Disease-free survival; FDUSCC: Fudan University Shanghai Cancer Center; MS: Mass spectrometry; OS: Overall survival; RIP: RNA immunoprecipitation

Funding

This study was supported by grants from the National Natural Science Foundation of China (81472222, 81772583, 81572254, 81472220, 81602269, 81602078, and 81272299), the Science and Technology Commission of the Shanghai Municipality (15495810300 and 17ZR1406500), the Shanghai Hospital Development Centre Emerging Advanced Technology joint research project (HDC12014105), the Shanghai Key Developing Disciplines (2015ZB0201), the Shanghai Science and Technology Development Fund (no. 15ZR1407400), the Domestic Science and Technology Cooperation Project (no. 14495800300), and the Hospital Foundation of the Fudan University Shanghai Cancer Center (YJ201504).

Authors' contributions

MZ, PW, and XD participated in the research design and coordination and helped draft the manuscript. MZ and WW conducted the experiments. MZ, QZ, and YW performed the immunoassays. SN, CT, and HS contributed to clinical sample collection. MZ, MX, and CL performed the data analysis. All authors read and approved the final manuscript.

Consent for publication

Informed consent for publication was obtained from all participants.

Competing interests

The authors declare that they have no competing interests.

Author details

¹Department of Pathology, Fudan University Shanghai Cancer Center, Shanghai 200032, China. ²Department of Pathology, Shanghai Medical College, Fudan University, Shanghai, China. ³Institute of Pathology, Fudan University, Shanghai, China. ⁴Department of Oncology, Shanghai Medical College, Fudan University, Shanghai, China. ⁵Institutes of Biomedical Sciences, Fudan University, Shanghai, China. ⁶Cancer Institute, Fudan University Shanghai Cancer Center, Shanghai, China.

References

1. Siegel R, Desantis C, Jemal A. Colorectal cancer statistics, 2014. CA Cancer J Clin. 2014;64(2):104–17.
2. Dow LE, O'Rourke KP, Simon J, Tschaharganeh DF, van Es JH, Clevers H, et al. Apc restoration promotes cellular differentiation and reestablishes crypt homeostasis in colorectal cancer. Cell. 2015;161(7):1539–52.
3. Kong J, Sun W, Li C, Wan L, Wang S, Wu Y, et al. Long non-coding RNA LINC01133 inhibits epithelial-mesenchymal transition and metastasis in colorectal cancer by interacting with SRSF6. Cancer Lett. 2016;380(2):476–84.
4. Lee JT. Epigenetic regulation by long noncoding RNAs. Science. 2012; 338(6113):1435–9.
5. Huang X, Xiao R, Pan S, Yang X, Yuan W, Tu Z, et al. Uncovering the roles of long non-coding RNAs in cancer stem cells. J Hematol Oncol. 2017;10(1):62.
6. Ulitsky I, Bartel DP. lincRNAs: genomics, evolution, and mechanisms. Cell. 2013;154(1):26–46.
7. Necsulea A, Soumillon M, Warnefors M, Liechti A, Daish T, Zeller U, et al. The evolution of lncRNA repertoires and expression patterns in tetrapods. Nature. 2014;505(7485):635–40.
8. Guttman M, Rinn JL. Modular regulatory principles of large non-coding RNAs. Nature. 2012;482(7385):339–46.
9. Clemson CM, Hutchinson JN, Sara SA, Ensminger AW, Fox AH, Chess A, et al. An architectural role for a nuclear noncoding RNA: NEAT1 RNA is essential for the structure of paraspeckles. Mol Cell. 2009;33(6):717–26.
10. Sunwoo H, Dinger ME, Wilusz JE, Amaral PP, Mattick JS, Spector DL. MEN epsilon/beta nuclear-retained non-coding RNAs are up-regulated upon muscle differentiation and are essential components of paraspeckles. Genome Res. 2009;19(3):347–59.
11. Tripathi V, Ellis JD, Shen Z, Song DY, Pan Q, Watt AT, et al. The nuclear-retained noncoding RNA MALAT1 regulates alternative splicing by modulating SR splicing factor phosphorylation. Mol Cell. 2010;39(6):925–38.
12. Li Y, Li Y, Chen W, He F, Tan Z, Zheng J, et al. NEAT expression is associated with tumor recurrence and unfavorable prognosis in colorectal cancer. Oncotarget. 2015;6(29):27641–50.
13. Wu Y, Yang L, Zhao J, Li C, Nie J, Liu F, et al. Nuclear-enriched abundant transcript 1 as a diagnostic and prognostic biomarker in colorectal cancer. Mol Cancer. 2015;14:191.
14. Xiong DD, Feng ZB, Cen WL, Zeng JJ, Liang L, Tang RX, et al. The clinical value of lncRNA NEAT1 in digestive system malignances: a comprehensive investigation based on 57 microarray and RNA-seq datasets. Oncotarget. 2017;8(11):17665–83.

15. Fodde R, Smits R, Clevers H. APC, signal transduction and genetic instability in colorectal cancer. Nat Rev Cancer. 2001;1(1):55–67.

16. Yamada N, Noguchi S, Mori T, Naoe T, Maruo K, Akao Y. Tumor-suppressive microRNA-145 targets catenin delta-1 to regulate Wnt/beta-catenin signaling in human colon cancer cells. Cancer Lett. 2013;335(2):332–42.

17. He TC, Sparks AB, Rago C, Hermeking H, Zawel L, da Costa LT, et al. Identification of c-MYC as a target of the APC pathway. Science. 1998; 281(5382):1509–12.

18. Shtutman M, Zhurinsky J, Simcha I, Albanese C, D'Amico M, Pestell R, et al. The cyclin D1 gene is a target of the beta-catenin/LEF-1 pathway. Proc Natl Acad Sci U S A. 1999;96(10):5522–7.

19. Clevers H, Nusse R. Wnt/beta-catenin signaling and disease. Cell. 2012; 149(6):1192–205.

20. Xu MD, Wang Y, Weng W, Wei P, Qi P, Zhang Q, et al. A positive feedback loop of lncRNA-PVT1 and FOXM1 facilitates gastric cancer growth and invasion. Clin Cancer Res. 2017;23(8):2071–80.

21. Chen Q, Cai J, Wang Q, Wang Y, Liu M, Yang J, et al. Long noncoding RNA NEAT1, regulated by the EGFR pathway, contributes to glioblastoma progression through the WNT/beta-catenin pathway by scaffolding EZH2. Clin Cancer Res. 2018;24(3):684–95.

22. Shin S, Rossow KL, Grande JP, Janknecht R. Involvement of RNA helicases p68 and p72 in colon cancer. Cancer Res. 2007;67(16):7572–8.

23. Qi P, Du X. The long non-coding RNAs, a new cancer diagnostic and therapeutic gold mine. Mod Pathol. 2013;26(2):155–65.

24. Chakravarty D, Sboner A, Nair SS, Giannopoulou E, Li R, Hennig S, et al. The oestrogen receptor alpha-regulated lncRNA NEAT1 is a critical modulator of prostate cancer. Nat Commun. 2014;5:5383.

25. Lo PK, Zhang Y, Wolfson B, Gernapudi R, Yao Y, Duru N, et al. Dysregulation of the BRCA1/long non-coding RNA NEAT1 signaling axis contributes to breast tumorigenesis. Oncotarget. 2016;7(40):65067–89.

26. Sun C, Li S, Zhang F, Xi Y, Wang L, Bi Y, et al. Long non-coding RNA NEAT1 promotes non-small cell lung cancer progression through regulation of miR-377-3p-E2F3 pathway. Oncotarget. 2016;7(32):51784–814.

27. Adriaens C, Standaert L, Barra J, Latil M, Verfaillie A, Kalev P, et al. p53 induces formation of NEAT1 lncRNA-containing paraspeckles that modulate replication stress response and chemosensitivity. Nat Med. 2016;22(8):861–8.

28. Blume CJ, Hotz-Wagenblatt A, Hullein J, Sellner L, Jethwa A, Stolz T, et al. p53-dependent non-coding RNA networks in chronic lymphocytic leukemia. Leukemia. 2015;29(10):2015–23.

29. Idogawa M, Ohashi T, Sasaki Y, Nakase H, Tokino T. Long non-coding RNA NEAT1 is a transcriptional target of p53 and modulates p53-induced transactivation and tumor-suppressor function. Int J Cancer. 2017;140(12): 2785–91.

30. Anantharaman A, Jadaliha M, Tripathi V, Nakagawa S, Hirose T, Jantsch MF, et al. Paraspeckles modulate the intranuclear distribution of paraspeckle-associated Ctn RNA. Sci Rep. 2016;6:34043.

31. Chiu HS, Somvanshi S, Patel E, Chen TW, Singh VP, Zorman B, et al. Pan-cancer analysis of lncRNA regulation supports their targeting of cancer genes in each tumor context. Cell Rep. 2018;23(1):297–312. e212

32. Yoon JH, Abdelmohsen K, Kim J, Yang X, Martindale JL, Tominaga-Yamanaka K, et al. Scaffold function of long non-coding RNA HOTAIR in protein ubiquitination. Nat Commun. 2013;4:2939.

33. Heinlein UA. Dead box for the living. J Pathol. 1998;184(4):345–7.

34. Stevenson RJ, Hamilton SJ, MacCallum DE, Hall PA, Fuller-Pace FV. Expression of the "dead box" RNA helicase p68 is developmentally and growth regulated and correlates with organ differentiation/maturation in the fetus. J Pathol. 1998;184(4):351–9.

35. Jacob J, Favicchio R, Karimian N, Mehrabi M, Harding V, Castellano L, et al. LMTK3 escapes tumour suppressor miRNAs via sequestration of DDX5. Cancer Lett. 2016;372(1):137–46.

36. Causevic M, Hislop RG, Kernohan NM, Carey FA, Kay RA, Steele RJ, et al. Overexpression and poly-ubiquitylation of the DEAD-box RNA helicase p68 in colorectal tumours. Oncogene. 2001;20(53):7734–43.

37. Fu Q, Song X, Liu Z, Deng X, Luo R, Ge C, et al. miRomics and proteomics reveal a miR-296-3p/PRKCA/FAK/Ras/c-Myc feedback loop modulated by HDGF/DDX5/beta-catenin complex in lung adenocarcinoma. Clin Cancer Res. 2017;23(20):6336–50.

38. Guturi KK, Sarkar M, Bhowmik A, Das N, Ghosh MK. DEAD-box protein p68 is regulated by beta-catenin/transcription factor 4 to maintain a positive feedback loop in control of breast cancer progression. Breast Cancer Res. 2014;16(6):496.

3

Immune cell subset differentiation and tissue inflammation

Pu Fang[1], Xinyuan Li[2], Jin Dai[1], Lauren Cole[1], Javier Andres Camacho[1], Yuling Zhang[4], Yong Ji[5], Jingfeng Wang[4], Xiao-Feng Yang[1,3] and Hong Wang[1,3]*

Abstract

Immune cells were traditionally considered as major pro-inflammatory contributors. Recent advances in molecular immunology prove that immune cell lineages are composed of different subsets capable of a vast array of specialized functions. These immune cell subsets share distinct duties in regulating innate and adaptive immune functions and contribute to both immune activation and immune suppression responses in peripheral tissue. Here, we summarized current understanding of the different subsets of major immune cells, including T cells, B cells, dendritic cells, monocytes, and macrophages. We highlighted molecular characterization, frequency, and tissue distribution of these immune cell subsets in human and mice. In addition, we described specific cytokine production, molecular signaling, biological functions, and tissue population changes of these immune cell subsets in both cardiovascular diseases and cancers. Finally, we presented a working model of the differentiation of inflammatory mononuclear cells, their interaction with endothelial cells, and their contribution to tissue inflammation. In summary, this review offers an updated and comprehensive guideline for immune cell development and subset differentiation, including subset characterization, signaling, modulation, and disease associations. We propose that immune cell subset differentiation and its complex interaction within the internal biological milieu compose a "pathophysiological network," an interactive cross-talking complex, which plays a critical role in the development of inflammatory diseases and cancers.

Keywords: Immune cell subset differentiation, T cell, B cell, Dendritic cell, Monocyte, Macrophage, Cardiovascular disease, Cancer

Background

The innate and adaptive immune system have been traditionally recognized mostly as the cellular response of immune cells, including T cells (TC), B cells (BC), dendritic cells (DC), monocytes (MC), and macrophages (MØ). During recent decades, molecular immunology research advanced this classical immunology concept with the discovery of subsets of each immune cell lineage. Between 1983 and 1992, the first major immune cell subsets were discovered [1–5]. Following these important breakthroughs, immune subset cell heterogeneity was proposed and its research has been continually flourishing. To date, more than 80 immune cell subsets are recognized [6]. Multiple cytokines and transcription factors have been discovered to control immune cell subset development. Moreover, the concept of immune cell subset plasticity was proposed. For example, pathological conditions could re-shape physiological regulatory T cells (Treg) into pathological Treg that have weakened immunosuppressive functions [7]. Here, we summarize our current knowledge regarding immune cell heterogeneity with an emphasis on their molecular characteristics and potential contributions to cardiovascular diseases (CVD) and cancers. We hypothesize that different immune cell subsets compose a "pathophysiological network" and an interactive cross-talking complex, which is crucial in the development of human diseases.

* Correspondence: hongw@temple.edu
[1]Center for Metabolic Disease Research, Lewis Kats School of Medicine, Temple University, Medical Education and Research Building, Room 1060, 3500 N. Broad Street, Philadelphia, PA 19140, USA
[3]Department of Pharmacology, Lewis Kats School of Medicine, Temple University, Philadelphia, PA, USA
Full list of author information is available at the end of the article

General processes of hematopoietic stem cell differentiation

The classical hematopoietic process has been updated in recent years, with the addition of committed common monocyte progenitors (CMoP) and granulocyte–macrophage progenitor (GMP)-independent monocyte-macrophage/dendritic lineage-restricted progenitor (MDP) arising from common myeloid progenitors (CMP) [8]. Nevertheless, it remains in agreement that the hematopoietic process is conserved among vertebrates [9] and that all hematopoietic lineages are derived from the long-term hematopoietic stem cell (LT-HSC) in bone marrow (BM) (Fig. 1). LT-HSC divisions can result in self-renewal or differentiation into multipotent and lineage-committed hematopoietic progenitor cells, such as common lymphoid progenitors (CLP), CMP, and GMP, all of which lack or have limited self-renewal capacity. CLP differentiate into lymphoid cells (T, B, and natural killer cells), while CMP give rise to megaerythroid cells (platelets and erythrocytes) when GATA-1 is highly expressed. CMP can differentiate into GMP with the expression of "myeloid factor" C/EBPα [10], or differentiate into MDP [8]. GMP could produce "neutrophil-like" inflammatory MC as well as granulocytes. By contrast, MDP could differentiate into common dendritic cell progenitor (CDP) and then DC. MDP also give rise to cMoP, which is a clonogenic, MC and MØ-restricted progenitor cell type [11]. cMoP further develop into MC, MC-derived MØ, and MC-derived DC. The balance among different immune cell subset differentiation is tightly controlled, the dysregulation of which contributes to both CVDs and cancers. However, significant future studies are still needed to identify more accurate markers for theses immune cell subsets and analyze their differentiation process systemically. Moreover, novel unidentified progenitor subsets still await discovery.

Lymphoid genesis and subset differentiation
TC development and subset differentiation

CLP migrates from BM to the thymus and differentiate into TC (Fig. 2a). Upon entering the thymus, CLP first become double-negative (DN) thymocytes which do not express the TC co-receptors CD4 and CD8, or T cell receptor (TCR). During the DN stage, CD4$^-$CD8$^-$ thymocytes gradually lose expression of adhesion molecule CD44 and gain expression of α chain of the IL-2 receptor CD25 on their cell surface, which selects cells that have successfully rearranged their TCR-β chain locus. Then, the DN TC starts to express pre-TCR, which is composed of the re-arranged β chain and pre-α chain. Pre-TCR expression leads to the double-positive (DP) transition with the expression of both CD4 and CD8 (CD4$^+$CD8$^+$) and the subsequent replacement of pre-TCR with TCR (both α chain and β chain re-arranged) [12].

The fate of the DP TC depends on signaling that is mediated by interaction of TCR with self-peptide presented by major histocompatibility complex (MHC)

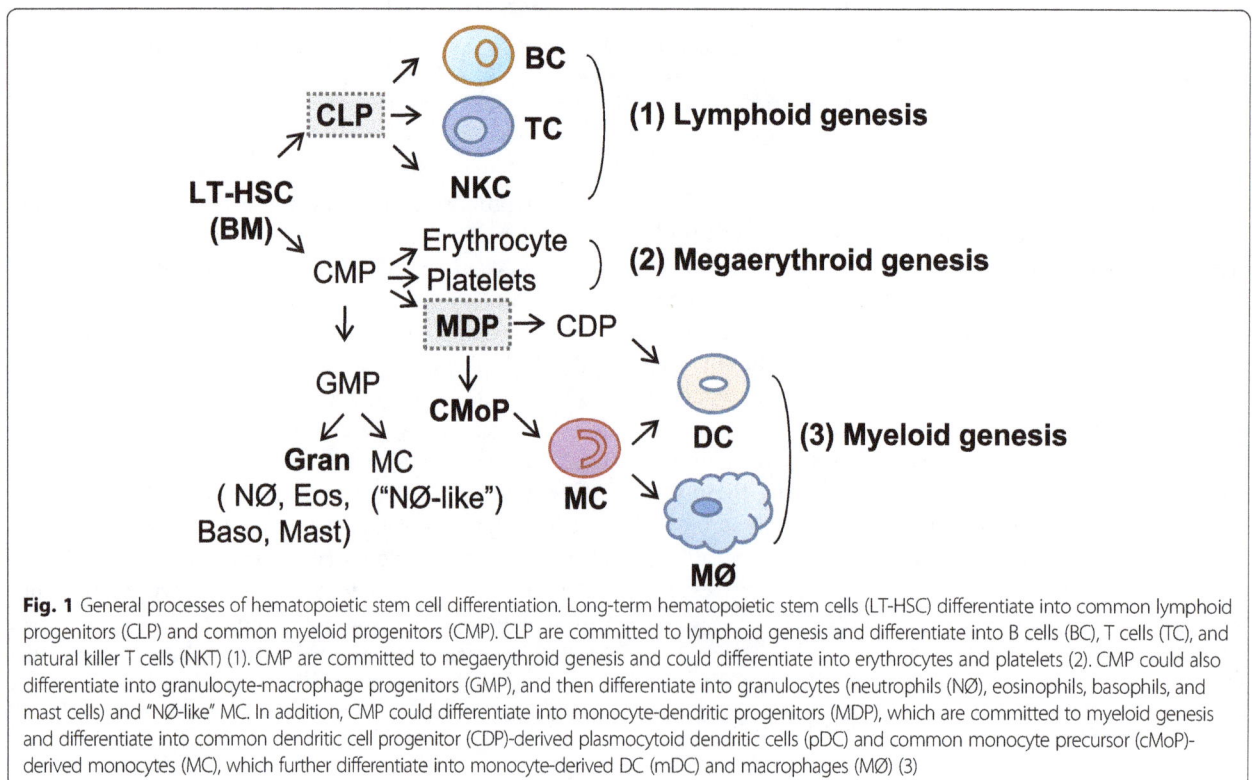

Fig. 1 General processes of hematopoietic stem cell differentiation. Long-term hematopoietic stem cells (LT-HSC) differentiate into common lymphoid progenitors (CLP) and common myeloid progenitors (CMP). CLP are committed to lymphoid genesis and differentiate into B cells (BC), T cells (TC), and natural killer T cells (NKT) (1). CMP are committed to megaerythroid genesis and could differentiate into erythrocytes and platelets (2). CMP could also differentiate into granulocyte-macrophage progenitors (GMP), and then differentiate into granulocytes (neutrophils (NØ), eosinophils, basophils, and mast cells) and "NØ-like" MC. In addition, CMP could differentiate into monocyte-dendritic progenitors (MDP), which are committed to myeloid genesis and differentiate into common dendritic cell progenitor (CDP)-derived plasmocytoid dendritic cells (pDC) and common monocyte precursor (cMoP)-derived monocytes (MC), which further differentiate into monocyte-derived DC (mDC) and macrophages (MØ) (3)

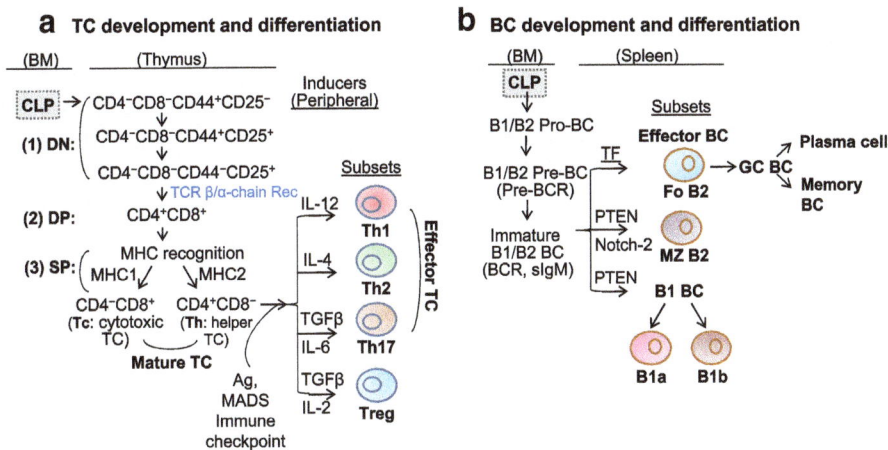

Fig. 2 Lymphoid genesis and subset differentiation. **a** Differentiation of T cells (TC). Common lymphoid progenitors (CLP) migrate from bone marrow (BM) to thymus entering double-negative (DN, CD4-CD8-) stage (1). These cells initially express adhesion molecule CD44 and then α-chain of the interleukin (IL)-2 receptor (CD25), eventually lose CD44 and maintain CD25, rearrange T cell receptor (TCR) β chain, and then enter double-positive (DP, CD4+CD8+) stage (2), a transition stage of TC maturation. The DP TC then lose their membrane expression of CD25, rearrange their α chain, generate a complete αβ TCR, which has the capacity to recognize host major histocompatibility complex (MHC) molecules (positive selection), therefore survives and enters single positive (SP, CD4+, or CD8+) stage (3). After TC bind to MHCI, they become CD8+ TC and are termed as cytotoxic TC (Tc), whereas those binding to self-peptide–MHCII become CD4+ TC and are called as Naïve TC (T0). These SP TC then undergo "negative selection" to eliminate those that recognize MHC that bound to self-peptides, thereby completing the process of TC maturation. T0 cells can differentiate into effector TC (T helper cells Th1, Th2, Th17) and regulatory T cells (Treg) under the regulation of antigen (Ag) presentation, immune checkpoint, cytokine inducers, and metabolite-associated danger signal (MADS), and produce functional cytokines. **b** Differentiation of B cells (BC). In BM, B1/B2-specific CLP first differentiate into B1/B2 progenitor BC (pro-BC), B1/B2 precursor BC (pre-BC) with assembled pre-B cell receptor (BCR) and then became immature B1/B2 BC that express BCR and secrete IgM. Immature B1/B2 BC then migrate to spleen and differentiate into follicular (Fo) B2 BC, marginal zone (MZ) B2 BC, or mature B1 BCs, depending on the transcription factors that are induced by different signals. Fo BC can generate GC BC with follicular DC (a stromal cell) retained-Ag encounter and Tfh help. An affinity-matured Ab response then produce durable memory BC with high affinity to foreign Ag, as well as long lived plasma cells, which can secrete large quantities of Ab. B2 BC constitute the majority of splenic BCs. Mature B1 BC further differentiate into B1a secreting IgM and IL-10, and B1b producing IgM

classes. Too little signaling results in delayed apoptosis (death by neglect, positive selection), while too much signaling can promote acute apoptosis (negative selection) [13, 14]. These DP TC then interact with thymus cortical epithelial cells that express a high density of self-peptide-MHC complexes. DP TC that bind to self-peptide–MHCI complexes become cytotoxic CD8+ TC, which lose CD4 expression because of signal-interrupted CD8 downregulation. Whereas those that bind to self-peptide–MHCII ligands become naïve CD4+ TC which lose CD8 expression because of continued CD8 downregulation. These single-positive (SP) TC are now mature and migrate to peripheral lymphoid sites. Cytotoxic CD8+ TC destroy virus-infected cells and tumor cells, and they are also implicated in transplant rejection. Helper CD4+ TC assist other leukocytes in immunologic processes, while regulatory CD4+ TC maintain immunological tolerance.

The pro-inflammatory Th1 and anti-inflammatory Th2 were discovered in 1989 by Mosmann and Coffman [1]. Then, this Th1/Th2 paradigm was expanded after the discovery of the additional subsets of Th cells, including Treg [15] and IL-17-producing Th17 [16], in the mid-1990s and 2005, respectively.

The subset differentiation of naïve CD4+ TC is determined by antigen presented by the antigen presenting cell (APC), immune checkpoints co-signaling, cytokines, and metabolism-associated danger signal (MADS) [17]. Different cytokines direct TC to polarize into subtypes. Interleukin (IL)-12 was discovered in the early 1990s to play a major role for the generation of Th1 cells [18]. At the same time, IL-4 was discovered as a critical cytokine for the generation of Th2 cells in vitro [19]. In 2006, CD4+ TC was found to express IL-17 (designated Th17 cells, a third subset of T helper cells) in response to the combination of IL-6 and transforming growth factor beta (TGF-β) [20]. Treg are generated when naïve CD4+ TC are primed with IL-2 and TGF-β [21]. Treg express high levels of forkhead box P3 (FOXP3) and acquire the capacity to suppress TC response. Due to limited information on other CD4+ TC subsets, including Th9, follicular T (Tfh), and Th22 cells, we only include their characterization information (Table 1).

Interestingly, the differentiation of CD4+ TC into lineages with distinct effector functions is not an irreversible event. Among all these CD4 subsets, Th2, Treg, and Th17 cells are more plastic than Th1 and they may not be stable [7]. For example, Th2 can convert to Th9 in

Table 1 Characterization of lymphoid cell subsets

Subsets		Markers	Frequency	Cytokines	Functions
TC	Th1	IL-2$^+$TNF-β$^+$IFN-γ$^+$	20% in blood CD4+ TC	IL-2, IL-12IFN-γ, TNF-α	↑MØ↑Cell-mediated immunity
	Th2	IL-4$^+$IL-5$^+$IL-10$^+$IL-13$^+$	2% in blood CD4+ TC	IL-4, IL-5, IL-10 IL-25, IL-13	↑Ab, Eos↓MØ function
	Th17	IL-17$^+$RORγt$^+$	0.5% in blood CD4+ TC	IL-21, IL-22, IL-24IL-26, IL-17A, IL-17F	Defend host↑Autoimmune disease
	Treg	Foxp3$^+$IL-10$^+$	5% in PBMC	IL-10, TGF-β	↓Autoimmune disease
	Tfh	CXCR5$^+$	13.5%in blood CD4+ TC	IL-21	↑BC activation and functional differentiation
	Th22	AHR$^+$CCR4$^+$CCR6$^+$CCR10$^+$	0.05%In blood CD4+ TC	IL-17, IL-22	↓Immune activation
BC	Fo B2	CD21/35^{int}CD23$^+$CD24^{low} CD62L$^+$CD93- IgM^{low}IgD^{high}	4.3% in blood CD19+ BC	IgD, IgM	↑Adaptive response
	MZ B2/B1-like	CD21/35^{high}CD23- CD24$^+$CD93$^-$IgM^{high}IgD^{low}	17% in blood BC	IgM	Respond toblood-borne pathogen

CD4+ helper T cells (TC) can be subdivided into seven groups, which include T helper cells Th1, Th2, Th17, regulatory T cells (Treg), Th9, T follicular helper cells (Tfh), and Th22. Th1 drive autoimmune diseases, while Th2 synthesize interleukin (IL)-4, IL-5, IL-6, and IL-1, and facilitate antibody production. Th17 produce IL-17 and play critical roles in autoimmunity and inflammatory diseases. Treg are in charge of suppressing potentially deleterious activities of Th cells. Th9 protect hosts against helminthic infection and also mediate allergic disease. Tfh are known to regulate BC activation and functional differentiation. Th22-secreted IL-22 maintains intestinal epithelial barrier integrity and stimulates the secretion of antimicrobial peptides that limit bacterial dissemination and intestinal inflammation. Bone marrow (BM)-derived B cells (BC) develop into either follicular (Fo) BC or marginal zone (MZ) BC in the spleen. Fo BC participate in TC-dependent immune responses to protein antigens. MZ BC express high levels of CD21 and CD1d, and respond vigorously to blood borne pathogens. Both B-1a and B-1b BC seed the peritoneal and pleural cavities. While B-1a BC contribute to innate-like immune responses, B-1b BC contribute to adaptive immunity

response to TGF-β stimulation. Treg can switch to Th1 by T-bet, Th2 by interferon regulatory factor 4 (IRF4), Th17 by IL-6+IL21/STAT3, or Tfh by B cell CLL/lymphoma 6 (BCL-6). Similarly, Th17 can convert into interferon gamma (IFN-γ)-producing Th1 cells or IL-4-producing Th2 cells when stimulated with IL-12 or IL-4, respectively.

BC development and subset differentiation
The stages of BC developmental pathway have been extensively characterized over the past years, revealing important growth factors and regulatory interactions. It was initially described by Lee Herzenberg in 1983 that murine B1 cells are a unique CD5$^+$ BC subpopulation [2] distinguished from conventional B2 cells by their phenotype, anatomic localization, self-renewing capacity, and production of natural antibodies. As our understanding progresses, interesting differences between B1 and B2 cell subsets have become apparent (Fig. 2b). B1 and B2 development occurs in BM and spleen [22]. In BM, CLP develop through B1- or B2-specific pro-BC, pre-BC, and immature BC. During this differentiation process, rearrangements at the immunoglobulin locus result in the generation and surface expression of the pre-B cell receptor (pre-BCR), and finally a mature BCR (comprised of rearranged heavy- and light-chain genes) that is capable of binding antigen. During this stage, BC undergo a selection process to prevent any self-reactive cells. Cells successfully completing this checkpoint leave bone marrow, eventually maturing into predominant follicular B2 (Fo BC), marginal-zone B2 (MZ BC), B1a, and B1b BC. Fo BC can further develop into germinal center (GC) BC with

follicular DC-retained antigen encounter and Tfh help [23]. An affinity-matured antibody response will produce durable memory BC with high affinity to foreign antigen, as well as long-lived plasma cells, which can secrete large quantities of antibody.

NKC development and subset differentiation
Both human [24] and mouse [25] studies have shown that NKC can be differentiated from CLP. Three major human NK cell subsets can be distinguished in peripheral blood based on the expression levels of low-affinity Fc-receptor γ IIIA (CD16) and neural cell adhesion molecule (NCAM, CD56), namely, CD56^{high}CD16$^{high/low}$, CD56^{low}CD16^{low}, and CD56^{low}CD16^{high}. These subsets are more likely to be NKC at a different stage of maturation. CD56^{high}CD16$^{high/low}$ can be firstly differentiated from BM-derived CLP [26]. These CD56^{high}CD16$^{high/low}$ NKC stay within the lymph node and interact with DC or further mature into CD56^{low}CD16^{low}, and then became cytotoxic CD56^{low}CD16^{high} NKC [27].

Myeloid genesis and subset differentiation
DC development and subset differentiation
In 1973, Ralph Steinman and Zanvil Cohn [28, 29] discovered dendritic cells (DC). DC diversity was first acknowledged in 1992 [3]. Murine lymphoid organ DC consist of two subsets, defined by the presence or absence of CD8 expression, each with distinct immune functions [30]. After around another 20 years, CD103$^+$ DC in nonlymphoid tissues was found to be lymphoid CD8$^+$ DC equivalents, sharing several phenotypic features [31]. More recently, plasmacytoid DC (pDC) were

uncovered. pDC morphologically resemble plasma cells but, upon exposure to viral stimuli, produce enormous amounts of IFN-α [32]. Importantly, pDC also differentiate upon stimulation into immunogenic DC that can prime TC against viral antigens. To distinguish pDC from the DC that are characterized by Steinman, the latter were renamed classical DC (cDC) and remain so today. Two main subsets of classical cDC along with pDC and MC-derived dendritic cell (mDC) all originate from MDP in BM (Fig. 3a). MDP firstly give rise to CDP and MC in BM. CDP can differentiate into pre-DC, and then become pDC and cDC. Pre-DC migrate from BM, via blood, to lymphoid and nonlymphoid tissues, and constantly replenish CD103+ and CD11b+ cDC [33]. In BM, pre-DC give rise to immature-pDC, and then pDC [34]. The basic helix-loop-helix (bHLH) transcription factor E2-2 is essential for pDC development in both mice and humans [35]. mDC can be generated by culturing human or mouse MC with granulocyte-macrophage colony-stimulating factor (GM-CSF) and other cytokines (IL-4, IL-1β, IL-6, tumor necrosis factor α [TNF-α], PGE2), which express high levels of CD11c and MHCII, and act as potent antigen-presenting cells [36].

MC/MØ development and subset differentiation

Human MC are classified by the levels of their surface expression of CD14, CD16, and CD40 (CD14++CD16−, CD14++CD16+, CD14+CD16++, CD14+CD40+), which differ in their function and phenotype [37]. CD14++CD16− MC, also called the classical MC, are the most prevalent MC subset in human blood. The CD14++CD16+ MC are intermediate MC that contribute significantly to atherosclerosis. The CD14+CD16++ MC are referred to as non-classical MC, which perform a

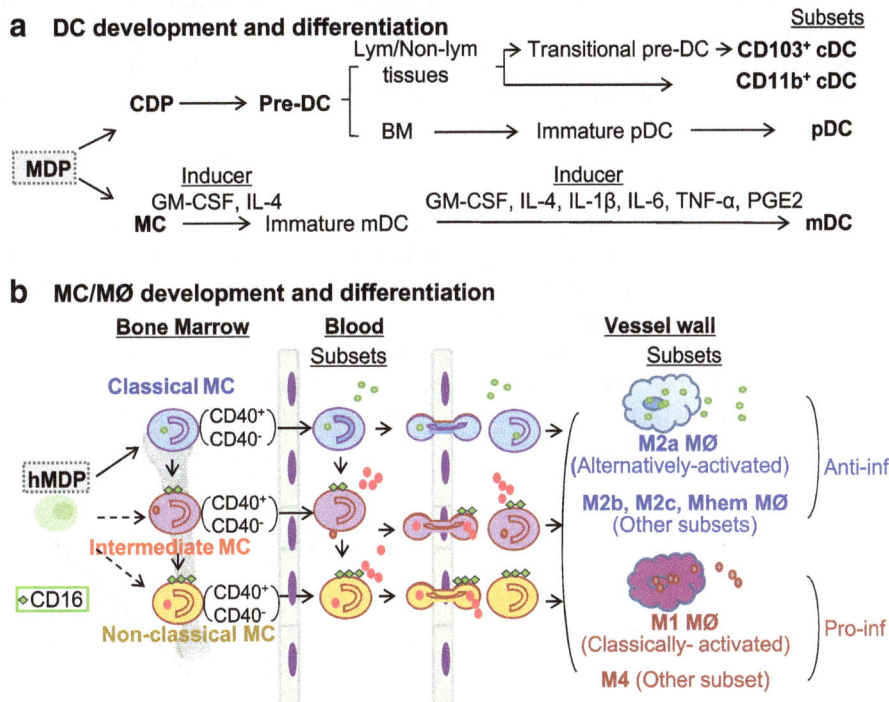

Fig. 3 Myeloid genesis and subset differentiation. **a** Differentiation of dendritic cells (DC). Monocyte-dendritic progenitors (MDP) are the direct precursors to common dendritic cell progenitors (CDP) and monocytes (MC), which both give rise to DC lineages. In bone marrow (BM), CDP become precursor DC (pre-DC) and differentiate into immature plasmocytoid DC (pDC) and mature pDCs, and then exit the BM traveling through the blood to secondary lymphoid organs and non-hematopoietic tissues. In the lymphoid or non-lymphoid tissues, pre-DC become CD103+ classical/conventional DC (cDC) through transitional pre-cDC stage and CD11b+ cDC directly. In cultured system, MC differentiate into immature monocyte-derived DC (mDC) in the presence of interleukin (IL)-4 and granulocyte macrophage colony-stimulating factor (GM-CSF). Terminal differentiated mDC are induced upon stimulation with inflammatory cytokines (IL-1, IL-6, and tumor necrosis factor (TNF)) and prostaglandin E2 (PGE2). **b** Differentiation of monocytes (MC)/macrophages (MØ) in human. In the steady state, human classical MC can differentiate into intermediate MC, then patrolling non-classical MC. Classical MC have a high antimicrobial capability due to their potent capacity of phagocytosis. Intermediate MC secrete inflammatory cytokines and have inflammatory properties, whereas non-classical MC mainly patrol along endothelium. During inflammation, all the MC subsets are tethered and penetrate vessel wall and then mature into anti-inflammatory MØ (M2a, M2b, M2c, and Mhem) and inflammatory MØ (M1 and M4) in tissue. Classical, intermediate and non-classical MC can be further divided into CD40+ and CD40- MC subsets. CD40+ classical/intermediate MC are induced in cardiovascular disease (CVD) and further elevated with the progress of chronic kidney disease (CKD). Dashed arrows indicate potential differentiation pathways, while solid arrows indicate experimentally verified differentiation pathways

patrolling function. In the steady state, classical MC can differentiate into intermediate MC, and then further differentiate into patrolling non-classical MC in circulation [38]. During inflammation, all MC subsets invade tissue and then mature to various MØ subsets according to environmental stimuli. Classical, intermediate, and non-classical MC can be further divided into CD40$^+$ and CD40$^-$ MC subsets. CD40$^+$ classical/intermediate MC are induced in CVD and further elevated with the progress of chronic kidney disease (CKD) [39] (Fig. 3b).

Although in 1989, it was thought that human peripheral blood MC are a heterogeneous population of leukocytes, distinguishable by the expression of lipopolysaccharide (LPS) receptor CD14 and Fc-receptor γ IIIA CD16 [4], it was not confirmed in the murine circulation until 2001 [40]. Mouse MC subsets were originally defined by surface expression of CD11b, lymphocyte antigen 6 complex locus C1 (Ly6C), and CD62L and lacking CD11c and MHCII [41]. A second MC subset was discovered based on the higher expression of chemokine receptor CX3CR1 in *Cx3cr1*$^{GFP/+}$ mice [42]. The expression of CX3CR1 was found to be opposite with granulocytic marker Gr1. Later, CX3CR1^{low} and CX3CR1^{high} MC (also termed as Gr-1^{high} and Gr-1^{low} MC) were defined as Ly6C^{high} and Ly6C^{low} MC, respectively. Ly6C is a glycosylphosphatidylinositol-anchored glycoprotein associated with homing to lymph nodes function. Gr-1 is composed of Ly6C and Ly6G subunits and its antibody recognize both Ly6C and Ly6G molecules. Ly6C is expressed on both MC and granulocytes, while Ly6G is exclusively expressed on granulocytes. Therefore, a better-justified approach to define mouse MC subsets is to use Ly6C$^+$Ly6G$^-$. This is also the reason that Ly6C, but not Gr-1, is used as mouse MC subset marker [43]. Currently, Ly6C^{high} MC is determined to be an inflammatory MC subset, corresponding to human conventional MCs. This subset can also be characterized with a set of surface markers and defined as CX3CR1^{low}CCR2$^+$CD62L$^+$CCR5$^-$. In contrast, the Ly6C^{low} MC is determined as a patrolling MC subset, corresponding to human non-classical MC and can be characterized as CX3CR1^{high}, CCR2$^-$, CD62L$^-$, and CCR5$^+$ [44]. The Ly6C^{high} and Ly6C^{middle} subsets perform pro-inflammatory functions and are considered the counterpart of human classical MC. The Ly6C^{low} subsets patrol along the vascular endothelium. They are involved in tissue repair, which resemble human non-classical MC. In steady state, Ly6C$^+$ MC differentiate into Ly6C$^-$ MC in the circulation. During inflammation, Ly6C$^+$ MC are preferentially recruited into inflamed tissue and mature to different MØ subsets, based on various stimuli.

In 1973, Van Furth reported that pro-inflammatory stimuli elicit MC recruitment and MØ differentiation in tissue [45]. In1992, a new MØ subset, termed "alternative activation" of MØ, was identified from IL-4 induced differential gene expression [5]. By contrast, IFN-γ and LPS induced "classical activation" of MØ [46]. As shown in Fig. 3b myeloid precursor MDP give rise to MC within BM. Afterwards, MC exit to the blood, migrate to the tissues under inflammatory conditions, and further differentiate into MØ. Although BM-originated MC could be the precursors of MØ lineage, tissue MØ could also be derived from embryonic tissue [47], or converted from somatic cells, such as smooth muscle cells [48]. However, different developmental origins of MØ and their functional specificity remain largely unknown.

Granulocyte development and subset differentiation

Mature granulocytes include neutrophils, eosinophils, basophils, and mast cells, which all develop from GMP. The maturation of neutrophil, eosinophil, and basophil proceeds from GMP to myeloblasts. When primary granules are visible, myeloblasts develop into neutrophil, eosinophil, and basophil myelocytes. When cell division ceases and secondary or specific granules begin to appear, they finally become mature neutrophils, eosinophils, and basophils [49]. Originally described in 1879 by Paul Ehrlich, the origin of mast cell is still a matter of debate [50]. Recently, researchers identified a mast cell progenitor that is derived from BM GMP [51]. The mast cell progenitors transiently circulate in the bloodstream and are capable of migrating to the peripheral tissues, where they mature into connective tissue mast cells or mucosal mast cells, following instructive signals from the tissue environment.

Characterization of immune cell subsets

Most of the human immune cell subsets have mouse counterparts that share similar functions. We summarized the molecular and functional characterization of currently recognized immune cell subset.

Characterization of lymphoid cell subsets (Table 1)
TC subset
The CD4$^+$ TC subsets (Th1, Th2, Th17, Treg, Th9, Th22, and Tfh) differ in their extra-cellular and intracellular markers. Each TC subset releases specific cytokines that can have either pro- or anti-inflammatory functions, and they play either pathogenic or protective functions in human diseases. Th1 produce IFN-γ and TNF, and they can activate MØ, enhance cell-mediated cytotoxicity, mediate delayed-type hypersensitivity responses, and effectively respond to intracellular pathogens; Th2 release IL-4 (an important survival factor for BC and required for IgG1 and IgE production), IL-5, and IL-13; Th17 produce IL-17 (a strong inducer of autoimmune conditions, such as experimental encephalomyelitis (EAE)); Treg are characterized by the expression of FOXP3 (maintaining expression of FOXP3 transcription factor is needed for the suppressive function of Treg),

and they secrete immunosuppressive cytokines IL-10 and TGF-β; Tfh are CD4+CXCR5+ TC [52, 53], and they are known to regulate the activation and differentiation of BC. They preferentially select BC that present high levels of peptide-MHCII and promote their extensive proliferation or differentiation to antibody-forming cells [54]; Th22 were recently distinguished from Th1 and Th17 by its unique IFNγ- and IL-17-independent IL-22 secretion [55]. It is characterized by the expression of CCR4, CCR6, CCR10, and aryl hydrocarbon receptor (AHR). Similar to Th17, Th22 have the capacity to acquire functional features of Th1 [56]. Moreover, within Th22, three more subsets were delineated in human liver, indicating the complexity of the immune cell subset system [57]; Th9 are defined by their production of IL-9 [58], although IL-9 is not unique to Th9. IL-9 is associated with host defense against intestinal nematode infection and the development of allergic responses. They could mediate protection against parasitic infections, while they could also induce allergic inflammation, asthma, and other autoimmune disease.

BC subset

Fo BC are activated in the spleen follicular niche by TC-dependent antigens of microbial origin. They receive synergistic signals via BCR, CD40, and toll-like receptors (TLRs) [59]. Activated Fo BC can further differentiate into GC BC, which express MHC-II and CD27 [60]. GC BC selection can lead to differentiation of antibody secreting plasma cells and memory BC [61]. Marginal zone B2 (MZ BC) are innate-like cells and appear to mediate TC-independent responses to antigens from blood-borne pathogens. MZ BC can also mediate the transport of antigen from immune complexes into splenic follicles, which is involved in TC-dependent BC responses. Moreover, MZ BC may participate in the immune responses to lipid antigen. Furthermore, they can shuttle between splenic follicle and marginal sinus, and the high level of CD21 expressed on MZ BC is presumably evolved to facilitate immune complex capture [59]. B1 BC population has not been clearly defined in humans [62], so our knowledge about the function of B1 BC is based on studies in rodents. B1 BC can contribute to the generation of IgM responses to TC-independent antigens such as phosphorylcholine, an antigen on many pathogenic bacteria [59]. While B-1a BC contribute to innate-like immune responses, B-1b BC contribute to adaptive immunity [63].

Characterization of myeloid cell subsets (Table 2)
DC subset

DC express both MHCI and MHCII molecules [64], and they are unrivaled stimulators of TC. They process protein antigen and initiate antigen-specific cellular immune responses. Recent work has established that tissue DC consist of developmentally and functionally distinct subsets, including mDC, pDC, and cDC. As genetically distinct DC subsets, they arise from different bone marrow precursors. mDC are rapidly differentiated from MC and infiltrate into tissues in response to inflammation. Their role is therefore likely to be more specialized in expediting immune responses [65]. Recently, mDC are developed as immunotherapy target for treating cancer [66]. pDC accumulate mainly in blood and lymphoid tissues and they enter lymph node through blood circulation. Upon recognition of foreign nucleic acids, they produce massive amounts of type I IFN and acquire the capacity to present foreign antigens [67]. However, chronic inflammatory settings will exhaust pDC through IFN-I and TLR7 [68]. Human and murine cDC consist of two subsets as defined by the presence or absence of CD103, Xcr1, CD11b, and CD11c expression (CD11c+Xcr1+CD103+ or CD11c+CD11b+) [30]. CD11c is also expressed on MC and MØ, which complicates cDC characterization. CD11c+Xcr1+CD103+ cDC have superior ability over other cDC to present microbial antigens [69] and cell-associated antigens [69, 70] to CD8+ TC. CD11c+CD11b+ cDC are thought to have a predominant role in MHCII presentation to CD4+ TC [71].

MC subset

Contemporary studies have demonstrated that four subsets of MC reside in the peripheral circulation. These subsets are distinct in their functions and fates [72].

Human MC subpopulations include CD14++CD16− (classical, which account for 80–90% of peripheral blood MC), CD14++CD16+ (intermediate), CD14+CD16++ (non-classical) subpopulations [73], and CD14+CD40+ (CD40) MC [39]. Classical MC are phagocytic with no inflammatory attributes. The intermediate subtype constitutes a very small percentage in circulation (under physiological conditions); they appear to be transitional MC that display both phagocytic and inflammatory function. The non-classical subtype displays inflammatory characteristics upon activation and presents antigen [74]. Our lab recently identified CD40+ MC as a stronger inflammatory MC subset and a better marker for CKD severity stage compared with intermediate MC subset [39]. We provided evidence suggesting that metabolic risk factors, such as hyperhomocysteinemia (HHcy), induced CD40 in MC, in a reverse (towards APC) co-stimulation manner [17].

The mouse Ly6C^middle+high inflammatory subset corresponds to human CD14++CD16− classical MC, while the mouse Ly6C^low patrolling subset corresponds to human CD14+CD16++ non-classical MC [75]. Microarray-based gene expression profiling has confirmed that differential gene expression profiles observed in mouse monocyte subsets are conserved in human monocyte subpopulations [73, 76]. Mouse Ly6C^middle+high inflammatory MC

Table 2 Characterization of myeloid cell subsets

Subsets		Markers	Frequency	Cytokines	Functions
DC	cDC	CD11c$^+$MHCII$^+$CD141$^+$(BDCA3$^+$)XCR1$^+$CLEC9A$^+$FLT3$^+$CD103$^+$	5~10% in blood	IL-12, IFN-III	↑IFN-IIICross-present Ag
		CD11c$^+$MHCII$^+$(BDCA1$^+$)CD172a$^+$CD11b$^+$FLT3$^+$	45–50% in blood	IL-23?	Present Ag
	pDC	BDCA2$^+$LILRA4$^+$CD45RA$^+$	45–50% in blood	IFNα	Sense pathogenActivate IC
	mDC	MHCII$^+$CD11c$^+$CD86$^+$CD40$^+$CD80$^+$CD83$^+$CCR7$^+$CD14$^-$	Induced by inflammation	TNFα, iNOSIL-12, IL-23	Cross-present Ag
MC	Classical	CD14$^+$CD16$^-$CXCR1$^+$ CXCR2$^+$CD62L$^+$	80–95% in MNC	ROS, NO, MPOIFN-I, IL-1α, TNFIL-6, IL-8, CCL2	Phagocytosis↑Inflammation
	Intermediate	CD14$^+$CD16^{+C}D64^{int}CCR1^{int}CCR2^{int} CX3CR1^{int} CD11b^{int} CD33^{int} CD115^{int} CD40$^+$ CD54$^+$ HLA-DR$^+$	2–11% in MNC	ROS, NO, MPOIFN-I, IL-1α, TNFIL-6, IL-8 CCL2	↑Inflammation
	Non-classical	CD14$^-$CD16$^+$	2–8% in MNC	TNF, IL-1β, CCL3	Patrol, repair tissue
	CD40	CD14$^+$CD40$^+$	64% in PBMC	TNFα, IL-6	↑Inflammation
MØ	M1	iNOS$^+$CXCL11$^+$IL-12high IL-23^{high}IL-10^{low}	1% in gastric tissue	IL-6, TNFαiNOS, IL-12	Microbicidal↑Inflammation
	M2a	FIZZ1$^+$Arg1$^+$IL-12^{low}IL-23^{low}	1% in gastric tissue	IL-10	↓InflammationHeal woundRepair tissue
	M2b	CD80^{high}CD14^{high}HLA-DR^{low}IL-12^{low}IL-23^{low}	0 in PBMC	IL-10	Activate Th2↓Inflammation
	M2c	CD86^{low}HLA-DR^{low}CD163$^+$TLR4^{high}IL-12^{low}IL-23^{low}	2.4% in CD68$^+$ MØ	CCL18	↓InflammationDeposit matrixRemodel tissue
	M4	MMP7$^+$MR$^+$S100A8$^+$CD68$^+$	31.7% in CD68$^+$ MØ from coronary artery	CD86, IL-6, TNFα	↑Inflammation
	Mhem	HOMX1$^+$CD163$^+$	25% in thrombosis	IL-10	↓Lipid accumulationRetain iron, ↓Inflammation

Four kinds of dendritic cells (DC) can be defined in human based in part on their functional specialization: monocyte-derived DC (mDC), CD103+ classical/ conventional dendritic cell (cDC), CD11b + cDC, and plasmocytoid dendritic cell (pDC). mDC exhibit a strong costimulatory capacity for TC activation. cDC are the most efficient cell type for priming and functional polarization of TC. pDCs can secrete high concentrations of interferon (IFN)-I (mainly IFN-α). In humans, there are three populations of monocytes (MC), as defined by the expression of CD14 and CD16 (CD14++CD16−, CD14+CD16+, and CD14+CD16++). The CD14++CD16− MC represent 80% to 90% of blood MC, express high levels of the chemokine receptor C-C chemokine receptor type 2 (CCR2) and low levels of CX3C chemokine receptor 1 (CX3CR1), and produce IL-10 rather than TNF and IL-1 in response to lipopolysaccharide (LPS) in vitro. CD14+CD16+ MC express the Fc receptors CD64 and CD32, have phagocytic activity, and are entirely responsible for the production of tumor necrosis factor-α (TNF-α) and IL-1 in response to LPS. In contrast, CD14+CD16++ MC lack the expression of other Fc receptors, are poorly phagocytic, and do not produce TNF-α or IL-1 in response to LPS. Our lab recently identified CD40+ MC as a stronger inflammatory subset related to chronic kidney disease (CKD). Macrophages (MØ) also display phenotypic heterogeneity. Depending on the stimuli, M0 MØ could polarize towards the pro-inflammatory M1 subset by lipopolysaccharide or IFN-γ, or towards the alternative M2a type by IL-4. M2b MØs are induced upon combined exposure to immune complexes and Toll-like receptor (TLR) ligands or IL-1 receptor agonists. M2c MØs are induced by IL-10 and glucocorticoids. Atheroprotective Mhem subset could be induced by hemoglobin, and highly express haem oxygenase 1 and CD163. Chemokine (C-X-C motif) ligand 4 drives differentiation of human specific M4 MØ, with unique expression of surface markers such as S100A8, mannose receptor CD206, and matrix metalloproteinase 7

circulate in the blood and egress into tissues following pathological insult, at which point they differentiate into MØ and DC, producing inflammatory cytokines and reactive oxygen species, stimulating effector TC proliferation, and mediating tissue repair [75]. Ly6C^{low} MC are characterized by long-range crawling along the luminal surface of small vessels, which allows them to survey for dying and infected cells and mediate their disposal [75]. They also play an important role in mediating live vaccine's protective effects by dictating Tfh differentiation, germinal center formation, and protective antibody production via IL-1β [77]. Furthermore, both Ly6C$^+$ and Ly6C$^-$ MC can have two sources including GMP and MDP, with distinct gene expression signatures and functions [8].

MØ subset

MØ are highly heterogeneous cells that can rapidly change their function in response to local microenvironmental signals [78]. *Classically activated MØ* (M1 MØ) are activated by cytokines such as IFN-γ [79]. M1 MØ protect the host from a variety of bacteria, protozoa, and viruses, and they also play critical a role in antitumor immunity [78]. *Alternatively activated MØ* (M2a MØ) have anti-inflammatory function and regulate wound healing [78]. M2a MØ can secrete large amounts of IL-10 in response to Fc receptor-γ (FcγR) ligation [80]. Interestingly, M2a MØ resembles tumor-associated macrophages (TAM) in cancer, which promote tumor progression by stimulating tumor proliferation, invasion, and metastasis, and inhibiting TC-mediated antitumor immune response [81]. The *third subset M2b* are activated when their FcγRs bind to LPS [82, 83]. M2b MØ turn off their production of IL-12 and secrete IL-10. In addition, M2b MØ upregulate antigen presentation and, importantly, promote Th2 responses. The *fourth subset M2c* is induced by IL-10/TGF-β, which exhibit anti-inflammatory functions in vitro and protect against renal injury in vivo due to their ability to induce Treg [84]. The activation of the *fifth subset M4* MØ is M-CSF/CXCL4-dependent [85]. M4 MØ are weakly phagocytic and unable to efficiently phagocytize acetylated LDL (acLDL) or oxidized LDL (oxLDL) [86]. In the context of atherosclerosis, atherosclerotic lesions have been demonstrated to contain M4 MØ, suggesting that M4 MØ may play important roles in the pathology of atherosclerosis [85]. The *sixth subset Mox* is polarized upon oxidized phospholipid (ox-PL) 1-palmitoyl-2arachidonoyl-sn-glycero-3-phosphorylcholine treatment, which upregulate the expression of oxygenase-1 (HO-1) and thioredoxin reductase 1 (Txnrd1) [87]. This unique Mox MØ comprised 23% of the aortic CD11b$^+$F4/80$^+$ population from 30-week western diet-fed low-density lipoprotein receptor-deficient (*Ldlr$^{-/-}$*) mice [87]. As Mox MØ express anti-oxidant enzymes HO-1 and Txnrd1, they exert anti-inflammatory actions on vasculature in vivo [85]. This proposed phenotype of Mox MØ closely resembles the phenotypes of the *seventh subset Mhem* MØ, which generated from hapto-hemoglobin complexes or oxidized red blood cells treatment [88]. CD163 and IL-10 are upregulated in an Nrf2-dependent manner in Mhem MØ [88]. Mhem MØ promote atherosclerosis development due its angiogenic, vessel permeability causing, and leukocyte attracting properties, through hemoglobin:haptoglobin/CD163/HIF1α-mediated VEGF induction [89].

Representative immune cell subset changes in diseases (Table 3)

Immune cell subsets play a significant role in the development of various inflammatory diseases and cancers and we have summarized their changes during various disease development (Table 3). Atherosclerosis is a chronic inflammatory pathogenic process of arteries, which leads to cardiovascular diseases (CVDs), including myocardial infarction and stroke [90]. Here, we focused on the discussion of the immune cell changes in atherosclerosis-related diseases. In human studies, the percentage of TC was found to be higher in blood samples from carotid atherosclerotic patients than those from healthy subjects [91, 92]. Similarly, a higher number of subintimal TCs was observed in those patients with carotid atherosclerotic plaque (CAP) [92]. This is also the case in rheumatoid arthritis (RA) [93]. Consistently, the number of natural killer T cell (NKT) was increased in the blood from patients that underwent

endarterectomy [91] and those that had colorectal cancer [94]. At the same line, elevated neutrophil count was found to be correlated with increased mortality in patients with acute myocardial infarction (AMI) [95] and stable coronary artery disease (CAD) [96]. In mouse studies, atherosclerotic plaques of *ApoE$^{-/-}$* mice showed an increase in CD45$^+$ leukocyte content [97]. More specifically, more TC and less BC were found in ApoE$^{-/-}$ mice, indicating the functions of these immune cells [98].

TC subsets

Antigen-specific CD8$^+$ TC shows impressive anti-tumor effects [99]. Similarly, there is increasing evidence that both CD4$^+$ [93] and CD8$^+$ [6, 93, 100] TC are involved in atherosclerosis. More specifically, Th1 and Th17 cell numbers and their related gene expression (T-bet, IFN-γ, STAT4, RORγt, STAT3, and IL-17) were significantly increased in acute coronary syndrome (ACS) patients, whereas the Treg cell population, Foxp3 levels, and plasma IL-10 and TGF-β1 were decreased in ACS patients [6]. NKT-like and NKT cells are a small but significant population of T lymphocytes, and they play an essential role at the very early stages of atherosclerotic plaque development [101]. In atherosclerosis-inducing hyperglycemic diseases (diabetes type 2 or pre-diabetes) [101], endarterectomy at the carotid [91] and colorectal cancer patients [94], the counts of CD3$^+$ 56$^+$ NKT-like and NKT cells were significantly higher than those of healthy controls. Moreover, there was an increase of the production of granzyme and perforin in these patients.

In atherosclerotic mice, elevated levels of CD4$^+$ TC were found in lesions [97, 98]. CD8$^+$ TC expressing pro-inflammatory cytokines (IFN-γ, TNF-α, and IL-12) were also found in the atherosclerotic lesions and spleens of high-fat diet-fed *Ldlr$^{-/-}$*[102] or *ApoE$^{-/-}$* mice [97]. Importantly, antibody-mediated CD8$^+$ TC depletion significantly decreased atherosclerotic plaque formation [102]. More specifically, Th1 were significantly increased in *Ldlr$^{-/-}$* mice, correlating with increased lesion formation and smooth muscle cell content [103]. Moreover, the amount of Th2 was reduced in atherosclerotic *Ldlr$^{-/-}$* mice [103]. Furthermore, Th17 quantities were increased in the lesions from *ApoE$^{-/-}$* mice [104] and in the spleens from obesity mice [105]. In addition, *ApoE–/–* mice exhibit significantly lower numbers of splenic Treg than their wild-type counterparts [106]. Additionally, there was a strong positive correlation between CD4$^+$ NKT numbers and markers of inflammation in the plaque (including CD3, T-bet, CCR5, and CCR7), indicating that they promote atherogenesis [91]. Finally, effector memory T cells, including CD4$^+$ Th1 and CD8$^+$ TC, were associated with increased atherosclerosis and CAD [6].

Table 3 Representative immune cell subset changes in human diseases

Cells	Changes	Tissues	PMID#
Atherosclerosis (carotid/coronary atherosclerosis, stenosis, cardiovascular death, nonhemorrhagic stroke)			
TC	TC↑, PD-1+Tim-3+CD8+ TC↑, Th17/Th1 TC↑Th1 TC↑, CD4+LAP+ or CD4+CD25+ Treg TC↓CD3+CD4+CD45RA− CD45RO+CCR7− T(EM) TC↑	PBMC	260352072152475023130116
BC	TC/BC↑	Fibro-fatty (aorta, coronary)	24122585
	MC	CD14++CD16+ MC↑, CD14++CD16−CCR2+ MC↑CD14+CD16++CCR2- MC↑	PBMC
	2299972825012963	MØ	CD86+ M1 MØ↑, M2 MØ↑
	PBMC, rupture-prone shoulder regions, Adventitial tissue	23078881	
Acute myocardial infarction			
TC	CD3+CD4+CD45RA−CD45RO+CCR7− T(EM) TC↑HLA-DR+ T(EM) TC↑	PBMC	23121518
	MC	CD14++CD16-CCR2+TLR4+ MC↑CD14+CD16++CCR2+TLR4+ MC↑	PBMC
	23121518	Hypercholesterolemia (total serum C levels > 200 mg/dl or 6.5 mmol/L, LDL-C > 160 mg/dl, serum TG ≤ 300 mg/dl)	
TC	CD3+ TC↑, CD4+ TC↑, CD8+ TC↑	PBMC	8546748
	MC	CD14dimCD16+ non-classical MC↑CD64−CD16+ non-classical MC↑	PBMC
	103812988977447	Infection (HCMV with CAP, HIV on stable ART with CAC)	
TC	Lymphocyte↑, CD3+ TC↑, CD4+ TC↑, CD8+ TC↑, Th1 TC↑, CD4+CD25+Foxp3+ Treg TC↓CD8+IL-6Ralow T(EM) TC↑, CD8+CD57+ TC↑	Subintimal PBMC	239689792636053027062409
	MC	CD14++CD16+ MC↑, CD14++CD16- MC↑CD14+CD16++ MC↓, CD14+CD16++ MC↑	PBMC
	2636053024118494	Chronic kidney diseases	
	MC	CD14+CD16+ non-classical MC↑	PBMC
	26,877,933	Early rheumatoid arthritis, systemic lupus erythematosus	
TC	CD8+CD31+CXCR4+ TC↑	PBMC	1780453027065298
Obese, pre-diabetes, diabetes mellitus type 2			
TC	NKT-like TC↑, CD3+CD56+ NKT TC↑	PBMC	24554505
	MC	CD14++CD16+ MC↑, CD14+CD16++ MC↑	PBMC
	21799175	Endarterectomy (CEA and endarterectomy at the femoropopliteal level)	
TC	NKTs↑, TC↑	PBMC, plaques	27051078
	DC	CD11b+ cDC↑	PBMC, plaques
	27051078	MØ	MMP-12+CD68+ MØ↑
	Culprit sections	23316311	
Colorectal cancer			
TC	NKT cells↑	PBMC	22220404

BC subsets

Consistent with TC subset changes, TC/BC ratios were found to be positively correlated with fibro-fatty percentage in the plaque [107]. While B2 BC aggravated atherosclerosis, B1a and B1b BC were atheroprotective by secreting natural IgM that increased IgM deposits and reduced necrotic cores in atherosclerotic lesions [108].

Follicular DC (stromal cells) are an important cell type that help with BC maturation. They present antigen in activated germinal centers of primary (BM and thymus), secondary (lymph node and spleen), and artery tertiary lymphoid organs, and contribute to innate and adaptive immune responses in atherosclerosis [109].

NKC

The CD56^{low}CD16^{high} cells comprise the majority of all NKC and are potent mediators of cytotoxicity. By contrast, the CD56^{high}CD16$^{high/low}$ cells have low or no cytotoxicity but produce large amounts of various immunoregulating cytokines. Thus, it is not surprising to observe a significant reduction of CD56^{low}CD16^{high} NKC and a concomitant loss of NKC function in patients with CAD [110].

DC

CD11b$^+$ cDC, CD11c$^+$MHCII$^+$CD103$^-$CD11b$^+$F4/80$^-$ cDC, CD11c$^+$MHCII$^+$CD103$^+$CD11b$^-$F4/80$^-$ cDC, CD11c$^+$MHCII$^+$CD103$^-$CD11b$^+$F4/80$^+$ mDC, and CD11c$^+$CD8$^-$CD4$^-$ cDC were all found to be expanded in atherosclerotic plaque [91, 111]. In addition, the number of pDC decreased [97].

MC

MC are the most abundant immune cell type found in atherosclerotic plaques, indicating that they are crucial promoters of atherogenesis. Classical CD14^{++}CD16$^+$ MC independently predicted cardiovascular events in coronary atherosclerotic subjects [100, 112, 113]. Based on flow cytometry results, the intermediate monocyte subset (CD14^{++}CD16$^+$) was increased in atherosclerotic patients when compared with that of healthy subjects [93, 100, 112, 114, 115]. Contradictory results were found for non-classical MC subset (CD14$^+$CD16^{++}): it was observed that they were reduced in patients with CAD, compared with those in healthy donor group [113]; however, a majority of studies showed that they were increased in the patients with coronary plaque vulnerability [115], CKD [116], obesity [114], and hypercholesterolemia [117]. Furthermore, CD40$^+$ MC number was found to be a useful biomarker for CKD severity [39] and they were induced in metabolic diseases [17].

We and the others have reported that in mice, CD11b$^+$Ly6G$^-$Ly6C$^{middle+high}$ MC were consistently and dramatically increased in hypercholesterolemic ApoE$^{-/-}$ mice that were fed with a high-fat diet [118], in Ldlr$^{-/-}$ mice [119], in HHcy mice [120], in miR155$^{-/-}$ mice [121], and in type 1 diabetes mellitus (T1DM) mice [122]. In addition, resident CD11b$^+$Ly6G$^-$Ly6C^{low} MC subset in the circulation was reduced in atherosclerotic mice [121].

MØ

Specific macrophage subsets have been implicated in atherosclerosis, with M1 MØ dominating the rupture-prone shoulder regions of the plaque and M2 MØ dominating the vascular adventitial tissue [123]. In mouse studies, enhanced M1 MØ polarization was observed in left ventricular remodeling after myocardial infarction (MI) [124] as well as in immune organs from hyperglycemic and HHcy mice [122].

Granulocytes

Over the past couple of years, studies have provided convincing evidence for the presence of neutrophils in atherosclerotic plaques. It was further revealed that neutrophils aggravate endothelial dysfunction [125], recruit MC [126], activate MØ [127], and destabilize plaque [128], which may be attributed to neutrophil-derived reactive species and proteases. Eosinophils may also have a significant role in coronary atherosclerosis since consistent studies have shown a positive association between eosinophil count and increased risk for future cardiovascular events [129]. Eosinophils may exert their pro-atherosclerotic actions through proteins stored in prominent cytoplasmic granules, which may modulate the acute phase response and innate inflammatory response [130]. Similarly, basophils also promote atherosclerosis via these actions [131]. Mast cells are potent immune cells known for their functions in host defense responses and they drive the development of diseases such as asthma and allergies. Mast cells can exert its effects on atherosclerotic plaque progression and destabilization through their release of mast cell-specific proteases chymase and tryptase, growth factors, histamine, and chemokines [132].

Representative signaling pathways of immune cell subset differentiation
TC subset differentiation signaling

It is now well established that CD4$^+$ TC differentiate into four subsets, which are characterized by their distinct cytokine secretion patterns (Fig. 4a). Among the factors controlling such differentiation are the cytokines present in the milieu of the TC during initial priming. In the case of murine Th1 differentiation, APC-derived IL-12 plays a key role in this respect, as shown by the fact that either IL-12 p40 or IL-12R chain knockout mice had highly impaired Th1 responses [133]. In addition, downregulation of the IL-12Rβ2 chain and thus cessation of IL-12 signaling resulted in alternative differentiation into Th2 cells [134]. IL-12/IL-12R activates STAT4, presumably giving rise to IFN-γ [135]. IFN-γ then activates STAT1/STAT4 and T-bet, which are essential transcription factors for Th1 cell development [136].

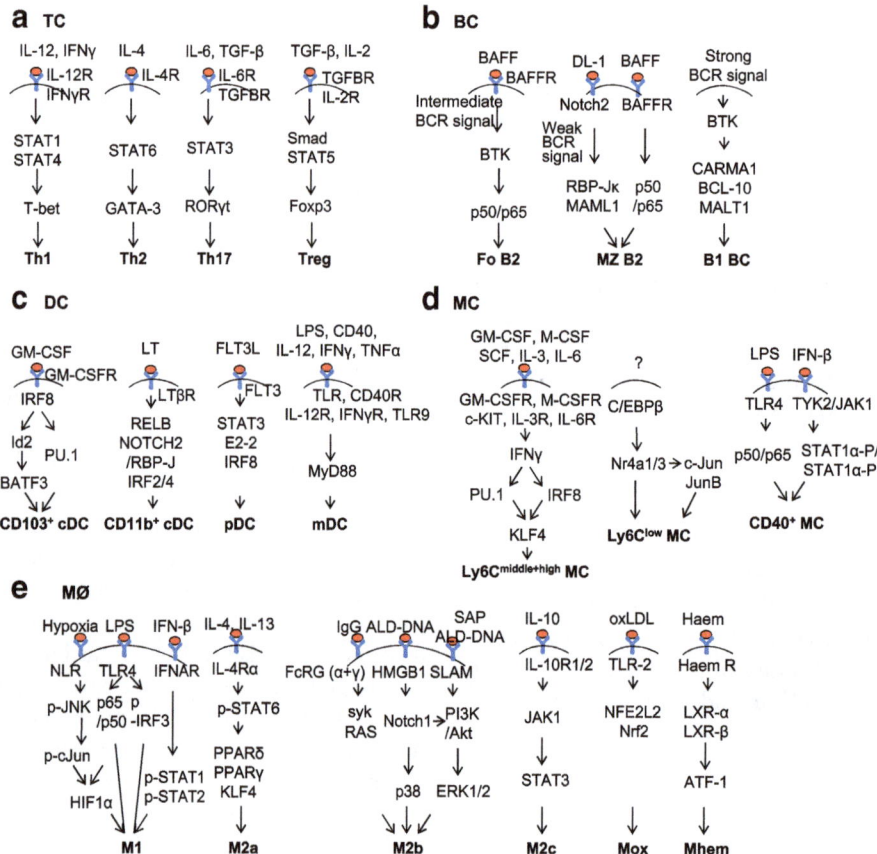

Fig. 4 Representative signaling pathways of immune cell subset differentiation. **a** TC. **b** BC. **c** DC. **d** MC. **e** MØ

IL-4 is the hallmark cytokine that directs Th2 development, since mice deficient in IL-4 or IL-4R failed to develop a potent population of effector Th2 cells [137]. Ligation of IL-4R by IL-4 results in activation of STAT6, which upregulates expression of the Th2 specific transcription factor GATA-3 [138].

The cytokines that are responsible for the differentiation of naïve mouse TC into Th17 are IL-6 and TGF-β [139]. The combination of IL-6 and TGFβ preferentially activates Stat3, which upregulates RORγt, a critical transcription factor for Th17 cells [140]. Multiple functional RORγt binding sites are present in the *Il17A* promoter. Using chromatin immunoprecipitation, RORγt was also found to bind the *Il17A* gene [141].

TGFβ plays an important role in Treg differentiation [142]. It induces phosphorylation of Smad3, which stimulates *Foxp3* transcription by binding to the transcription control elements of *Foxp3* [143]. Treg differentiation is also mediated by IL-2/IL-2R, as IL-2 signaling pathway has been associated with accumulation of Treg in vivo [144]. Upon IL-2/IL-2R activation, phosphorylation of the transcription factor STAT5 appears to play a key role in the generation and expansion of Treg.

BC subset differentiation signaling

For the transition from immature BC to Fo BC, intermediate level of BCR signal is required (Fig. 4b) [145]. After BCR ligation by antigen, TEC-family protein tyrosine kinase (PTK) BTK5 is recruited and activated [146]. Nuclear factor-κB (NF-κB) is an important downstream effector of BCR/BTK5 signaling [145]. The NF-κB transcription-factor family consists of heterodimers or homodimers of the subunits p50 (NF-κB1), p52 (NF-κB2), c-REL, p65 (RELA), and RELB. The p50/p65 pair determines Fo BC fate. BAFF (B cell-activating factor of the tumor-necrosis-factor family) is also required for Fo BC differentiation. Overexpression of BAFF in transgenic mice induces the production of Fo BC. BAFF engagement activates BTK, which then facilitates BCR-induced activation of the canonical NF-κB pathway.

During MZ BC differentiation, Notch2 interacts with its ligand, Delta-like 1 (DL1), which is specifically expressed by the endothelial cells of red pulp venules in mice [147]. This interaction initiates the cleavage of Notch2, which is not inhibited by weak BCR signaling. The intracellular domain of Notch2 enters the nucleus where it interacts with Mastermind-like 1 (MAML1) and RBP-Jκ transcription factors. This transcriptional complex induces the commitment of BC towards MZ BC [147]. BAFF/BAFF-R interaction also delivers survival signals through canonical NF-KB activation in MZ BCs [148].

A stronger BCR/BTK signal is required for the generation of B1 BC [145], which is supported by the phenotypes of *Btk*-deficient mice [149]. BTK signals through CARMA1, BCL-10 (B cell lymphoma 10), and MALT1 (mucosa-associated lymphoid tissue lymphoma translocation protein 1), which are critical in the development of B1 cells [150]. Interestingly, B1 cell formation is unaffected by impaired BAFF signaling, raising the possibility that elevated BCR signaling in these cells or other microenvironmental factors in the pleural cavity where B1 BC reside may be important for BAFF-independent survival [151].

DC subset differentiation signaling

Development of CD103$^+$ cDC is orchestrated by the transcription factors including inhibitor of DNA binding 2 (ID2), interferon regulatory factor 8 (IRF8), basic leucine zipper ATF-like 3 transcription factor (BATF3), BCL2, and PU.1 (Fig. 4c) [152, 153]. Deletion of any of these genes leads to a severe developmental defect of CD103$^+$ DC [70, 154, 155]. The hierarchy and sequential involvement of these specific transcription factors is emerging [153]: IRF8 is required for CD103$^+$ cDC differentiation [156]. It was shown that *Irf8*-deficient DC progenitors had reduced expression of several important transcription factors, including ID2 and BCL2 [157]. Id2 is induced in vitro by granulocyte-macrophage colony-stimulating factor (GM-CSF) and is required in vivo for the development of CD103$^+$ DC [155]. IRF8 is obligatory for the development of ID2-expressing DC precursors, while BATF3 is induced at later maturation stages of CD103$^+$ cDC [70]. It is not clear if all of IRF8's actions in regulating CD103$^+$ cDC development are mediated by BATF3. More likely, IRF8 acts to control both PU.1-dependent and BATF3-dependent target genes in cDC development [153]. Notably, CD103$^+$ DC are required for the recruitment of tumor-infiltrating lymphocytes (TILs). It has been shown that melanoma-intrinsic WNT/β-catenin signaling pathway was responsible for inhibiting the crosstalk between TILs and CD103$^+$ DC [158]. It was later found that in a tumor model resembling non-T cell-inflamed human tumors, adoptive transferred T cells failed to traffic into tumor site due to the absence of CD103$^+$ DC secreting CXCL9 and CXCL10. As a result, TILs highly expressing CXCR3, which is the receptor for CXCL9 and CXCL10, could not be recruited to the tumor site [159]. Taken together, these results indicated that absence of CD103$^+$ DC from the tumor microenvironment may be a dominant mechanism of resistance to cancer immunotherapies.

The transcription factors that control general CD11b$^+$ cDC development include RELB [160], NOTCH2 [161], RBP-J [162], IRF2 [163], and IRF4 [164]. Of note, IRF4 also controls functional aspects of CD11b$^+$ DC, such as their MHC presentation [165] and migration [166]. Consistent with the notion that CD11b$^+$ cDC are heterogeneous, deficiency of IRF4 or NOTCH2 only partially impaired CD11b$^+$ DC development [161, 166]. In contrast to CD103$^+$ cDC, the hierarchy of transcription factors required for CD11b$^+$ cDC development is less known [152]. Splenic CD11b$^+$ DC were recognized to comprise two subpopulations that are distinguished by ESAM expression [153]. Only the ESAM$^+$ subsets of CD11b$^+$ cDC are dependent on signaling from the lymphotoxin (LT) β receptor/Notch2/RBP-J, as deletion of *Rbp-J*, using a CD11c-Cre deleter strain in mice led to a 50% reduction in the CD11b$^+$ subset of splenic DC [153].

FLT3L and FLT3 constitute the best-characterized growth factor–receptor axis for pDC [167]. STAT3, a key component of the Flt3 signaling pathway, plays a nonredundant role in pDC development [168]. Mice lacking STAT3 have profound reductions in pDC that cannot be rescued by Flt3L administration. In addition, transcription factor IRF8 plays a critical role in pDC differentiation since *Irf8*$^{-/-}$ animals lack pDC [156]. Furthermore, E2-2 directly controls the expression of pDC signature genes, while antagonizing several cDC genes, including *Id2* [169].

The cytokines and factors that control the differentiation of MCs into mDC are less well defined, but key requirements appear to be the recognition of bacterial products through TLR and MyD88 [170] or TC activation signals [171].

MC subset differentiation signaling

IFN-I signaling in hematopoietic cells is required for the generation of Ly6C$^+$ MC (Fig. 4d) [172]. A critical transcription factor that plays a key role in Ly6C$^+$ MC differentiation is PU.1. PU.1 is critical for early steps of both myeloid and lymphoid development because PU.1-deficient mice lack MC, granulocytes, and BC [173]. Overexpression of PU.1 leads to activation of IRF8 and Kruppel-like factor 4 (KLF4), which are also key transcription factors involved in Ly6C$^+$ MC development [174, 175]. KLF4 is directly regulated by IRF8. Chromatin immunoprecipitation sequencing analysis of the *Klf4* gene locus showed multiple IRF8 peaks [176]. Moreover, it was found that *Irf8*$^{-/-}$ MC progenitors did not express *Klf4* mRNA, and rescue of *Klf4* in *Irf8*$^{-/-}$ mouse myeloid progenitor cells restored MC differentiation. In addition, KLF4 deficiency abolished CCR2 on Ly6C^{high} MC that is a homing chemokine receptor associated with Ly6C^{high}

MC migration to tissues upon the sensing of inflammatory stimuli [175].

Transcription factor nuclear receptor subfamily 4, group A, member 1 (NR4A1) is required for Ly6C$^-$ MC development [177, 178]. NR4A1 was highly expressed in Ly6C$^-$ MC, and Ly6C$^-$ nonclassical MC were missing in the blood, BM, and other tissues of $Nr4a1^{-/-}$ mice [177, 178]. NR4A1 (also called TR3 or Nur77) is a member of the NR4A family of nuclear receptors, which is considered to function in an anti-inflammatory manner in the vasculature. It was also found that MC from $Nr4a1^{-/-}Nr4a3^{-/-}$ mice contained lower levels of c-Jun and JunB compared with wild-type mice, indicating that the NR4A family likely regulates expression of c-Jun and JunB, which are both proto oncogenes, in MC development [174]. The few non-inflammatory Ly6C$^-$ MC remaining in the BM of $Nr4a1^{-/-}$ mice are arrested in S phase of the cell cycle and undergo apoptosis, implying that NR4A1 functions as a master regulator to control the differentiation and survival of anti-inflammatory Ly6C$^-$ monocytes [178].

LPS is a potent inducer of CD40$^+$ MC differentiation. The induction of CD40 expression by LPS occurs at the transcriptional level and involves activation of the transcription factors NF-κB and STAT1α. More specifically, LPS directly activates NF-κB and induces endogenous production of IFN-β, which then leads to STAT1α activation, and ultimately CD40 gene expression [179].

MØ subset differentiation signaling

In respond to various environmental cues, MØ can acquire distinct functional phenotypes via different phenotypic polarization programs (Fig. 4e). M1 differentiation signaling results in the proteosomal degradation of I-κB and the release of NF-κB p65/p50 heterodimer from the NF-κB/I-κB complex [180]. The NF-κB p65/p50 heterodimer is then translocated to the nucleus and binds to the promoters of inflammatory genes. LPS/TLR4 also phosphorylates and activates the transcription factor interferon-responsive factor 3 (IRF3), which are involved in M1 polarization and M1-associated gene induction [181]. These M1-associated genes include type I interferon, such as IFN-β. Secreted type I interferons bind to the type I interferon receptor (IFNAR), which leads to phosphorylation and activation of the transcription factor STAT1 and STAT2. The induced STAT1 and STAT2 then mediate the gene expression of CXCL9 and CXCL10 chemokines [182], which are characteristic of classical M1 MØ activation. In addition to binding to TLRs, some pathogen-associated molecular patterns (PAMPs) and danger-associated molecular patterns (DAMPs), such as hypoxia, are also recognized by a family of cytosolic nucleotide-binding receptors and NOD-like receptors (NLRs) [183]. Upon ligand recognition, NLRs

undergo conformational changes and self-oligomerization, which is followed by phosphorylation and activation of JNK and c-Jun MAPKs, both of which are essential for activating hypoxia-inducible factor (HIF) 1α [184]. The crucial role of hypoxia in regulating MØ inflammatory response has been confirmed in mice with myeloid cell-specific deletion of HIF-1α [185], in which HIF-1α was found to be essential in regulating myeloid cell glycolytic capacity, survival and function in the inflammatory microenvironment, which are usually avascular and hypoxic [180]. This is in line with the finding that HIF-1α was induced by NF-κB p65/p50 [186] and plays an important role in modulating MØ phagocytosis of bacteria under sepsis conditions [187].

M2a MØ can be driven by canonical M2a stimuli, such as IL-4 and IL-13 [188]. IL-4 and IL-13 polarize MØs to M2a phenotype via phosphorylation and activation of STAT6 through the IL-4 receptor alpha (IL-4Rα) [180]. The M2a MØ phenotype is then promoted by several transcription factors, including peroxisome proliferator activated receptor γ (PPARγ) [189], PPARδ, and KLF4 [190]. Myeloid-specific deficiency of either PPARγ or KLF-4 resulted in decreased M2a polarization of MØ, leading to accelerated lesion formation in ApoE$^{-/-}$ [191] or Ldlr$^{-/-}$ mice [192]. Moreover, ligation of PPARγ by specific PPARγ ligands preferentially resulted in M2a polarization in mice and in humans [189]. Furthermore, IL-4 and IL-13 strongly increase the production of several different endogenous PPAR ligands, which include 13-HODE, 15-HETE, 15d-GPalpha, and PPAR coactivators (PGC-1), thereby stimulating the PPAR trans-activating activity. Indeed, many of the hallmark IL-4/IL-13-inducible M2 marker genes, such as macrophage mannose receptor (MMR), Arginase I, CD36, dectin-1, depend on PPAR expression [193].

Activated lymphocyte-derived (ALD)-DNA confer MØ M2b polarization via Notch-1/p38 signaling activation [194]. Notch-1 signaling also facilitates ALD-DNA–induced M2b differentiation via PI3K and ERK1/2 pathway [195]. In addition, the M2c MØ phenotype arises in the presence of anti-inflammatory cytokine IL-10 [196]. IL-10 binds to the IL-10R, which is composed of two chains: IL-10R1 and IL-10R2 [197]. IL-10 binding to the receptor activates the tyrosine kinase JAK1, which leads to the phosphorylation of transcription factor STAT3. STAT3 then dimerizes, enters the nucleus, and activates the transcription of anti-inflammatory genes [198]. In murine atherosclerotic plaques, Kadl et al. described a phenotypically distinct MØ subset called Mox [87]. This subset is induced by oxidized phospholipids, such as oxLDL, and protects the organisms from oxidative stress through nuclear factor (erythroid-derived 2)-like 2 (NFE2L2)-mediated expression of antioxidant enzymes such as HMOX1, thioredoxin reductase 1 (Txnrd1), and sulfiredoxin-1 (Sxrn-1). Finally, in human and mouse, haem induces Mhem MØs, which are characterized by increased production of LXRα, LXRβ, haem-induced cyclic AMP-dependent transcription factor 1 (ATF1), HMOX1, and ABCA1 [199].

All the immune cell subsets may interact and communicate with each other. For example, when TGF-β signaling is deficient in CD11c⁺ mDC, there would be increased CD4⁺, CD8⁺, Th1, and Th17 activation and maturation as a result [97]. CD8⁺ TC could also increase monopoiesis and circulating MC levels [102], while Th1 could reduce E06 antibodies that are produced by B1 BC [103]. Moreover, Th17 differentiation relies on IL-6, which is significantly contributed by MØ [105]. Lastly, DC-mediated TLR4/IL-12/IL-10 signaling could polarize Treg, which control GC Tfh-BC axis [200, 201].

Molecular and cellular modulation of immune cell subsets and its impact on atherosclerosis

Diverse immune cell subsets in the atherosclerotic plaque strongly contribute to the development of atherosclerotic vascular disease in humans and mice (Fig. 5). During an inflammatory response, increased Th1 TC, Th17 TC, B2 BC, mDC, cDC, Ly6C⁺ MC, and M1 MØ drive atherogenesis. On the other side, atherosclerotic disease risk factors also promote the differentiation of Treg TC, Ly6C⁻ MC, M2a/b/c MØ, Mox MØ, and Mhem MØ, Th2 TC, B1 BC, and pDC, which regulate the inflammatory response and play anti-atherogenic roles during resolution phase [178].

There are many factors that could interfere with immune cell subset functions. Many in vivo and in vitro studies have established a clear role for IL-4 in inhibiting Th1 cell development [202], while Th1-derived cytokine

IFN-γ inhibits Th2 proliferation by interfering with Th2 costimulator, IL-1 [203]. IL-2 signaling via STAT5 constrains Th17 cell generation [204], while IL-6 inhibits TGF-β-induced Treg differentiation [205]. Specialized subsets of TC, including follicular Treg and Qa-1-restricted CD8⁺ Treg control Fo BC responses [206]. Humanized LL2 (Epratuzumab), an IgG1 monoclonal antibody, delivers antibody-dependent cellular cytotoxicity to MZ B2 when it binds CD22, which is strongly expressed on MZ BC in lymphoid tissues ("Epratuzumab in Non-Hodgkin's Lymphomas", [207]). BC-specific deletion of Shp-1 promotes the development of B1a cells and their expansion in the secondary lymphoid organs [208], indicating that Shp-1 is a key negative regulator of B1a BC activation. Ezh2 was shown to be recruited to the promoters of CCL2 and CCL8 genes in human blood MC, resulting in their gene silencing by H3K27me3, thus controlling the number of inflammatory Ly6C⁺ MC [209]. West Nile virus infection accelerated migrating BM Ly6C⁻ MC differentiation into DC [210]. p21 reprograms M1 MØ by shifting activating p65-p50 to inhibitory p50-p50 NF-κB pathways, and an M2-like status [211]. M2a polarization induced by IL-4 are subject to several negative regulation mechanisms: the SH2-containing tyrosine phosphatases (PTPs) can modulate IL-4 signaling by dephosphorylating JAKs and STAT6 [212], whereas the suppressor of cytokine signaling (SOCS) family, such as SOCS1 and SOCS3, can inhibit the activity of JAKs by blocking the interaction of the JAK catalytic domain with their STAT protein substrates [213]. Importantly, increased IL-10 secretion, accompanied by anti-inflammatory effect exerted by M2a MØ, was found to predominantly impede macrophage M2b polarization [194]. miR-155 represses C/EBP-β/arginase-1 signaling,

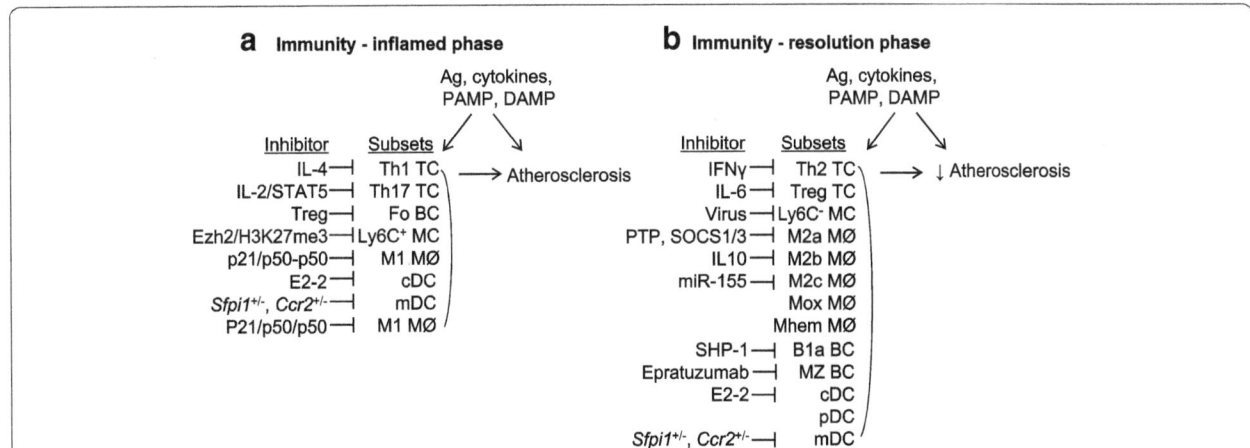

Fig. 5 Molecular and cellular modulation of immune cell subsets and its impact on atherosclerosis. Immune cell subsets play different roles in atherosclerosis and can be suppressed by individual endogenous inhibitors as indicated. **a** Inflamed phase in immunity. Inflammatory subsets are induced by antigens (Ag), inflammatory cytokines, pathogen-associated molecular patterns (PAMP), danger-associated molecular patterns (DAMP), in inflamed phase of disease and promote atherosclerosis. **b** Resolution phase in immunity. Anti-inflammatory subsets are induced in resolution phase of disease and suppress atherosclerosis. There are many inhibitors can could interfere with immune cell subset functions

which is a hallmark of M2c MØ [214]. Transcription factor E2–2 actively maintains the cell fate of mature pDCs and opposes the "default" cDC fate, in part through direct regulation of lineage-specific gene expression programs [169]. Lastly, *Sfpi1*$^{+/-}$ or *Sfpi1*$^{+/-}$ mice had reduced differentiation of GM-CSF-dependent mDCs [215].

Molecular and cellular modulation of immune cell subsets and its impact on cancer

Tumor-entrained neutrophils (TENs) play a crucial pathophysiological role during cancer development. It has been shown that TENs that are distributed in the pre-metastatic niche in the lung tissues could inhibit metastatic tumor seeding in the lung tissues by generating reactive oxygen species [216]. Mechanistically, tumor-secreted CCL2 was shown to be a critical mediator in this process, which is required for optimal anti-metastatic entrainment of G-CSF-stimulated TENs. In addition, TENs are present in the peripheral blood of breast cancer patients prior to surgical resection, but not in healthy individuals. Importantly, the above mechanism is why CD44 variant-positive ROS-resistant cancer stem-like cells tend to be accumulated in the invasive front of the gastric and breast cancer tissues [217].

Immune-checkpoint inhibitors (ICI) have already emerged as successful therapeutic approaches against

multiple cancers [218]. Novel strategies which include promoting immunogenic cell death (such as chemotherapy and radiation) and enhancing antigen presentation by stimulating innate immune responses and dendritic cell function (such as IFN-I and TLR ligands) could potentially promote the formation or the presentation of suitable neo-antigens in tumor tissues that have a non-inflamed, immune cell poor tumor microenvironment. In addition, when combined with ICI, blockage of immunosuppressive factors (such as VEGF, IL-10, and TGF-β), which promotes dendritic cell migration, maturation, and function, might lead to better T cell priming and better immunotherapy against cancers [219].

Myeloid-derived suppressor cells (MDSCs) are a heterogeneous subpopulation of immune cells that are important for inflammatory diseases and cancers [220, 221]. Although MDSCs are present in low quantities in healthy individuals, their numbers are dramatically increased in patients with chronic inflammatory diseases such as cancer, cardiovascular diseases, and autoimmune diseases [220, 222]. MDSCs are generated as a result of sustained and aberrant myeloid cell differentiation. MDSCs are different from terminally differentiated myeloid cells (such as macrophages, dendritic cells, and neutrophils), and they have an activation program that is different from that of mature myeloid cells [223]. MDSCs are characterized by both Gr1 and CD11b

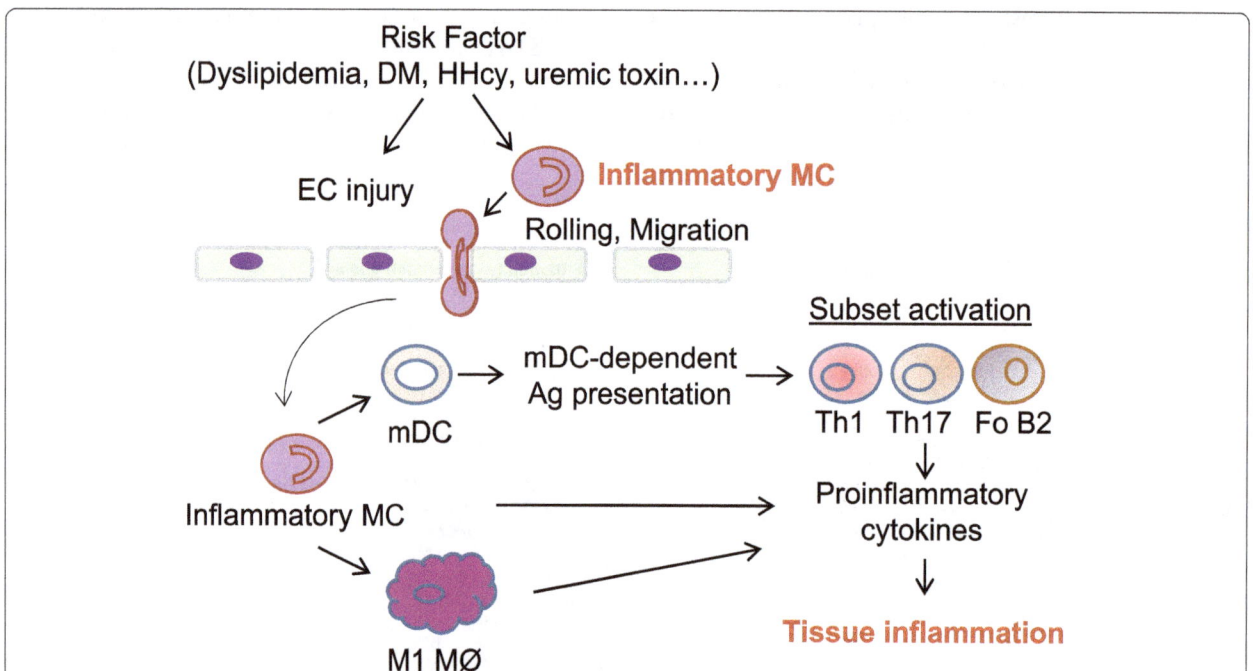

Fig. 6 Model of differentiation of inflammatory mononuclear cell, their interaction with endothelial cells and contribution to lymphocyte subset differentiation and tissue inflammation. In early stage of atherosclerosis, Ly6Cmiddle + high monocytes (MC) transmigrate to sub-endothelial space of vessel and further differentiate to M1 macrophages (MØ) and monocyte-derived dendritic cells (mDC). mDC activate T helper cells Th1, Th17, and B2 cells, resulting in chronic inflammation in atherosclerotic plaque. All of these inflammatory mononuclear cell subsets promote atherosclerosis development partially through production of proinflammatory cytokines

markers in mice, which can be used to categorize MDSCs into two subpopulations, which include granulocytic (G)-MDSCs (CD11b$^+$Ly6G$^+$Ly6C^{low}) and monocytic (M)-MDSCs (CD11b$^+$Ly6G$^-$Ly6C^{high}). In humans, G-MDSCs are characterized by CD11b$^+$CD14$^-$CD15$^+$ or CD11b$^+$CD14$^-$CD66b$^+$, whereas M-MDSCs are defined as CD11b$^+$CD14$^+$HLA-DR^{low}CD15$^-$ [223]. MDSCs, rather than MC or neutrophils, potently suppress immune responses [220]. It has been shown that depletion of MDSCs results in markedly enhanced anti-tumor immune responses [224, 225]. Thus, MDSCs are promising targets of cancer immunotherapy.

IL-6 is a pleiotropic cytokine with varied systemic functions and it plays a critical role in hematopoiesis as a cofactor in stem cell differentiation and amplification [226]. Clinical studies have shown that upregulated serum IL-6 levels in patients were associated with advanced stages of a number of tumors and short survival in patients [227]. Thus, anti-IL-6 antibodies have been used in the treatment of patients with various cancers and inflammatory diseases. Clinically registered IL-6 inhibitors include anti-IL-6 monoclonal antibody (mAb) (siltuximab) and anti-IL6R mAb (tocilizumab). Blocking IL-6 was proven beneficial towards patients with Castleman disease and inflammatory diseases, and it was well tolerated in cancer patients as well. Nevertheless, IL-6 inhibitors showed no efficacy in large randomized trials of various cancers, in particular plasma cell cancers [228]. One possibility of such failure may be related to our incomplete understanding of the role of IL-6 in regulating the differentiation and function of immune cell subtypes. Future studies are warranted to develop better cytokine-based cancer immunotherapy methods.

Summary

Compelling evidence in human and mouse immune cell heterogeneity research points towards a scenario in which immune cell subsets actively change and modulate the development of CVD and cancers. In this review article, we addressed several issues regarding immune cell subset differentiation, which include general hematopoietic cell differentiation processes, subset development, differentiation process and signaling, characterization, disease relevance, and modulation. We elaborated a working model to elucidate the differentiation of pro-inflammatory mononuclear cells, their interaction with endothelial cells, and their contribution to lymphocyte subset differentiation and tissue inflammation (Fig. 6).

Conclusion

Immune cells can be sub-divided into various subsets that play specialized roles in innate and adaptive immune responses. Immune cell subset differentiation and its complex interaction within the internal biological milieu compose a "pathophysiological network," an interactive cross-talking complex, which determines and regulates vital conditions of life. Continued research in the understanding of immune cell subsets will provide crucial insights for the etiology, pathobiology, prognosis, and treatment of human CVD and cancers.

Abbreviations

Ab: Antibody; acLDL: Acetylated low density lipoprotein; ACS: Acute coronary syndrome; Ag: Antigen; AHR: Aryl hydrocarbon receptor; ALD: Activated lymphocyte-derived; Anti-inf: Anti-inflammatory; AP-1: Activator protein 1; APC: Antigen presenting cell; ApoE: Apolipoprotein E; ApoE$^{-/}$ $^-$CD11cDNR: Functional inactivation of TGFβ receptor II (TGFβRII) signaling in CD11c + cells; Arg1: Arginase 1; Arg2: Arginase 2; ART: Antiretroviral therapy; ASK1: Apoptosis signal regulating kinase 1; ATF: Activating transcription factor; BAFF: B cell-activating factor of the tumor-necrosis-factor family; Baso: Basophil; BATF3: Basic leucine zipper ATF-like 3 transcription factor; BC: B cell; BCL: B cell lymphoma; BCR: B cell receptor; BDCA2: Blood DC antigen 2; BHA: Butylated hydroxyanisole; BM: Bone marrow; BST2: Bone marrow stromal antigen 2; BTK: Bruton's tyrosine kinase; C: Cholesterol; C/EBP: CCAAT-enhancer-binding protein; CAC: Coronary artery calcification; CAD: Coronary artery disease; CAP: Carotid atherosclerotic plaque; CCR2: C-C chemokine receptor type 2; CD11cDNR: Functional inactivation of TGFβ receptor II signaling in CD11c + cells; cDC: Classical/conventional dendritic cell; Cdkn2a: Cyclin-dependent kinase inhibitor 2A; CDP: Common dendritic cell progenitor; CEA: Carotid endarterectomy; chol: Cholesterol; CKD: Chronic kidney disease; CLP: Common lymphoid progenitor; CMoP: Common monocyte precursor; CMP: Common myeloid progenitor; CRE: Creatinine; CSF-1: Colony stimulating factor 1; CSFR: Colony-stimulating factor receptor; CVD: Cardiovascular disease; CX3CR1: CX3C chemokine receptor 1; CXCL4: Chemokine (C-X-C motif) ligand 4; DC: Dendritic cell; DC-SIGN: Dendritic cell-specific intercellular adhesion molecule-3-grabbing non-integrin; DIO: Diet-induced obesity; DL-1: Delta-like 1; Dnmt1: DNA methyltransferase 1; EAE: Encephalomyelitis; Eos: Eosinophil; FcγR: Fc receptor-γ receptor; FIZZ1: Found in inflammatory zone 1; Fli-1: Friend leukemia integration 1; Fo: Follicular; FoxP3: Forkhead box P3; Gata-3: GATA binding protein; GC: Germinal center; GM-CSF: Granulocyte macrophage colony-stimulating factor; GMP: Granulocyte-macrophage progenitor; Gran: Granulocyte; haem: Hemoglobin; HCMV: Human cytomegalovirus; HFD: High-fat diet; HHcy: Hyperhomocysteinemia; HIF1α: Hypoxia-inducible factor 1-α; HLA-DR: Human leukocyte antigen – antigen D related; Hlx: H2.0-like homeobox protein; hMDP: Human monocyte-dendritic progenitor; HMGB1: High mobility group box 1; HMOX-1: Heme oxygenase 1; HOX-1: Homeobox-leucine zipper protein; HSV1: Herpes simplex virus 1; IC: Immunocomplex; ICOSL: Inducible T cell costimulatory ligand; ID2: DNA-binding protein inhibitor 2; ID2: Inhibitor of DNA binding 2; IFN: Interferon; IGF: Insulin-like growth factor; IL: Interleukin; IL-1Rα: Interlukin-1 receptor antagonist; Inf: Inflammatory; iNOS: Inducible nitric oxide synthase; IRF: Interferon regulatory factor; KLF: Kruppel-like factor; LCMV: Lymphocytic choriomeningitis virus; Ldlr: Low density lipoprotein receptor; LILRA4: Leukocyte immunoglobulin-like receptor, subfamily A, member 4; LPS: Lipopolysaccharide; LT: Lymphotoxin; LT-HSC: Long-term hematopoietic stem cell; Ly6C: Lymphocyte antigen 6 complex locus C1; lym: Lymphoid; MADS: Metabolite-associated danger signal; MALT1: Mucosa-associated lymphoid tissue lymphoma translocation protein 1; MAML: Mastermind like transcriptional coactivator; MAPK: Mitogen-activated protein kinase; MC: Monocyte; MCMV: Murine cytomegalovirus; mDC: Monocyte-derived DC; MDP: Monocyte-dendritic progenitor; MHC: Major histocompatibility complex; MI: Myocardial infarction; miR: MicroRNA; MM: Multiple myeloma; MMP-7: Matrix metalloproteinase-7; MNC: Mononuclear cell; MØ: Macrophage; MR: Mannose receptor; MZ: Marginal zone; NFAT: Nuclear factor of activated T cells; NFE2L2: Nuclear factor (erythroid-derived 2)-like 2; NF-κB: Nuclear factor κB; NKC: Natural killer cell; NKT: Natural killer T; NØ: Neutrophil; NOI: Nitric oxide intermediates; Nr4a1: Nuclear Receptor

Subfamily 4, Group A, Member 1; NSTEACS: Non-ST-elevation acute coronary syndromes; NSTEMI: Non-ST-elevation myocardial infarction; O: Obese; OW: Overweight; oxLDL: Oxidized low density lipoprotein; oxPL: Oxidized phospholipid; PBMC: Peripheral blood mononuclear cell; pDC: Plasmocytoid dendritic cell; PGE2: Prostaglandin E2; PMID: PubMed ID; PPAR: Peroxisome proliferator-activated receptor; PTK: Protein tyrosine kinase; PTP: Phosphatase; RA: Rheumatoid arthritis; RBP-J: Recombination signal binding protein for immunoglobulin kappa J region; Rec: Recombination; ROI: Radical oxygen intermediates; RORγt: Retinoic acid receptor-related orphan receptor γt; SA: Stable angina; SAP: Serum amyloid P component; Siglec: Sialic acid-binding immunoglobulin-like lectin; SIRPα: Signal regulatory protein α; SLE: Systemic lupus erythematosus; SOCS: Suppressor of cytokine signaling; STAT: Signal transducer and activator of transcription; STEAMI: ST-elevation acute myocardial infarction; STEMI: ST segment elevation myocardial infarction; T(EM): Effector memory T cell; T1DM: Type 1 diabetes mellitus; T2DM: Type 2 diabetes mellitus; TC: T cell; TCR: T cell receptor; TD: T cell dependent; Tfh: T follicular helper; TG: Triglyceride; TGFβ: Transforming growth factor β; Th: T helper cell; TH0: Naïve T cell; THBS1: Thrombospondin 1; Throm: Thrombosed; TI: T cell independent; TLR: Toll-like receptor; TNF-α: Tumor necrosis factor-α; Treg: Regulatory T cell; Txnrd1: Thioredoxin reductase 1; UA: Unstable angina; UAP: Unstable angina pectoris; VEGF: Vascular endothelial growth factor; VSV: Vesicular stomatitis virus; α: Anti

Funding
This work was supported in part by the NIH grants HL117654, HL-110764, HL130233, HL131460, DK104116, and DK113775 to Hong Wang, HL132399, HL138749 to Xiaofeng Yang, T32 Hematopoiesis Training Grant 5T32DK007780 to Xinyuan Li, and AHA SDG 17SDG33671051 to Pu Fang.

Authors' contributions
PF and HW drafted the manuscript. XL and XFY participated in the discussion. LC provided the immune cell subset in disease table and language editing. JAC contributed to MC subset differentiation pathways. Other authors revised the manuscript. All authors read and approved the final manuscript.

Consent for publication
Not applicable.

Competing interests
The authors declare that they have no competing interests.

Author details
[1]Center for Metabolic Disease Research, Lewis Kats School of Medicine, Temple University, Medical Education and Research Building, Room 1060, 3500 N. Broad Street, Philadelphia, PA 19140, USA. [2]Department of Pathology and Laboratory Medicine, University of Pennsylvania, Philadelphia, PA, USA. [3]Department of Pharmacology, Lewis Kats School of Medicine, Temple University, Philadelphia, PA, USA. [4]Cardiovascular Medicine Department, Sun Yat-Sen Memorial Hospital, Sun Yat-Sen University, Guangzhou 510120, China. [5]Key Laboratory of Cardiovascular Disease and Molecular Intervention, Nanjing Medical University, Nanjing, China.

References
1. Mosmann TR, Coffman RL. TH1 and TH2 cells: different patterns of lymphokine secretion lead to different functional properties. Annu Rev Immunol. 1989;7:145–73.
2. Hayakawa K, et al. The "Ly-1 B" cell subpopulation in normal immunodefective, and autoimmune mice. J Exp Med. 1983;157(1):202–18.
3. Vremec D, et al. The surface phenotype of dendritic cells purified from mouse thymus and spleen: investigation of the CD8 expression by a subpopulation of dendritic cells. J Exp Med. 1992;176(1):47–58.
4. Passlick B, Flieger D, Ziegler-Heitbrock HW. Identification and characterization of a novel monocyte subpopulation in human peripheral blood. Blood. 1989;74(7):2527–34.
5. Stein M, et al. Interleukin 4 potently enhances murine macrophage mannose receptor activity: a marker of alternative immunologic macrophage activation. J Exp Med. 1992;176(1):287–92.
6. Ammirati E, et al. Effector memory T cells are associated with atherosclerosis in humans and animal models. J Am Heart Assoc. 2012;1(1):27–41.
7. Yang WY, et al. Pathological conditions re-shape physiological Tregs into pathological Tregs. Burns Trauma. 2015;3(1)
8. Yanez, A., et al. Granulocyte-monocyte progenitors and monocyte-dendritic cell progenitors independently produce functionally distinct monocytes. Immunity, 2017. 47(5): p. 890–902 e4.
9. Jagannathan-Bogdan M, Zon LI. Hematopoiesis. Development. 2013;140(12): 2463–7.
10. Orkin SH, Zon LI. Hematopoiesis: an evolving paradigm for stem cell biology. Cell. 2008;132(4):631–44.
11. Hettinger J, et al. Origin of monocytes and macrophages in a committed progenitor. Nat Immunol. 2013;14(8):821–30.
12. Germain RN. T-cell development and the CD4-CD8 lineage decision. Nat Rev Immunol. 2002;2(5):309–22.
13. Hogquist KA, Baldwin TA, Jameson SC. Central tolerance: learning self-control in the thymus. Nat Rev Immunol. 2005;5(10):772–82.
14. Cho JH, Sprent J. TCR tuning of T cell subsets. Immunol Rev. 2018;283(1): 129–37.
15. Sakaguchi S, Wing K, Miyara M. Regulatory T cells—a brief history and perspective. Eur J Immunol. 2007;37(Suppl 1):S116–23.
16. Harrington LE, et al. Interleukin 17-producing CD4+ effector T cells develop via a lineage distinct from the T helper type 1 and 2 lineages. Nat Immunol. 2005;6(11):1123–32.
17. Dai J, et al. Metabolism-associated danger signal-induced immune response and reverse immune checkpoint-activated CD40(+) monocyte differentiation. J Hematol Oncol. 2017;10(1):141.
18. Hsieh CS, et al. Development of TH1 CD4+ T cells through IL-12 produced by Listeria-induced macrophages. Science. 1993;260(5107):547–9.
19. Schmitt N, Ueno H. Regulation of human helper T cell subset differentiation by cytokines. Curr Opin Immunol. 2015;34:130–6.
20. Littman DR, Rudensky AY. Th17 and regulatory T cells in mediating and restraining inflammation. Cell. 2010;140(6):845–58.
21. Tran DQ, Ramsey H, Shevach EM. Induction of FOXP3 expression in naive human CD4+FOXP3 T cells by T-cell receptor stimulation is transforming growth factor-beta dependent but does not confer a regulatory phenotype. Blood. 2007;110(8):2983–90.
22. Cambier JC, et al. B-cell anergy: from transgenic models to naturally occurring anergic B cells? Nat Rev Immunol. 2007;7(8):633–43.
23. Jacobi AM, Diamond B. Balancing diversity and tolerance: lessons from patients with systemic lupus erythematosus. J Exp Med. 2005;202(3):341–4.
24. Galy A, et al. Human T, B, natural killer, and dendritic cells arise from a common bone marrow progenitor cell subset. Immunity. 1995;3(4):459–73.
25. Kondo M, Weissman IL, Akashi K. Identification of clonogenic common lymphoid progenitors in mouse bone marrow. Cell. 1997;91(5):661–72.
26. Gasteiger G, Rudensky AY. Interactions between innate and adaptive lymphocytes. Nat Rev Immunol. 2014;14(9):631–9.
27. Bostik P, et al. Innate immune natural killer cells and their role in HIV and SIV infection. HIV Ther. 2010;4(4):483–504.
28. Steinman RM, Cohn ZA. Identification of a novel cell type in peripheral lymphoid organs of mice. II. Functional properties in vitro. J Exp Med. 1974; 139(2):380–97.
29. Steinman RM, Cohn ZA. Identification of a novel cell type in peripheral lymphoid organs of mice. I. Morphology, quantitation, tissue distribution. J Exp Med. 1973;137(5):1142–62.
30. Shortman K, Heath WR. The CD8+ dendritic cell subset. Immunol Rev. 2010; 234(1):18–31.
31. Helft J, et al. Origin and functional heterogeneity of non-lymphoid tissue dendritic cells in mice. Immunol Rev. 2010;234(1):55–75.
32. Colonna M, Trinchieri G, Liu YJ. Plasmacytoid dendritic cells in immunity. Nat Immunol. 2004;5(12):1219–26.
33. Liu K, et al. In vivo analysis of dendritic cell development and homeostasis. Science. 2009;324(5925):392–7.
34. Murphy TL, et al. Transcriptional control of dendritic cell development. Annu Rev Immunol. 2016;34:93–119.
35. Cisse B, et al. Transcription factor E2-2 is an essential and specific regulator of plasmacytoid dendritic cell development. Cell. 2008;135(1): 37–48.

36. Bender A, et al. Improved methods for the generation of dendritic cells from nonproliferating progenitors in human blood. J Immunol Methods. 1996;196(2):121–35.

37. Appleby LJ, et al. Sources of heterogeneity in human monocyte subsets. Immunol Lett. 2013;152(1):32–41.

38. Yang J, et al. Monocyte and macrophage differentiation: circulation inflammatory monocyte as biomarker for inflammatory diseases. Biomark Res. 2014;2(1):1.

39. Yang J, et al. Chronic kidney disease induces inflammatory CD40+ monocyte differentiation via homocysteine elevation and DNA hypomethylation. Circ Res. 2016;119(11):1226–41.

40. Palframan RT, et al. Inflammatory chemokine transport and presentation in HEV: a remote control mechanism for monocyte recruitment to lymph nodes in inflamed tissues. J Exp Med. 2001;194(9):1361–73.

41. Leon B, et al. Dendritic cell differentiation potential of mouse monocytes: monocytes represent immediate precursors of CD8- and CD8+ splenic dendritic cells. Blood. 2004;103(7):2668–76.

42. Jung S, et al. Analysis of fractalkine receptor CX(3)CR1 function by targeted deletion and green fluorescent protein reporter gene insertion. Mol Cell Biol. 2000;20(11):4106–14.

43. Fleming TJ, Fleming ML, Malek TR. Selective expression of Ly-6G on myeloid lineage cells in mouse bone marrow. RB6-8C5 mAb to granulocyte-differentiation antigen (Gr-1) detects members of the Ly-6 family. J Immunol. 1993;151(5):2399–408.

44. Nahrendorf M, et al. The healing myocardium sequentially mobilizes two monocyte subsets with divergent and complementary functions. J Exp Med. 2007;204(12):3037–47.

45. Van Furth R, Diesselhoff-den Dulk MC, Mattie H. Quantitative study on the production and kinetics of mononuclear phagocytes during an acute inflammatory reaction. J Exp Med. 1973;138(6):1314–30.

46. Nathan CF, et al. Identification of interferon-gamma as the lymphokine that activates human macrophage oxidative metabolism and antimicrobial activity. J Exp Med. 1983;158(3):670–89.

47. Ginhoux F, et al. Fate mapping analysis reveals that adult microglia derive from primitive macrophages. Science. 2010;330(6005):841–5.

48. Rosenfeld ME. Converting smooth muscle cells to macrophage-like cells with KLF4 in atherosclerotic plaques. Nat Med. 2015;21(6):549–51.

49. Hong CW. Current understanding in neutrophil differentiation and heterogeneity. Immune Netw. 2017;17(5):298–306.

50. Arock M. Mast cell differentiation: still open questions? Blood. 2016;127(4): 373–4.

51. Dahlin JS, et al. Lineage- CD34hi CD117int/hi FcepsilonRI+ cells in human blood constitute a rare population of mast cell progenitors. Blood. 2016; 127(4):383–91.

52. Shan Y, et al. Increased frequency of peripheral blood follicular helper T cells and elevated serum IL21 levels in patients with knee osteoarthritis. Mol Med Rep. 2017;15(3):1095–102.

53. Morita R, et al. Human blood CXCR5(+)CD4(+) T cells are counterparts of T follicular cells and contain specific subsets that differentially support antibody secretion. Immunity. 2011;34(1):108–21.

54. Victora GD, et al. Germinal center dynamics revealed by multiphoton microscopy with a photoactivatable fluorescent reporter. Cell. 2010;143(4): 592–605.

55. Duhen T, et al. Production of interleukin 22 but not interleukin 17 by a subset of human skin-homing memory T cells. Nat Immunol. 2009;10(8): 857–63.

56. Sallusto F, Zielinski CE, Lanzavecchia A. Human Th17 subsets. Eur J Immunol. 2012;42(9):2215–20.

57. Kuang DM, et al. B7-H1-expressing antigen-presenting cells mediate polarization of protumorigenic Th22 subsets. J Clin Invest. 2014;124(10): 4657–67.

58. Dardalhon V, et al. IL-4 inhibits TGF-beta-induced Foxp3+ T cells and, together with TGF-beta, generates IL-9+ IL-10+ Foxp3(−) effector T cells. Nat Immunol. 2008;9(12):1347–55.

59. Allman D, Pillai S. Peripheral B cell subsets. Curr Opin Immunol. 2008;20(2): 149–57.

60. Moller B, et al. Class-switched B cells display response to therapeutic B-cell depletion in rheumatoid arthritis. Arthritis Res Ther. 2009;11(3):R62.

61. Genestier L, et al. TLR agonists selectively promote terminal plasma cell differentiation of B cell subsets specialized in thymus-independent responses. J Immunol. 2007;178(12):7779–86.

62. Thiriot A, et al. The Bw cells, a novel B cell population conserved in the whole genus Mus. J Immunol. 2007;179(10):6568–78.

63. Haas KM, et al. B-1a and B-1b cells exhibit distinct developmental requirements and have unique functional roles in innate and adaptive immunity to S. pneumoniae. Immunity. 2005;23(1):7–18.

64. Nussenzweig MC, et al. Dendritic cells are accessory cells for the development of anti-trinitrophenyl cytotoxic T lymphocytes. J Exp Med. 1980;152(4):1070–84.

65. Wakim LM, et al. Dendritic cell-induced memory T cell activation in nonlymphoid tissues. Science. 2008;319(5860):198–202.

66. Gardner A, Ruffell B. moDCs, less problems. Immunity. 2018;48(1):6–8.

67. Reizis B, et al. Plasmacytoid dendritic cells: recent progress and open questions. Annu Rev Immunol. 2011;29:163–83.

68. Macal, M., et al., Self-renewal and toll-like receptor signaling sustain exhausted plasmacytoid dendritic cells during chronic viral infection. Immunity, 2018. 48(4): p. 730–744 e5.

69. Bedoui S, et al. Cross-presentation of viral and self antigens by skin-derived CD103+ dendritic cells. Nat Immunol. 2009;10(5):488–95.

70. Hildner K, et al. Batf3 deficiency reveals a critical role for CD8alpha+ dendritic cells in cytotoxic T cell immunity. Science. 2008;322(5904):1097–100.

71. Merad M, et al. The dendritic cell lineage: ontogeny and function of dendritic cells and their subsets in the steady state and the inflamed setting. Annu Rev Immunol. 2013;31:563–604.

72. Yona S, Jung S. Monocytes: subsets, origins, fates and functions. Curr Opin Hematol. 2010;17(1):53–9.

73. Cros J, et al. Human CD14dim monocytes patrol and sense nucleic acids and viruses via TLR7 and TLR8 receptors. Immunity. 2010;33(3):375–86.

74. Mukherjee R, et al. Non-classical monocytes display inflammatory features: validation in sepsis and systemic lupus erythematous. Sci Rep. 2015;5:13886.

75. Boyette, L.B., et al., Phenotype, function, and differentiation potential of human monocyte subsets. PLoS One, 2017. 12(4): p. e0176460.

76. Robbins SH, et al. Novel insights into the relationships between dendritic cell subsets in human and mouse revealed by genome-wide expression profiling. Genome Biol. 2008;9(1):R17.

77. Barbet, G., et al., Sensing microbial viability through bacterial RNA augments T follicular helper cell and antibody responses. Immunity, 2018. 48(3): p. 584–598 e5.

78. Murray PJ, Wynn TA. Protective and pathogenic functions of macrophage subsets. Nat Rev Immunol. 2011;11(11):723–37.

79. Yang L, Zhang Y. Tumor-associated macrophages: from basic research to clinical application. J Hematol Oncol. 2017;10(1):58.

80. Sutterwala FS, et al. Reversal of proinflammatory responses by ligating the macrophage Fcgamma receptor type I. J Exp Med. 1998;188(1):217–22.

81. Yang L, Zhang Y. Tumor-associated macrophages: potential targets for cancer treatment Biomark Res. 2017;5:25.

82. Edwards JP, et al. Biochemical and functional characterization of three activated macrophage populations. J Leukoc Biol. 2006;80(6):1298–307.

83. Anderson CF, Mosser DM. A novel phenotype for an activated macrophage: the type 2 activated macrophage. J Leukoc Biol. 2002;72(1):101–6.

84. Lu J, et al. Discrete functions of M2a and M2c macrophage subsets determine their relative efficacy in treating chronic kidney disease. Kidney Int. 2013;84(4):745–55.

85. Butcher MJ, Galkina EV. Phenotypic and functional heterogeneity of macrophages and dendritic cell subsets in the healthy and atherosclerosis-prone aorta. Front Physiol. 2012;3:44.

86. Gleissner CA, et al. CXC chemokine ligand 4 induces a unique transcriptome in monocyte-derived macrophages. J Immunol. 2010;184(9):4810–8.

87. Kadl A, et al. Identification of a novel macrophage phenotype that develops in response to atherogenic phospholipids via Nrf2. Circ Res. 2010;107(6): 737–46.

88. Boyle JJ, et al. Coronary intraplaque hemorrhage evokes a novel atheroprotective macrophage phenotype. Am J Pathol. 2009;174(3):1097–108.

89. Pourcet B, Staels B. Alternative macrophages in atherosclerosis: not always protective! J Clin Invest. 2018;128(3):910–2.

90. Li X, et al. Mitochondrial reactive oxygen species mediate lysophosphatidylcholine-induced endothelial cell activation. Arterioscler Thromb Vasc Biol. 2016;36(6):1090–100.

91. Rombouts, M., et al., Linking CD11b (+) dendritic cells and natural killer T cells to plaque inflammation in atherosclerosis. Mediat Inflamm, 2016. 2016: p. 6467375.

92. Martinez-Rodriguez JE, et al. Expansion of the NKG2C+ natural killer-cell subset is associated with high-risk carotid atherosclerotic plaques in seropositive patients for human cytomegalovirus. Arterioscler Thromb Vasc Biol. 2013;33(11):2653–9.

93. Winchester R, et al. Association of elevations of specific T cell and monocyte subpopulations in rheumatoid arthritis with subclinical coronary artery atherosclerosis. Arthritis Rheumatol. 2016;68(1):92–102.

94. Mrakovcic-Sutic I, et al. Cross-talk between NKT and regulatory T cells (Tregs) in modulation of immune response in patients with colorectal cancer following different pain management techniques. Coll Antropol. 2011;35(Suppl 2):57–60.

95. Dragu R, et al. Predictive value of white blood cell subtypes for long-term outcome following myocardial infarction. Atherosclerosis. 2008; 196(1):405–12.

96. Li S, et al. Association of plasma PCSK9 levels with white blood cell count and its subsets in patients with stable coronary artery disease. Atherosclerosis. 2014;234(2):441–5.

97. Lievens D, et al. Abrogated transforming growth factor beta receptor II (TGFbetaRII) signalling in dendritic cells promotes immune reactivity of T cells resulting in enhanced atherosclerosis. Eur Heart J. 2013;34(48):3717–27.

98. Caligiuri G, et al. Protective immunity against atherosclerosis carried by B cells of hypercholesterolemic mice. J Clin Invest. 2002;109(6):745–53.

99. Liu X, et al. Is CD47 an innate immune checkpoint for tumor evasion? J Hematol Oncol. 2017;10(1):12.

100. Tapp LD, et al. TLR4 expression on monocyte subsets in myocardial infarction. J Intern Med. 2013;273(3):294–305.

101. Dworacka M, et al. Circulating CD3+56+ cell subset in pre-diabetes. Exp Clin Endocrinol Diabetes. 2014;122(2):65–70.

102. Cochain C, et al. CD8+ T cells regulate monopoiesis and circulating Ly6C-high monocyte levels in atherosclerosis in mice. Circ Res. 2015; 117(3):244–53.

103. Buono C, et al. T-bet deficiency reduces atherosclerosis and alters plaque antigen-specific immune responses. Proc Natl Acad Sci U S A. 2005;102(5): 1596–601.

104. Taleb S, Tedgui A, Mallat Z. IL-17 and Th17 cells in atherosclerosis: subtle and contextual roles. Arterioscler Thromb Vasc Biol. 2015;35(2):258–64.

105. Winer S, et al. Obesity predisposes to Th17 bias. Eur J Immunol. 2009;39(9): 2629–35.

106. Pastrana JL, et al. Regulatory T cells and atherosclerosis. J Clin Exp Cardiolog. 2012;2012(Suppl 12):2.

107. Satoh S, et al. Relationships between inflammatory mediators and coronary plaque composition in patients with stable angina investigated by ultrasound radiofrequency data analysis. Cardiovasc Interv Ther. 2011;26(3): 193–201.

108. Rosenfeld SM, et al. B-1b cells secrete atheroprotective IgM and attenuate atherosclerosis. Circ Res. 2015;117(3):e28–39.

109. Mohanta SK, et al. Artery tertiary lymphoid organs contribute to innate and adaptive immune responses in advanced mouse atherosclerosis. Circ Res. 2014;114(11):1772–87.

110. Jonasson L, Backteman K, Ernerudh J. Loss of natural killer cell activity in patients with coronary artery disease. Atherosclerosis. 2005;183(2):316–21.

111. Busch M, et al. Dendritic cell subset distributions in the aorta in healthy and atherosclerotic mice. PLoS One. 2014;9(2):e88452.

112. Jaipersad AS, et al. Expression of monocyte subsets and angiogenic markers in relation to carotid plaque neovascularization in patients with pre-existing coronary artery disease and carotid stenosis. Ann Med. 2014;46(7):530–8.

113. Czepluch FS, et al. Increased proatherogenic monocyte-platelet cross-talk in monocyte subpopulations of patients with stable coronary artery disease. J Intern Med. 2014;275(2):144–54.

114. Poitou C, et al. CD14dimCD16+ and CD14+CD16+ monocytes in obesity and during weight loss: relationships with fat mass and subclinical atherosclerosis. Arterioscler Thromb Vasc Biol. 2011;31(10):2322–30.

115. Imanishi T, et al. Association of monocyte subset counts with coronary fibrous cap thickness in patients with unstable angina pectoris. Atherosclerosis. 2010;212(2):628–35.

116. Lee JW, et al. Proinflammatory CD14(+)CD16(+) monocytes are associated with vascular stiffness in predialysis patients with chronic kidney disease. Kidney Res Clin Pract. 2013;32(4):147–52.

117. Rothe G, et al. A more mature phenotype of blood mononuclear phagocytes is induced by fluvastatin treatment in hypercholesterolemic patients with coronary heart disease. Atherosclerosis. 1999;144(1):251–61.

118. Li, T., et al., Huanglian jiedu decoction regulated and controlled differentiation of monocytes, macrophages, and foam cells: an experimental study. Zhongguo Zhong Xi Yi Jie He Za Zhi, 2014. 34(9): p. 1096–1102.

119. Medina I, et al. Hck/Fgr kinase deficiency reduces plaque growth and stability by blunting monocyte recruitment and intraplaque motility. Circulation. 2015;132(6):490–501.

120. Zhang, D., et al., Severe hyperhomocysteinemia promotes bone marrow-derived and resident inflammatory monocyte differentiation and atherosclerosis in LDLr/CBS-deficient mice. Circ Res, 2012. 111(1): p. 37–49.

121. Donners MM, et al. Hematopoietic miR155 deficiency enhances atherosclerosis and decreases plaque stability in hyperlipidemic mice. PLoS One. 2012;7(4):e35877.

122. Fang P, et al. Hyperhomocysteinemia potentiates hyperglycemia-induced inflammatory monocyte differentiation and atherosclerosis. Diabetes. 2014; 63(12):4275–90.

123. Stoger JL, et al. Distribution of macrophage polarization markers in human atherosclerosis. Atherosclerosis. 2012;225(2):461–8.

124. Hu Y, et al. Class A scavenger receptor attenuates myocardial infarction-induced cardiomyocyte necrosis through suppressing M1 macrophage subset polarization. Basic Res Cardiol. 2011;106(6):1311–28.

125. Alipour A, et al. Leukocyte activation by triglyceride-rich lipoproteins. Arterioscler Thromb Vasc Biol. 2008;28(4):792–7.

126. Soehnlein O, Lindbom L, Weber C. Mechanisms underlying neutrophil-mediated monocyte recruitment. Blood. 2009;114(21):4613–23.

127. Gombart AF, et al. Aberrant expression of neutrophil and macrophage-related genes in a murine model for human neutrophil-specific granule deficiency. J Leukoc Biol. 2005;78(5):1153–65.

128. Ionita MG, et al. High neutrophil numbers in human carotid atherosclerotic plaques are associated with characteristics of rupture-prone lesions. Arterioscler Thromb Vasc Biol. 2010;30(9):1842–8.

129. Tanaka M, et al. Eosinophil count is positively correlated with coronary artery calcification. Hypertens Res. 2012;35(3):325–8.

130. Serhan CN, Savill J. Resolution of inflammation: the beginning programs the end. Nat Immunol. 2005;6(12):1191–7.

131. Soylu K, et al. The effect of blood cell count on coronary flow in patients with coronary slow flow phenomenon. Pak J Med Sci. 2014;30(5):936–41.

132. Bot I, Shi GP, Kovanen PT. Mast cells as effectors in atherosclerosis. Arterioscler Thromb Vasc Biol. 2015;35(2):265–71.

133. Wu, C., et al., Characterization of IL-12 receptor beta1 chain (IL-12Rbeta1)-deficient mice: IL-12Rbeta1 is an essential component of the functional mouse IL-12 receptor. J Immunol, 1997. 159(4): p. 1658–65.

134. Letimier FA, et al. Chromatin remodeling by the SWI/SNF-like BAF complex and STAT4 activation synergistically induce IL-12Rbeta2 expression during human Th1 cell differentiation. EMBO J. 2007;26(5):1292–302.

135. Afkarian M, et al. T-bet is a STAT1-induced regulator of IL-12R expression in naive CD4+ T cells. Nat Immunol. 2002;3(6):549–57.

136. Athie-Morales V, et al. Sustained IL-12 signaling is required for Th1 development. J Immunol. 2004;172(1):61–9.

137. Wurster AL, Tanaka T, Grusby MJ. The biology of Stat4 and Stat6. Oncogene. 2000;19(21):2577–84.

138. Kelly-Welch AE, et al. Interleukin-4 and interleukin-13 signaling connections maps. Science. 2003;300(5625):1527–8.

139. Bettelli E, et al. Reciprocal developmental pathways for the generation of pathogenic effector TH17 and regulatory T cells. Nature. 2006;441(7090): 235–8.

140. O'Shea JJ, et al. Signal transduction and Th17 cell differentiation. Microbes Infect. 2009;11(5):599–611.

141. Ichiyama K, et al. Foxp3 inhibits RORgammat-mediated IL-17A mRNA transcription through direct interaction with RORgammat. J Biol Chem. 2008;283(25):17003–8.

142. Li MO, Rudensky AY. T cell receptor signalling in the control of regulatory T cell differentiation and function. Nat Rev Immunol. 2016;16(4):220–33.

143. Tone Y, et al. Smad3 and NFAT cooperate to induce Foxp3 expression through its enhancer. Nat Immunol. 2008;9(2):194–202.

144. Webster KE, et al. In vivo expansion of T reg cells with IL-2-mAb complexes: induction of resistance to EAE and long-term acceptance of islet allografts without immunosuppression. J Exp Med. 2009;206(4):751–60.

145. Niiro H, Clark EA. Regulation of B-cell fate by antigen-receptor signals. Nat Rev Immunol. 2002;2(12):945–56.

146. Kurosaki T. Genetic analysis of B cell antigen receptor signaling. Annu Rev Immunol. 1999;17:555–92.

147. Garraud O, et al. Revisiting the B-cell compartment in mouse and humans: more than one B-cell subset exists in the marginal zone and beyond. BMC Immunol. 2012;13:63.

148. Cariappa A, et al. The follicular versus marginal zone B lymphocyte cell fate decision is regulated by Aiolos, Btk, and CD21. Immunity. 2001; 14(5):603–15.

149. Croker BA, et al. The Rac2 guanosine triphosphatase regulates B lymphocyte antigen receptor responses and chemotaxis and is required for establishment of B-1a and marginal zone B lymphocytes. J Immunol. 2002; 168(7):3376–86.

150. Thome M. CARMA1, BCL-10 and MALT1 in lymphocyte development and activation. Nat Rev Immunol. 2004;4(5):348–59.

151. Rickert RC, Jellusova J, Miletic AV. Signaling by the tumor necrosis factor receptor superfamily in B-cell biology and disease. Immunol Rev. 2011; 244(1):115–33.

152. Mildner A, Jung S. Development and function of dendritic cell subsets. Immunity. 2014;40(5):642–56.

153. Murphy KM. Transcriptional control of dendritic cell development. Adv Immunol. 2013;120:239–67.

154. Ginhoux F, et al. The origin and development of nonlymphoid tissue CD103 + DCs. J Exp Med. 2009;206(13):3115–30.

155. Hacker C, et al. Transcriptional profiling identifies Id2 function in dendritic cell development. Nat Immunol. 2003;4(4):380–6.

156. Tamura T, et al. IFN regulatory factor-4 and -8 govern dendritic cell subset development and their functional diversity. J Immunol. 2005;174(5):2573–81.

157. Becker AM, et al. IRF-8 extinguishes neutrophil production and promotes dendritic cell lineage commitment in both myeloid and lymphoid mouse progenitors. Blood. 2012;119(9):2003–12.

158. Spranger S, Bao R, Gajewski TF. Melanoma-intrinsic beta-catenin signalling prevents anti-tumour immunity. Nature. 2015;523(7559):231–5.

159. Spranger, S., et al., Tumor-residing Batf3 dendritic cells are required for effector T cell trafficking and adoptive T cell therapy. Cancer Cell, 2017. 31(5): p. 711–723 e4.

160. Wu L, et al. RelB is essential for the development of myeloid-related CD8alpha- dendritic cells but not of lymphoid-related CD8alpha+ dendritic cells. Immunity. 1998;9(6):839–47.

161. Lewis KL, et al. Notch2 receptor signaling controls functional differentiation of dendritic cells in the spleen and intestine. Immunity. 2011;35(5):780–91.

162. Caton ML, Smith-Raska MR, Reizis B. Notch-RBP-J signaling controls the homeostasis of CD8- dendritic cells in the spleen. J Exp Med. 2007;204(7): 1653–64.

163. Ichikawa E, et al. Defective development of splenic and epidermal CD4+ dendritic cells in mice deficient for IFN regulatory factor-2. Proc Natl Acad Sci U S A. 2004;101(11):3909–14.

164. Suzuki, S., et al., Critical roles of interferon regulatory factor 4 in CD11bhighCD8alpha- dendritic cell development. Proc Natl Acad Sci U S A, 2004. 101(24): p. 8981–6.

165. Vander Lugt B, et al. Transcriptional programming of dendritic cells for enhanced MHC class II antigen presentation. Nat Immunol. 2014;15(2):161–7.

166. Bajana S, et al. IRF4 promotes cutaneous dendritic cell migration to lymph nodes during homeostasis and inflammation. J Immunol. 2012; 189(7):3368–77.

167. Naik SH, et al. Cutting edge: generation of splenic CD8+ and CD8- dendritic cell equivalents in Fms-like tyrosine kinase 3 ligand bone marrow cultures. J Immunol. 2005;174(11):6592–7.

168. Laouar Y, et al. STAT3 is required for Flt3L-dependent dendritic cell differentiation. Immunity. 2003;19(6):903–12.

169. Ghosh HS, et al. Continuous expression of the transcription factor e2-2 maintains the cell fate of mature plasmacytoid dendritic cells. Immunity. 2010;33(6):905–16.

170. Serbina NV, et al. Sequential MyD88-independent and -dependent activation of innate immune responses to intracellular bacterial infection. Immunity. 2003;19(6):891–901.

171. De Trez C, et al. iNOS-producing inflammatory dendritic cells constitute the major infected cell type during the chronic Leishmania major infection phase of C57BL/6 resistant mice. PLoS Pathog. 2009;5(6):e1000494.

172. Seo SU, et al. Type I interferon signaling regulates Ly6C(hi) monocytes and neutrophils during acute viral pneumonia in mice. PLoS Pathog. 2011;7(2): e1001304.

173. Iwasaki H, Akashi K. Myeloid lineage commitment from the hematopoietic stem cell. Immunity. 2007;26(6):726–40.

174. Zhu YP, Thomas GD, Hedrick CC. 2014 Jeffrey M. Hoeg award lecture: transcriptional control of monocyte development. Arterioscler Thromb Vasc Biol. 2016;36(9):1722–33.

175. Alder JK, et al. Kruppel-like factor 4 is essential for inflammatory monocyte differentiation in vivo. J Immunol. 2008;180(8):5645–52.

176. Kurotaki D, et al. Essential role of the IRF8-KLF4 transcription factor cascade in murine monocyte differentiation. Blood. 2013;121(10):1839–49.

177. Carlin LM, et al. Nr4a1-dependent Ly6C(low) monocytes monitor endothelial cells and orchestrate their disposal. Cell. 2013;153(2):362–75.

178. Hanna RN, et al. The transcription factor NR4A1 (Nur77) controls bone marrow differentiation and the survival of Ly6C- monocytes. Nat Immunol. 2011;12(8):778–85.

179. Qin H, et al. LPS induces CD40 gene expression through the activation of NF-kappaB and STAT-1alpha in macrophages and microglia. Blood. 2005; 106(9):3114–22.

180. Wang N, Liang H, Zen K. Molecular mechanisms that influence the macrophage m1-m2 polarization balance. Front Immunol. 2014;5:614.

181. Krausgruber T, et al. IRF5 promotes inflammatory macrophage polarization and TH1-TH17 responses. Nat Immunol. 2011;12(3):231–8.

182. Donlin LT, et al. Modulation of TNF-induced macrophage polarization by synovial fibroblasts. J Immunol. 2014;193(5):2373–83.

183. Tschopp J, Martinon F, Burns K. NALPs: a novel protein family involved in inflammation. Nat Rev Mol Cell Biol. 2003;4(2):95–104.

184. Imtiyaz HZ, Simon MC. Hypoxia-inducible factors as essential regulators of inflammation. Curr Top Microbiol Immunol. 2010;345:105–20.

185. Cramer T, et al. HIF-1alpha is essential for myeloid cell-mediated inflammation. Cell. 2003;112(5):645–57.

186. Rius J, et al. NF-kappaB links innate immunity to the hypoxic response through transcriptional regulation of HIF-1alpha. Nature. 2008;453(7196):807–11.

187. Nizet V, Johnson RS. Interdependence of hypoxic and innate immune responses. Nat Rev Immunol. 2009;9(9):609–17.

188. O'Farrell AM, et al. IL-10 inhibits macrophage activation and proliferation by distinct signaling mechanisms: evidence for Stat3-dependent and -independent pathways. EMBO J. 1998;17(4):1006–18.

189. Bouhlel MA, et al. PPARgamma activation primes human monocytes into alternative M2 macrophages with anti-inflammatory properties. Cell Metab. 2007;6(2):137–43.

190. Liao X, et al. Kruppel-like factor 4 regulates macrophage polarization. J Clin Invest. 2011;121(7):2736–49.

191. Sharma N, et al. Myeloid Kruppel-like factor 4 deficiency augments atherogenesis in ApoE-/- mice—brief report. Arterioscler Thromb Vasc Biol. 2012;32(12):2836–8.

192. Babaev VR, et al. Conditional knockout of macrophage PPARgamma increases atherosclerosis in C57BL/6 and low-density lipoprotein receptor-deficient mice. Arterioscler Thromb Vasc Biol. 2005;25(8):1647–53.

193. Van Ginderachter JA, et al. Macrophages, PPARs, and cancer. PPAR Res. 2008;2008:169414.

194. Zhang W, Xu W, Xiong S. Macrophage differentiation and polarization via phosphatidylinositol 3-kinase/Akt-ERK signaling pathway conferred by serum amyloid P component. J Immunol. 2011;187(4):1764–77.

195. Zhang W, Xu W, Xiong S. Blockade of Notch1 signaling alleviates murine lupus via blunting macrophage activation and M2b polarization. J Immunol. 2010;184(11):6465–78.

196. Sica A, Mantovani A. Macrophage plasticity and polarization: in vivo veritas. J Clin Invest. 2012;122(3):787–95.

197. Moore KW, et al. Interleukin-10 and the interleukin-10 receptor. Annu Rev Immunol. 2001;19:683–765.

198. Murray PJ. Understanding and exploiting the endogenous interleukin-10/ STAT3-mediated anti-inflammatory response. Curr Opin Pharmacol. 2006; 6(4):379–86.

199. Boyle JJ, et al. Activating transcription factor 1 directs Mhem atheroprotective macrophages through coordinated iron handling and foam cell protection. Circ Res. 2012;110(1):20–33.

200. Hayashi C, et al. Protective role for TLR4 signaling in atherosclerosis progression as revealed by infection with a common oral pathogen. J Immunol. 2012;189(7):3681–8.

201. Clement M, et al. Control of the T follicular helper-germinal center B-cell axis by CD8(+) regulatory T cells limits atherosclerosis and tertiary lymphoid organ development. Circulation. 2015;131(6):560–70.

202. Choi P, Reiser H. IL-4: role in disease and regulation of production. Clin Exp Immunol. 1998;113(3):317–9.

203. Oriss, T.B., et al., Crossregulation between T helper cell (Th)1 and Th2: inhibition of Th2 proliferation by IFN-gamma involves interference with IL-1. J Immunol, 1997. 158(8): p. 3666–72.

204. Laurence, A., et al., Interleukin-2 signaling via STAT5 constrains T helper 17 cell generation. Immunity, 2007. **26**(3): p. 371–81.

205. Kimura A, Kishimoto T. IL-6: regulator of Treg/Th17 balance. Eur J Immunol. 2010;40(7):1830–5.

206. Chang JH, Chung Y. Regulatory T cells in B cell follicles. Immune Netw. 2014;14(5):227–36.

207. Wilson GL, et al. cDNA cloning of the B cell membrane protein CD22: a mediator of B-B cell interactions. J Exp Med. 1991;173(1):137–46.

208. Pao LI, et al. B cell-specific deletion of protein-tyrosine phosphatase Shp1 promotes B-1a cell development and causes systemic autoimmunity. Immunity. 2007;27(1):35–48.

209. Nguyen KD, et al. Circadian gene Bmal1 regulates diurnal oscillations of Ly6C(hi) inflammatory monocytes. Science. 2013;341(6153):1483–8.

210. Davison AM, King NJ. Accelerated dendritic cell differentiation from migrating Ly6C(lo) bone marrow monocytes in early dermal West Nile virus infection. J Immunol. 2011;186(4):2382–96.

211. Rackov, G., et al., p21 mediates macrophage reprogramming through regulation of p50-p50 NF-kappaB and IFN-beta. J Clin Invest, 2016. 126(8): p. 3089–3103.

212. Myers MP, et al. TYK2 and JAK2 are substrates of protein-tyrosine phosphatase 1B. J Biol Chem. 2001;276(51):47771–4.

213. Dickensheets H, et al. Suppressor of cytokine signaling-1 is an IL-4-inducible gene in macrophages and feedback inhibits IL-4 signaling. Genes Immun. 2007;8(1):21–7.

214. Liu G, Abraham E. MicroRNAs in immune response and macrophage polarization. Arterioscler Thromb Vasc Biol. 2013;33(2):170–7.

215. Menezes S, et al. The heterogeneity of Ly6C(hi) monocytes controls their differentiation into iNOS(+) macrophages or monocyte-derived dendritic cells. Immunity. 2016;45(6):1205–18.

216. Granot Z, et al. Tumor entrained neutrophils inhibit seeding in the premetastatic lung. Cancer Cell. 2011;20(3):300–14.

217. Yoshida GJ. The heterogeneity of cancer stem-like cells at the invasive front. Cancer Cell Int. 2017;17:23.

218. Ok CY, Young KH. Checkpoint inhibitors in hematological malignancies. J Hematol Oncol. 2017;10(1):103.

219. Jenkins RW, Barbie DA, Flaherty KT. Mechanisms of resistance to immune checkpoint inhibitors. Br J Cancer. 2018;118(1):9–16.

220. Kumar V, et al. The nature of myeloid-derived suppressor cells in the tumor microenvironment. Trends Immunol. 2016;37(3):208–20.

221. Foks AC, et al. CD11b+Gr-1+ myeloid-derived suppressor cells reduce atherosclerotic lesion development in LDLr deficient mice. Cardiovasc Res. 2016;111(3):252–61.

222. Ostrand-Rosenberg S. Myeloid derived-suppressor cells: their role in cancer and obesity. Curr Opin Immunol. 2018;51:68–75.

223. Bronte V, et al. Recommendations for myeloid-derived suppressor cell nomenclature and characterization standards. Nat Commun. 2016;7:12150.

224. Srivastava MK, et al. Myeloid suppressor cell depletion augments antitumor activity in lung cancer. PLoS One. 2012;7(7):e40677.

225. Stromnes IM, et al. Targeted depletion of an MDSC subset unmasks pancreatic ductal adenocarcinoma to adaptive immunity. Gut. 2014;63(11):1769–81.

226. Trikha M, et al. Targeted anti-interleukin-6 monoclonal antibody therapy for cancer: a review of the rationale and clinical evidence. Clin Cancer Res. 2003;9(13):4653–65.

227. Guo Y, et al. Interleukin-6 signaling pathway in targeted therapy for cancer. Cancer Treat Rev. 2012;38(7):904–10.

228. Rossi JF, et al. Interleukin-6 as a therapeutic target. Clin Cancer Res. 2015; 21(6):1248–57.

4

Recombination of a dual-CAR-modified T lymphocyte to accurately eliminate pancreatic malignancy

Erhao Zhang[1,2], Peiwei Yang[1], Jieyi Gu[1], Heming Wu[3], Xiaowei Chi[1], Chen Liu[1], Ying Wang[1], Jianpeng Xue[1,4], Weiyan Qi[1,4], Qingbo Sun[1], Shengnan Zhang[1], Jialiang Hu[1,4*†] and Hanmei Xu[1,4,5*†]

Abstract

Background: The therapeutic application of T cells endowing with chimeric antigen receptors (CARs) is faced with "on-target, off-tumor" toxicity against solid tumors, particularly in the treatment of the pancreatic cancer. To our best knowledge, the pancreatic cancer cell line AsPC-1 often highly expressed some distinct tumor-associated antigens, such as carcino-embryonic antigen (CEA) and mesothelin (MSLN). Therefore, in this research, we have characterized dual-receptor CAR-modified T cells (dCAR-T) that exert effective and safe cytotoxicity against AsPC-1 cells.

Methods: Based on the dual signaling pathway of wild T cells, we designed a novel dCAR diagram specific for CEA and MSLN, which achieved comparable activity relative to that of conventional CAR-T cells (CEA-CAR T or MSLN-CAR T). In this dCAR, a tandem construct containing two physically separate structures, CEA-CD3ζ and MSLN-4/1BB signaling domains were effectively controlled with tumor antigens CEA and MSLN, respectively. Finally, the activity of dCAR-T cells has been verified via in vitro and in vivo experiments.

Results: In the presence of cognate tumor cells (AsPC-1) expressing both CEA and MSLN, dCAR-T cells exerted high anti-tumor activity relative to that of other single-receptor CAR-T cells bearing only one signaling pathway (e.g., Cζ-CAR and MBB-CAR). In a xenograft model, dCAR-T cells significantly inhibited the growth of AsPC-1 cells yet no effect on the growth of non-cognate tumor cells. Furthermore, the released cytokines and T cell persistence in mice were comparable with that of conventional CAR-T cells, obtaining specific and controllable cytotoxicity.

Conclusions: A novel type of CAR-T cells, termed dCAR-T, was designed with specific activities, that is, significant cytotoxicity for two antigen-positive tumor cells yet no cytotoxicity for single antigen-positive tumor cells. Dual-targeted CAR-T cells can be precisely localized at the tumor site and can exert high cytotoxicity against tumor cells, alleviating "on-target, off-tumor" toxicity and enabling accurate application of CAR-T cell therapy.

Keywords: Cancer immunotherapy, Dual-receptor CAR, Pancreatic cancer, Carcino-embryonic antigen, Mesothelin

* Correspondence: haobo89@163.com; 13913925346@126.com
†Jialiang Hu and Hanmei Xu contributed equally to this work.
[1]The Engineering Research Center of Peptide Drug Discovery and Development, China Pharmaceutical University, Nanjing 210009, People's Republic of China
Full list of author information is available at the end of the article

Background

Chimeric antigen receptor (CAR) T cell therapy is a cancer treatment that uses a patient's T cells modified to express specific proteins allowing T cells to better recognize cancer cells as well as become highly activated to exert cytotoxicity against tumors [1–4]. Once in the body, this type of cancer immunotherapy is capable of immediately providing ongoing tumor control and possible protection against recurrence in some clinical trials, a promising approach to adoptive T cell therapy for cancer treatment [5–9]. Although this type of immunotherapy holds a tremendous response for tumor elimination, especially in some hematological malignancies [10–12], it has recently been faced with a serious limitation caused by treatment-induced adverse effects in some clinical trials, such as "on-target, off-tumor" toxicity [13, 14]. In general, this toxicity derived from CAR-T cell therapy can lead to killing of non-tumor cells as a result of tumor-associated antigens expressed on normal tissues [15–17]. For example, infusion of CD19-specific CAR-T cells in one patient with B cell malignancies often caused long-term B cell aplasia symptoms, resulting from eradication of normal B cells [18, 19]. For another case, after infusion of T cells endowed with a CAR specific for human epidermal growth factor receptor 2 (HER-2), a patient with the breast cancer underwent lethal inflammatory cytokine release due to HER-2 expression on lung epithelial cells [20]. Therefore, some new approaches to treat solid tumors with sustained tumor elimination and reduced side effects are needed.

Pancreatic cancer with a metastatic property is the most lethal human cancer with poor prognosis, which the average 5-year survival rate is only 5%, with standard treatment based on surgery, radiotherapy, and chemotherapy promoting an overall survival of about 6 months, highlighting the need for more effective treatments [21–23]. Cancer immunotherapy involving T cells with redirected specificity via expression of CAR may complement such treatments, resulting in complete elimination. To further improve safety and efficacy of CAR-T cell therapy for pancreatic cancer treatment, here, we designed a novel CAR structure to render engineered T cells specific for pancreatic cancer cells in an antigen-dependent manner. Based on the dual signaling pathway of natural T cells, the dual-targeting CAR facilitates T cell immune response against dual antigen-expressing tumors compared to single-positive tumors, resulting from the two signaling domains of CAR structure controlled by the distinct tumor antigens. To our best knowledge, some previous papers reported that carcino-embryonic antigen (CEA) and mesothelin (MSLN) are tumor-associated antigens (TAAs), which are simultaneously overexpressed in the majority of pancreatic cancers, ovarian cancers, and other cancers, resulting in the pancreatic cancer

AsPC-1 expressing MSLN and CEA as a cognate tumor cell in this work [24–27]. Theoretically, in this study, engineering T cells with a dual-receptor chimeric antigen receptor (dCAR) requires CAR-mediated recognition of one antigen, here being CEA, for activation, and then, their co-stimulation must be mediated by the other CAR engaging a second antigen, which is MSLN.

Herein, we demonstrate, for the first time to our knowledge, that dCAR-modified T cell exerts effective and safe cytotoxicity for the treatment of pancreatic cancer cell expressing the tumor antigens CEA and MSLN in vitro and in vivo. In this study, we proposed a novel CAR-T cell therapy that not only discriminates tumor tissues and normal tissues, but also promotes effector cell localization, thereby preventing the tumor escape from immune surveillance. Compared with the single-positive antigen-expressing tumor, T cells endowing with a dCAR could eradicate some tumors that express two antigens. Finally, the "two tumor antigen-input" strategy may accurately control the activity of dCAR-T cells, which ultimately helps broaden the applicability of this cancer immunotherapy and decrease some serious side effects of CAR-modified T cell therapies in the field of solid tumor treatment.

Methods
Cell lines and culture conditions

Fresh blood was obtained from healthy volunteers after informed consent on protocols was approved by the China Pharmaceutical University Institutional Review Board. Peripheral blood mononuclear cells (PBMCs) were purified from the blood by gradient centrifugation using Lymphoprep™ (Axis-Shield), and then, human T cell subtypes (i.e., CD4$^+$ T cells and CD8$^+$ T cells) were enriched by positive selection using the magnetic bead separation (Miltenyi Biotec). Isolated T cells were cultured in X-VIVO15 medium (Lonza) supplemented with 5% human AB serum (vol/vol, Valley Biomedical Inc.), and 10 mM N-acetyl L-Cysteine (Sigma-Aldrich). Lastly, the T cell medium was supplemented with 30 IU/mL or 100 IU/mL human IL-2 (PeproTech) for CD4$^+$ T cell or CD8$^+$ T cell growth, respectively.

The pancreatic cancer cell line, AsPC-1 cells and PANC-1 cells, the colorectal cancer cell line, HT29 cells, and the glioma cell line, U87 cells, were obtained from the American Type Culture Collection (ATCC). AsPC-1 cells were cultured in RPMI 1640-media (Hyclone), while PANC-1 cells, HT29 cells, and U87 cells were grown in Dulbecco's modified Eagle's medium (DMEM) media (Hyclone). All of the tumor cell culture media were supplemented with 10% fetal bovine serum (FBS), 2 mmol/L-glutamine (Gibco), 100 U/mL penicillin, and 100 μg/mL streptomycin (Sangong Biotech).

Cell line 293 T was also acquired from ATCC and maintained in DMEM medium supplemented with 10% FBS, 10 mM HEPES (Gibco), 2 mmol/L-glutamine, 100 U/mL penicillin, and 100 μg/mL streptomycin. All cell lines were incubated at 37 °C in a humidified atmosphere with 5% carbon dioxide.

Construction of plasmids

The lentiviral vector encoding various CARs or red fluorescence protein (RFP) was constructed based on the pLV-puro vector (Hanbio Biotechnology Co., Ltd.). Briefly, for modifying T cells, the dCAR vector consisted of the following components in frame from 5′ end to 3′ end: a XhoIsite, Kozak and signaling peptide sequences, anti-MSLN scFv, hinge and transmembrane of CD8α molecule, cytoplasmic domain of 4/1BB, internal ribosome entry site (IRES) sequence and signaling peptide sequence, anti-CEA scFv, hinge and transmembrane of CD8α molecule, cytoplasmic domain of CD3ζ, P2A and green fluorescence protein (GFP) sequences, and a XbaI-site. The Cζ-CAR plasmid included some gene elements as follows (5′ end to 3′ end): a XhoIsite, Kozak and signaling peptide sequences, anti-CEA scFv, hinge and transmembrane of CD8α molecule, cytoplasmic domain of CD3ζ, P2A and GFP sequences, and a XbaIsite. The MBB-CAR plasmid included some gene elements as follows (5′ end to 3′ end): a XhoIsite, Kozak and signaling peptide sequences, anti-MSLN scFv, hinge and transmembrane of CD8α molecule, cytoplasmic domain of 4/1BB, P2A and GFP sequences, and a XbaIsite. The second-generation CAR plasmids, CEA-CAR or MSLN-CAR, had some gene elements as follows (5′ end to 3′ end): a XhoIsite, Kozak and signaling peptide sequences, anti-CEA scFv or anti-MSLN scFv, hinge and transmembrane of CD8α molecule, cytoplasmic domains of 4/1BB and CD3ζ, P2A and GFP sequences, and a XbaIsite. For modifying target cells, the RFP vector included the following components (5′ end to 3′ end): a XhoIsite, Kozak and signaling peptide sequences, RFP sequence, and a XbaIsite.

The anti-MSLN scFv portion or anti-CEA scFv portion in the CAR vector was derived from the amino acid sequence of the second generation of CAR specific for MSLN or CEA, respectively, which was kindly provided by Prof. Hanmei Xu of China Pharmaceutical University, China. The sequences of other gene elements were obtained from the National Center for Biotechnology Information. The corresponding DNA sequence was synthesized by GENEWIZ® after codon optimization and then ligated into the pLV-puro vector via XhoIand XbaI.

Lentiviral engineering of T cells and target cells

Twenty-four hours prior to viral transduction, isolated T subtype cells were activated with human CD3/CD28 beads (Life Technologies) at a 1:3 cell to bead ratio in human T cell medium as described above. Activated T cells were transduced with the engineered virus in the presence of 1 μg/mL protamine sulfate (Sigma) by spinfection (800×g, 60 min) and were incubated overnight with the virus at 37 °C, 5% CO_2 until the medium was replaced with fresh medium. Five days after transduction, modified T cells were harvested and CAR expression was detected by flow cytometry and western blot analyses.

All tumor cells, including AsPC-1, PANC-1, HT29, and U87, were cultured 36 h in advance to ensure that target cells would be in log phase at the time of lentivirus transduction. In a six-well plate, the fresh complete medium containing 6 μg/mL polybrene and the appropriate amount of virus were added to each well. After a 24-h incubation, the transduction medium was replaced with fresh complete medium to remove lentivirus and polybrene. Five days after transduction, transduced cells expressing RFP were selected with medium containing appropriate concentration of puromycin. Expression of transgenes in transduced tumor cells was confirmed by detecting fluorescent reporter proteins with flow cytometry and western blot analyses.

Flow cytometry and western blot assays

For the flow cytometry assays, all cells were harvested and washed three times with FACS wash buffer (1 × PBS containing 0.5% BSA and 0.03% sodium azide) prior to flow cytometry. Surface staining of cells was performed with monoclonal antibodies directed against CD4, CD8, and CEA, which were purchased from Becton Dickinson (BD), while the monoclonal antibody against MSLN was purchased from R&D Systems. Transgenic populations with GFP expression for T cells or with RFP expression for tumor cells were analyzed on the fluorescein isothiocyanate (FITC) channel or the PerCP channel, respectively. For T cell activation, after overnight incubation, the T cell surface markers, CD25 and CD69, were detected using the APC-conjugated CD25 antibody (Biolegend) and APC-conjugated CD69 antibody (Biolegend), respectively. After a 30-min incubation period at 4 °C, protected from light, all cells were washed and analyzed by flow cytometry.

For western blot analysis, the proteins were extracted from modified cells and stored at − 80 °C. Western blots were performed using GFP primary antibody (abcam) and RFP primary antibodies (abcam).

Enzyme-linked immunosorbent assays

For in vitro trials, primary T cells expressing CARs were mixed with various target cells at a 2:1 T cell to target cell ratio in a U-bottom 96-well plate. After overnight incubation, supernatants were harvested and assayed for the released IL-2, IFN-γ, TNFα, IL-4, IL-13, and IL-15 by ELISA assays, following manufacturer's instruction (MultiSciences).

For in vivo trials, 100 μL of peripheral blood was collected from the treated mice at the designed time points and cytokines in blood serum, such as IL-2, IFNγ, TNFα, and IL-6, were analyzed by ELISA assays, according to the manufacturer's instruction (MultiSciences).

Quantitation of T cell proliferation

For proliferation assays, primary CD4$^+$ T cells expressing the CARs or control CD4$^+$ T cells were washed with PBS and then labeled with CellTrace Violet Kit (Life Technologies) at the final concentration of 5 μM, according to the manufacturer's instructions. Cognate target cells (AsPC-1) expressing desired antigens and non-cognate target cells (HT29, U87, or PANC-1) were treated with 25 μg/mL mitomycin C (MedChem Express), resulting in target cells with a replication-incompetent state. Then, labeled T cells were co-cultured with treated target cells at a 2:1 effector/target ratio in human T cell medium and mixtured cells were collected for flow cytometry analysis. Lastly, the proliferation of CAR-T cells was assayed by monitoring the CellTrace Violet dilution after incubation for 3 days.

Cytotoxicity assays

Primary CD8$^+$ T cells endowing with CARs were co-cultured with target cells at a 2:1 effector/target ratio in 100 μL of T cell culture media supplemented with 10% FBS for 24 h at 37 °C. Cytolytic activity of modified T cells was determined by the level of lactate dehydrogenase (LDH) using Lactate Dehydrogenase Cytotoxicity Assay Kit (Cayman). The experimental groups and the control groups were designed according to the manufacturer's protocol. Determination of LDH activity present in the sample was performed by the absorbance at 490 nm for each sample using a Multiskan FC plate reader (Thermo Scientific). Finally, T cell cytotoxicity was calculated by the following formula: specific cytotoxicity (%) = (mixture cell experiment − effector cell spontaneous − target cell spontaneous − medium control)/(target cell maximum − target cell spontaneous − medium control) × 100.

Xenograft mouse models and living imaging assays

Female nude mice, 7–9 weeks of age, were housed in the Laboratory Animal Research Center of China Pharmaceutical University (CPU), and all protocols were performed as approved by the CPU Institutional Animal Care and Use Committee. To carry out the xenograft models, nude mice were randomly divided into six groups ($n = 5$) and were intravenously inoculated with 5×10^5 engineered tumor cells per mouse (day 0),

including AsPC-1 cells, HT29 cells, U87 cells, or PANC-1 cells. After 7 days, 2×10^6 CAR-T cells or wild T cells per mouse were infused intravenously.

To characterize the tumor killing effect in vivo, tumor burden of each mouse was measured using the In-Vivo Imaging System Fx Pro (Carestream Health) following the instrument's instructions at 7 days, 14 days, 21 days, 28 days, and 35 days after tumor injection. In this experiment, the cytotoxicity of modified T cells was calculated according to the radiance intensity in the region of the tumor site. Finally, a ratio of the mean fluorescence intensity (MFI) of tumor cells in the mice treated with engineered T cells to that of the mice treated with wild T cells (No CAR T) was calculated to enumerate redirected cytotoxic activities of engineered T cells at 35 days after tumor injection.

Quantitation of T cell counts and cytokine production in vivo

Furthermore, 80 μL of peripheral blood of each nude mouse was drawn at 1 days, 7 days, 14 days, 21 days, and 28 days after modified T cell infusion (totally five times) to determine T cell expansion and persistence in the blood at the stated time points by flow cytometry detection of GFP expression. In this experiment, a ratio of the number of T cells at the indicated time in the mice treated with effector cells to T cell counts at 24 h after modified T cell infusion was calculated for each sample to enumerate the relative survival of injected T cells.

At the end of the experiment, serum cytokine concentrations were monitored in peripheral blood of each nude mouse using the Elisa Kit, including IL-2, IFNγ, IL-6, and TNFα.

Statistical analysis

Statistical significance were calculated using GraphPad software, version 6.0. Unless otherwise stated, in vitro and in vivo data were analyzed using the two-tailed Student's t test. Data acquired from in vitro assays using experimental replicates ($n = 3$) and other data acquired from in vivo assays using biological replicates ($n = 5$) are presented as mean ± SD. All graphs were also generated using GraphPad prism. A p value less than 0.05 was considered statistically significant. Significance of findings was defined as n.s. or not significant $p > 0.05$, *$p < 0.05$, **$p < 0.01$, and ***$p < 0.001$. For Figs. 2c and 3c, e, f, statistical significance was calculated using "experiment group" vs "No CAR T cell treatment group." For Fig. 2g and Additional file 1: Figure S4, statistical significance was calculated using "experiment group" vs "CEA-CAR T cell treatment group." For Additional file 1: Figure S3, statistical significance was calculated using "experiment group" vs "dCAR T cell incubated with AsPC-1 cell group."

Results

Construction of effector cells and target cells

To demonstrate that both T cell activation and co-stimulation signals can be supplied by two distinct receptors, we have constructed a novel CAR model, termed dual-receptor CAR (dCAR), according to the dual-signal pathway of natural T cells. Briefly, in this CAR, a CD3ζ-mediated activation signal was dependent upon recognition of the tumor antigen CEA and a 4/1BB co-stimulation signal domain was subjected to the second receptor specific for tumor antigen MSLN (Fig. 1a). Insertion of a GFP tag would facilitate detection of dCAR expression present on modified T cells. We also provided two negative controls, single-receptor CARs including CEA-CD3ζ CAR (Cζ-CAR) and MSLN-4/1BB CAR (MBB-CAR), and two positive controls, the second-generation CAR specific for CEA (CEA-CAR) and the second-generation CAR specific for MSLN (MSLN-CAR) (Fig. 1b, Additional file 1: Figure S1). After lentivirus transfection, modified T cells typically yielded expression of antigen receptors in 36–40% of T cells by detection of GFP expression with flow cytometry assays and WB assays (Fig. 1c, Additional file 1: Figure S2a). In all subsequent experiments, six groups of T cells, endowing with Cζ-CAR, MBB-CAR, dCAR, CEA-CAR, MSLN-CAR, or neither (mock), were analyzed and used to verify the effectiveness and safety of dCAR-T cell therapy.

In this study, we selected the pancreatic cancer cell line AsPC-1 as a target cell due to its high expression of both CEA and MSLN (Fig. 1d). In order to facilitate the detection of target cells in in vitro and in vivo trials, target cells highly expressed the RFP via lentivirus transfection. In addition, we also constructed some non-cognate target cells with expression of RFP, such as, HT29 cells expressing CEA yet lack of MSLN expression, U87 cells expressing MSLN yet lack of CEA expression, and PANC-1 cells without expression of CEA or MSLN (Fig. 1d). After screening with the puromycin-containing medium, the transduction efficiency of RFP-modified-AsPC-1 cells, RFP-modified-HT29 cells, and RFP-modified-U87 cells, RFP-modified-PANC-1 cells was 93.51%, 83.20%, 81.23% and 92.17%, respectively (Fig. 1e). The data obtained from WB assays were consistent with that of the flow cytometry assays, indicating that cognate and non-cognate target cells have been successfully constructed (Additional file 1: Figure S2b).

Determination of the effector/target ratio

Cytotoxicity against cognate target cells expressing both CEA and MSLN was, as expected, endowed by dCAR expression. To minimize the effect of differential CAR expression, CAR-T cells after each transfection were measured by flow cytometry assays prior to in vitro and in vivo efficacy studies. To effectively characterize the CAR-modified T cell activity, we first performed a 24-h cytotoxicity assay at varying effector-to-target (E:T) cell ratios. In these experiments, the cytotoxicity of modified T cells was measured by detection of the level of lactic dehydrogenase (LDH) release from the apoptotic target cells in the supernatant. Our data showed that dCAR cells, CEA-CAR T cells and MSLN-CAR T cells specifically lysed 81–87% cognate target cells at the 2:1 effector/target ratio, whereas Cζ-CAR T cells had approximately 18% cytotoxicity yet MBB-CAR T cells did not lyse cognate target cells (Fig. 2a). Therefore, the optimal effector-to-target ratio in this research was determined to be 2:1, which was used in subsequent experiments.

In addition, for the CEA-expressing tumor cell line, HT29 cells, CEA-CAR T cells could achieve significant target cell killing (approximately 70%), whereas other modified effector cells have no ability to eliminate target cells. For U87 cells, which have MSLN expression yet not CEA expression, results showed that only MSLN-CAR T cells could achieve remarkable target cell killing. For PANC-1 cells that are lack of both CEA and MSLN, data showed that all CAR-modified T cells and wild T cells did not exert significant cytotoxicity. In summary, the novel dual-targeting modified T cells, dCAR-T cells, yielded significant anti-tumor activity only when two antigen receptors were simultaneously targeted; however, dCAR-T cells cannot cause the target cell apoptosis when only the single pathway (e.g., Cζ or MBB) was activated. dCAR-T cells achieved significant cytotoxicity only in the presence of AsPC-1 cells expressing both CEA and MSLN, which rivaled that obtained with conventional CAR-T cells, CEA-CAR T cells, or MSLN-CAR T cells. Therefore, CAR-T cells endowed with a dual-targeting receptor have significant specificity and safe activity, mitigating "on-target, off-tumor" toxicity derived from conventional CAR-T cell therapy.

Combinatorial antigen requirement for T cell activation

We next tested the activation of dCAR in modified T cells exposed to target cells, including AsPC-1 cells and PANC-1 cells. All of the tested CD4⁺ T cell responses, including cytokine production (such as IL-2, IFNγ, TNFα, IL-4, IL-13, and IL-15) and expression of activation markers on T cell surface (such as CD69 and CD25), showed the requirement for T cell activation with the two distinct antigens (Fig. 2b).

Production of various cytokines was maximal when dCAR-T cells were co-cultured with AsPC-1 cells expressing both CEA and MSLN, compared with that of Cζ-CAR or MBB-CAR-modified T cells stimulated by AsPC-1 cells. In addition, cytokine production of activated dCAR-T cells was comparable with that obtained with modified T cells expressing the conventional CAR

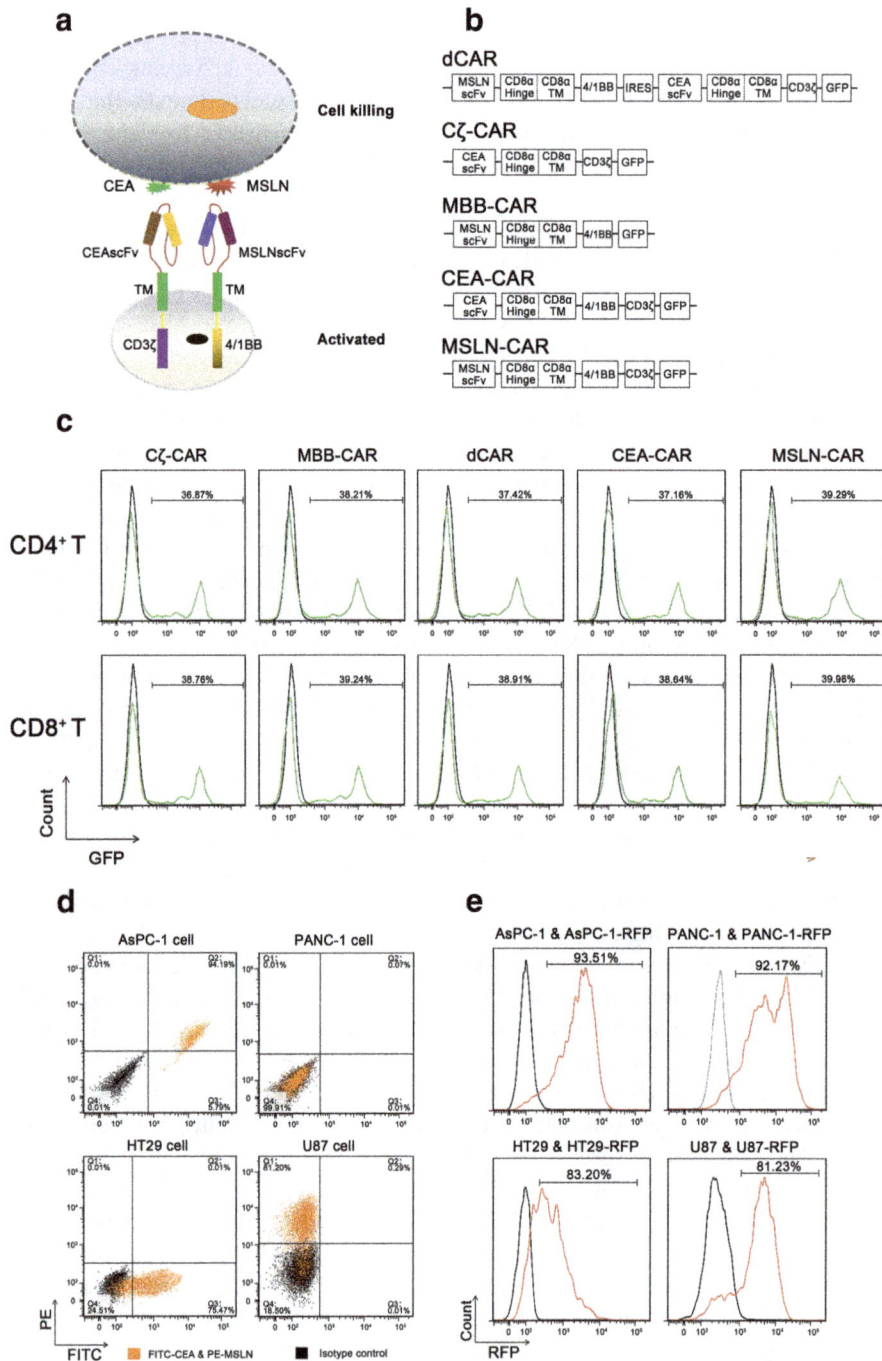

Fig. 1 Construction of effector cells and target cells. **a** Schematic representation of dCAR-engineered T cells. Engineered T cells endowed with the dCAR structure are activated in the presence of CEA and MSLN and eliminate target cells. **b** Structure of the plasmids used to construct modified T cells. After lentivirus transfection, effector cells yield expression of the novel dCAR structure consisting of anti-MSLN scFv, cytoplasmic domain of 4/1BB, anti-CEA scFv, cytoplasmic domain of CD3ζ, and green fluorescence protein (GFP) sequences. Simultaneously, we also constructed two negative controls, Cζ-CAR and MBB-CAR, and two positive controls, CEA-CAR and MSLN-CAR. **c** CAR-engineered T cells were successfully constructed by lentivirus transfection. With endogenous GFP expression, we measured the transduction efficiency by flow cytometry assays, quantifying fractions of CAR positive-CD4$^+$ T and CAR positive-CD8$^+$ T cells in different CAR groups. **d** Antigen expression on the cognate and non-cognate tumor cells. By flow cytometry assays, AsPC-1 cells highly expressed both CEA and MSLN while PANC-1 cells did not express the above antigens. In addition, HT29 cells could only highly express CEA and U87 cells only express MSLN. **e** Detection of the transfection efficacy of modified tumor cells. After puromycin screening, the transduction efficiencies were determined to be 93.51%, 92.17%, 83.20%, and 81.23% by flow cytometry assays for AsPC-1-RFP cells, PANC-1-RFP cells, HT29-RFP, and U87-RFP, respectively

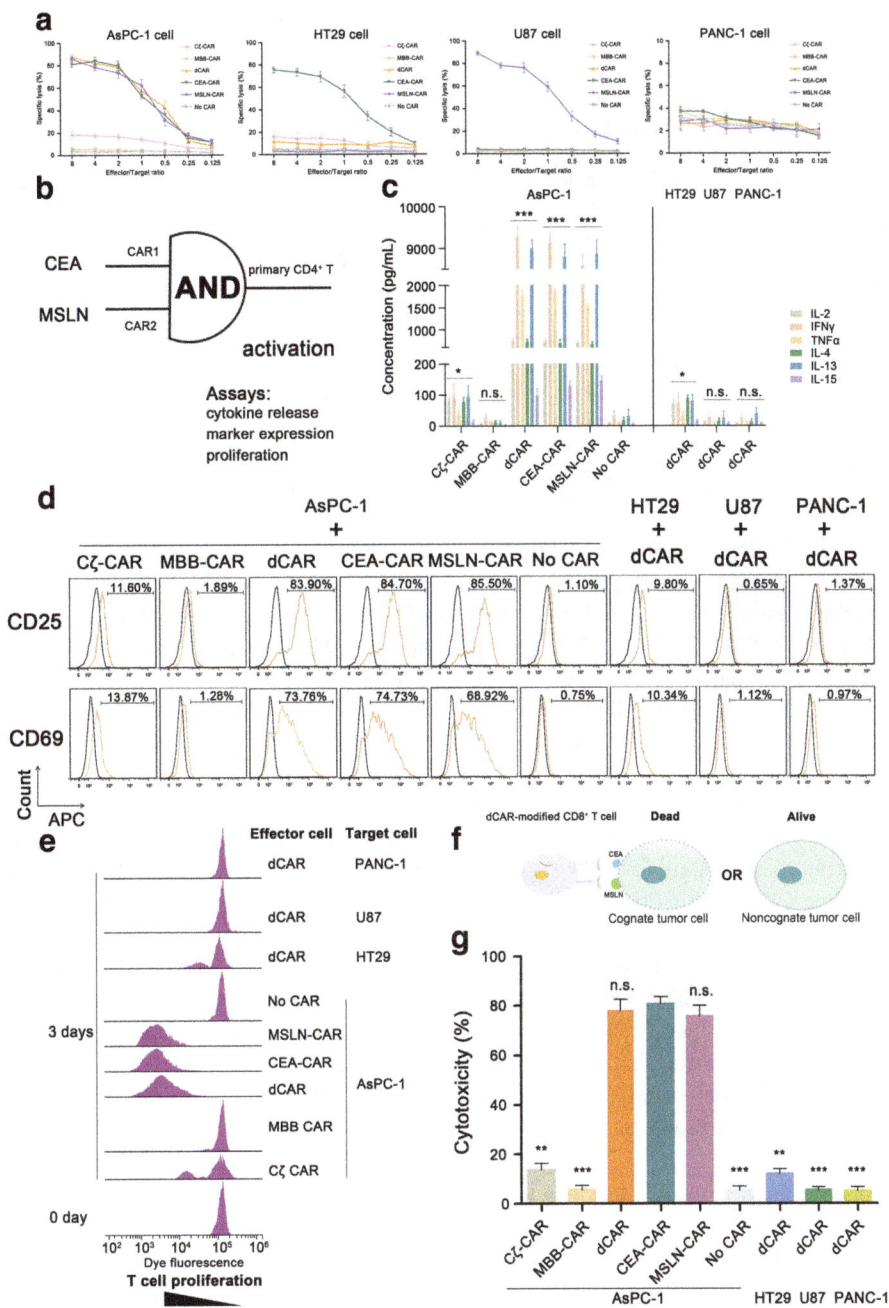

Fig. 2 (See legend on next page.)

Fig. 2 Combinatorial antigen requirement for T cell activity in vitro. **a** Modified T cells or wild T cells were incubated at indicated with various tumor cells at an effector/target rations of 8:1, 4:1, 2:1, 1:1, 1:2, 1:4, or 1:8. After a 24-h incubation, target cell lysis was measured by LDH release in the supernatant. The optimal effector/target ratio in this research was determined to be 2:1. In addition, dCAR-T cells could specifically lyse AsPC-1 cells yet do not eliminate HT29 cells, U87 cells, and PANC-1 cells ($n = 3$, error bars denote standard deviation). **b** Activation of dCAR-engineered CD4$^+$ T cells required cognate target cells. The primary CD4$^+$ T cells were modified with dCARs by lentivirus transfection, and cell activation assays were performed with an "AND logic gate" strategy, including cytokines release, marker expression, and T cell proliferation. **c** Released cytokines in each sample were quantified by enzyme-linked immunosorbent assay, including IL-2, IFNγ, TNFα, IL-4, IL-13, and IL-15. All cytokines were significantly produced when dCAR-T cells were exposed to AsPC-1 cells yet not when exposed to non-cognate tumor cells (HT29 cells, U87 cells, or PANC-1 cells). For conventional CAR-T (CEA-CAR or MSLN-CAR) cell treatment, similar cytokines were obtained ($n = 3$, error bars denote standard deviation). **d** Monitoring T cell activation by CD25 and CD69 expression. T cell activation marker, CD25 or CD69, was significantly expressed on dCAR-T cells or conventional CAR-T cells compared with that of other single-receptor modified T cells in the presence of AsPC-1 cells ($n = 3$). **e** Combinatorial antigen-dependent T cell proliferation. Data showed that dCAR-T cells have a high proliferation activity in the presence of cognate tumor cells expressing CEA and MSLN, which was similar to that of conventional CAR-T cells against target cells. Interestingly, Cζ-CAR-modified T cells showed a lower proliferation capacity, indicating that the CD3ζ signaling pathway is not sufficient to trigger T cell activation ($n = 3$). **f** dCAR-engineered CD8$^+$ T cells yield specific target cell killing in vitro. **g** Cytotoxicity mediated by dCAR-CD8$^+$ T cells in a 24-h experiment. After an overnight incubation, significant cytotoxicity was observed in dCAR-T cells co-cultured with AsPC-1 cells, approximately 85% of target cell apoptosis ($n = 3$, error bars denote standard deviation)

(CEA-CAR or MSLN-CAR) (Fig. 2c). Briefly, during the experiment, dCAR-T cells could release significant levels of cytokines only in the presence of cognate tumor cells expressing both CEA and MSLN, including 751 pg/mL IL-2, 9297 pg/mL IFNγ, 1777 pg/mL TNFα, 732 pg/mL IL-4, 8991 pg/mL IL-13, and 99 pg/mL IL-15. For the single-receptor CARs, Cζ-CAR and MBB-CAR, cognate tumor cells stimulate modified T cells to release low level of cytokines, which is similar with that of wild T cells (No CAR).

In addition, T cells could significantly express the activation markers, including CD69 and CD25, within hours after cell activation. In this study, as was observed with the conventional CAR-T cells, T cells expressing the dCAR displayed a high CD69 and CD25 expression pattern upon activation compared with single-receptor modified T cells (Fig. 2d). Data showed that the modified T cells required an activated dual-signal pathways, including CD3ζ and 4/1BB, for activation in the presence of cognate tumor cells.

In summary, the novel mode of dCAR renders T cells with significant activity through targeting the distinct tumor-associated antigens, improving the specificity and safety of CAR-modified T cells against tumor cells.

Combinatorial antigen control over T cell proliferation
Cognate tumor cell-induced proliferation of CAR-T cells is an indispensable prerequisite for amplification of T cell therapeutic activities; however, uncontrolled T cell proliferation leads to some severe toxicities. We next examined whether the proliferation of dCAR-T cells was dependent upon the cognate tumor cells expressing both CEA and MSLN.

Modified CD4$^+$ T cells were labeled with an intracellular fluorescent dye to monitor T cell proliferation and then were co-cultured with replication-incompetent target cells. In a flow cytometry experiment, data

showed that dCAR-T cells had a high proliferation activity in the presence of cognate tumor cells expressing CEA and MSLN, which was similar to that of conventional CAR-T cells (CEA-CAR T or MSLN-CAR T) (Fig. 2e). On the contrary, MBB-CAR-modified T cells or wild T cells had no significant cell proliferation in the presence of cognate target cells, while Cζ-CAR-modified T cells showed a lower proliferation capacity, indicating that the CD3ζ signaling pathway is vital for the T cell activation yet by itself is not sufficient to completely initiate T cell activity. Additionally, data showed that dCAR-T cells incubated with non-cognate tumor cells (HT29 cells, U87 cells, and PANC-1 cells) had no remarkable proliferation.

In summary, proliferation of dCAR-T cells indeed required two distinct tumor antigens, whereas only one antigen did not thoroughly induce dCAR-T cell proliferation. Therefore, controlling the degree of modified T cell expansion by targeting the two tumor-associated antigens may be an effective approach to control the strength of the immune response, mitigating the serious "on-target, off-tumor" toxicity.

Combinatorial antigen control over tumor killing in vitro
Next, we evaluated the ability of two distinct tumor-associated antigens (i.e., CEA and MSLN) to redirect dCAR-T cells to cognate tumor cell AsPC-1, using antigen-negative PANC-1 cell line as a control. In general, a major purpose of CARs is to redirect human CD8$^+$ T cell to selectively recognize tumor cells expressing antigens of interest, thereby improving therapeutic accuracy and tumor elimination. Thus, we examined whether primary human CD8$^+$ T cells expressing the dCAR could mount a cytotoxic response that was still antigen specific but gated by the two tumor-associated antigens. The cytotoxic activity of CD8$^+$ T cells expressing the dCAR was then quantified based on the level of

LDH released from apoptotic target cells in the supernatant (Fig. 2f).

After an overnight incubation, significant cell-mediated cytotoxicity was observed in dCAR-T cells co-cultured with cognate tumor cells expressing both CEA and MSLN, with approximately 80% of target cell apoptosis which was similar to that of conventional CAR-T cells (CEA-CAR T or MSLN-CAR T) (Fig. 2g). Efficient killing of the cognate target cells was not observed when single-receptor CAR-T cells (i.e., Cζ-CAR-T cells and MBB-CAR-T cells) or wild T cells were added. In addition, killing of non-cognate target cells (HT29, U87, or PANC-1) was not observed in co-culture with dCAR-modified T cells, confirming that dCAR-T cell have a specific activity.

In summary, the results with primary human CD8$^+$ T cells confirmed that dCAR-T cells showed highly potent cytotoxicity for cognate tumor cells expressing two distinct tumor-associated antigens, suggesting that complete tumor eradication had been achieved. However, based on our data, we envision that the single antigen-expressing tumor do not initiate dCAR-T cell with significant activity, providing a precise cell-based therapeutic approach in a dual-targeting combinatorial antigen manner (Additional file 1: Figure S3). In addition, dCAR-modified CD4$^+$ T cells also have cytotoxicity against cognate tumor cells (approximately 30%); therefore, CD4$^+$ T cells possess lower target cell killing capacity compared with CD8$^+$ T cells (Additional file 1: Figure S4).

dCAR-engineered T cells on tumor clearance in vivo

To investigate the activity of dCAR-T cells in vivo, we evaluated tumor regression in a xenograft model using RFP-modified tumor cells. In this model, mice were treated with various effector cells at 7 days after tumor injection (Fig. 3a). Briefly, to demonstrate the efficacy and safe of the novel structure of dual-receptor CAR in vivo, mice were inoculated with various cancer cells, including AsPC-1 (MSLN$^+$ CEA$^+$), HT29 (MSLN$^-$ CEA$^+$), U87 (MSLN$^+$ CEA$^-$), or PANC-1 (MSLN$^-$ CEA$^-$), followed by intravenous injection of modified T cells or mock T cells 7 days later. The tumor regression was followed by in vivo living image of the mean fluorescence intensity from RFP-engineered tumor cells. Based on our in vivo results, 28 days after T cell infusion, mice that received dCAR-T cells showed a marked reduction in tumor burden and even complete tumor remission, which was similar to that of the conventional CAR (CEA-CAR or MSLN-CAR) T cell treatment (Fig. 3b). However, for cognate tumor cells (AsPC-1), the tumor burden in mice treated with MBB-CAR T cells or mock T cells gradually increased. In addition, mice injected Cζ-CAR T cells did not show a significant decrease in tumor burden, suggesting that the tumor eradication

had not been achieved. Meanwhile, mice bearing non-cognate tumor cells (HT29, U87, or PANC-1) had underwent substantial increase in tumor burden even after dCAR-T cell infusion.

Next, the cytotoxic activities of engineered T cells were characterized based on the mock T cell cytotoxicity at 35 days after tumor injection. In mice that were injected with AsPC-1 cells followed by dCAR-T cells, the relative cytotoxic activity of effector cells is approximately 93.8%, having a significant differences relative to that of mock T cells ($p < 0.001$) (Fig. 3c). Similar results were obtained in mice treated with conventional CAR T cells, such as CEA-CAR T cells (93.2%) or MSLN-CAR T cells (91%). Taken together, in agreement with our in vitro results, dCAR-T cells can eliminate cognate tumor cells with comparable efficacy to conventional CAR-T cells in vivo; however, other mice treated with Cζ-CAR cells or MBB-CAR cells failed in inhibiting the cognate tumor cell growth.

T cell proliferation and cytokine production in vivo

We next investigated modified T cell proliferation during target cell elimination in mice. After effector cell infusion, increased T cell counts in the peripheral blood were detected at 24 h and every other 7 days for 4 weeks during tumor burden decrease. Results revealed that dCAR-T cells provided significantly greater proliferation compared with Cζ-CAR T cells or MBB-CAR T cells (Fig. 3d).

In general, effector cells rejected the tumor cells, accompanying with cytokine release, including IL-2, TNFα, IL-6, and IFNγ. In our experiment, production of various cytokines had achieved in mice infused with the dCAR or conventional CAR-T cells (Fig. 3e, f). Briefly, dCAR-T cells in mice bearing the cognate tumor cells (AsPC-1) released high levels of cytokines, including 2320 pg/mL IL-2, 609 pg/mL TNFα, 2486 ng/mL IL-6, and 67 ng/mL IFNγ, which was similar to that observed for cytotoxicity. The significant cytokine production had also been observed in response to CEA-CAR T cells or MSLN-CAR T cells. Furthermore, other engineered T cells did not produce significant levels of cytokines.

Collectively, the above experiments demonstrated that the activity of dCAR-T cells requires both the first signal pathway (antigen recognition signaling domain, CD3ζ) and the second signal pathway (co-stimulation signaling domain, 4/1BB). Based on the data, dCAR-T cell cytotoxicity is comparable to that of conventional CAR-T cells. For the single-receptor CAR bearing one signal pathway in this research, including Cζ-CAR and MBB-CAR, effector cells had no significant activation activity and did not exert remarkable cytotoxicity even in the presence of cognate tumor cells (AsPC-1) expressing both MSLN and CEA. Therefore, the dual signaling pathway is a

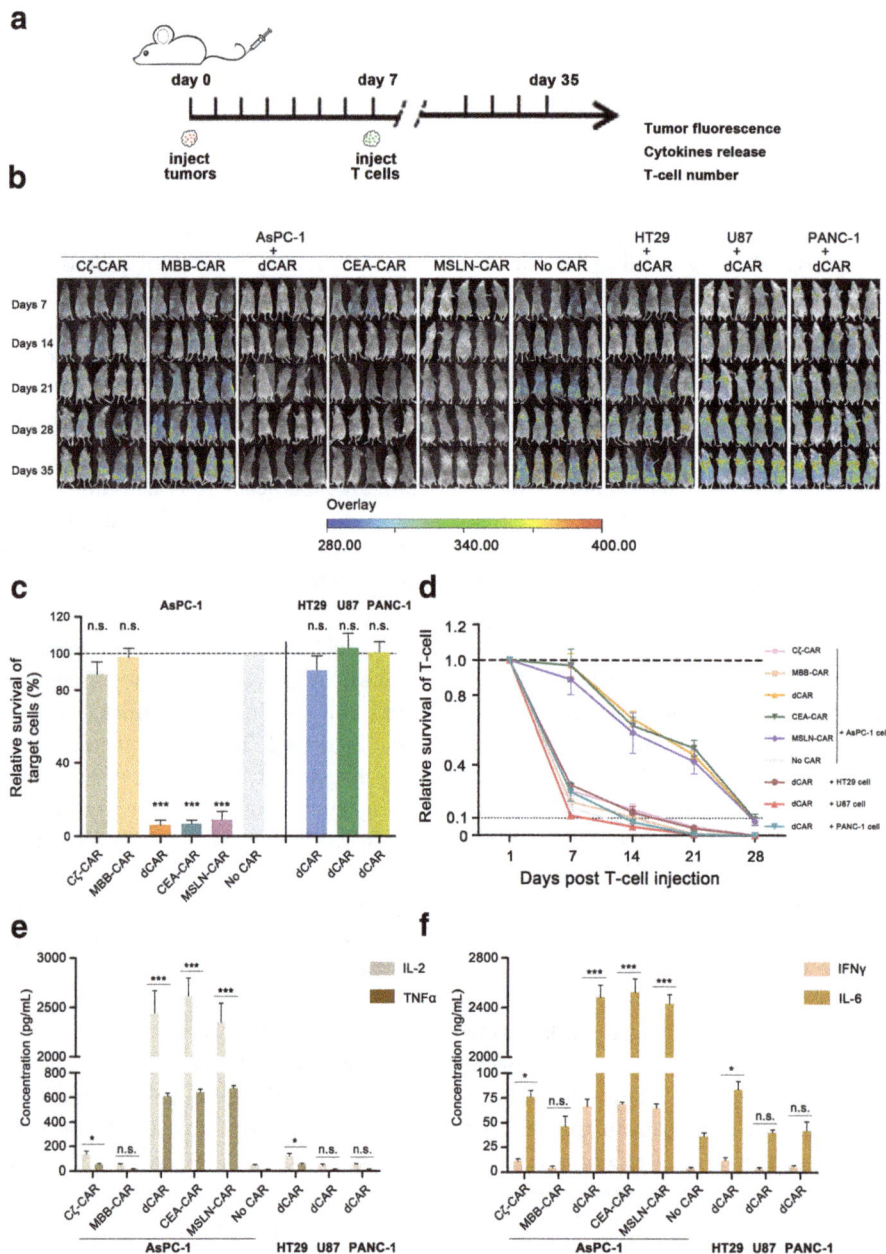

Fig. 3 dCAR-engineered T cells on tumor clearance in vivo. To investigate the activity of dCAR-T cells in vivo, we evaluated the pancreatic cancer regression in immunodeficient mice. **a** Schematic of the mouse treatment strategy. Day 0, all tumor cells, including AsPC-1 cells, HT29 cells, U87 cells, or PANC-1 cells, were injected into nude mice intravenously (*i.v.*). Mice treated with various effector cells at 7 days after tumor injection, and then the survival of target cells, cytokine release, and T cell number were detected. **b** After effector cell injection, the tumor regression was followed by in vivo living image of the mean fluorescence intensity from RFP-engineered tumor cells ($n = 5$). **c** Cytotoxic activities of engineered T cells were characterized based on the mock T cell cytotoxicity at 35 days after tumor injection. Data showed that the relative cytotoxic activity of effector cells is approximately 93.8%, having a significant difference relative to that of mock T cells ($n = 5$, error bars denote standard deviation). **d** The proliferation of modified T cells was measured in vivo. Data showed that dCAR-T cells provided significantly greater proliferation compared with the single-receptor structure, including CÇ-CAR and MBB-CAR ($n = 5$, error bars denote standard deviation). **e**, **f** Effector cells released various cytokines, including IL-2, TNFα, IL-6, and IFNγ. In our experiment, significant cytokine production had achieved in mice treated with dCAR-T cells, which was similar to that of conventional CAR-T cells (CEA-CAR T or MSLN-CAR T) ($n = 5$, error bars denote standard deviation)

prerequisite for T cell activity, whereas the CAR containing a single-signaling pathway endows T cells with resting state, including activation, proliferation, and cytotoxicity.

Excitingly, a novel type of CAR-T cells, termed dCAR-T, was designed with high specificity, that is, significant cytotoxicity for tumor cells that express both distinct antigens yet no cytotoxicity for single antigen-positive tumor cells. Finally, this novel CAR model has a good safety and high activity, alleviating "on-target, off-tumor" toxicity in the presence of the known tumor-associated antigens.

Discussion

Chimeric antigen receptor modified T cells have achieved promising clinical responses in the treatment of the hematological malignancies in recent years [28, 29]. With advance in tumor microenvironment, some approaches have been developed to enhance the efficacy of CAR-T cells against various solid tumors, resulting in some ongoing clinical trials [30]. While achieving significant therapeutic effects with the immune cell therapy, patients are often accompanied with severe side effects, especially "on-target, off-tumor" toxicity [16, 18]. The antigens used for CAR structure are often tumor-associated antigens co-expressed both on cancerous tissues and adjacent tissues; therefore, conventional CAR-T cells effectively rejected the tumor cells while damaging the normal tissues expressing the targeted antigen. In general, the two signaling domains derived from the intracellular part of T cell receptors are connected in a tandem manner and controlled by a targeted-antigen receptor; therefore, one antigen can control the two signaling domains, which increases the chance of damaging normal cells expressing interested antigens specific for CAR structure present on T cells [31].

To achieve safe cytotoxicity of CAR-T cells, several strategies have been described that use a novel CAR structure or a tumor-specific antigen to control the activation of T cell receptor. In the present study, the activity of CAR-engineered T cells was significantly improved through the action of a dual-receptor CAR paradigm. For the first time, we designed a dual-receptor CAR model that contains two physically separate structures, CEA-CD3ζ and MSLN-4/1BB signaling domains specific for CEA and MSLN, respectively (Fig. 4a). The dCAR-engineered T cell cytotoxicity was effectively controlled with cognate tumor cells (AsPC-1) expressing CEA and MSLN, thereby mitigating "on-target, off-tumor" toxicity and improving the safety of T cell therapy. In addition, dCAR-T cells cleared cognate tumor cells with a similar cytotoxicity comparable to that of conventional CAR-T cells (CEA-CAR T or MSLN-CAR T) in in vitro and in vivo experiments, thereby promoting their applications.

Based on our results, cognate tumor cells expressing MSLN and CEA are required for dCAR-T cell activity, including activation, proliferation, and cytotoxicity. Engineered T cells designed here are not activated when a single-receptor of dCAR-T cells interacts with the corresponding antigen, which triggers phosphorylation of the intracellular 4/1BB signal domain yet is not able to initiate T cell activation because the first signaling pathway (CD3ζ) is vital for the activity of T cells. Hence,

dCAR-engineered T cells have no any cytotoxicity for normal tissues expressing only the tumor-associated antigen MSLN. Similar with the first generation of CAR-T cells, dCAR-T cells designed here have low-level activation in the presence of CEA antigen, resulting in lower cytotoxicity against target cells. However, the activation of dCAR-T cells targeted by CEA is not sufficient to achieve significant cytotoxicity (Fig. 4b). Theoretically, targeting the CEA receptor expressed on T cell surfaces triggers phosphorylation of the intracellular CD3ζ signal domain and then initiates T cell activation with slight and transient characteristics. Therefore, the novel dCAR-T cells can have slight damage for normal tissues expressing only the antigen CEA, or even no damage. Our experiments showed that the modified T cell activity derived from this model where only the CEA-CD3ζ signaling pathway was activated is very limited, resulting from the fact that the intracellular phosphorylation may fail to exert the persistent T cell activity. Therefore, the co-stimulatory signaling pathway (MSLN-4/1BB) in the novel dCAR is also crucial for the activity of engineered T cells. As expected, dCAR-T cells can exert strong cytotoxicity for dual antigen-expressing tumor cells (AsPC-1), which is comparable with that of conventional CAR-T cells. The synergistical phosphorylation of the CD3ζ and 4/1BB signal domains in the presence of cognate tumor cells expressing CEA and MSLN ultimately rendered T cells with complete activation and significant cytotoxicity. Thus, the dCAR-T cell activity was strictly dependent on cognate tumor cells, mitigating the "on-target, off-tumor" toxicity.

In fact, engineered T cells bearing the activated CD3ζ signaling pathway have a potential to exert cytotoxicity for CEA single-positive target cells. To further improve the safety of dCAR-T cell therapy, we envision that the CD3ζ signaling pathway of dCAR structure could be characterized to a novel model that can be precisely regulated. With the advance of a CAR diagram and a switch molecule, the dCAR model could be regulated via the first signaling pathway (CD3ζ) in the presence or absence of the exogenous factors, achieving the precise control of injected dCAR-T cells [32–34] (Fig. 4c). According to the characteristics of the solid tumor microenvironment, the new CAR structure, termed masked CAR, rendered the CD3ζ signaling pathway with an activated state only at the tumor site as a result of the proteases, thereby enabling dCAR-T cells to recognize the tumor tissue [35] (Fig. 4d).

In conclusion, because TAAs widely are expressed in many kinds of human solid carcinomas, this dCAR strategy offers a conception toward the design of CARs capable of targeting cancer cells lacking the tumor-specific antigens. Dual-targeted CAR-T cells can be precisely localized at the tumor site and can exert high cytotoxicity against tumor cells while the

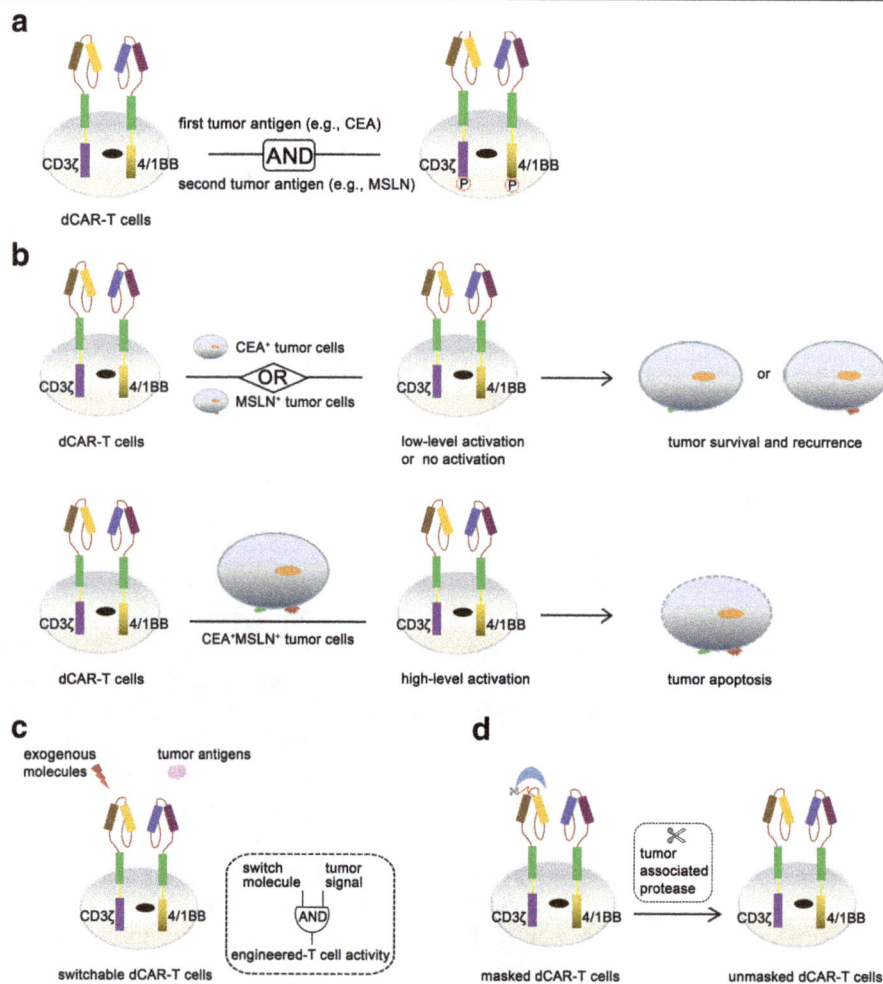

Fig. 4 General strategies that improve the therapeutic safety of engineering dCAR-T cells. **a** In the presence of the first tumor antigen (e.g., CEA) >and the second tumor antigen (e.g., MSLN), the intracellular CD3ζ and 4/1BB signal domain were phosphorylated, resulting in the fact that cognate tumor cells expressing MSLN and CEA are required for dCAR-T cell activity. **b** For tumor cells expressing a single tumor-associated antigen, dCAR-T cells have low-level activation in the presence of CEA yet no activation in the presence of MSLN, resulting in tumor survival and recurrence. For dual antigen-expressing tumor cells, dCAR-T cells have high-level activation and exert significant cytotoxicity, resulting in tumor apoptosis. **c** To achieve the accurate control of dCAR-T cells in vitro and in vivo, the CD3ζ signaling pathway of dCAR structure was regulated by an exogenous molecular. Therefore, switchable dCAR-T cells eliminate cognate tumor cells expressing the tumor antigens specific for the second CAR of this model only in the presence of the switch molecule. **d** To decrease normal tissue damage, a cleavable masking peptide could be re-engineered into the N-terminal of CEA-CD3ζ pathway domain, thereby blocking the antigen recognition domain of the CEA scFv. Thus, masked dCAR-T cells eradicate cognate tumor cells only in the presence of the tumor-associated protease locally active in tumor environment, thus enabling dCAR-T cell to differentiate tumor tissue and normal tissue

adjacent tissues are not damaged, enabling accurate application of CAR-T cell therapy.

Conclusions

Based on our data, a novel type of CAR-T cells, dCAR-T cells, can exert significant cytotoxicity only in the presence of cognate tumor cells (AsPC-1) expressing both CEA and MSLN, which is comparable with that obtained with conventional CAR-T cells and alleviates "on-target, off-tumor" toxicity. In summary, the combination therapy using two distinct TAAs to regulate dCAR-T cell activity is becoming

increasingly prospective in the field of cell-based cancer immunotherapy.

Additional file

Additional file 1: Figure S1. Schematic representation of CAR-engineered T cells in this research. **Figure S2.** Detection of effector cells and target cells. **Figure S3.** dCAR-mediated activation and co-stimulation of CD8+ T cells facilitates significant cytotoxicity and specific activity. **Figure S4.** dCAR-engineered CD4+ T cells could yield slight cytotoxicity compared with CAR-modified CD8+ T cells. (DOCX 911 kb)

Abbreviations

APC: Allophycocyanin; BSA: Bovine serum albumin; CARs: Chimeric antigen receptors; CEA: Carcino-embryonic antigen; dCAR: Dual-receptor chimeric antigen receptor; FBS: Fetal bovine serum; FITC: Fluorescein isothiocyanate; GFP: Green fluorescence protein; HER-2: Human epidermal growth factor receptor 2; IRES: Internal ribosome entry site; LDH: Lactate dehydrogenase; MFI: Mean fluorescence intensity; MSLN: Mesothelin; PBMCs: Peripheral blood mononuclear cells; PBS: Phosphate buffer saline; RFP: Red fluorescence protein; TAAs: Tumor-associated antigens

Funding

This work was supported by the Project Program of State Key Laboratory of Natural Medicines (No. SKLNMBZ201403) and the National Science and Technology Major Projects of New Drugs (No. 2014ZX09508007) in China. This project was also funded by the Priority Academic Program Development of Jiangsu Higher Education Institutions (PAPD) and Natural Science Foundation of Jiangsu Province (BK20160757).

Authors' contributions

EZ designed the experiment and contributed to the writing of the manuscript. PY, JG, HW, XC, CL, YW, JX, WQ, QS, SZ, and JH analyzed data. HX contributed to the revision of the manuscript. All authors read and approved the final manuscript.

Consent for publication

Not applicable.

Competing interests

The authors declare that they have no competing interests.

Author details

[1]The Engineering Research Center of Peptide Drug Discovery and Development, China Pharmaceutical University, Nanjing 210009, People's Republic of China. [2]Basic Medical Research Center, School of Medicine, Nantong University, Nantong 226001, People's Republic of China. [3]Jiangsu Key Laboratory of Oral Diseases, Department of Oral and Maxillofacial Surgery, Affiliated Hospital of Stomatology, Nanjing Medical University, Nanjing 211166, People's Republic of China. [4]State Key Laboratory of Natural Medicines, Ministry of Education, China Pharmaceutical University, Nanjing 210009, People's Republic of China. [5]Nanjing Anji Biotechnology Co., Ltd, Nanjing 210046, People's Republic of China.

References

1. Fesnak AD, June CH, Levine BL. Engineered T cells: the promise and challenges of cancer immunotherapy. Nat Rev Cancer. 2016;16:566–81.
2. Pagel JM, West HJ. Chimeric antigen receptor (CAR) T-cell therapy. JAMA Oncol. 2017;3:1595.
3. Lim WA, June CH. The principles of engineering immune cells to treat cancer. Cell. 2017;168:724–40.
4. Rivière I, Sadelain M. Chimeric antigen receptors: a cell and gene therapy perspective. Mol Ther. 2017;25:1117–24.
5. Maude SL, Frey N, Shaw PA, Aplenc R, Barrett DM, Bunin NJ, et al. Chimeric antigen receptor T cells for sustained remissions in leukemia. N Engl J Med. 2014;371:1507–17.
6. Ramos CA, Ballard B, Zhang H, Dakhova O, Gee AP, Mei Z, et al. Clinical and immunological responses after CD30-specific chimeric antigen receptor-redirected lymphocytes. J Clin Invest. 2017;127:3462–71.
7. Gardner RA, Finney O, Annesley C, Brakke H, Summers C, Leger K, et al. Intent-to-treat leukemia remission by CD19 CAR T cells of defined formulation and dose in children and young adults. Blood. 2017;129:3322–31.
8. Locke FL, Neelapu SS, Bartlett NL, Siddiqi T, Chavez JC, Hosing CM, et al. Phase 1 results of ZUMA-1: a multicenter study of KTE-C19 anti-CD19 CAR T cell therapy in refractory aggressive lymphoma. Mol Ther. 2017;25:285–95.
9. Schuster SJ, Svoboda J, Chong EA, Nasta SD, Mato AR, Anak Ö, et al. Chimeric antigen receptor T cells in refractory B-cell lymphomas. N Engl J Med. 2017;377:2545–54.
10. Lee DW, Kochenderfer JN, Stetler-Stevenson M, Cui YK, Delbrook C, Feldman SA, et al. T cells expressing CD19 chimeric antigen receptors for acute lymphoblastic leukaemia in children and young adults: a phase 1 dose-escalation trial. Lancet. 2015;385:517–28.
11. Porter DL, Levine BL, Kalos M, Bagg A, June CH. Chimeric antigen receptor-modified T cells in chronic lymphoid leukemia. N Engl J Med. 2011;365:725–33.
12. Garfall AL, Maus MV, Hwang WT, Lacey SF, Mahnke YD, Melenhorst JJ, et al. Chimeric antigen receptor T cells against CD19 for multiple myeloma. N Engl J Med. 2015;373:1040–7.
13. Brudno JN, Kochenderfer JN. Toxicities of chimeric antigen receptor T cells: recognition and management. Blood. 2016;127:3321–30.
14. Neelapu SS, Tummala S, Kebriaei P, Wierda W, Gutierrez C, Locke FL, et al. Chimeric antigen receptor T-cell therapy - assessment and management of toxicities. Nat Rev Clin Oncol. 2017;15:47–62.
15. Gross G, Eshhar Z. Therapeutic potential of T cell chimeric antigen receptors (CARs) in cancer treatment: counteracting off-tumor toxicities for safe CAR T cell therapy. Annu Rev Pharmacol Toxicol. 2016;56:59–83.
16. Fisher J, Abramowski P, Wisidagamage Don ND, Flutter B, Capsomidis A, Cheung GW, et al. Avoidance of on-target off-tumor activation using a co-stimulation-only chimeric antigen receptor. Mol Ther. 2017;25:1234–47.
17. Turtle CJ, Riddell SR, Maloney DG. CD19-targeted chimeric antigen receptor-modified T-cell immunotherapy for B-cell malignancies. Clin Pharmacol Ther. 2016;100:252–8.
18. Kochenderfer JN, Dudley ME, Feldman SA, Wilson WH, Spaner DE, Maric I, et al. B-cell depletion and remissions of malignancy along with cytokineassociated toxicity in a clinical trial of anti-CD19 chimeric-antigen-receptor-transduced T cells. Blood. 2012;119:2709–20.
19. Davila ML, Riviere I, Wang X, Bartido S, Park J, Curran K, et al. Efficacy and toxicity management of 19-28z CAR T cell therapy in B cell acute lymphoblastic leukemia. Sci Transl Med. 2014;6:224ra25.
20. Morgan RA, Yang JC, Kitano M, Dudley ME, Laurencot CM, Rosenberg SA. Case report of a serious adverse event following the administration of T cells transduced with a chimeric antigen receptor recognizing ERBB2. Mol Ther. 2010;18:843–51.
21. Rosales-Velderrain A, Bowers SP, Goldberg RF, Buchanan MA, Stauffer JA, Asbun HJ. National trends in resection of the distal pancreas. World J Gastroenterol. 2012;18:4342–9.
22. Li D, Xie K, Wolff R, Abbruzzese JL. Pancreatic cancer. Lancet. 2004;363:1049–57.
23. Lin QJ, Yang F, Jin C, Fu DL. Current status and progress of pancreatic cancer in China. World J Gastroenterol. 2015;21:7988–8003.
24. Morello A, Sadelain M, Adusumilli PS. Mesothelin-targeted CARs: driving T cells to solid tumors. Cancer Discov. 2016;6:133–46.
25. O'Hara M, Stashwick C, Haas AR, Tanyi JL. Mesothelin as a target for chimeric antigen receptor-modified T cells as anticancer therapy. Immunotherapy. 2016;8:449–60.
26. Parkhurst MR, Yang JC, Langan RC, Dudley ME, Nathan DA, Feldman SA, et al. T cells targeting carcinoembryonic antigen can mediate regression of metastatic colorectal cancer but induce severe transient colitis. Mol Ther. 2011;19:620–6.
27. Imaoka H, Mizuno N, Hara K, Hijioka S, Tajika M, Tanaka T, et al. Prognostic impact of carcinoembryonic antigen (CEA) on patients with metastatic pancreatic cancer: a retrospective cohort study. Pancreatology. 2016;16:859–64.
28. Kenderian SS, Ruella M, Gill S, Kalos M. Chimeric antigen receptor T-cell therapy to target hematologic malignancies. Cancer Res. 2014;74:6383–9.
29. Gill S, June CH. Going viral: chimeric antigen receptor T-cell therapy for hematological malignancies. Immunol Rev. 2015;263:68–89.
30. Zhang E, Gu J, Xu H. Prospects for chimeric antigen receptor-modified T cell therapy for solid tumors. Mol Cancer. 2018;17:7.

31. Sadelain M, Brentjens R, Rivière I. The basic principles of chimeric antigen receptor design. Cancer Discov. 2013;3:388–98.

32. Wu CY, Roybal KT, Puchner EM, Onuffer J, Lim WA. Remote control of therapeutic T cells through a small molecule–gated chimeric receptor. Science. 2015;350:aab4077.

33. Kim MS, Ma JS, Yun H, Cao Y, Kim JY, Chi V, et al. Redirection of genetically engineered CAR-T cells using bifunctional small molecules. J Am Chem Soc. 2015;137:2832–5.

34. Zhang E, Gu J, Xue J, Lin C, Liu C, Li M, et al. Accurate control of dual-receptor-engineered T cell activity through a bifunctional anti-angiogenic peptide. J Hematol Oncol. 2018;11:44.

35. Han X, Bryson PD, Zhao Y, Cinay GE, Li S, Guo Y, et al. Masked chimeric antigen receptor for tumor-specific activation. Mol Ther. 2017;25:274–84.

5

The CCR4-NOT complex is a tumor suppressor in *Drosophila melanogaster* eye cancer models

Carmen Vicente[1,2,6*†], Rocco Stirparo[1,2†], Sofie Demeyer[1,2], Charles E. de Bock[1,2], Olga Gielen[1,2], Mardelle Atkins[1,3], Jiekun Yan[2,4], Georg Halder[1,3], Bassem A. Hassan[2,4,5] and Jan Cools[1,2*]

Abstract

Background: The CNOT3 protein is a subunit of the CCR4-NOT complex, which is involved in mRNA degradation. We recently identified CNOT3 loss-of-function mutations in patients with T-cell acute lymphoblastic leukemia (T-ALL).

Methods: Here, we use different *Drosophila melanogaster* eye cancer models to study the potential tumor suppressor function of *Not3*, the CNOT3 orthologue, and other members of the CCR4-NOT complex.

Results: Our data show that knockdown of *Not3*, the structural components *Not1/Not2*, and the deadenylases *twin/Pop2* all result in increased tumor formation. In addition, overexpression of *Not3* could reduce tumor formation. *Not3* downregulation has a mild but broad effect on gene expression and leads to increased levels of genes involved in DNA replication and ribosome biogenesis. *CycB* upregulation also contributes to the *Not3* tumor phenotype. Similar findings were obtained in human T-ALL cell lines, pointing out the conserved function of Not3.

Conclusions: Together, our data establish a critical role for *Not3* and the entire CCR4-NOT complex as tumor suppressor.

Keywords: CCR4-NOT, Leukemia, mRNA stability, Tumor suppressor, *Drosophila melanogaster*

Background

The CCR4-NOT complex is an essential and conserved multi-subunit complex that regulates gene expression [1]. Although it is implicated in many different cellular functions, it has been mainly studied for its mRNA deadenylation activity, a first step in mRNA degradation [1, 2]. In humans, the CCR4–NOT complex consists of at least nine conserved "canonical" subunits: CNOT1, CNOT2, CNOT3, CNOT6, CNOT6L, CNOT7, CNOT8, CNOT9, and CNOT10. Among these subunits, CNOT6, CNOT6L, CNOT7, and CNOT8 have deadenylase activity and are directly responsible for the removal of the poly-A tail from the target mRNA [3].

Besides, other subunits of the complex are also important for mRNA degradation. For instance, deadenylation is suppressed by *CNOT1* depletion and *CNOT2*

downregulation affects the length of mRNA poly-A tails [4, 5]. Recent data indicate that CNOT3 is also involved in the control of mRNA stability. *Cnot3* haplodeficiency in ob/ob mice ameliorated the obese phenotype through the regulation of the CCR4–NOT-mediated deadenylation of specific mRNAs involved in energy metabolism [6]. Furthermore, CNOT3 regulates bone mass through regulation of *Rank* mRNA stability [7]. Recently, it has been shown that CNOT3 contributes to early B cell development by controlling *Igh* rearrangement and *p53* mRNA stability [8].

Escape from post-transcriptional regulation of gene expression is a crucial step in the pathogenesis of cancer. Aberrant polyadenylation site usage, leading to a truncated 3′UTR, has been detected in many human malignancies and might allow malignant cells to escape regulation by both microRNA and RNA binding proteins [9, 10]. The RNA-binding protein TTP has been shown to impair MYC-driven lymphoma development [11]. Deletion of the genes *Zfp36L1* and *Zfp36L2*, which encode RNA-binding proteins, was shown to cause T-cell acute lymphoblastic

* Correspondence: cvicente@unav.es; jan.cools@kuleuven.be
†Carmen Vicente and Rocco Stirparo contributed equally to this work.
[1]Center for Cancer Biology, VIB, Leuven, Belgium
Full list of author information is available at the end of the article

leukemia (T-ALL) in mice due to impaired *Notch1* mRNA degradation [12].

We recently identified loss-of-function mutations on the *CNOT3* gene in patients with T-ALL [13]. Other studies have confirmed *CNOT3* mutations in T-ALL and have also identified mutations in *CNOT1* and *CNOT2* [14–16]. Furthermore, T-ALL patients with HOXA-rearrangements and terminal 5q deletions show CNOT6 downregulation and high incidence of CNOT3 mutations [17]. These data suggest that the CCR4-NOT complex is involved in cancer, although it remains unclear how it is contributing to tumor development.

Here, we explored how loss of *Not3*, the CNOT3 orthologue, is involved in tumor development using loss-of-function and gain-of-function analyses in *Drosophila melanogaster* eye cancer models. We established that *Not3* behaves as a tumor suppressor gene. Reduction of *Not3* expression resulted in a significant increase in tumor incidence, while its overexpression suppressed tumor formation. Downregulation of other subunits of the CCR4-NOT complex also enhanced tumor formation. Our results indicate that the entire complex and its deadenylase activity are required for tumor suppression, which is linked with *CycB* upregulation and the regulation of genes implicated in DNA replication and ribosome biogenesis.

Methods
Fly husbandry
All crosses were raised on standard fly food at 25 °C. All fly lines used are listed in Additional file 1: Table S1. For the generation of eyeless>UAS-RNAi Not3, eyeless>UAS-Dl>UAS-RNAi Not3 and eyeless>UAS-Dl>UAS-RNAi twin animals standard methods were used to recombine UAS-RNAi Not3 (VDRC KK102144, v105990) or UAS-RNAi twin (VDRC KK108897, v104442) with an eyeless-Gal4 or an eyeless-Gal4>UAS-Dl insertion on the second chromosome. To perform experiments for quantifying proliferation, apoptosis, and differentiation, control crosses were established using eyeless>UAS-Dl stock virgins and males carrying UAS-RNAi *white*. This chromosome was maintained in a stock balanced over CyO, GFP. Three independent crosses were established per experimental condition tested, and five transfers from each cross into new fly food flasks were performed.

Analyses of eye tumor burden
Adult animals of the correct genotypes were imaged using a Zeiss Apotome microscope. To analyze tumor burden, each eye was scored separately on flies with the genotype of interest (positive F1 progeny). The score of the eye tumor burden was performed double-blind (except for those experiments in which we investigated the function of the seven selected target genes, shown in Fig. 6). Eyes were counted as hyperplastic when showing at least one

fold. Metastases were observed as masses of amorphous red-pigmented cells outside of the eye field (head, thorax, and abdomen). The percentages shown on the bar graphs represent the average percentage of three independent crosses, and the mean number of eyes analyzed is indicated on each graph (*Y*-axis). In the experiments involving (1) the downregulation of *Not3/twin* on the sensitized, the *Ras*-V12, or the wild-type genetic backgrounds and (2) the overexpression of *Not3* or the *Not3* mutant construct on the eyeful genetic background, the whole eye area (region with presence of differentiated photoreceptors) was measured on representative adult eyes. Image processing and eye measurements were performed with ImageJ. Control eyes measured values were considered as 100%. Values for eight individual discs were plotted. Data was analyzed using GraphPad Prism v6.

Immunohistochemistry, imaging, and quantification
Dissections and stainings were performed as previously described [18]. Primary antibodies used were rat anti-ELAV (1:100, DSHB), rabbit anti-Phospho-Histone-3 (1:1000, Millipore), and rabbit anti-cleaved-DCP1a (1:150, Cell signaling). All secondary antibodies were used at 1:500. Samples were mounted in Prolong antifade mounting media. Fluorescence imaging was performed using a Leica confocal microscope. Images were processed (Z-projection) using ImageJ/FIJI. Phospho-histone H3 (pH3), cleaved-DCP1a, and BrdU positive cells within the posterior part of eye discs from the appropriate genotypes (GFP negative larvae) were counted. Values for 10 individual discs were plotted. Data was graphed and analyzed using GraphPad Prism v6.

RNA-sequencing sample preparation and analyses
Dissection tools and surfaces were treated with RNAseq Away, and RNA was isolated using the RNAqueous-Micro Kit (Ambion). Eye-antennal imaginal discs were dissected from 30 L3 wandering larvae and transferred into RNAse-free ependorfs containing lysis buffer on ice. Following dissection, either RNA was extracted immediately or discs on lysis buffer were snap-frozen and kept at – 80 °C for later extraction. All the RNA samples showed high quality on the Bioanalyzer (Agilent Technologies). Next-generation sequencing libraries were constructed from 500 ng of total RNA using the Truseq RNA sample prep kit v2, and RNA-seq libraries were subjected to 1 × 50 bp single-end sequencing on a HiSeq2500 instrument (Illumina). For each condition, three replicates were sequenced. The reads were cleaned with fastq-mcf, and a quality control was performed with FastQC (http://www.bioinformatics.babraham.ac.uk/projects/fastqc). Reads were then mapped to the *Drosophila melanogaster* genome (dm6) with TopHat2 [19]. Subsequently, HTSeq-count [20] was used to count the number of reads per gene. For

differential gene expression analysis, the Bioconductor package DESeq2 [21] was used. The lists of differential genes were then further analyzed using FlyMine [22].

Drosophila Not3 overexpression and S2 cell transfection experiments

All Not3 constructs were cloned into the pUASTattB vector. We used Canton S L3 wandering larval eye discs cDNA as template. Fragments were PCR amplified using the primers shown in Additional file 1: Table S2. All constructs were verified by Sanger sequencing. The transgenic flies were generated by BestGene (Strain #9744, 89E11 acceptor site). Drosophila S2 cells were co-transfected with a pMT-Gal4 plasmid and a flag-tagged version of each of the UAS-Not3 plasmids. Gal4 expression was induced 24 h post-transfection by adding $CuSO_4$. Cells were treated with cycloheximide (50 µg/ml, 3 h treatment) 24 h after gene expression induction. Lysates were immunoblotted with anti-Flag antibodies. To test the stability of Cycb, fancl, or upd2 mRNAs in Drosophila S2 cells, co-transfections of the pMT-Gal4 plasmid and the RNAi plasmid targeting Not3 (construct ID 4068, dna4068 from the VDRC) or a UAS-YFP plasmid (as a negative control) were performed using an Amaxa nucleofector. Gal4 expression (thus, Not3 RNAi or YFP expression) was induced 24 h post-transfection by adding CuSO4. After 24 h of Not3 RNAi or YFP expression induction, transcription was stopped by addition of 5 µg/ml actinomycin D. Cells were harvested, and RNA was purified after 0, 10, 20, 40, 80, and 160 min and quantified by qPCR. Three independent experiments were performed. Expression of the CG1239 gene was used as a control of no stabilization, since its expression was not significantly changed on our RNA-sequencing experiments after Not3 downregulation.

cDNA synthesis and qPCR analyses

cDNA synthesis from eye discs was performed using the QuantiTec Reverse Transcription kit following manual instructions. cDNA synthesis from S2 cells experiments was performed using the GoScript Reverse Transcription system protocol (Promega). Real-time qPCR reactions were performed using the GoTaq Real-Time kit, and reactions were run in a Lightcycler 480 device (Roche). Primers are listed in Additional file 1: Table S2.

T-ALL cell lines electroporation and RNA stability assay

Jurkat and CCRF-CEM cells were cultured under standard conditions. Electroporations were performed using the gene pulser Xcell™ electroporation system as previously described [23]. The negative control siRNA (D-001810-01-20), CNOT3 siRNA 326 (J-020319-06), and CNOT3 siRNA 328 (J-020319-08) were purchased from Dharmacon. Cells were treated with 5 µg/ml Actinomycin D (Sigma Aldrich) 24 h after electroporation.

RNA was immediately extracted at 0 h, 2 h, and 4 h with Maxwell® simplyRNA Cells Kit. Regarding the RNA-sequencing analysis pipeline, reads were mapped to the human genome (GRCh37/hg19). For the differential gene expression analysis (DESeq2), a linear model was applied, as we needed to compare all conditions with each other (instead of a one-to-one comparison). The data was modeled as TP + KD + TP:KD, in which the term TP (time point) represents the mRNA degradation over time, the term KD (knockdown) is related to the knockdown of CNOT3, and the combined term TP:KD shows the impact of the CNOT3 knockdown on mRNA degradation. The differential genes resulting from this last term, which are the more stable mRNAs (less degraded), were then used for further analysis with DAVID [24].

Results

Not3 behaves as a tumor suppressor gene in Drosophila melanogaster eye cancer models

To investigate the tumor suppressor role of Not3, we downregulated or overexpressed it in various genetic backgrounds. As a first model, we used flies with overexpression of the Notch ligand Delta (Dl) in the eye (driven by ey-Gal4) which results in hyper-activation of the Notch signaling pathway, thereby, leading to an increase in eye size but no tumor development [18, 25]. We refer to these flies as "sensitized" flies. We downregulated the expression of Not3 in this genetic background using three different UAS-RNAi Not3 lines, and a line with a P-element transposon insertion, in which the expression of one of the Not3 alleles has been shown to be disrupted [26]. Reduction of Not3 expression resulted in a remarkable increase in tumor incidence, from 7% of the eyes with control RNA interference (UAS-RNAi white) to up to 90% with the three different Not3 RNAi lines (Fig. 1a). Strikingly, inactivation of one allele of Not3 by the P-element insertion (which results in modest downregulation of Not3) was sufficient to induce tumor formation in 50% of the eyes (Fig. 1a). In all cases, tumor development was observed without metastases. These data support the hypothesis that loss of Not3 is sufficient to transform a sensitized lesion into a tumor, possibly by interfering with patterning and cell fate determination.

Next, we performed immunofluorescence stainings on sensitized L3 larval eye discs to investigate changes on the number of proliferative and differentiated cells upon Not3 downregulation. To do that, we used the phospho-Histone3 (pH3) and BrdU as markers of proliferation and ELAV as a marker of differentiation. Knockdown of Not3 expression was first confirmed by qPCR (Fig. 1b) and resulted in a significant increase of pH3 and BrdU positive cells (Fig. 1c). Downregulation of Not3 expression did not cause a significant loss of ELAV expressing cells (differentiated cells), although it did

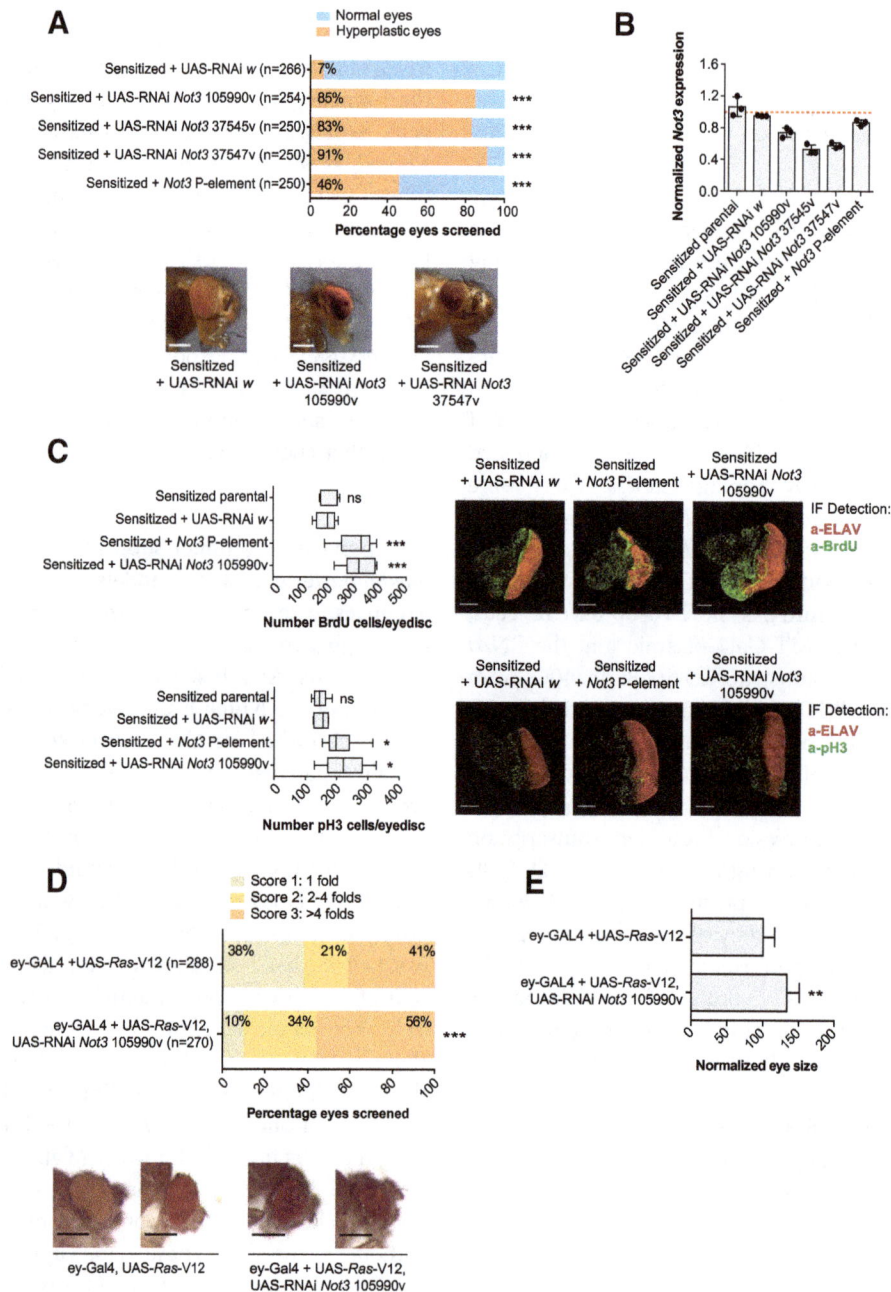

Fig. 1 Reduced expression of *Not3* increases tumor formation in *Drosophila melanogaster* eye cancer models. **a** Qualitative and quantitative representation of the tumor burden upon downregulation of *Not3* on sensitized flies. Bars show the percentage of eyes screened: blue, normal eyes; orange, hyperplastic eyes; *** $p < 0.001$. Three independent experimental crosses were established. The mean number of eyes screened is shown on the graph (Y-axis). Microscopy images show eyes of adult flies from representative genotypes, scale bars are 200 µM. **b** qPCR analyses showing the *Not3* expression levels from each genotype. Expression values are calculated from three independent crosses. From each cross, 30 eye-antennal imaginal discs were dissected. The red dotted bar represents the expression value = 1. **c** Quantification of BrdU and pH3 positive cells on the posterior portion of eye-antennal imaginal discs. Values for 10 individual discs were plotted. Representative confocal images of eye-antennal imaginal discs of the indicated genotypes. Green staining: BrdU or pH3 positive cells; red staining: ELAV protein. Scale bars are 70 µM; ns, not significant; * $p < 0.05$; *** $p < 0.001$. **d** Qualitative and quantitative representation of the tumor burden upon downregulation of *Not3* on the *Ras*-V12 background. Bars show the average percentage of eyes screened: light orange, eyes classified as score 1 (presence of 1 fold); yellow, eyes classified as score 2 (presence of 2–4 folds); dark orange, eyes classified as score 3 (presence of more than 4 folds); *** $p < 0.001$. Three independent experimental crosses were established. The mean number of eyes screened is shown on the graph (Y-axis). Microscopy images show eyes of adult flies from representative genotypes, scale bars are 200 µM. **e** Quantitative representation of the whole eye area (region with presence of differentiated photoreceptors) on representative adult eyes ($n = 8$) with downregulation of *Not3* on the *Ras*-V12 genetic background. Control eyes measured values were considered as 100%; ** $p < 0.01$

markedly disrupt the pattern of ELAV expression when compared to parental and control eye discs (Fig. 1c).

To further confirm the tumor suppressor activity of *Not3* in a different context, we used a fly model that specifically overexpresses *Ras*-V12 in the eye. Overexpression of only *Ras*-V12 resulted in increased eye size and also in hyperplastic tissue with a penetrance of 62%. Reduction of *Not3* in this oncogenic background resulted in a marked increase in tumor incidence (90%) and more aggressive phenotype as indicated by increased folds observed on the eye (Fig. 1d, e). Thus, reduction of *Not3* expression increases proliferation of retinal precursors in the *Dl*-sensitized and the *Ras*-V12 backgrounds.

Downregulation of Not3 abrogates normal retinal differentiation

We next aimed to dissect the physiological role of *Not3* in eye development. We observed that reduction of *Not3* expression in wild-type eyes (driven by *ey*-Gal4) resulted in a significant decrease of eye size (small rough phenotype) with a penetrance of 100% in adult flies (Fig. 2a). Expression of a UAS-RNAi *white* construct (control) did not change the external morphology of the eye. The *Not3* P-element mutant line showed no obvious defects in retinal differentiation, maybe because the reduction of *Not3* expression levels was not enough to cause defects on a wild-type tissue (Fig. 2b). These data indicate that *Not3* expression is essential for proper retinal development.

We also performed immunofluorescence stainings on larval eye discs to investigate the number of pH3/BrdU, cleaved-DCP1a (marker of apoptosis), and ELAV positive cells. Although not significant, we observed that reduction of *Not3* resulted in less cell proliferation, measured by pH3 and BrdU. Our results also showed that loss of *Not3* led to induction of apoptosis. Differentiation was strongly inhibited, although some photoreceptors could still form in *Not3*-downregulated eye discs (Fig. 2c–e).

Next, we tested if downregulation of other subunits of the CCR4-NOT complex could cause similar effects. Reduction of *twin* (deadenylase, CNOT6/CNOT6L orthologue) or *Pop2* (deadenylase, CNOT7/CNOT8 orthologue) expression led to a phenotype similar to the one observed among *Not3*-defective eye discs (rough small eyes) (Fig. 2d–e, Additional file 2: Figure S1A). Downregulation of *Not1* (scaffold protein of the complex, *CNOT1* orthologue) and *Not2* (*CNOT2* orthologue) was not significant, and as a consequence, the effects of *Not1* or *Not2* downregulation could not be assessed (Additional file 3: Figure S2A).

These results show that reduction of *Not3* or the CCR4-NOT complex subunits beyond a certain threshold disrupts normal retinal differentiation and causes subsequent loss of the differentiated tissue in a wild-type background.

Overexpression of Not3 suppresses tumor formation

To investigate whether *Not3* overexpression could suppress tumor formation, we first generated transgenic flies carrying a UAS-*Not3* construct. Ectopic expression of *Not3* was able to rescue the small rough eye phenotype previously observed in wild-type *Not3*-downregulated eyes, indicating that both UAS-*Not3* overexpression and the effects observed upon *Not3* downregulation are specific (Fig. 3a).

For subsequent experiments, we used the so-called "eyeful" flies. These flies have overexpression of the Notch ligand *Dl*, together with overexpression of the epigenetic regulators *lola* and *psq*. Eyeful flies display excessively enlarged eyes and eye tumors and macroscopically visible metastases derived from the developing retina [18, 25]. Overexpression of *Not3* in this model significantly suppressed formation of eye tumors: 43% vs. 21% ($p < 0.01$) when compared with UAS-GFP or 43% vs. 14% ($p < 0.001$) when compared with UAS-LacZ. When hyperplastic eyes were detected, the tumorigenic phenotypes observed were also milder than the ones observed in the control crosses (Fig. 3b).

In the eyeful eye discs, disorganization of the epithelium as well as defects in the pattern of differentiated cells were evident (Fig. 3c). Eyeful L3 larval eye discs with *Not3* overexpression had significantly less proliferating cells (less pH3/ BrdU positive cells) than control eye discs (Fig. 3c). Ectopic expression of *Not3* did not significantly affect the number of apoptotic cells (cleaved-DCP1a), although it seemed there were fewer apoptotic cells when compared to the control conditions. In addition, upregulation of *Not3* expression resulted in the re-establishment of the typical epithelial organization, accordingly to ELAV stainings.

Taken together, our data show that *Not3* acts as a classical tumor suppressor in *Drosophila melanogaster* eye cancer models, with its downregulation enhancing tumor formation and its overexpression suppressing tumor formation/progression.

The tumor suppressor function of Not3 is related to its function within the CCR4-NOT complex

Since *Not3* is a subunit of the CCR4-NOT complex, we asked whether downregulation of other subunits in the sensitized background causes similar effects. Reduction of expression of *Not1*, *Not2*, *twin*, or *Pop2* all caused increased tumor formation (Fig. 4a, b, Additional file 2: Figure S1B, and Additional file 3: Figure S2B). Of interest, reduction of *twin* also caused metastatic tumors (Fig. 4a). These data confirm that not only *Not3*, but also the entire CCR4-NOT complex functions as a tumor suppressor.

CNOT3, the human *Not3* orthologue, contains three important domains. The N-terminal region contains two coiled-coil (CC) domains, while the C-terminal region harbors a Not-box domain (NB). ClustalW2 alignment analysis

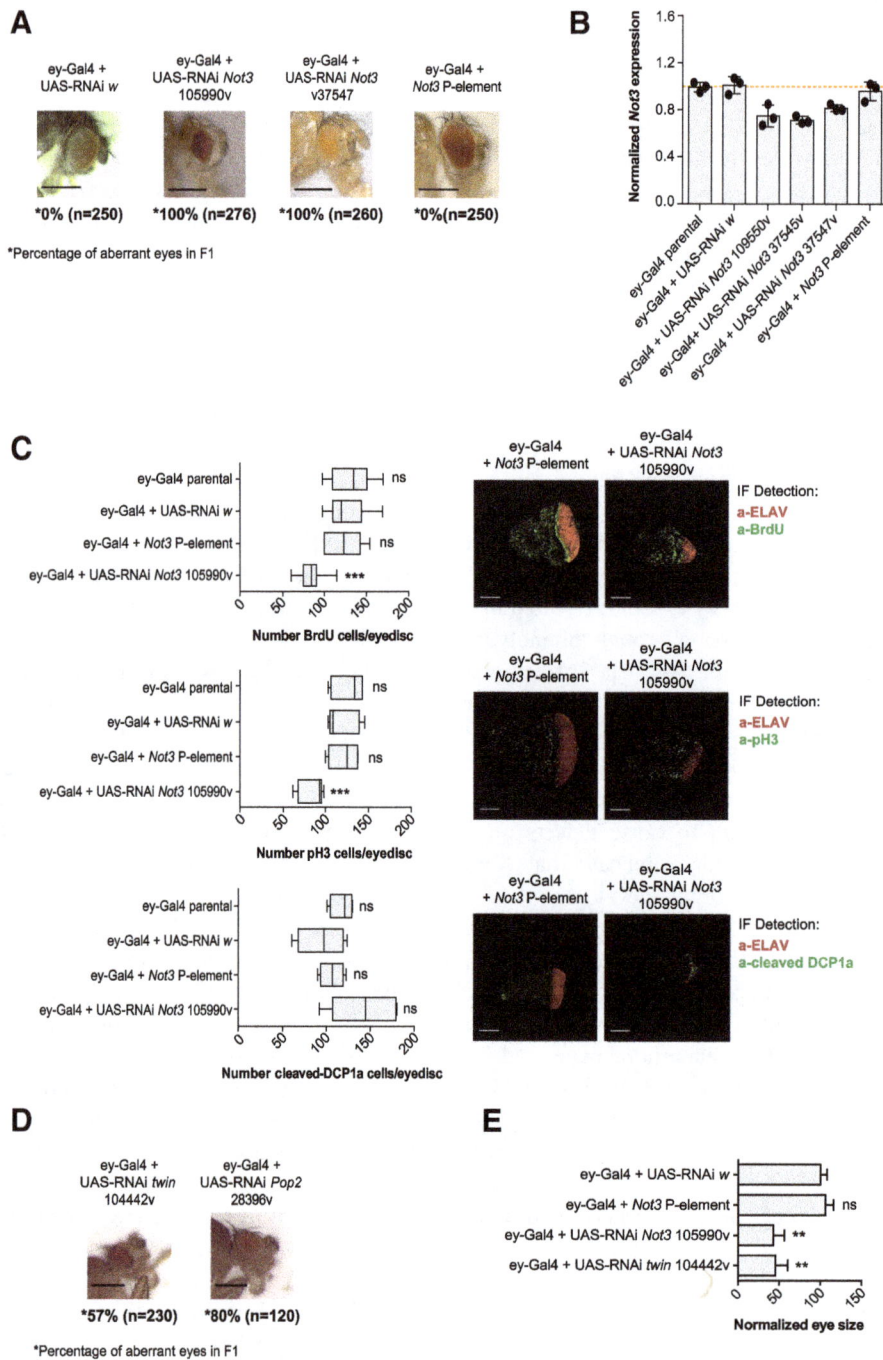

Fig. 2 Reduced expression of *Not3* in a wild-type genetic background abolishes normal retinal differentiation. **a** Microscopy images show eyes of adult flies with *Not3* reduced expression levels from representative genotypes, scale bars are 200 μM. The percentage of F1 "small rough" defective eyes and the mean number of eyes screened are indicated on the bottom side of each image. Three independent crosses were performed for each experimental condition. **b** qPCR analyses showing the *Not3* expression levels from each genotype. Expression values are calculated from three independent crosses. From each cross, 30 eye-antennal imaginal discs were dissected. The red dotted bar represents the expression value = 1. **c** Quantification of BrdU, pH3, and cleaved-DCP1a positive cells on the posterior portion of eye-antennal imaginal discs (*n* = 10). Representative confocal images of eye-antennal imaginal discs of the indicated genotypes. Green staining: BrdU, pH3, or cleaved-DCP1a positive cells; red staining: ELAV protein. Scale bars are 70 μM; ns, not significant; *** *p* < 0.001. **d** Microscopy images show eyes of adult flies with downregulation of the *Pop2* and twin CCR4-NOT complex subunits on a wild-type background, scale bars are 200 μM. The percentage of F1 "small rough" defective eyes and the mean number of eyes screened are indicated on the bottom side of each image. **e** Quantitative representation of the whole eye area (region with presence of differentiated photoreceptors) on representative adult eyes (*n* = 8) with downregulation of *Not3* or *twin* on the wild-type genetic background. Control eyes measured values were considered as 100%; ns, not significant; ** *p* < 0.01

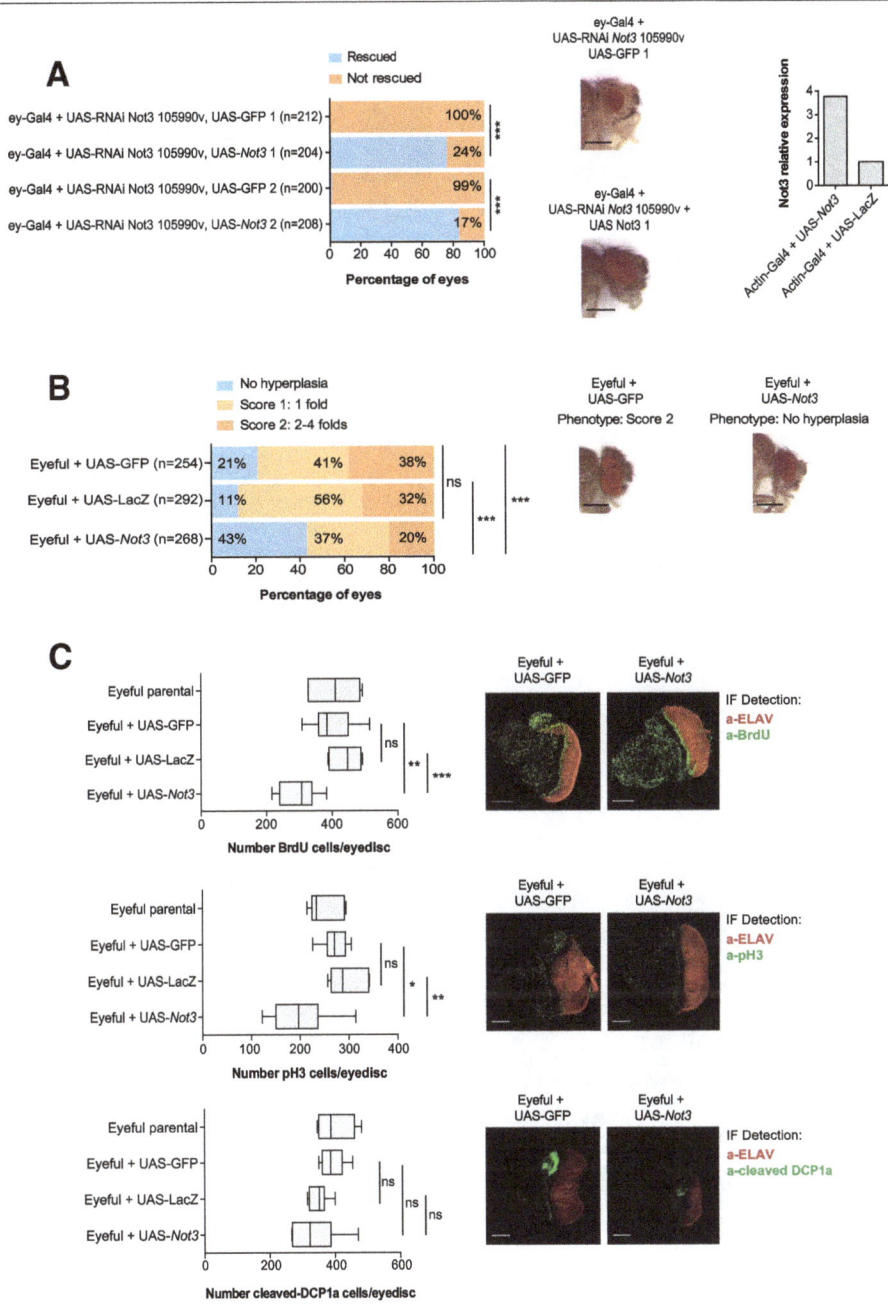

Fig. 3 Ectopic expression of *Not3* suppresses tumor formation in eyeful flies. **a** Qualitative and quantitative representation of the defective eyes upon ectopic expression of *Not3* on wild-type flies with reduced *Not3* expression. Bars show the percentage of eyes screened: blue, rescued eyes; orange, not rescued eyes; *** $p < 0.001$. Numbers 1 and 2 on each genotype represented on the graph refer to different recombinant clones. Three independent crosses were analyzed. The mean number of eyes screened is shown on the graph (*Y*-axis). Microscopy images show eyes of adult flies from representative genotypes, scale bars are 200 µM. qPCR analyses showing the *Not3* expression levels from each genotype. Each bar represents the expression value of a pool of 10 individuals. **b** Qualitative and quantitative representation of the hyperplastic eyes upon ectopic expression of *Not3* on eyeful flies. Bars show the percentage of eyes screened: blue, eyes with no hyperplasia; light orange, eyes classified as score 1 (presence of 1 fold); dark orange, eyes classified as score 2 (presence of 2–4 folds); ** $p < 0.01$, *** $p < 0.001$. Three independent crosses were analyzed. The mean number of eyes screened is shown on the graph (*Y*-axis). Microscopy images show eyes of adult flies from representative genotypes. Scale bars are 200 µM. **c** Quantification of BrdU, pH3, and cleaved-DCP1a positive cells on the posterior part of L3 larval eye-antennal imaginal discs. Values for 10 individual discs were plotted. Representative confocal images of eye-antennal imaginal discs of the indicated genotypes. Green staining: BrdU, pH3, or cleaved-DCP1a positive cells; red staining: ELAV protein. Scale bars are 70 µM; ns, not significant; * $p < 0.05$; ** $p < 0.01$; ***$p < 0.001$

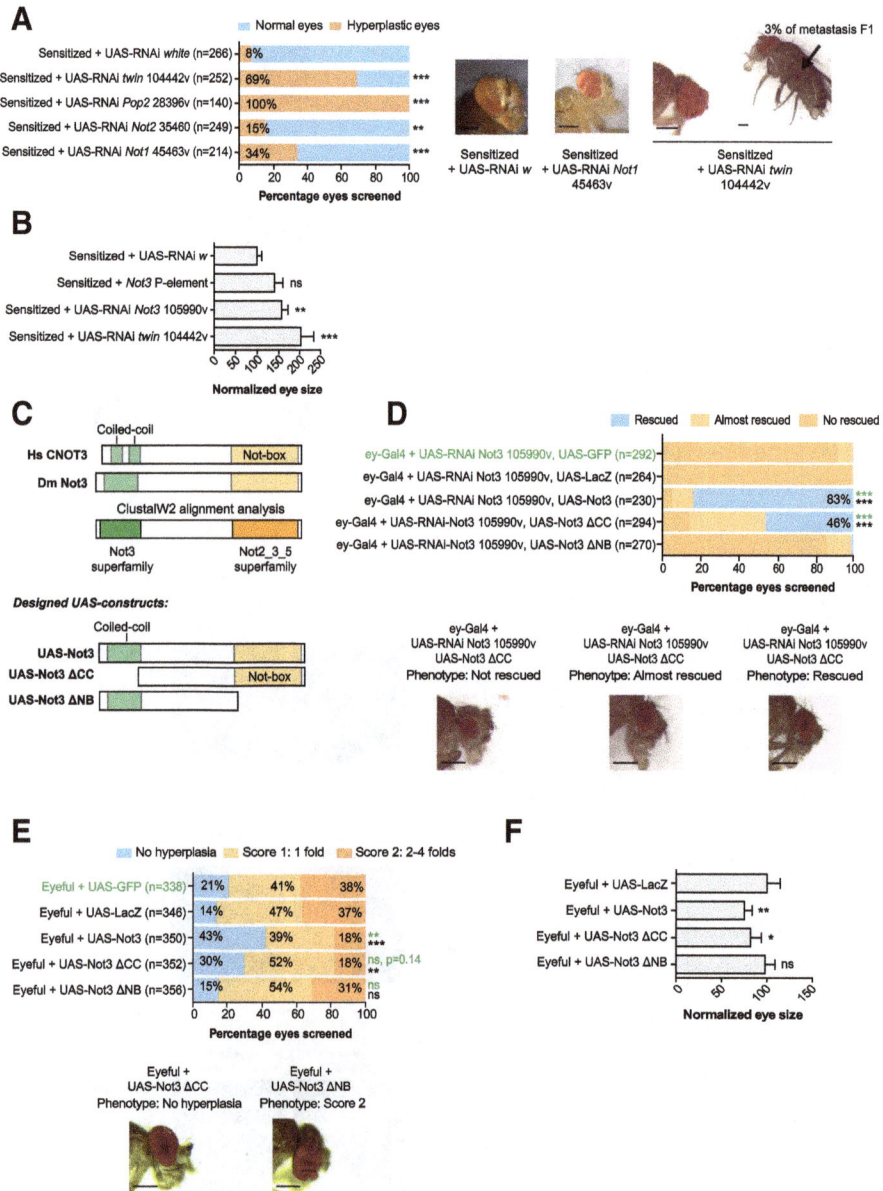

Fig. 4 (See legend on next page.)

Fig. 4 The *Not3* Not-box domain is important for normal protein functionality. **a** Qualitative and quantitative representation of the tumor burden upon downregulation of different CCR4-NOT complex subunits on the sensitized background. Bars show the percentage of eyes screened: blue, normal eyes; orange, hyperplastic eyes; ** $p < 0.01$; *** $p < 0.001$. The mean number of eyes screened is shown on the graph (*Y*-axis) and three independent crosses were established. Microcopy images show the eyes of adult flies from representative genotypes. Scale bars are 200 μM. Black arrow indicates the presence of metastasis. **b** Quantitative representation of the whole eye area (region with presence of differentiated photoreceptors) on representative adult eyes (*n* = 8) with downregulation of *Not3* or *twin* on the sensitized genetic background. Control eyes measured values were considered as 100%; ns, not significant; ** $p < 0.01$; *** $p < 0.001$. **c** Schematic representation of the human CNOT3 and the fly Not3 proteins. ClustalW2 alignment analyses show that the coiled-coil (green) and Not-box (orange) regions are present in both species. Designed UAS constructs are also shown: UAS-Not3 (wild-type Not3), UAS-Not3 ΔCC (deletion of the coiled-coil domain region), UAS-Not3 ΔNB (deletion of the Not-box domain). **d** Qualitative and quantitative representation of the defective eyes upon ectopic expression of Not3, Not3-ΔCC, and Not3-ΔNB on wild-type flies with reduced Not3 expression. The mean number of eyes screened is shown on the graph (*Y*-axis), and three independent crosses were established. Bars show the percentage of eyes screened: blue, normal eyes; light orange, eyes classified as "almost rescued"; dark orange, eyes classified as "not rescued"; *** $p < 0.001$. In green color, comparisons to UAS-GFP control flies; black color, comparison to UAS-LacZ control flies. Microscopy images show the eyes of adult flies from each category. Scale bars are 200 μM. **e** Qualitative and quantitative representation of the defective eyes upon ectopic expression of Not3, Not3-ΔCC, and Not3-ΔNB on eyeful flies. Bars show the percentage of eyes screened: blue, normal eyes; light orange, eyes classified as score 1 (presence of 1 fold); dark orange, eyes classified as score 2 (presence of 2–4 folds); ns, means not significant, ** $p > 0.01$, *** $p < 0.001$. The mean number of eyes screened is shown on the graph (*Y*-axis). In green color, comparisons to UAS-GFP control flies; black color, comparison to UAS-LacZ control flies. Microscopy images show the eyes of adult flies from each category. Scale bars are 200 μM. **f** Quantitative representation of the whole eye area (region with presence of differentiated photoreceptors) on representative adult eyes (*n* = 8) with ectopic expression of *Not3* wild-type or *Not3* mutants on the eyeful genetic background. Control eyes measured values were considered as 100%; ns, not significant; * $p < 0.05$; ** $p < 0.01$

showed that the CC and NB domains are conserved in the Not3 protein from *Drosophila melanogaster* (Fig. 4c). We then characterized which Not3 domains are essential for tumor suppression in the eyeful background. We designed and cloned two versions of the wild-type *Not3* open reading frame in a pUASTattB vector: UAS-*Not3*-ΔCC (lacking the CC domain) and UAS-*Not3*-ΔNB (lacking the NB domain) (Fig. 4c). First, we measured whether the expression levels achieved by ectopic expression of these constructs were similar. Since a good antibody against the Not3 protein from *Drosophila melanogaster* was not available, we co-transfected S2 cells with a pMT-Gal4 plasmid and a flag-tagged version of each of the UAS-Not3 plasmids. Cycloheximide treatment of the transfected cells was also performed in order to investigate the stability of the translated proteins. Our results showed that similar expression levels were achieved with all plasmids and that the translated proteins were equally stable (Additional file 4: Figure S3A).

Next, we engineered transgenic flies expressing the different versions of the wild-type *Not3* open reading frame (without a flag-tag). Since *Not3* is on chromosome 2 on flies, we decided to insert our UAS-*Not3* transgenes on chromosome 3 (site 89E11). Our qPCR analyses showed that ectopic expression of UAS-*Not3* plasmids driven by Actin5C-Gal4 results in similar expression levels among all constructs used in these experiments (Additional file 4: Figure S3B).

Ectopic expression of UAS-*Not3*-ΔCC in *Not3*-defective flies rescued the *Not3* small rough eye phenotype previously observed, while no rescue was observed upon expression of UAS-*Not3*-ΔNB (Fig. 4d). Similar results were observed in the eyeful background. Overexpression of UAS-*Not3*-ΔCC had a mild effect tumor formation

with 30% penetrance, while UAS-*Not3*-ΔNB did not suppress the tumor phenotype at all (Fig. 4e, f).

Taken together, our results show that the NB domain is essential to rescue developmental and cancer phenotypes observed upon downregulation of *Not3*. Since the NB domain is essential for the association of *Not3* with the CCR4-NOT complex [27, 28], these data further indicate that the effects observed with downregulation of *Not3* are linked to its function within the CCR4-NOT complex.

Not3 disruption in the sensitized background causes an aberrant gene expression program

The major role of the CCR4-NOT complex is to regulate mRNA stability through deadenylation of mRNA. To determine which mRNA transcripts are affected by *Not3* knockdown, we carried out RNA-sequencing analysis (Fig. 5a) on L3 larvae eye discs isolated from the sensitized parental, sensitized control (sensitized + UAS-RNAi *white*), and sensitized *Not3-tumor* eye discs: sensitized + *Not3*-Pelement and sensitized + UAS-RNAi *Not3* knockdowns. Correlations were calculated between the mRNA expression profiles of the different samples. High correlations were observed between the different *Not3* knockdown samples. The sensitized + *Not3* P-element samples were more closely related to the control samples, which is in agreement with mild reduction of *Not3* in this model and mild phenotypic effects observed (Fig. 5b).

A differential gene expression analysis was performed between the different *Not3* knockdown models and the sensitized parental, confirming the significant downregulation of *Not3* mRNA levels with an average log2 fold change of − 0.2270. Moreover, these analyses revealed that

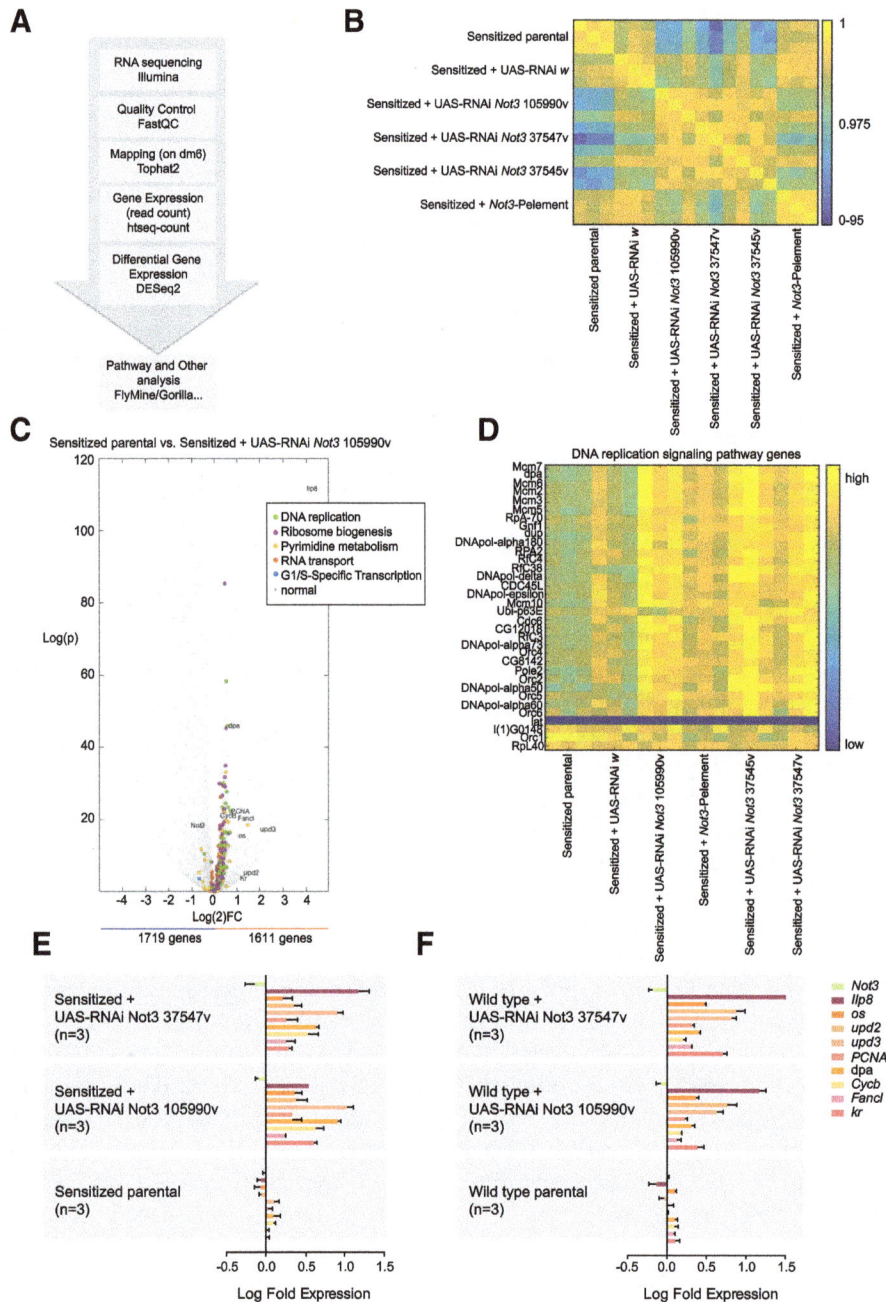

Fig. 5 *Not3* reduced expression in the sensitized background drives oncogenic altered gene expression. **a** Workflow for the analysis of the RNA-sequencing experiments performed on fly eye-antennal eye discs. **b** Correlation matrix between the different samples, calculated on the normalized mRNA expression levels. **c** Volcano plot of all differential genes between sensitized + UAS-RNAi *Not3* 105990v and sensitized parental, which represents the results of three biological replicates. The other *Not3* knockdowns show similar results. The genes belonging to one of the most enriched signaling pathways are marked in color. **d** Matrix showing the normalized mRNA expression levels of those genes that belong to the DNA replication signaling pathway. **e** qPCR validation experiments of selected genes on the sensitized + *Not3* defective tumor models. Data were normalized accordingly to the expression levels on the sensitized + UAS-RNAi *white* eye-antennal discs. Results are plotted as mean ± standard deviation. **f** qPCR validation experiments of selected genes on the ey-Gal4 *Not3* defective models. Data were normalized accordingly to the expression levels on the ey-Gal4 + UAS-RNAi *white* eye-antennal discs. Results are plotted as mean ± standard deviation

approximately 3000 significant differential genes were found on each of the *Not3* knockdowns performed (Additional file 1: Tables S3–S6). Combining the different gene lists revealed 1028 misregulated genes, with 448 and 580 significantly up- and downregulated, respectively (Additional file 1: Table S7).

Gene set enrichment analysis (GSEA) identified DNA replication and ribosome biogenesis as significantly enriched signaling pathways ($p = 4.81E{-}6$ and $p = 9.68E{-}4$, respectively) (Fig. 5c). Notably, we found that 30 out of 34 genes from the DNA replication pathway were significantly upregulated (Fig. 5d). Metabolic, RNA transport and cell cycle signaling pathways were also highly enriched (Additional file 1: Table S8). Of importance, we only identified significantly enriched signaling pathways among the upregulated genes (Fig. 5e). These findings strongly support that the upregulated genes are specific effects of *Not3* knockdown, while downregulated genes may represent secondary effects.

Besides, we also detected upregulation of genes that could be linked to tumorigenesis. These included the pupation regulator insulin-like peptide 8 (*Ilp8*), the three unpaired (*upd*) genes (which encode the ligands for the JAK/STAT pathway), the cyclin B (*Cycb*) cell cycle regulator, and the discs proliferation abnormal (*dpa*) and the *PCNA* genes (Additional file 1: Table S7). Increased expression of those selected genes was further validated by using qPCR on the sensitized and the wild-type models. These results show that downregulation of *Not3* causes the upregulation of those genes specifically and independently of *Dl* ectopic expression (Fig. 5f).

In order to clarify whether Not3 regulates mRNA decay of those target genes or controls the transcription of those genes, we performed an i-CisTarget analysis on the upregulated genes to determine if Not3 DNA-binding sites were present in the promoters of the upregulated genes. We did not see any enrichment of the described Not3 motif [29] (NES = 0.72). Moreover, with PWMtools, we looked for occurrences of the Not3 motif in the promoter sites of these upregulated genes and we found that only a small portion of the genes, not more than expected by chance, has Not3 binding motifs. Next, we tested the stability of some target genes in vitro using Drosophila S2 cells (Additional file 5: Figure S4A–C). Our results show a clear knockdown of the *Not3* mRNA expression (almost 50% efficiency) at time point 0 h, which was associated with significant upregulation of *Cycb*, *fancl*, and *upd2* (Additional file 5: Figure S4B). No significant changes were detected on the expression level of *CG1239*, a gene we used as a control, since its expression was not significantly changed on our RNA-sequencing experiments after *Not3* downregulation (Additional file 5: Figure S4B). Analysis after transcription block provided a view on mRNA stability and changes induced by *Not3* downregulation. *Cycb*, *fancl*, and *upd2* mRNAs showed a moderate increase in stability after *Not3* downregulation when compared with the control condition (YFP expression). Again, no effects were observed on the mRNA stabilization of *CG1239* (Additional file 5: Figure S4C), indicating that the

effects observed are specific. In conclusion, our results show that *Not3* downregulation causes an upregulation of *Cycb*, *fancl*, and *upd2* transcripts in S2 cells and that this can be linked to increased mRNA stability.

Upregulation of CycB contributes to the Not3 tumor phenotype

We decided to investigate the function of seven selected target genes (*Cycb*, *os*, *upd2*, *upd3*, *Fancl*, *PCNA*, and *dpa*) on tumor development by knocking down their expression in the sensitized + *Not3*-tumor model (independent RNAi constructs/loss-of-function mutants were tested per gene). Before doing that, we excluded the possibility that downregulation of the selected genes could already cause defects on the wild-type retina. Downregulation of *PCNA* and *dpa* led to significant developmental defects on the fly's retina, preventing their study in the eye tumor models.

For the other genes, we quantified effects on eye tumor rescue. Knockdown of *CycB* on the sensitized + *Not3*-tumor model yielded the strongest effects. The *cycB* [2] mutant rescued the tumor phenotype to over 50% compared to the control RNAi construct (~ 15% for *white* RNAi). Knockdown of *fancl* and JAK-STAT ligands had minor effects. For instance, knockdown of *upd2*/*upd3* showed rescue of tumor formation in 28% of eyes screened. A trend towards significance ($p = 0.06$) was observed on tumor rescue upon knockdown of *upd3* only (Fig. 6a). Genetic suppression of *os* and *upd3* on the sensitized + *Not3*-tumor animals caused pupal lethality, precluding its analysis. If tumor development associated with *Not3* disruption is linked to the CCR4-NOT complex functionality, downregulation of selected genes could also rescue tumor development in the sensitized + *twin*-tumors. Again, genetic suppression of *Cycb* yielded the strongest effects, with the *cycb* [2] mutant rescuing tumor phenotype to over 50% compared to the control RNAi construct (~ 10% for *white* RNAi) (Fig. 6a). Knockdown of *fancl* and genetic suppression of the JAK-STAT ligands on the sensitized + *twin* background showed a significant effect on tumor rescue (Fig. 6a).

Examination of expression of a 10xSTAT92E-GFP reporter for JAK-STAT pathway activation [30] by immunofluorescence upon *Not3* or *twin* downregulation on the sensitized model was then performed. We observed a significant increase of the 10xSTAT92E-GFP expression domains (Fig. 6b–d). However, since knockdown of JAK-STAT ligands had minor effects on tumor growth rescue, especially upon *Not3* downregulation, it might be that the pathway is active due to alternative mechanisms.

Taken together, our results show that upregulation of *CycB* contributes to the tumor phenotype in our sensitized *Not3* and *twin* tumor models.

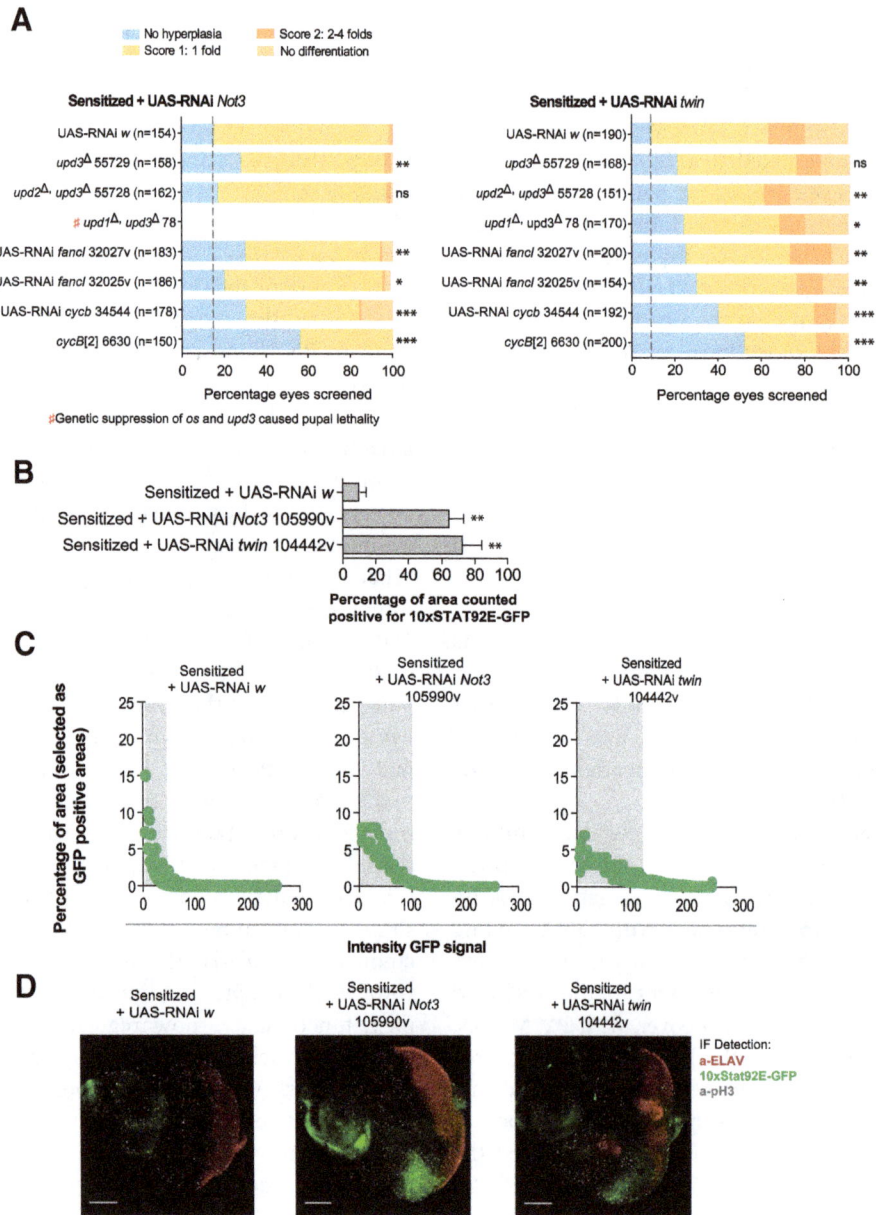

Fig. 6 Upregulation of *cycB* contributes to the tumor phenotype in *Not3* and *twin* sensitized tumor models. **a** Sensitized + *Not3* defective tumor model and sensitized + *twin* defective tumor model. Bar graphs showing rescue scoring results for tumor model or tumor plus knockdown for the indicated gene. Two independent RNAis/mutant lines are shown. Three independent crosses were screened on each experimental condition. The mean number of eyes analyzed is shown on the graph (*Y*-axis). Genetic suppression of *os* and *upd3* on the sensitized + Not3 tumor animals caused pupal lethality precluding its analysis. Blue, no hyperplasia; yellow, score 1: 1 fold; light orange, score 2: 2–4 folds; dark orange, no differentiation; gray, no data available. ns, not significant; * $p < 0.05$; ** $p < 0.01$; *** $p < 0.001$. **b** Quantification of 10xSTAT92E-GFP expression domains on the posterior part of L3 wandering larval eye-antennal discs using the color inspector 3D ImageJ plugin. GFP expression domains were measured by analysis of confocal micrographs and expressed as a percentage of the posterior eye-disc area. Bar graphs show the percentage of areas positive for GFP signal (thus, areas with JAK-STAT signaling activation) from the different genotypes; ** $p < 0.01$. Six eye-antennal discs were analyzed per experimental condition. Experimental crosses were performed in triplicate. Graph shows results from one representative experiment. **c** Dot graphs show the green signal intensity of those areas previously selected as GFP positive areas. We observed that both the area of GFP expression domains and the green intensity of those areas are increased in sensitized + *Not3* ($n = 6$) or sensitized + *twin* tumor eye-antennal discs ($n = 6$). Experimental crosses were performed in triplicate; graph shows results from one representative experiment. **d** Representative confocal images of eye-antennal imaginal discs of the indicated genotypes. Green signal: 10xSTAT92E-GFP; red signal: ELAV protein; white signal: pH3 positive cells. Scale bars are 50 μM

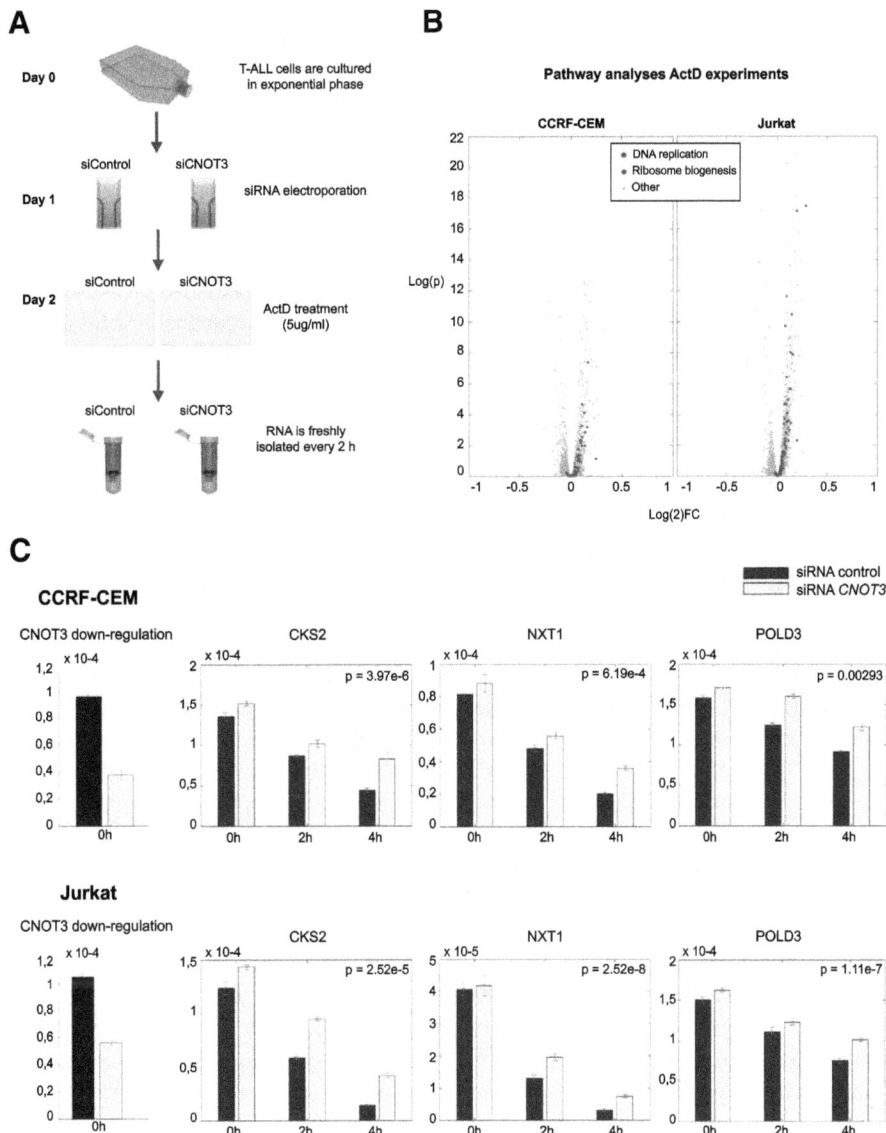

Fig. 7 Loss of CNOT3 leads to stabilization of DNA replication and ribosome biogenesis signaling components in human T-ALL cell lines. **a** Workflow for the Actinomycin D experiments upon CNOT3 downregulation on T-ALL cell lines. Experiments were performed in three independent series. **b** Volcano plots from Jurkat and CCRF-CEM T-ALL cell lines. Those genes belonging to one of the most enriched signaling pathways are marked in color. **c** mRNA expression levels of CNOT3 in all conditions and mRNA expression levels of three exemplary genes that become more stable upon CNOT3 knockdown, i.e., they show an increasing difference between the knockdown and the wild-type. Experiments were performed in three independent series

Loss of CNOT3 leads to stabilization of DNA replication and ribosome biogenesis signaling components in human T-ALL cell lines

Thereafter, we tested if the results obtained in Drosophila could be translated to human T-ALL, since CNOT3 mutations were described in this tumor type. We knocked down *CNOT3* in human T-ALL cell lines JURKAT and CCRF-CEM by using siRNAs (two *CNOT3* specific and a negative control siRNA). We determined effects on steady-state mRNA expression levels and also assessed the effect on RNA stability by blocking transcription and measuring the half-life of mRNA's in a global way by

RNA-seq. We stopped the transcription of newly synthesized mRNA by treating cells with Actinomycin D 24 h after electroporation. RNA was isolated at 0 h (reference time point), 2 h, and 4 h time points after Actinomycin D treatment and submitted to RNA-sequencing (Fig. 7a).

As expected, we observed a clear knockdown of the CNOT3 mRNA expression (almost 50% efficiency) at time point 0 h (Fig. 7b), which was associated with the upregulation of 975 and 1611 transcripts in JURKAT and CCRF-CEM cells, respectively (Additional file 1: Tables S9 and S10). Pathway analysis with DAVID revealed that, similar to our findings in Drosophila, the DNA replication pathway and the ribosome biogenesis pathways were significantly enriched (Fig. 7c, Additional file 1: Tables S11–S13) in both cell lines. RNA-seq analysis at 2 h and 4 h after transcription block provided a genome-wide view on mRNA stability and changes induced by CNOT3 downregulation. Among the significantly upregulated and more stable genes were genes involved in DNA replication pathway and the ribosome biogenesis including *NXT1*, *POLD3*, and *CKS2* (Fig. 7c, Additional file 1: Tables S12 and S13).

Discussion

Mutations on CNOT3, and more rarely in other members of the CCR4-NOT complex, have recently been identified in T-ALL and chronic lymphoblastic leukemia [13, 31]. In solid tumors, recent reports show that CNOT3 and other CCR4-NOT subunits could be involved in tumor formation/progression. Downregulation of *Cnot2* expression results in a significant increase of breast cancer pulmonary metastasis in vivo [32]. Instead, *CNOT3* confers an aggressive behavior in colorectal cancer cells through a self-renewal transcriptional program [33]. Mutations on *CNOT3* have been found in T-ALL patients experiencing treatment failure after first relapse, although this observation needs to be confirmed in a larger cohort of patients [34]. Thus, it seems that depending on the cellular context, those proteins can have either tumor suppressor or oncogenic properties. However, it still remains unclear how mutations on CNOT3 or other CCR4-NOT subunits can contribute to tumor development.

In this report, we show that *Not3* behaves as a classical tumor suppressor, with reduction of *Not3* expression leading to increased tumor formation and overexpression of *Not3* leading to suppressed tumor formation. Interestingly, and in agreement with sequencing data in human cancers, we also observed increased tumor formation upon knockdown of other members of the CCR4-NOT complex, including the deadenylases. These data make clear that the entire CCR4-NOT complex functions as a tumor suppressor complex and that this is likely, at least in part, through its function in mRNA metabolism.

In human cancer, only one allele of CNOT3 is mutated, suggesting that this is sufficient to contribute to tumor development and that complete loss of CNOT3 is not viable for the cells. In fact, our results show that little reduction on *Not3* expression levels in a sensitized/pre-neoplastic background is sufficient to initiate and dramatically increase tumor formation. Conversely, a little reduction on *Not3* expression is not enough to cause defects on wild-type tissues. This is consistent with previous data showing that the presence of only one *Cnot3* allele is enough to sustain normal cell development [6].

Recent structure-function analyses have revealed that CNOT2 and CNOT3 bind to the CCR4-NOT complex through the Not-box domain [27, 28]. We demonstrate that overexpression of a *Not3* mutant lacking the Not-box domain does not rescue neither the *Not3*--downregulated nor the eyeful tumor phenotype. These data confirm that the defects observed in our models are related to the function of *Not3* within the CCR4-NOT complex. In agreement, it has been shown that expression of a CNOT3 mutant lacking the Not-box domain in CNOT3-depleted mouse embryonic fibroblasts was not able to rescue proper formation of the CCR4-NOT complex and the decreased cell viability [35].

To further determine the exact consequences of downregulation of *Not3*, we performed RNA-sequencing on Drosophila eye discs. CNOT3 was described to be involved in transcriptional regulation [26, 32, 35]. However, we did not find evidence that Not3 is directly involved in the transcription of the genes that were upregulated upon Not3 knockdown, as the Not3 DNA-binding motif was not enriched in the promoters of that gene set. Our findings revealed an important role for Cyclin B (*CycB*), a gene known to be upregulated in various cancers [36, 37]. We observed that *CycB* was upregulated upon *Not3* downregulation and stabilized upon *Not3* downregulation in S2 cells in vitro. Moreover, downregulation of *CycB* counteracted tumor formation, illustrating an important role for *CycB* in these tumors.

Our RNA-sequencing analyses also revealed that genes involved in DNA replication and ribosome biogenesis are significantly increased upon *Not3* downregulation. Moreover, we confirmed on human cell lines that the increased mRNA expression level of those genes is due to mRNA stabilization, and not to a significant increased on gene transcription rates. Increased expression of genes involved in DNA replication has been found in cancer cells [38] and might result in increased replication initiation activity at a global level. There is growing evidence that an upregulated ribosome biogenesis might provide an increased risk of cancer onset [39]. Aberrant ribosome synthesis contributes to increased cellular proliferation [40, 41]. Differential expression of several ribosomal protein genes has been observed in cancer [39, 42]. Thus, *Not3/CNOT3* loss could contribute to cancer development through those two signaling pathways.

Conclusions

- We establish for the first time that *Not3* and other members of the CCR4-NOT complex act as tumor suppressor genes.
- Our results indicate that the entire CCR4-NOT complex serves as a tumor suppressor, in part by suppressing transcripts implicated in DNA replication and RNA biogenesis.

Additional files

Additional file 1: Table S1. Fly stocks used in the present study. Table S2 Primers used for cloning and real-time PCR. Table S3 Differential gene analysis. Comparison using the sensitized + UAS-RNAi Not3 105990v as target. Table S4 Differential gene analysis. Comparison using the sensitized + UAS-RNAi Not3 37547v as target. Table S5 Differential gene analysis. Comparison using the sensitized + UAS-RNAi Not3 37545v as target. Table S6 Differential gene analysis. Comparison using the sensitized + Not3 P-element as target. Table S7 List of core differential genes in all 4 comparisons. Table S8 Pathway analyses derived from the gene eye tumor signature, results from a FlyMine analysis. Table S9. Differential genes in Actinomycin D experiments on JURKAT cells. Table S10 Differential genes in Actinomycin D experiments on CCRF-CEM cells. Table S11 Description of the KEGG gene sets. Table S12 KEGG analyses on JURKAT cells. Table S13 KEGG analyses on CCRF-CEM cells. (XLSX 14974 kb)

Additional file 2: Figure S1. Reduced expression levels of twin lead to a change on the number of positive pH3 on eye discs from ey-Gal4 wild type and sensitized fly models. Quantification of the number of pH3 positive cells on the posterior portion of eye-antennal imaginal discs ($n = 10$) from sensitized + twin larvae. Representative confocal images of eye-antennal imaginal discs of the indicated genotypes. Green staining: BrdU, pH3 or cleaved-DCP1a positive cells; red staining: ELAV protein. Results are compared with data of the other genotypes shown in Figs. 2c and 4a. Scale bars are 70 μM. (PDF 4225 kb)

Additional file 3 Figure S2. Expression of the different CCR4-NOT subunits after downregulation on ey-Gal4 wild-type and sensitized fly models. Downregulation of Not1, Not2, Pop2, and twin on wild-type eye-antennal discs and B) Downregulation of Not1, Not2, Pop2, and twin on sensitized eye-antennal discs. Bars represent expression mRNA levels, normalized using Rps13 as house-keeping gene and ey-Gal4 (wild-type) + UAS-RNAi white as reference sample. Each bar represents pool of 40 eye-antennal discs isolated from 40 L3 wandering larvae from two independent crosses. (PDF 390 kb)

Additional file 4: Figure S3. Similar expression levels are achieved and translated proteins are equally stable when we ectopically express the different Not3 constructs. A) The yellow graph bar represents the percentage of transfection achieved on S2 cells. Western blot analyses show protein levels of the different Not3 proteins 24 h after gene expression induction, with or without cycloheximide treatment. No differences on protein expression/stability among the UAS-Not constructs were observed. Asterisks indicate unspecific protein bands. B) qPCR analyses showing the Not3 expression levels on each genotype. Each bar represents the expression value of a pool of 10 individuals. (PDF 422 kb)

Additional file 5: Figure S4. Stabilization of mRNA expression levels of Cycb, fancl, and upd2 upon Not3 downregulation and transcription inhibition on Drosophila S2 cells in vitro. **A)** Percentage of YFP expressing cells upon addition of CuSO4 on the cell media. **B)** Expression of the different genes at time-point 0. Our results show a clear knockdown of the Not3 mRNA expression (almost 50% efficiency) at time point 0 h, which was associated with upregulation of Cycb, fancl, and upd2. **C)** Cycb, fancl, and upd2 mRNAs showed a moderate increase in stability after Not3 downregulation when compared with the control condition (YFP expression). In all figure panels, results are shown as mean ± S.D. Three independent experiments were performed. (PDF 418 kb)

Abbreviations
CC: Coiled coil; Cycb: Cyclin B; Dl: Notch ligand Delta; dpa: Discs proliferation abnormal; GSEA: Gene set enrichment analysis; NB: Not-box; pH3: Phospho-Histone3; T-ALL: T-cell acute lymphoblastic leukemia; upd: Unpaired

Acknowledgements
The rat anti-Elav 7E8A10 antibody developed by Gerald Rubin was obtained from the Developmental Studies Hybridoma Bank. Stocks were obtained from the Bloomington Drosophila Stock Center and the Vienna Drosophila Resource Center. This study was supported by grants from the European Research Council and the Interuniversity Attraction Poles granted by the Federal Office for Scientific, Technical and Cultural Affairs, Brussels, Belgium (JC); the FWO-Vlaanderen (RS); and the European Hematology Association (CV).

Funding
This study was supported by grants from the European Research Council (JC), KU Leuven project financing SymBioSys (JC), the FWO-Vlaanderen (RS), and the European Hematology Association (CV).

Authors' contributions
CV, JC, BH, MA, and GH contributed to the conceptualization of the study. CV, RS, SD, OG, and JY contributed to the methodology and analysis. CV, RS, SD, JC, and BH contributed to the investigation. CV, RS, SD, BH, GH, and JC wrote the manuscript. All authors read and approved the final manuscript.

Consent for publication
This is not applicable for this study.

Competing interests
The authors declare that they have no competing interests.

Author details
[1]Center for Cancer Biology, VIB, Leuven, Belgium. [2]Center for Human Genetics, KU Leuven, Herestraat 49, box 912, B-3000 Leuven, Belgium. [3]Department of Oncology, KU Leuven, Leuven, Belgium. [4]Center for Brain & Disease Research, VIB, Leuven, Belgium. [5]Institut du Cerveau et de la Moelle Epinière (ICM) - Hôpital Pitié-Salpêtrière, UPMC, Sorbonne Universités, Inserm, CNRS, Paris, France. [6]Centro de Investigación Médica Aplicada, Av. de Pío XII, 55, 31008 Pamplona, Spain.

References
1. Collart MA, Panasenko OO. The Ccr4--not complex. Gene. 2012;492:42–53.
2. Shirai Y-T, Suzuki T, Morita M, Takahashi A, Yamamoto T. Multifunctional roles of the mammalian CCR4-NOT complex in physiological phenomena. Front Genet. 2014;5:286.
3. Wahle E, Winkler GS. RNA decay machines: deadenylation by the Ccr4-not and Pan2-Pan3 complexes. Biochim Biophys Acta. 1829;2013:561–70.
4. Ito K, Inoue T, Yokoyama K, Morita M, Suzuki T, Yamamoto T. CNOT2 depletion disrupts and inhibits the CCR4-NOT deadenylase complex and induces apoptotic cell death. Genes Cells. 2011;16:368–79.
5. Ito K, Takahashi A, Morita M, Suzuki T, Yamamoto T. The role of the CNOT1 subunit of the CCR4-NOT complex in mRNA deadenylation and cell viability. Protein Cell. 2011;2:755–63.
6. Morita M, Oike Y, Nagashima T, Kadomatsu T, Tabata M, Suzuki T, et al. Obesity resistance and increased hepatic expression of catabolism-related mRNAs in Cnot3+/− mice. EMBO J. 2011;30:4678–91.
7. Watanabe C, Morita M, Hayata T, Nakamoto T, Kikuguchi C, Li X, et al. Stability of mRNA influences osteoporotic bone mass via CNOT3. Proc Natl Acad Sci U S A. 2014;111:2692–7.
8. Inoue T, Morita M, Hijikata A, Fukuda-Yuzawa Y, Adachi S, Isono K, et al. CNOT3 contributes to early B cell development by controlling Igh rearrangement and p53 mRNA stability. J Exp Med. 2015;212:1465–79.
9. Mayr C, Bartel DP. Widespread shortening of 3′UTRs by alternative cleavage and polyadenylation activates oncogenes in cancer cells. Cell. 2009;138:673–84.
10. Wiestner A, Tehrani M, Chiorazzi M, Wright G, Gibellini F, Nakayama K, et al. Point mutations and genomic deletions in CCND1 create stable truncated cyclin D1 mRNAs that are associated with increased proliferation rate and shorter survival. Blood. 2007;109:4599–606.

11. Rounbehler RJ, Fallahi M, Yang C, Steeves MA, Li W, Doherty JR, et al. Tristetraprolin impairs myc-induced lymphoma and abolishes the malignant state. Cell. 2012;150:563–74.

12. Hodson DJ, Janas ML, Galloway A, Bell SE, Andrews S, Li CM, et al. Deletion of the RNA-binding proteins ZFP36L1 and ZFP36L2 leads to perturbed thymic development and T lymphoblastic leukemia. Nat Immunol. 2010;11:717–24.

13. De Keersmaecker K, Atak ZK, Li N, Vicente C, Patchett S, Girardi T, et al. Exome sequencing identifies mutation in CNOT3 and ribosomal genes RPL5 and RPL10 in T-cell acute lymphoblastic leukemia. Nat Genet. 2013;45:186–90.

14. Vicente C, Schwab C, Broux M, Geerdens E, Degryse S, Demeyer S, et al. Targeted sequencing identifies associations between IL7R-JAK mutations and epigenetic modulators in T-cell acute lymphoblastic leukemia. Haematologica. 2015;100:1301–10.

15. Seki M, Kimura S, Isobe T, Yoshida K, Ueno H, Nakajima-Takagi Y, et al. Recurrent SPI1 (PU.1) fusions in high-risk pediatric T cell acute lymphoblastic leukemia. Nat Genet. 2017;49:1274–81.

16. Liu Z, Hornakova T, Hornakova T, Li F, Staerk J, Staerk J, et al. Acute lymphoblastic leukemia-associated JAK1 mutants activate the Janus kinase/STAT pathway via interleukin-9 receptor alpha homodimers. J Biol Chem. 2009;284:6773–81.

17. La Starza R, Barba G, Demeyer S, Pierini V, Di Giacomo D, Gianfelici V, et al. Deletions of the long arm of chromosome 5 define subgroups of T-cell acute lymphoblastic leukemia. Haematologica. 2016;101:951–8.

18. Bossuyt W, De Geest N, Aerts S, Leenaerts I, Marynen P, Hassan BA. The atonal proneural transcription factor links differentiation and tumor formation in Drosophila. PLoS Biol. 2009;7:e40.

19. Kim D, Pertea G, Trapnell C, Pimentel H, Kelley R, Salzberg SL. TopHat2: accurate alignment of transcriptomes in the presence of insertions, deletions and gene fusions. Genome Biol. 2013;14:R36.

20. Anders S, Pyl PT, Huber W. HTSeq--a Python framework to work with high-throughput sequencing data. Bioinformatics. 2015;31:166–9.

21. Love MI, Huber W, Anders S. Moderated estimation of fold change and dispersion for RNA-seq data with DESeq2. Genome Biol. 2014;15:550.

22. Lyne R, Smith R, Rutherford K, Wakeling M, Varley A, Guillier F, et al. FlyMine: an integrated database for Drosophila and Anopheles genomics. Genome Biol. 2007;8:R129.

23. Dagklis A, Pauwels D, Lahortiga I, Geerdens E, Bittoun E, Cauwelier B, et al. Hedgehog pathway mutations in T-cell acute lymphoblastic leukemia. Haematologica. 2015;100:e102–5.

24. Jiao X, Sherman BT, Huang DW, Stephens R, Baseler MW, Lane HC, et al. DAVID-WS: a stateful web service to facilitate gene/protein list analysis. Bioinformatics. 2012;28:1805–6.

25. Ferres-Marco D, Gutierrez-Garcia I, Vallejo DM, Bolivar J, Gutierrez-Aviño FJ, Dominguez M. Epigenetic silencers and Notch collaborate to promote malignant tumours by Rb silencing. Nature. 2006;439:430–6.

26. Neely GG, Kuba K, Cammarato A, Isobe K, Amann S, Zhang L, et al. A global in vivo Drosophila RNAi screen identifies NOT3 as a conserved regulator of heart function. Cell. 2010;141:142–53.

27. Basquin J, Roudko VV, Rode M, Basquin C, Séraphin B, Conti E. Architecture of the nuclease module of the yeast Ccr4-not complex: the Not1-Caf1-Ccr4 interaction. Mol Cell. 2012;48:207–18.

28. Petit A-P, Wohlbold L, Bawankar P, Huntzinger E, Schmidt S, Izaurralde E, et al. The structural basis for the interaction between the CAF1 nuclease and the NOT1 scaffold of the human CCR4-NOT deadenylase complex. Nucleic Acids Res. 2012;40:11058–72.

29. Hu G, Kim J, Xu Q, Leng Y, Orkin SH, Elledge SJ. A genome-wide RNAi screen identifies a new transcriptional module required for self-renewal. Genes Dev. 2009;23(7):837–48.

30. Bach EA, Ekas LA, Ayala-Camargo A, Flaherty MS, Lee H, Perrimon N, et al. GFP reporters detect the activation of the Drosophila JAK/STAT pathway in vivo. Gene Expr Patterns. 2007;7:323–31.

31. Puente XS, Beà S, Valdés-Mas R, Villamor N, Gutiérrez-Abril J, Martín-Subero JI, et al. Non-coding recurrent mutations in chronic lymphocytic leukaemia. Nature. 2015;526:519–24.

32. Faraji F, Hu Y, Wu G, Goldberger NE, Walker RC, Zhang J, et al. An integrated systems genetics screen reveals the transcriptional structure of inherited predisposition to metastatic disease. Genome Res. 2014;24:227–40.

33. Cejas P, Cavazza A, Yandava CN, Moreno V, Horst D, Moreno-Rubio J, et al. Transcriptional regulator CNOT3 defines an aggressive colorectal cancer subtype. Cancer Res. 2017;77:766–79.

34. Richter-Pechańska P, Kunz JB, Hof J, Zimmermann M, Rausch T, Bandapalli OR, et al. Identification of a genetically defined ultra-high-risk group in relapsed pediatric T-lymphoblastic leukemia. Blood Cancer J. 2017;7:e523.

35. Suzuki T, Kikuguchi C, Sharma S, Sasaki T, Tokumasu M, Adachi S, et al. CNOT3 suppression promotes necroptosis by stabilizing mRNAs for cell death-inducing proteins. Sci Rep. 2015;5:14779.

36. Song Y, Zhao C, Dong L, Fu M, Xue L, Huang Z, et al. Overexpression of cyclin B1 in human esophageal squamous cell carcinoma cells induces tumor cell invasive growth and metastasis. Carcinogenesis. 2008;29:307–15.

37. Yuan J, Yan R, Krämer A, Eckerdt F, Roller M, Kaufmann M, et al. Cyclin B1 depletion inhibits proliferation and induces apoptosis in human tumor cells. Oncogene. 2004;23:5843–52.

38. Kauffmann A, Rosselli F, Lazar V, Winnepenninckx V, Mansuet-Lupo A, Dessen P, et al. High expression of DNA repair pathways is associated with metastasis in melanoma patients. Oncogene. 2008;27:565–73.

39. Ruggero D, Pandolfi PP. Does the ribosome translate cancer? Nat Rev Cancer. 2003;3:179–92.

40. Boon K, Caron HN, van Asperen R, Valentijn L, Hermus MC, van Sluis P, et al. N-myc enhances the expression of a large set of genes functioning in ribosome biogenesis and protein synthesis. EMBO J. 2001;20:1383–93.

41. Shenoy N, Kessel R, Bhagat TD, Bhattacharyya S, Yu Y, McMahon C, et al. Alterations in the ribosomal machinery in cancer and hematologic disorders. J Hematol Oncol. 2012;5:32.

42. Kim J-H, You K-R, Kim IH, Cho B-H, Kim C-Y, Kim D-G. Over-expression of the ribosomal protein L36a gene is associated with cellular proliferation in hepatocellular carcinoma. Hepatology. 2004;39:129–38.

6

Past, present, and future of Bcr-Abl inhibitors: from chemical development to clinical efficacy

Federico Rossari[1,2]*, Filippo Minutolo[3] and Enrico Orciuolo[4]

Abstract

Bcr-Abl inhibitors paved the way of targeted therapy epoch. Imatinib was the first tyrosine kinase inhibitor to be discovered with high specificity for Bcr-Abl protein resulting from t(9, 22)-derived Philadelphia chromosome. Although the specific targeting of that oncoprotein, several Bcr-Abl-dependent and Bcr-Abl-independent mechanisms of resistance to imatinib arose after becoming first-line therapy in chronic myelogenous leukemia (CML) treatment.

Consequently, new specific drugs, namely dasatinib, nilotinib, bosutinib, and ponatinib, were rationally designed and approved for clinic to override resistances. Imatinib fine mechanisms of action had been elucidated to rationally develop those second- and third-generation inhibitors. Crystallographic and structure-activity relationship analysis, jointly to clinical data, were pivotal to shed light on this topic. More recently, preclinical evidence on bafetinib, rebastinib, tozasertib, danusertib, HG-7-85-01, GNF-2, and 1,3,4-thiadiazole derivatives lay promising foundations for better inhibitors to be approved for clinic in the near future.

Notably, structural mechanisms of action and drug design exemplified by Bcr-Abl inhibitors have broad relevance to both break through resistances in CML treatment and develop inhibitors against other kinases as targeted chemotherapeutics.

Keywords: Bcr-Abl, Structure-activity relationship, Leukemia, Targeted therapy, Tyrosine kinase inhibitors (TKIs), Imatinib, Dasatinib, Nilotinib, Bosutinib, Ponatinib

Background

The vast majority of chronic myelogenous leukemia (CML) cases and 20–30% of those of acute lymphoblastic leukemia (ALL) are caused by a reciprocal chromosomal translocation between chromosome 9 and 22—t(9, 22)—thus forming the so-called Philadelphia chromosome (Ph) [1]. The product of this genetic rearrangement consists in Bcr-Abl fusion protein with deregulated tyrosine kinase activity that leads immune precursors to divide endlessly. That was the first innovative prove of a disease to be caused and marked by an acquired chromosomal translocation.

As the fusion protein was recognized to be the *primum movens* of those leukemias in the 1980s, the

therapeutic effort was directed towards that specific target, trying to emulate the successful breakthrough of tamoxifen in breast cancer, the very first "targeted therapy" [2]. Imatinib (STI571) was therefore discovered as the first selective Bcr-Abl tyrosine kinase inhibitor (TKI) by means of drug screening approach [3, 4].

Despite the increase in overall survival allowed by imatinib [5], drug resistance onset led scientists to investigate imatinib fine structural mechanism of action to develop new and more effective compounds against mutated forms of Bcr-Abl. Most of resistances rely on Bcr-Abl aminoacidic substitutions, mainly within the kinase domain. One of the most frequent mutations, ranging from 2 to 20% of CML cases [6], is T315I (isoleucine replaces threonine in position 315 of Bcr-Abl), which is also the deadliest case since it leads to resistance to second-generation TKIs, such as nilotinib and dasatinib [7, 8]. Only with the advent of ponatinib has it been possible to overcome that further therapeutic

* Correspondence: f.rossari@santannapisa.it
[1]Institute of Life Sciences, Scuola Superiore Sant'Anna, Piazza Martiri della Libertà, 33, 56127 Pisa, PI, Italy
[2]University of Pisa, Pisa, Italy
Full list of author information is available at the end of the article

hurdle [9]. Therefore, Bcr-Abl inhibitors represent a model for paving the way towards the development of new small molecules for targeted therapy.

Here, we review the rational development of the latter TKIs that allow the already-high CML survival to become even higher, approaching totality of cases [10]. Specific in vitro potency of TKIs will be compared in term of IC_{50} in cell proliferation assays testing target kinases (50% inhibitory concentration (IC_{50})is defined as the drug concentration resulting in 50% cell growth inhibition that corresponds to the fraction affected of 0.5). IC_{50} values of the debated TKIs are summarized in Table 1. Clinical effects will instead be reported accordingly to the end points of the most authoritative trials on the subject.

Main text
Structural data of Bcr-Abl fusion protein
Crystallographic analysis of Bcr-Abl protein highlights a two-lobe catalytic domain: N- and C-lobes towards N- and C-terminus of the sequence, respectively (Fig. 1). β-Sheets compose the former, whereas α-helices prevail in the latter. An important Wolker loop (also known as phosphate-binding or P-loop) links two β-sheets of N-lobe. Thanks to its high flexibility, a P-loop residue can interpose between β- and γ-phosphates of bound adenosine triphosphate (ATP), thus promoting phosphoric anhydride bond break after nucleophilic attack from Asp363 of the so-called catalytic loop [11]. The hinge region, which links the two lobes, also participates in ATP binding by two hydrogen bonds. Within the ATP-binding pocket, a "gatekeeper" residue, Thr315, interacts with ATP, too; furthermore, it plays a key role in conferring selectivity to some of the Bcr-Abl inhibitors. Indeed, Thr315 is located at the peak of one of the multiple hydrophobic "spikes" connecting C- and N-lobes in active conformation [12].

At one portion of the C-lobe, a pivotal loop with regulatory function stems out. Thanks to its mobility, this "activation loop" can alter its conformation to activate and inactivate the kinase. On a structural point of view, the activation loop has in turn three key portions: a DFG (Asp-Phe-Gly) motif at the N-terminus, a central tyrosine residue (Tyr393), and the peptide substrate-binding C-terminus [11]. During active phase, the former contributes with its Asp381 residue in coordinating Mg^{2+} ions, key cofactors of catalysis, whereas the latter accommodates the peptide substrate to be phosphorylated. Tyr393, instead, is the Abl target residue whose phosphorylation leads to loop extension and assumption of kinase active conformation. This conformation shows a high grade of similarity among various kinase families, thus justifying the greater number of TKIs developed towards the conversely more

characteristic inactive conformation. In fact, the latter conformation displays the activation loop folding in towards ATP-binding site, hence avoiding ATP entrance. This arrangement dislocates the DFG motif out of the catalytic site (here the name "DFG-out" conformation) and prevents Mg^{2+}-mediated catalysis. Conversely, the active conformation is also known as "DFG-in," since the activation loop protrudes out from the ATP-binding pocket, confining DFG motif inside the catalytic site. While the latter conformation is shared by different kinases, the former defines a peculiar site among the dislocated activation loop, the gatekeeper residue, and the C-lobe, which has been set as the main target in the development of specific TKIs [13].

Counterintuitively, even if the chimeric oncoprotein is known to be hyperactive to cause leukemia, after each substrate phosphorylation step, the Asp363 residue gets transiently protonated (Fig. 2), leading to conformational changes and a consequent inactivation, which allows inhibitor binding. This represents the reason why the DFG-out inhibitors are effective despite the kinase hyperactivity in the tumor. As previously told, the Thr315 residue is pivotal in stabilizing active conformation: its replacement by isoleucine (T315I) prevents conformational changes to inactive form, therefore conferring resistance to several DFG-out inhibitors [12].

First-generation inhibitor: imatinib
In the early 1990s, a screening for protein kinase C (PKC) inhibitors was carried out and led to the identification of a phenylaminopyrimidine derivative as potential lead compound with high prospective for diversity, allowing simple chemistry to produce more potent and selective molecules against several kinases [14]. At first, a pyridyl group was added at the 3′-position of the pyrimidine to boost its cellular activity. Various functional groups were then tested as substituents in the phenyl ring, until the presence of an amide group was found to confer inhibitory action against tyrosine kinases. Furthermore, analysis of structure-activity relationships evidenced that a substitution in position 6 of the diaminophenyl ring abolished the activity against PKC. Conversely, the addition of a methyl group in an *ortho* position to the amino group increased selectivity for Bcr-Abl. However, the resulting molecule still showed poor oral bioavailability and solubility in water, which were considerably improved by the introduction of an N-methylpiperazine group. Nevertheless, in spite of the abovementioned improvements and of the increased affinity of the resulting molecule for its target, the N-methylypiperazine addition would have generated an aniline moiety in the structure. To abolish its mutagenic potential, the abovementioned amide group and a spacer benzene ring were introduced [14]. These structural

Table 1 Activity of tyrosine kinase inhibitors against wild-type and mutated kinases, expressed as IC$_{50}$ (nM) in cellular assays

Kinase		TKI										GNF-2 + dasatinib (dasatinib concentration)	GNF-5 + nilotinib (nilotinib concentration)
		Imatinib	Nilotinib	Dasatinib	Bosutinib	Ponatinib	Bafetinib	Rebastinib	Tozasertib	Danusertib	HG-7-85-01		
Abl													
P-loop	WT	100–500	<10–25	0.8–1.8	41.6	0.5	72	19–80	10–104	26–360	58.5	100 (2 nM)	30 (1 µM)
	M244V	1600–3100	38–39	1.3	147.4	2.2	240	78–90					
	L248V	1866–10,000	49.5–919	9.4	145.6	1.7							
	G250E	1350–>20,000	48–219	1.8–8.1	179.2	4.1	160	98–600	180				
	Q252H	734–3120	16–70	3.4–5.6	33.7	2.2	410	24–190	130		50–100		
	Y253F	>6400–8953	182–725	6.3–11	40	2.8	81	39	80				
	Y253H	>6400–17,700	450–1300	1.3–10	24.9	6.2		56–300	190		500–1000		
	E255K	3174–12,100	118–566	5.6–13	394	14	540	127–251	84	470	500–1000		
	E255V	6111–8953	430–725	6.3–11	230.1	36	1400	850					
C-helix	D276G	1147	35.3	2.6	25	1.05							
	E279K	1872	36.5–75	3	39.7	1.5							
ATP-binding region	V299L	540–814	23.7	15.8–18	1086	0.3		72	200		500–1000		
	F311L	480–1300	23	1.3				140					
	T315I	>6400–>20,000	697–>10,000	137–>1000	1890	11	>10,000	13–200	30–74	120	140	3300 (1 µM)	300 (1 µM)
	T315A	125	27–67.5	760	249.6	1.6		19–64	88				
	F317L	810–7500	39.2–91	7.4–18	100.7	1.1	760	36–280	84		500–1000		
	F317V	500	350	17–38	478.4	10		223					
Catalytic segment	M351T	880–4900	7.8–38	1.1–1.6	29.1	1.5	150	14–86	65	510	250–500		
	F359V	1400–1825	91–175	2.2–2.7	38.6	10	1300	138–350					
	V379I	1000–1630	51	0.8									
Activation loop	L384M	674–2800	39–41.2	4	19.5	1.1							
	L387M	1000–1100	49	2									
	H396R	1750–5400	41–55	1.3–3	33.7	2.95		290					
	H396P	850–4300	41–43	0.6–2	18.1	1.1	95	66–81	160				
C-term	F486S	2728–9100	32.8–87	5.6	96.1	1.05	470				500		
cKit (CD117)													
	WT	100–150	14.7	79	6313	12.5	840	424–538			>1000		
	D816V	3800	500	37	2772	72–143	3800		100				
	V560G	75	108	585	181	165	51		>2000				
	V559D	3927	297	432		11					250–500		

Handbook of Hematology and Oncology

Table 1 Activity of tyrosine kinase inhibitors against wild-type and mutated kinases, expressed as IC_{50} (nM) in cellular assays (Continued)

Kinase	TKI										GNF-2 + dasatinib (dasatinib concentration)	GNF-5 + nilotinib (nilotinib concentration)
	Imatinib	Nilotinib	Dasatinib	Bosutinib	Ponatinib	Bafetinib	Rebastinib	Tozasertib	Danusertib	HG-7-85-01		
PDGFR α												
WT	100	3–71	13–16	>10,000	1.1	56	60–80					
T674I	>5000	376	>500		9					6.25		
D842V	642	1310	62		154	1281				1000		
V561D	10	10				59				>1000		
PDGFR β												
WT	39	60.11	4	>10,000		>1000	103–123			<100		
T681I	>25,000									>1000		
Aurora A, B, C							>5000	4–27	13–79			
Src	>10,000		0.8	1.2	2.2	1700	34					
Lyn	352	1281				19	29					
References	[20, 69–72]	[20, 69, 71, 73–75]	[69, 76–78]	[69, 79, 80]	[69, 79, 81, 82]	[36, 70, 83]	[39, 40, 84]	[40, 85]	[48, 86]	[50]	[53]	[87]

Here, IC_{50} values related to cell growth assays of tyrosine kinase inhibitors (TKIs) against their main targets, both unmutated (WT) and mutated, are shown in nanomolar units. Regarding Abl kinase, domains harboring specific mutations are displayed on the left of the table. Range values represent either intra- or inter-study variability, while the missing ones are still unavailable to the best of our knowledge, representing putative objectives to be determined in future studies. The activity spectrum of the newest inhibitors, namely rebastinib, tozasertib, danusertib, HG-7-85-01, and GNF, should be characterized in further details to fill the current data gap

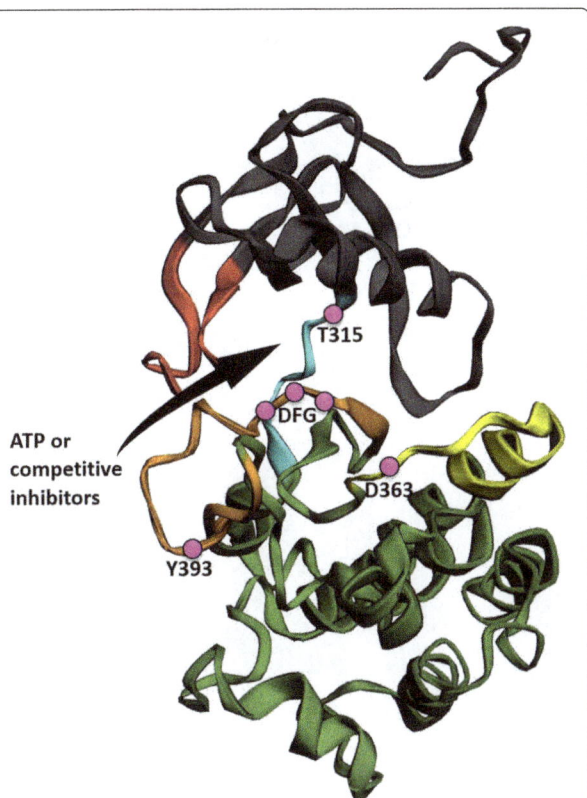

Fig. 1 Structural 3D model of Bcr-Abl catalytic domain. The ribbon diagram of crystal structure shows the *N*-lobe at the top (dark gray) and *C*-lobe at the bottom (green), rich in β-sheets and α-helices respectively. The catalytic segment (yellow), the P-loop (red), the activation loop (orange), and the hinge region (light blue) stand in the middle. Key amino acidic residues are indicated in magenta circles: Thr315 (T315) is the gatekeeper residue within the ATP-binding pocket (black arrow), Asp363 (D363) is pivotal for nucleophilic attack on peptide substrate during catalysis, Tyr393 (Y393) is the target of phosphorylation that controls Abl activation and inactivation, whereas the DFG (Asp-Phe-Gly) motif coordinates fundamental cofactors for catalysis, namely Mg^{2+} ions [88]

interacts with gatekeeper Thr315 through both hydrogen bond (H-b) and Van der Waals (VdW) interactions. The two substituents, instead, are splayed at about 120°, fitting the adenine-binding site and the abovementioned peculiar site of the DFG-out conformation, respectively. The former is shielded from the solvent in a hydrophobic cage delimited by Tyr253 of the P-loop (which is kinked during the inactive phase), Phe382 of the activation loop, together with Leu248, Phe317 and Leu370 residues; the latter preeminently establishes VdW interactions with the following Bcr-Abl residues: Val289 and Met290 of the *C*-lobe, Asp381 of the DFG motif, and Ile360 and His361 of the catalytic loop [11].

Overall, the majority of imatinib interactions are of weak VdW type, but also six highly energetic H-bs take place: each of these accounts for a relative high portion of the total binding energy of the complex kinase-inhibitor, thus providing a theoretical explanation for resistance due to mutations of H-b donor/acceptor residues. In fact, if one of these bonds and consequently its energetic contribution gets lost, free energy of dissociated state becomes highly competitive against that of the bound state, thus justifying the missed interaction between imatinib and the mutated kinase due to less favorable thermodynamic factors: that underlies resistance.

Mechanisms of resistance to imatinib

Imatinib treatment fails in approximately one third of patients [18]. Underlying mechanisms of resistance are classically divided into two types: Bcr-Abl-dependent and Bcr-Abl-independent mechanisms. The latter consists mainly in increased drug efflux/decreased uptake and activation of alternative onco-pathways. The former, instead, are mainly due to point mutations of Bcr-Abl that alter inhibitor binding or conformational changes; nevertheless, a residual amount of Bcr-Abl-dependent resistances are also due to gene amplification or hyperexpression [19].

Since the vast majority of cases are due to point mutations, new inhibitors have been developed with a rational drug design approach aimed at overriding resistances by loosening conformational and binding requirements without losing specificity. Second-generation inhibitors solve almost the entirety of mutations except for T315I. The substitution of the gatekeeper residue frustrates the action of inhibitors through two potent mechanisms: break of a H-b and strong stabilization of the active DFG-in conformation. This consistent obstacle has been overcome only thanks to third-generation inhibitors [20].

Clinically approved second-generation inhibitors

In order to break through mutations, several second-generation TKIs have been developed and approved for clinics, i.e., nilotinib and dasatinib as

developments led to the production of imatinib (STI571) (Fig. 3), the first known ATP competitor able to inhibit Bcr-Abl kinase with high selectivity (but not absolute specificity: wild-type (WT) platelet-derived growth factor receptor (PDGFR) and c-Kit are inhibited, too, as demonstrated by similar IC_{50} values of approximately 100–150 nM for all three kinases [15], see Table 1) and to be approved in the clinics in 2001, less than a decade later its experimental production [5, 16]. Docking studies and X-ray crystallography evidence that imatinib interacts with its target through binding the hinge region in its entire width [17].

Imatinib consists in a typical bisarylanilino core comprising a phenyl ring on one side and a pyridine-pyrimidine moiety on the other side, possessing a benzamide-piperazine group in the meta-position of the aniline-type nitrogen atom (Fig. 3). The core

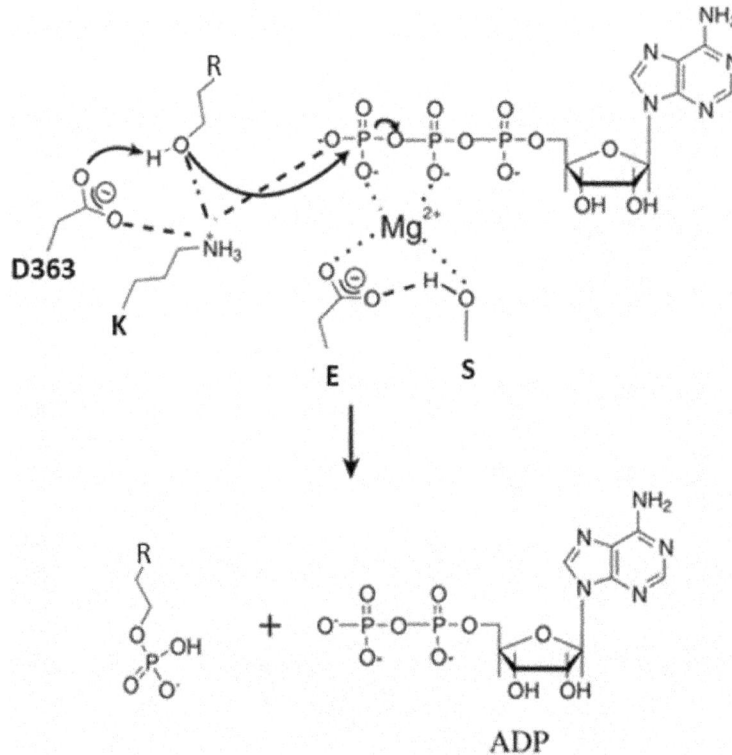

Fig. 2 Asp363 protonation during catalysis. Here, the reaction mechanism of substrate phosphorylation is shown. The nucleophilic attack of D363 on hydroxyl group of peptide substrate leads to its transient protonation that in turn causes conformational changes to inactive state. (R = peptide substrate, D = aspartate, K = lysine, E = glutamate, S = serine)

either first or second line of treatment, and bosutinib as second line only [21].

Nilotinib (AMN107) shows greater potency and effectiveness against almost the totality of resistance-conferring mutations (see Table 1 for IC$_{50}$ values), except for T315I and few others, in newly diagnosed Ph+ CML patients [22, 23]. This result has been reached starting from the structure of imatinib by inverting the amide linking group, by replacing the piperazine ring with 3-methylimidazole, and by adding trifluoro-methyl group to the anilinocarbonyl substituent, in order to increase the number of VdW interactions (Fig. 4a). Therefore, energetic contribution to the total of each H-b decreases, avoiding impairment of inhibitor binding in case of mutation of key residues involved in H-b interactions, although the overall number of H-bs was kept unchanged. In spite of these modifications, less stringent binding requirements did not compromise selectivity and potency of nilotinib, which conversely are even increased when compared to those of imatinib (IC$_{50}$ values of 10–25 and 100–500 nM, respectively—see Table 1). As previously told, nilotinib is active against DFG-out conformation only, and this accounts for T315I resistance. Interestingly, nilotinib is not substrate of neither influx transporter nor efflux P-glycoprotein pump, unlike imatinib and, therefore, is

not sensitive to Bcr-Abl-independent mechanisms of resistance [24].

Dasatinib (BMS-354825) is a peculiar DFG-in inhibitor, even though it is not effective in the case of T315I mutation [22]. Compared to imatinib, dasatinib enables patients with chronic phase CML to achieve faster and deeper treatment responses (i.e., median time to major molecular response (MMR) for dasatinib arm was 15 versus 36 months for the imatinib arm, and BCR-ABL transcript 4.5-log reduction was achieved by 17 versus 8% of patients by 24 months, respectively) [25]. Structurally, the core phenyl ring has been replaced by an aminothiazole group which occupies the adenine pocket of Abl (Fig. 4b). The pyridine group of imatinib is instead replaced by a hydroxyethyl piperazine, which remains solvent-exposed also after Bcr-Abl binding. Dasatinib is a smaller molecule than imatinib and it establishes less interactions with its targets: nuclear magnetic resonance studies have evidenced that dasatinib binds Bcr-Abl very versatilely, in both active and inactive conformations [26]. However, the free inactive DFG-out conformation has a higher entropy than the active conformation: the drop in entropy is less pronounced after dasatinib binding if the target is active, with enthalpy variation being very similar in both conformations. Thus, free energy

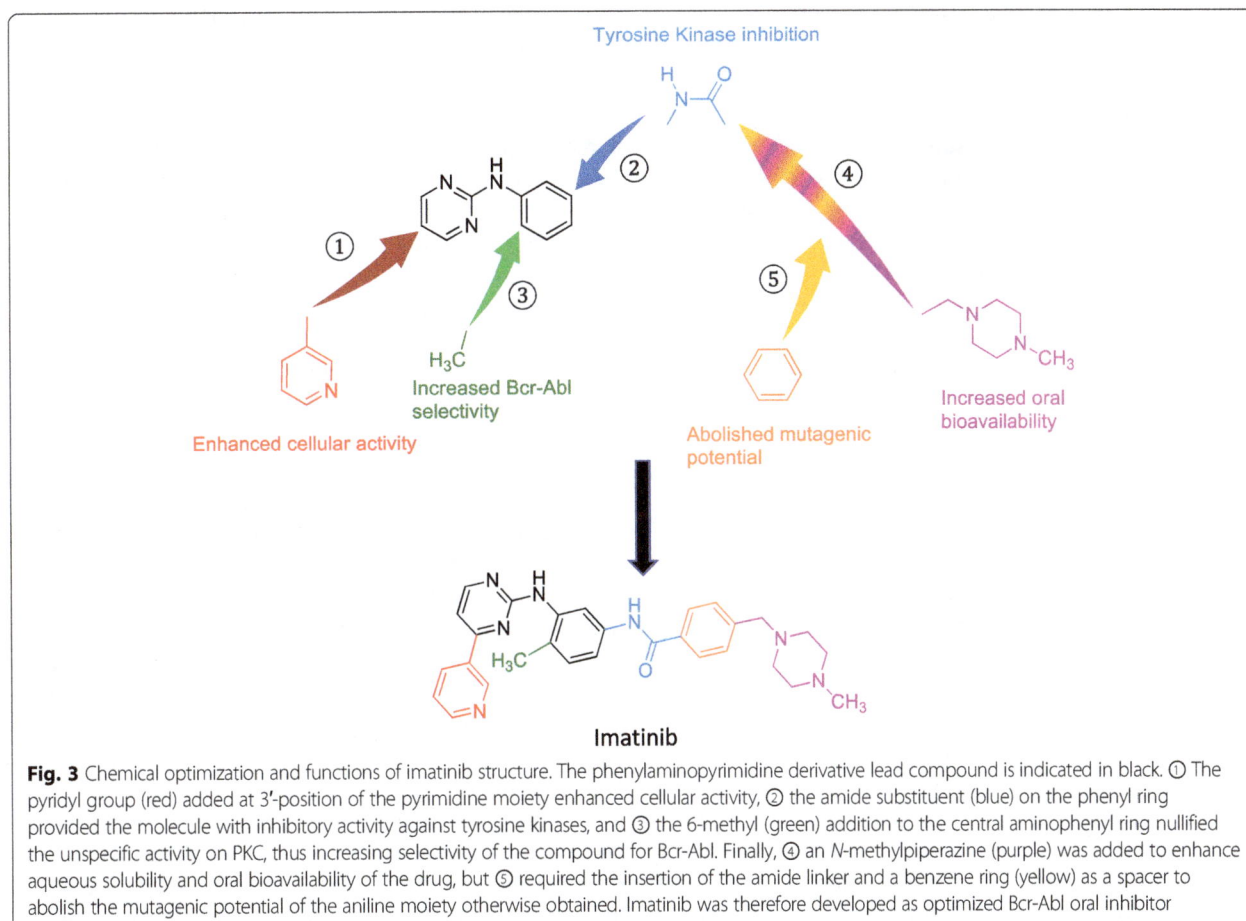

Fig. 3 Chemical optimization and functions of imatinib structure. The phenylaminopyrimidine derivative lead compound is indicated in black. ① The pyridyl group (red) added at 3'-position of the pyrimidine moiety enhanced cellular activity, ② the amide substituent (blue) on the phenyl ring provided the molecule with inhibitory activity against tyrosine kinases, and ③ the 6-methyl (green) addition to the central aminophenyl ring nullified the unspecific activity on PKC, thus increasing selectivity of the compound for Bcr-Abl. Finally, ④ an *N*-methylpiperazine (purple) was added to enhance aqueous solubility and oral bioavailability of the drug, but ⑤ required the insertion of the amide linker and a benzene ring (yellow) as a spacer to abolish the mutagenic potential of the aniline moiety otherwise obtained. Imatinib was therefore developed as optimized Bcr-Abl oral inhibitor

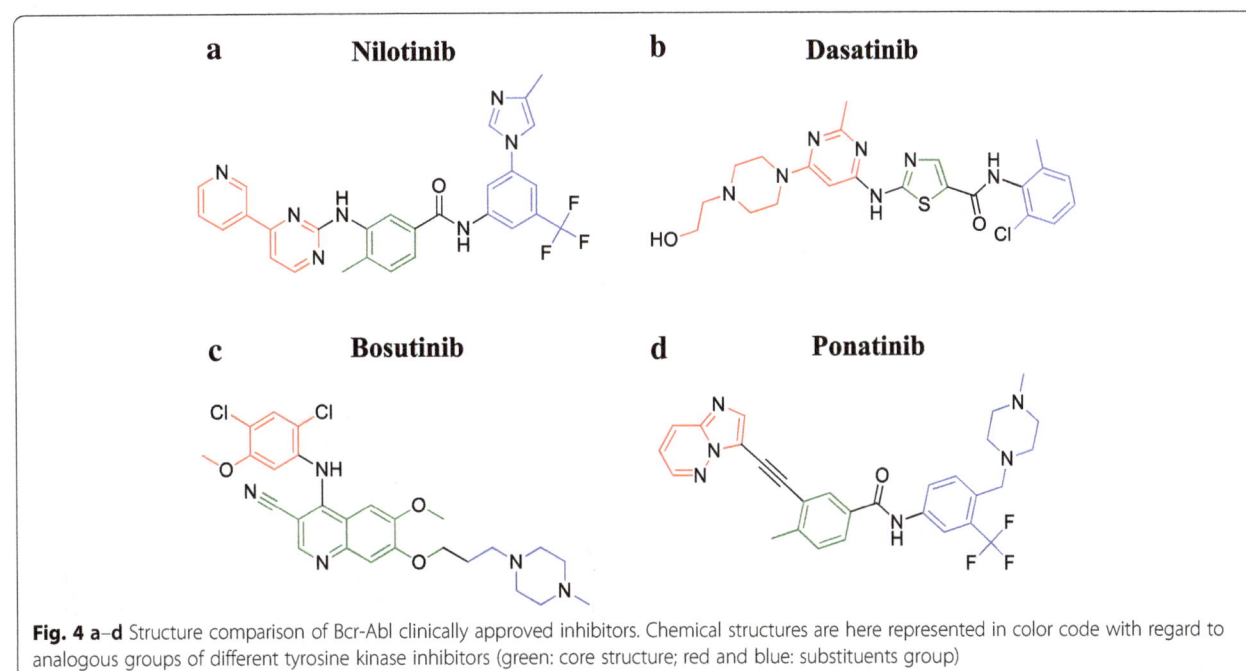

Fig. 4 a–d Structure comparison of Bcr-Abl clinically approved inhibitors. Chemical structures are here represented in color code with regard to analogous groups of different tyrosine kinase inhibitors (green: core structure; red and blue: substituents group)

decreases more in case of binding during DFG-in phase, which is therefore preferentially inhibited by dasatinib, because it is thermodynamically favored. Consequently, several conformation-altering mutations, except for T315I, are susceptible to dasatinib action, anyway [27].

Bosutinib (SKI-606) has a more different structure (Fig. 4c), since it has been developed from a leading Src inhibitor compound (4-[(2,4-dichlorophenyl)amino]-6,7-dimethoxy-3-quinolinecarbonitrile) [28]. The quinoline central core required the addition of a hydrophilic protonable N-methylpiperazino moiety. Though it is not effective against T315I mutation and does not show total selectivity for Bcr-Abl (see Table 1), it has the important advantage of being not efficiently excreted by multidrug resistance transporters [29, 30]. Bosutinib is currently approved as second-line treatment of CML [21]. Recent data suggest it can be an important alternative to imatinib for previously untreated patients with chronic phase CML, given its earlier and higher rate of responses (47.2 and 36.9% of MMR at 12 months for bosutinib and imatinib, respectively) [31].

Third-generation inhibitor: ponatinib

To date, the only approved third-generation TKI is ponatinib (AP24534), a dual Src/Abl inhibitor designed to especially overcome T315I mutation. In fact, isoleucine in position 315 complicates Bcr-Abl switching to inactive conformation and H-b formation with DFG-out inhibitors. Nonetheless, ethynyl linkage of ponatinib has indeed been inserted to accommodate isoleucine side chain without any steric interference also in inactive conformation (DFG-out) [32]. Structurally (Fig. 4d), it nicely overlaps to nilotinib with only small differences other than ethynyl linker: the methyl imidazole group is replaced by a methyl piperazine moiety (like in imatinib). Besides, instead of the pyridine-pyrimidine group of nilotinib, ponatinib has a terminal imidazo[1,2-b]pyridazin portion in the same position to optimize H-b formation within the hydrophilic pocket in which it gets accommodated. Other bonds are similar to those of nilotinib and so abundant that kinase point mutations have less effect on the overall binding affinity and the potency of the drug (see Table 1, ponatinib IC_{50} are the lowest for almost every Bcr-Abl point mutation) [33]. Clinically, all these structural modifications result in a high activity in heavily pretreated patients with Ph+ leukemias with resistance to other inhibitors, including patients with T315I mutation, other mutations, or no mutations (in [34], out of 43 patients with those characteristics, 98% had a complete hematologic response, 72% a major cytogenetic response, and 44% a MMR). Moreover, ponatinib has recently been demonstrated a valuable alternative to allogeneic stem cell transplantation in patients with T315I-positive advanced CML and Ph+ ALL [9].

Preclinically validated inhibitors: the targeted therapies of tomorrow?

Other molecules have been effectively tested since the advent of second-generation inhibitors, but have not entered common clinical practice for neither CML nor ALL, yet. Namely, they are bafetinib, rebastinib, tozasertib, danusertib, HG-7-85-01, GNF-2 and -5, and 1,3,4 thiadiazole derivatives. Furthermore, it is highly probable that new in silico and in vitro evidences may lead to new molecules to enter the clinics in the near future to overcome persistent resistances.

Bafetinib (INNO-406) development was aimed at extending the susceptibility spectrum of mutations to TKIs and increasing selectivity towards Bcr-Abl to reduce clinical adverse reactions during treatment, e.g., cardiovascular and metabolic toxicities of nilotinib [35]. That was pursued by increasing hydrophobic properties of the benzamide ring of imatinib (Fig. 5a): a trifluoro-methyl group, similarly to nilotinib, was added to increase VdW interactions in the abovementioned "hydrophobic cage" [36]. In the meantime, in light of X-ray crystallography predictions, the pyridine group of imatinib was replaced by a more hydrophilic pyrimidine ring, thus increasing aqueous solubility without impairing binding properties and potency against Bcr-Abl (IC_{50} 71 nM) [17]. Finally, the dimethylaminopyrrolidine portion took the place of the N-methylpiperazine ring, favoring H-b formation [36]. In this way, its activity is retained against several Bcr-Abl mutants (submicromolar IC_{50}, see Table 1), with the exception of a minority including T315I ($IC_{50} > 10$ μM) [37]. A phase I clinical trial evidenced that 19% of CML and Ph + ALL patients with imatinib resistance or intolerance reached the complete cytogenetic response after bafetinib as second-line treatment, suggesting its potential clinical efficacy [38]. Differently from some solid tumors, a phase II trial for CML and ALL is not ongoing, yet.

Rebastinib (DCC-2036) is a non-competitive conformational control inhibitor, designed to overcome Abl gatekeeper mutations, mainly T315I, that impede the occurrence of the DFG-out conformation and the inhibitory action of both first- and second-generation inhibitors [39]. It stabilizes a fundamental bond for inactive conformation between Glu282 and Arg386, regardless gatekeeper mutations. Structurally, the fluoro-substituted phenyl central core, possessing a ureic linker in *ortho* to the halogen atom, is also bound to a carboxamide-substituted pyridine on one side, and to a pyrazole, bearing 4-*tert*-butyl and 1-(6-quinolinyl) substituents, on the other side (Fig. 5b). Crystallography evidenced that the ureic and the carboxamide-pyridine groups establish five H-bs mainly with the aforementioned Glu282 and Arg386 residues, whereas the rest of the molecule optimizes VdW interactions with a hydrophobic cluster of

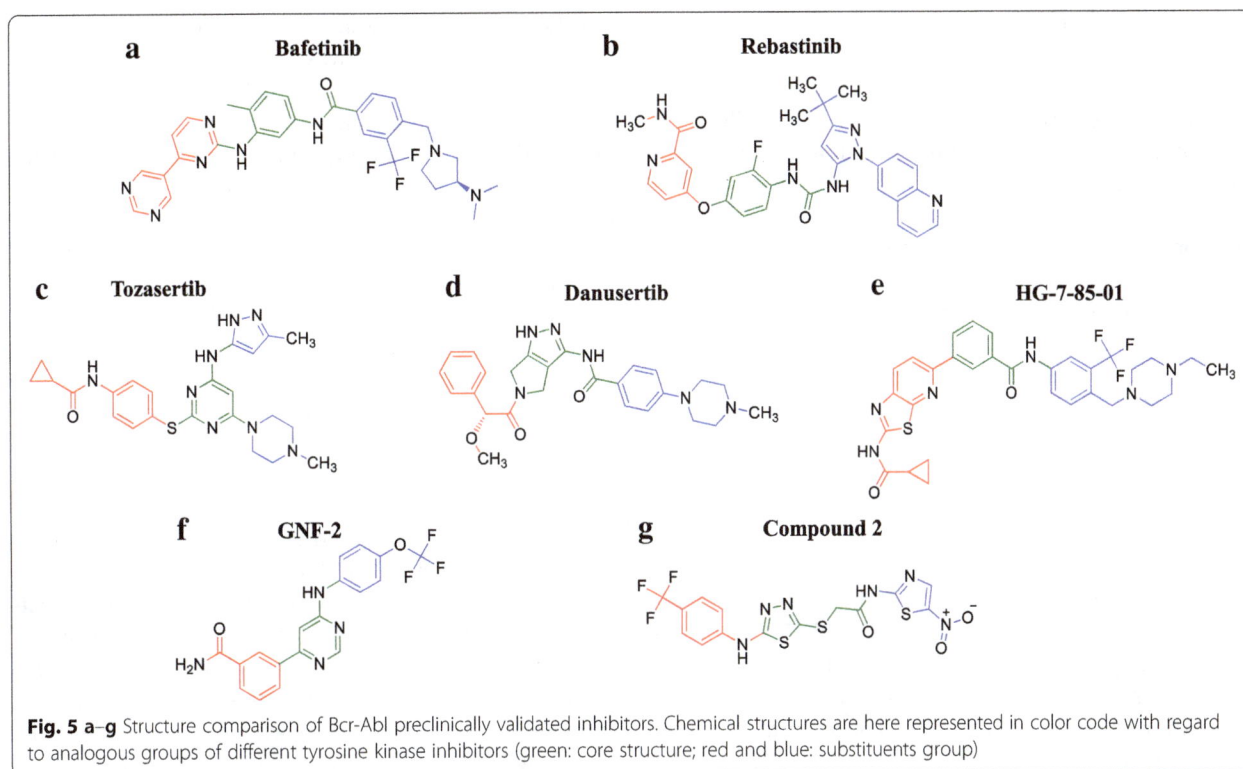

Fig. 5 a–g Structure comparison of Bcr-Abl preclinically validated inhibitors. Chemical structures are here represented in color code with regard to analogous groups of different tyrosine kinase inhibitors (green: core structure; red and blue: substituents group)

amino acids, forcing out the DFG motif from the catalytic site. In the case of T315I mutation, the hydrophobic interactions are even enhanced, justifying sensitivity to rebastinib in cellular assays with clones displaying this mutation (IC$_{50}$ 13 versus 19 nM for unmutated Abl) [40]. However, it is much less active against P-loop E255V mutation (IC$_{50}$ 800 nM), possibly due to destabilization of Bcr-Abl inactive conformation, but its molecular mechanism deserves further characterization [39]. Clinically, although rebastinib showed efficacy (of 40 CML patients, 8 complete hematologic responses were achieved, 4 of which had a T315I mutation) [41], benefit has been considered insufficient to justify continued development against leukemias since the advent of ponatinib, to date.

Tozasertib (MK-0457, VX-680) is a pan-Aurora Kinase inhibitor (IC$_{50}$ 4–27 nM) with activity also on Abl (IC$_{50}$ 10 nM) as ATP competitor [37, 42]. Peculiarly, Aurora kinases are inhibited in their inactive state, whereas Bcr-Abl, both WT and mutant T315I, in active conformation [37]. Indeed, co-crystal structures evidenced four H-bs established by the aminopyrazole pyrimidine inhibitor (Fig. 5c) with key residues of the ATP-binding pocket, including Asp381 of the DFG motif when folded in the ATP site. Neither bonds nor steric hindrance occur between tozasertib and the gatekeeper residue, accounting for vulnerability of both WT and T315I Bcr-Abl (with IC$_{50}$ of 30 nM) to this TKI [43]. All that led to a phase II clinical trial evidencing benefit for

patients with T315I Bcr-Abl CML (44% had hematologic responses), suggesting even more efficacy than ponatinib for accelerated phase disease or as bridge therapy for stem cell transplantation, given its higher myelosuppressive effect [44]. Further developments or combinational regimens seem to be amply justified for this promising compound.

Danusertib (PHA-739358) is a multikinase inhibitor with a selective spectrum extended to Aurora kinases, Ret, TrkA, FGFR1, and Abl (IC$_{50}$ of 13–79, 25, 31, 31, and 47 nM, respectively) [45, 46]. Similar to dasatinib and tozasertib, it is an ATP competitor for the active form of Bcr-Abl, as evidenced by crystallographic data [47]. Its pyrrolopyrazole core (Fig. 5d) provides three H-bs with the hinge region of Abl, whereas the benzyl group packs against Leu370 and the N-methyl-piperazine sticks out the kinase pocket to be solvated. No key interactions are established with the gatekeeper residue. Therefore, danusertib binding mode accommodates the T315I mutation, avoiding the steric clash that oppositely occurs between first-/second-generation inhibitors and the isoleucine 315 side chain. Actually, binding affinity for T315I mutant is even higher than that for WT Bcr-Abl (Kd 200 nM versus 2 μM, respectively [47]), possibly due to increase in VdW interactions between the inhibitor and the isoleucine residue. That accounts also for the higher potency shown in cellular assays against T315I mutant (IC$_{50}$ 120 vs 360 nM of WT Abl [48]). Clinically, danusertib has shown acceptable dose-dependent toxicities and promising activity in advanced and resistant ALL and CML patients within a phase II trial (4 out of 29 patients with accelerated or blast phase CML responded, all 4 with T315I Bcr-Abl) [49], paving the way for further preclinical and clinical advancements.

HG-7-85-01 is a hybrid compound, designed by superposition of nilotinib and dasatinib structures. The master concept of condensing in a unique molecule the advantages of a combinational therapy, i.e., overcoming resistances, led to its first design and synthesis [50]. Structurally, the aminothiazole moiety of dasatinib is condensed to a pyridine ring and the resulting portion is linked to the phenyl-benzamide group of nilotinib (Fig. 5e), conferring selectivity for DFG-out conformation of Bcr-Abl. In fact, this structural arrangement results in a very accommodating inhibitor molecule for the gatekeeper residue, showing activity also against T315I Bcr-Abl in cellular assays (IC$_{50}$ 140 nM, less than threefold higher than for WT, i.e., IC$_{50}$ 58.5 nM [50]). Furthermore, the target selectivity spectrum is narrower than that of ponatinib at a high-throughput screening [50, 51], suggesting less adverse reactions than ponatinib at a clinical level, especially those related to cardiovascular toxicity. However, no clinical data are currently available, nor are there ongoing trials, to the best of our knowledge.

Recently, new state-of-the-art molecules have been designed and tested at a preclinical level to sensitize T315I mutation to first and second-generation TKIs. Genetic, nuclear magnetic resonance, crystallography, mutagenesis and mass spectrometry studies identified GNF-2 (Fig. 5f) and GNF-5 (its analogue bearing a N-(2-hydroxyethyl) group at the amidic nitrogen atom) to be two allosteric interactors of Bcr-Abl [52]. They bind the myristylation site of C-lobe inducing a forced conformational change of the kinase to inactive state, even if its gatekeeper residue is mutated [53]. Co-administration of a classical inhibitor with these compounds may therefore be effective also against T315I mutant. However, mutations around the myristate binding site, e.g., C464Y, P465S and V506L, are known to induce resistance to GNF-2/5 activity, putatively by steric hindrance (IC$_{50}$ > 10 µM) [52]. This raises critical issues on some compound mutations of Bcr-Abl, i.e., the coexistence of different Bcr-Abl mutants in leukemic clones of a same patient, which necessarily need to be targeted by other approaches. Particularly, GNF-2 + dasatinib (IC$_{50}$ = 100 nM with 2 nM dasatinib concentration) and GNF-5 + nilotinib (IC$_{50}$ = 30 nM with 1 µM nilotinib concentration) resulted the most active and synergistic in vitro combinations [52, 53]. Clinical translation of these promising results could be found to be effective, especially for Ph+ ALL patients, since they often present the p190 Bcr-Abl variant on which these compounds seem to be more active.

A further way to inhibit Bcr-Abl could be paved by 1,3,4-thiadiazole derivatives, such as compound 2 (Fig. 5g), which emerged as putative DFG-in inhibitors from an in silico screening by molecular docking simulation studies [54]. Indeed, flexibility of its core is supposed to allow several conformations of the substances to bind the ATP site of Bcr-Abl active state [55]. As a matter of fact, compound 2 proved to be a better Bruton's tyrosine kinase-inhibitor than imatinib (IC$_{50}$ 1 vs 7 µM), but predictions about affinity while testing different substituents bound to the central thiadiazole core may lead to the development of even more effective Bcr-Abl inhibitors too, putatively also in the case of resistance to classical TKIs [54].

Conclusions

Treatment of Ph+ CML and ALL has dramatically changed since the advent of targeted therapy against the Bcr-Abl fusion protein at the turn of the twenty-first century, and so the prognosis has done. The development of targeted inhibitors started from a high-throughput screening to find out a leading pharmacophore that includes compounds able to bind and block the chimeric kinase, by impeding ATP binding in a competitive manner [16, 17]. After its rational development, according to structure-activity relationship analysis and enzymatic assays [16], imatinib was optimized and rapidly approved for the clinic [5]. Actually, the IRIS trial clearly demonstrated that imatinib presented much higher effectiveness and reduced toxicity if compared to the standard of care of that time, i.e., IFNα plus low-dose cytarabine regimen [56].

Although the radical increase in mean survival, new mutations and forms of resistance came upon in common clinical practice [57], requiring further development of inhibitors, similar to the process that led from the parent compound to imatinib. By means of imatinib modification or exploitation of totally different molecular scaffolds, several second- and third-generation TKIs were developed. Some have already been approved for clinic use, i.e., the second-generation nilotinib, dasatinib, and bosutinib, and the third-generation ponatinib, whereas other still need clinical validation, e.g., bafetinib, rebastinib, tozasertib, danusertib, HG-7-85-01, GNF-2 and GNF-5, and other 1,3,4-thiadiazole derivatives. The onset of new mechanisms of resistance, both Bcr-Abl dependent and independent, requires always new therapeutic strategies to be improved, in order to guarantee increasingly higher survival rates. Therefore, this continuous challenge makes the topic discussed in the present review undoubtedly up-to-date. Interestingly, most of the studies so far reported were carried out with high-throughput screening, cellular and enzymatic assays, crystallography, nuclear magnetic resonance, mass spectrometry, and in silico predictions to determine selectivity spectrum, activity against mutations, and bioavailability of the new inhibitors in view of clinical translation. Noteworthy, these approaches can be applied to other targeted therapies facing specific resistance-conferring mutations in different models, e.g., T790M mutation of epidermal growth factor receptor (EGFR) against gefitinib [58] or several anaplastic lymphoma kinase (ALK) point mutations against crizotinib [59].

The increasing number of approved and experimental inhibitors is slowly approaching the therapeutic solution of single specific mutations of Bcr-Abl, which were also highly deadly until recent past, e.g., T315I; nevertheless, compound mutations are a further emerging hurdle in the clinic, with only little knowledge about their prognostic and therapeutic meaning, to date [60]. Indeed, they may need innovative approaches to be dealt with, such as combination therapies, reevaluating discarded TKIs (in light of new therapeutic demands) or molecules with wider spectrum of targets, e.g., danusertib. In light of this, strategies other than Bcr-Abl targeting may be successfully exploited against refractory diseases, as recently evidenced for IL-15-mimetic ALT-803, Hsp90-inhibitor ganetespib, HDAC-inhibitor panabinostat, Ras-antagonist rigosertib, β-catenin-antagonist PRI-724, and MELK-inhibitor OTS167, reviewed elsewhere [61]. Moreover, the hurdle of developing therapeutic monoclonal antibodies against CML may be overcome by evolving promising detection tools, as TPγ B9-2 towards protein tyrosine phosphatase receptor gamma (PTPRG) [62].

Another caveat that should be kept in mind is that probably "CML not always simply relies on t(9,22) Ph chromosome": diverse translocations that activate Abl or other oncoproteins alternatively underlie very poor prognosis due to inefficacy of Bcr-Abl inhibitors [63, 64]. Conversely, other diseases characterized by hyperactivity of tyrosine kinases, such as PDGFRα in gastrointestinal stromal tumor (GIST) and hypereosinophilic syndrome or c-Kit in systemic mastocytosis, can benefit from imatinib and other inhibitors with wide selectivity spectrum [65]. Importantly, the mutational state of these kinases can drive the choice towards the most proper inhibitor: the commonly occurring imatinib-resistant PDGFRα D842V and c-Kit D816V mutants in GISTs and mastocytosis, respectively, are more strongly inhibited in vitro by dasatinib rather than imatinib (IC_{50} 62 vs 642 nM and 37 nM vs 3.8 μM, respectively—see Table 1 for these and other mutations), even though clinical benefits of dasatinib had been demonstrated only for the former [66]. However, the same therapy may work differently for diverse diseases, even if caused by similar genetic rearrangement: CML and Ph+ ALL are usually due to different Bcr-Abl forms, i.e., p210/p230 and p190,

respectively [67]. Actually, it has been reported that p190 and p210 have at least partially independent signaling cascades that are mediated by differential protein-protein interactions, which may help explain the observed association of p190 with Ph+ ALL and p210/p230 with CML. Notably, the differential signaling networks of Bcr-Abl p210 and p190 kinases in leukemia cells have very recently been identified by functional proteomics, e.g., demonstrating a strong and preferential binding of AP2 complex, a major regulator of clathrin-mediated endocytosis, with p190, whereas Bcr-Abl is likely to be inhibited by p210-selective interactor Sts2 tyrosine phosphatase [68].

All that may also account for different therapeutic efficacy of specific inhibitors, as noticed while describing GNF modulators previously in the main text of this review.

Overall, the developmental process of Bcr-Abl inhibitors perfectly exemplifies an important concept of biomedical research: translational medicine, aimed at lading scientific breakthroughs from bench to bedside, drove the development of imatinib starting from the identification of target and pharmacophore; nonetheless, the more innovative concept of reverse translational medicine, aimed at turning "bedside" problems to "bench" ones, has been followed during the rational development of second- and third-generation TKIs to effectively override the progressive onset of resistances and adverse drug reactions in the clinic.

In the context of tumor therapy, those lessons learned from Bcr-Abl inhibitors serve both as a model to overcome the still open issues about CML and Ph+ ALL and as a proof of concept for rationally developing novel small molecules against specific tumor types.

Finally, imatinib history may serve as a milestone of the developmental process of any inhibitor, driving drug discovery towards future chemotherapy-free and target-oriented treatments.

Abbreviations

ALK: Anaplastic lymphoma kinase; ALL: Acute lymphoblastic leukemia; ATP: Adenosine triphosphate; CML: Chronic myelogenous leukemia; DFG: Aspartate-phenylalanine-glycine; EGFR: Epidermal growth factor receptor; GIST: Gastrointestinal stromal tumor; H-b: Hydrogen bond; IC_{50}: 50% inhibitory concentration; MMR: Major molecular response; PDGFR: Platelet-derived growth factor receptor; Ph: Philadelphia chromosome; PKC: Protein kinase C; TKI: Tyrosine kinase inhibitor; VdW: Van der Waals; WT: Wild-type

Funding

This work was supported by the socially active non-profit organization A.I.L. (Associazione Italiana contro le leucemie-linfomi e mieloma)-Pisa section.

Authors' contributions

RF reviewed the state of the art on the topic and wrote the article; MF focused on the chemical aspect of the review and wrote the article; OE focused on the clinical aspect of the review and wrote the article. All authors read and approved the final manuscript.

Competing interests

The authors declare that they have no competing interests.

Author details

[1]Institute of Life Sciences, Scuola Superiore Sant'Anna, Piazza Martiri della Libertà, 33, 56127 Pisa, PI, Italy. [2]University of Pisa, Pisa, Italy. [3]Department of Pharmacy, University of Pisa, Pisa, Italy. [4]Department of Clinical and Experimental Medicine, Section of Hematology, Azienda Ospedaliero Universitaria Pisana, Pisa, Italy.

References

1. Burmeister T, Schwartz S, Bartram CR, Gökbuget N, Hoelzer D, Thiel E. Patients' age and BCR-ABL frequency in adult B-precursor ALL: a retrospective analysis from the GMALL study group. Blood. 2008;112:918–9.
2. Ward HW. Anti-oestrogen therapy for breast cancer: a trial of tamoxifen at two dose levels. Br Med J. 1973;1:13–4.
3. Druker BJ, Tamura S, Buchdunger E, Ohno S, Segal GM, Fanning S, et al. Effects of a selective inhibitor of the Abl tyrosine kinase on the growth of Bcr–Abl positive cells. Nat Med. 1996;2:561–6. https://doi.org/10.1038/nm0596-561.
4. Zimmermann J, Buchdunger E, Mett H, Meyer T, Lydon NB. Potent and selective inhibitors of the Abl-kinase: phenylaminopyrimidine (PAP) derivatives. Bioorganic Med Chem Lett. 1997;7:187–92.
5. O'Brien SG, Guilhot F, Larson RA, Gathmann I, Baccarani M, Cervantes F, et al. Imatinib compared with interferon and low-dose cytarabine for newly diagnosed chronic-phase chronic myeloid leukemia. N Engl J Med. 2003;348:994–1004. https://doi.org/10.1056/NEJMoa022457.
6. Nicolini FE, Mauro MJ, Martinelli G, Kim D-W, Soverini S, Müller MC, et al. Epidemiologic study on survival of chronic myeloid leukemia and Ph(+) acute lymphoblastic leukemia patients with BCR-ABL T315I mutation. Blood. 2009;114:5271–8. https://doi.org/10.1182/blood-2009-04-219410.
7. Jabbour E, Kantarjian H, Jones D, Breeden M, Garcia-Manero G, O'brien S, et al. Characteristics and outcomes of patients with chronic myeloid leukemia and T315I mutation following failure of imatinib mesylate therapy. Blood. 2008;112:53–5.
8. Bradeen HA, Eide CA, O'Hare T, Johnson KJ, Willis SG, Lee FY, et al. Comparison of imatinib mesylate, dasatinib (BMS-354825), and nilotinib (AMN107) in an N-ethyl-N-nitrosourea (ENU)-based mutagenesis screen: high efficacy of drug combinations. Blood. 2006;108:2332–8.
9. Nicolini FE, Basak GW, Kim DW, Olavarria E, Pinilla-Ibarz J, Apperley JF, et al. Overall survival with ponatinib versus allogeneic stem cell transplantation in Philadelphia chromosome-positive leukemias with the T315I mutation. Cancer. 2017;123:2875–80.
10. Wang W, Cortes JE, Tang G, Khoury JD, Wang S, Bueso-Ramos CE, et al. Risk stratification of chromosomal abnormalities in chronic myelogenous leukemia in the era of tyrosine kinase inhibitor therapy. Blood. 2016;127:2742–50.
11. Reddy EP, Aggarwal AK. The ins and outs of Bcr-Abl inhibition. Genes and Cancer. 2012;3:447–54.
12. Azam M, Seeliger MA, Gray NS, Kuriyan J, Daley GQ. Activation of tyrosine kinases by mutation of the gatekeeper threonine. Nat Struct Mol Biol. 2008;15:1109–18.
13. Schindler T. Structural mechanism for STI-571 inhibition of abelson tyrosine kinase. Science (80-). 2000;289:1938–42. https://doi.org/10.1126/science.289.5486.1938.
14. Capdeville R, Buchdunger E, Zimmermann J, Matter A. Glivec (ST1571, imatinib), a rationally developed, targeted anticancer drug. Nat Rev Drug Discov. 2002;1:493–502.
15. Buchdunger E, O'Reilly T, Wood J. Pharmacology of imatinib (STI571). Eur J Cancer. 2002;38(Suppl 5):S28–36.
16. Druker BJ, Lydon NB. Lessons learned from the development of an abl tyrosine kinase inhibitor for chronic myelogenous leukemia. J Clin Invest. 2000;105:3–7. https://doi.org/10.1172/JCI9083.
17. Rix U, Hantschel O, Dürnberger G, Remsing Rix LL, Planyavsky M, Fernbach NV, et al. Chemical proteomic profiles of the BCR-ABL inhibitors imatinib, nilotinib, and dasatinib reveal novel kinase and nonkinase targets. Blood. 2007;110:4055–63.
18. Hasford J, Baccarani M, Hoffmann V, Guilhot J, Saussele S, Rosti G, et al. Predicting complete cytogenetic response and subsequent progression-free survival in 2060 patients with CML on imatinib treatment: the EUTOS score. Blood. 2011;118:686–92.
19. Hochhaus A, Kreil S, Corbin AS, La Rosée P, Müller MC, Lahaye T, et al. Molecular and chromosomal mechanisms of resistance to imatinib (STI571) therapy. Leukemia. 2002;16:2190–6.
20. Weisberg E, Manley PW, Breitenstein W, Brüggen J, Cowan-Jacob SW, Ray A, et al. Characterization of AMN107, a selective inhibitor of native and mutant Bcr-Abl. Cancer Cell. 2005;7:129–41.
21. Hochhaus A, Saussele S, Rosti G, Mahon F-X, Janssen JJWM, Hjorth-Hansen H, et al. Chronic myeloid leukaemia: ESMO Clinical Practice Guidelines for diagnosis, treatment and follow-up. Ann Oncol. 2017;28(suppl_4):iv41–51. https://doi.org/10.1093/annonc/mdx219.
22. Hantschel O, Rix U, Superti-Furga G. Target spectrum of the BCR-ABL inhibitors imatinib, nilotinib and dasatinib. In: Leukemia and Lymphoma; 2008. p. 615–9.
23. Kantarjian HM, Hochhaus A, Saglio G, De SC, Flinn IW, Stenke L, et al. Nilotinib versus imatinib for the treatment of patients with newly diagnosed chronic phase, Philadelphia chromosome-positive, chronic myeloid leukaemia: 24-month minimum follow-up of the phase 3 randomised ENESTnd trial. Lancet Oncol. 2011;12:841–51.
24. Davies A, Jordanides NE, Giannoudis A, Lucas CM, Hatziieremia S, Harris RJ, et al. Nilotinib concentration in cell lines and primary CD34+ chronic myeloid leukemia cells is not mediated by active uptake or efflux by major drug transporters. Leukemia. 2009;23:1999–2006.
25. Kantarjian HM, Shah NP, Cortes JE, Baccarani M, Agarwal MB, Undurraga MS, et al. Dasatinib or imatinib in newly diagnosed chronic-phase chronic myeloid leukemia: 2-year follow-up from a randomized phase 3 trial (DASISION). Blood. 2012;119:1123–9.
26. Skora L, Mestan J, Fabbro D, Jahnke W, Grzesiek S. NMR reveals the allosteric opening and closing of Abelson tyrosine kinase by ATP-site and myristoyl pocket inhibitors. Proc Natl Acad Sci. 2013;110:E4437–45. https://doi.org/10.1073/pnas.1314712110.
27. Shah NP, Tran C, Lee FY, Chen P, Norris D, Sawyers CL. Overriding imatinib resistance with a novel ABL kinase inhibitor. Science. 2004;305:399–401.
28. Boschelli DH, Ye F, Wang YD, Dutia M, Johnson SL, Wu B, et al. Optimization of 4-phenylamino-3-quinolinecarbonitriles as potent inhibitors of Src kinase activity. J Med Chem. 2001;44:3965–77.
29. Boschelli F, Arndt K, Gambacorti-Passerini C. Bosutinib: a review of preclinical studies in chronic myelogenous leukaemia. Eur J Cancer. 2010;46:1781–9.
30. Redaelli S, Piazza R, Rostagno R, Magistroni V, Perini P, Marega M, et al. Activity of bosutinib, dasatinib, and nilotinib against 18 imatinib-resistant BCR/ABL mutants. J Clin Oncol. 2009;27:469–71.
31. Cortes JE, Gambacorti-Passerini C, Deininger MW, Mauro MJ, Chuah C, Kim D-W, et al. Bosutinib versus imatinib for newly diagnosed chronic myeloid leukemia: results from the randomized BFORE trial. J Clin Oncol. 2017:JCO2017747162. https://doi.org/10.1200/JCO. 2017.74.7162.
32. Zhou T, Commodore L, Huang WS, Wang Y, Thomas M, Keats J, et al. Structural mechanism of the Pan-BCR-ABL inhibitor ponatinib (AP24534): lessons for overcoming kinase inhibitor resistance. Chem Biol Drug Des. 2011;77:1–11.
33. Huang WS, Metcalf CA, Sundaramoorthi R, Wang Y, Zou D, Thomas RM, et al. Discovery of 3-[2-(imidazo[1,2- b]pyridazin-3-yl)ethynyl]-4-methyl-N -[4-[(4-methylpiperazin-1-yl)methyl]-3-(trifluoromethyl)phenyl]benzamide (AP24534), a potent, orally active pan-inhibitor of breakpoint cluster region-abelson (BCR-ABL) kinase including the T315I gatekeeper mutant. J Med Chem. 2010;53:4701–19.
34. Cortes JE, Kantarjian H, Shah NP, Bixby D, Mauro MJ, Flinn I, et al. Ponatinib in refractory Philadelphia chromosome–positive leukemias. N Engl J Med. 2012;367:2075–88. https://doi.org/10.1056/NEJMoa1205127.
35. Steegmann JL, Baccarani M, Breccia M, Casado LF, García-Gutiérrez V, Hochhaus A, et al. European LeukemiaNet recommendations for the management and avoidance of adverse events of treatment in chronic myeloid leukaemia. Leukemia. 2016;30:1648–71.

36. Kimura S, Naito H, Segawa H, Kuroda J, Yuasa T, Sato K, et al. NS-187, a potent and selective dual Bcr-Abl/Lyn tyrosine kinase inhibitor, is a novel agent for imatinib-resistant leukemia. Blood. 2005;106:3948–54.

37. Lambert GK, Duhme-Klair AK, Morgan T, Ramjee MK. The background, discovery and clinical development of BCR-ABL inhibitors. Drug Discov Today. 2013;18:992–9.

38. Kantarjian H, Le Coutre P, Cortes J, Pinilla-Ibarz J, Nagler A, Hochhaus A, et al. Phase 1 study of INNO-406, a dual Abl/Lyn kinase inhibitor, in Philadelphia chromosome-positive leukemias after imatinib resistance or intolerance. Cancer. 2010;116:2665–72.

39. Eide CA, Adrian LT, Tyner JW, Mac PM, David J, Wise SC, et al. ABL switch control inhibitor DCC 2036 active against CML mutant BCR ABL. Cancer Res. 2011;71:3189–95.

40. Chan WW, Wise SC, Kaufman MD, Ahn YM, Ensinger CL, Haack T, et al. Conformational control inhibition of the BCR-ABL1 tyrosine kinase, including the gatekeeper T315I mutant, by the switch-control inhibitor DCC-2036. Cancer Cell. 2011;19:556–68. https://doi.org/10.1016/j.ccr.2011.03.003.

41. Cortes J, Talpaz M, Smith HP, Snyder DS, Khoury J, Bhalla KN, et al. Phase 1 dose-finding study of rebastinib (DCC-2036) in patients with relapsed chronic myeloid leukemia and acute myeloid leukemia. Haematologica. 2017;102:519–28.

42. Bebbington D, Binch H, Charrier JD, Everitt S, Fraysse D, Golec J, et al. The discovery of the potent aurora inhibitor MK-0457 (VX-680). Bioorganic Med Chem Lett. 2009;19:3586–92.

43. Young MA, Shah NP, Chao LH, Seeliger M, Milanov ZV, Biggs WH, et al. Structure of the kinase domain of an imatinib-resistant Abl mutant in complex with the aurora kinase inhibitor VX-680. Cancer Res. 2006;66:1007–14.

44. Giles FJ, Swords RT, Nagler A, Hochhaus A, Ottmann OG, Rizzieri DA, et al. MK-0457, an Aurora kinase and BCR-ABL inhibitor, is active in patients with BCR-ABL T315I leukemia. Leukemia. 2013;27:113–7.

45. Gontarewicz A, Brümmendorf TH. Danusertib (formerly PHA-739358)—a novel combined Pan-aurora kinases and third generation Bcr-Abl tyrosine kinase inhibitor. In: Small molecules in oncology. Berlin Heidelberg: Springer Verlag; 2010. p. 199–214.

46. Meulenbeld HJ, Mathijssen RHJ, Verweij J, de Wit R, de Jonge MJ. Danusertib, an aurora kinase inhibitor. Expert Opin Investig Drugs. 2012;21:383–93. https://doi.org/10.1517/13543784.2012.652303.

47. Modugno M, Casale E, Soncini C, Rosettani P, Colombo R, Lupi R, et al. Crystal structure of the T315I Abl mutant in complex with the Aurora kinases inhibitor PHA-739358. Cancer Res. 2007;67:7987–90.

48. Gontarewicz A, Balabanov S, Keller G, Colombo R, Graziano A, Pesenti E, et al. Simultaneous targeting of Aurora kinases and Bcr-Abl kinase by the small molecule inhibitor PHA-739358 is effective against imatinib-resistant BCR-ABL mutations including T315I. Blood. 2008;111:4355–64.

49. Borthakur G, Dombret H, Schafhausen P, Brummendorf TH, Boisse N, Jabbour E, et al. A phase I study of danusertib (PHA-739358) in adult patients with accelerated or blastic phase chronic myeloid leukemia and Philadelphia chromosome-positive acute lymphoblastic leukemia resistant or intolerant to imatinib and/or other second generation c-ABL therapy. Haematologica. 2015;100:898–904.

50. Weisberg E, Choi HG, Ray A, Barrett R, Zhang J, Sim T, et al. Discovery of a small-molecule type II inhibitor of wild-type and gatekeeper mutants of BCR-ABL, PDGFRα, Kit, and Src kinases: novel type II inhibitor of gatekeeper mutants. Blood. 2010;115:4206–16.

51. Karaman MW, Herrgard S, Treiber DK, Gallant P, Atteridge CE, Campbell BT, et al. A quantitative analysis of kinase inhibitor selectivity. Nat Biotechnol. 2008;26:127–32.

52. Zhang J, Adrian FJ, Jahnke W, Cowan-jacob SW, Li AG, Iacob RE, et al. Targeting wild-type and T315I Bcr-Abl by combining allosteric with ATP-site inhibitors. Nature. 2010;463:501–6.

53. Khateb M, Ruimi N, Khamisie H, Najajreh Y, Mian A, Metodieva A, et al. Overcoming Bcr-Abl T315I mutation by combination of GNF-2 and ATP competitors in an Abl-independent mechanism. BMC Cancer. 2012;12:1. https://doi.org/10.1186/1471-2407-12-563.

54. Altintop MD, Ciftci HI, Radwan MO, Otsuka M, Özdemir A. Design, synthesis, and biological evaluation of novel 1,3,4-thiadiazole derivatives as potential antitumor agents against chronic myelogenous leukemia: striking effect of nitrothiazole moiety. Molecules. 2018 https://doi.org/10.3390/molecules23010059.

55. Jain AK, Sharma S, Vaidya A, Ravichandran V, Agrawal RK. 1,3,4-Thiadiazole and its derivatives: a review on recent progress in biological activities. Chem Biol Drug Des. 2013;81:557–76.

56. Kalmanti L, Saussele S, Lauseker M, Müller MC, Dietz CT, Heinrich L, et al. Safety and efficacy of imatinib in CML over a period of 10 years: data from the randomized CML-study IV. Leukemia. 2015;29:1123–32.

57. Shah NP, Nicoll JM, Nagar B, Gorre ME, Paquette RL, Kuriyan J, et al. Multiple BCR-ABL kinase domain mutations confer polyclonal resistance to the tyrosine kinase inhibitor imatinib (STI571) in chronic phase and blast crisis chronic myeloid leukemia. Cancer Cell. 2002;2:117–25.

58. Yu HA, Arcila ME, Hellmann MD, Kris MG, Ladanyi M, Riely GJ. Poor response to erlotinib in patients with tumors containing baseline EGFR T790M mutations found by routine clinical molecular testing. Ann Oncol. 2014;25:423–8.

59. Kim S, Kim TM, Kim DW, Go H, Keam B, Lee SH, et al. Heterogeneity of genetic changes associated with acquired crizotinib resistance in ALK-rearranged lung cancer. J Thorac Oncol. 2013;8:415–22.

60. Deininger MW, Hodgson JG, Shah NP, Cortes JE, Kim DW, Nicolini FE, et al. Compound mutations in BCR-ABL1 are not major drivers of primary or secondary resistance to ponatinib in CP-CML patients. Blood. 2016;127:703–12.

61. Kavanagh S, Nee A, Lipton JH. Emerging alternatives to tyrosine kinase inhibitors for treating chronic myeloid leukemia. Expert Opin Emerg Drugs. 2018; https://doi.org/10.1080/14728214.2018.1445717.

62. Vezzalini M, Mafficini A, Tomasello L, Lorenzetto E, Moratti E, Fiorini Z, et al. A new monoclonal antibody detects downregulation of protein tyrosine phosphatase receptor type γ in chronic myeloid leukemia patients. J Hematol Oncol. 2017;10(1):129.

63. Orciuolo E, Buda G, Galimberti S, Cervetti G, Cecconi N, Papineschi F, et al. Complex translocation t(6;9;22)(p21.1;q34;q11) at diagnosis is a therapy resistance index in chronic myeloid leukaemia. Leuk Res. 2008;32:190–1.

64. Orciuolo E, Buda G, Galimberti S, Cecconi N, Cervetti G, Petrini M. Concomitant translocation t(14;22)(q32;q11) in a case of chronic myeloid leukemia. Leuk Res. 2008;32:188–90.

65. Ogbogu PU, Bochner BS, Butterfield JH, Gleich GJ, Huss-Marp J, Kahn JE, et al. Hypereosinophilic syndrome: a multicenter, retrospective analysis of clinical characteristics and response to therapy. J Allergy Clin Immunol. 2009;124:1319–25.e3. https://doi.org/10.1016/j.jaci.2009.09.022.

66. Montemurro M, Cioffi A, Dômont J, Rutkowski P, Roth AD, von Moos R, et al. Long-term outcome of dasatinib first-line treatment in gastrointestinal stromal tumor: A multicenter, 2-stage phase 2 trial (Swiss Group for Clinical Cancer Research 56/07). Cancer. 2018;124:1449–54.

67. Chiarella P, Summa V, De Santis S, Signori E, Picardi E, Pesole G, et al. BCR/ABL1 fusion transcripts generated from alternative splicing: implications for future targeted therapies in Ph+ leukaemias. Curr Mol Med. 2012;12:547–65. https://doi.org/10.2174/156652412800619996.

68. Reckel S, Hamelin R, Georgeon S, Armand F, Jolliet Q, Chiappe D, et al. Differential signaling networks of Bcr-Abl p210 and p190 kinases in leukemia cells defined by functional proteomics. Leukemia. 2017;31:1502–12.

69. Breccia M, Alimena G. Second-generation tyrosine kinase inhibitors (Tki) as salvage therapy for resistant or intolerant patients to prior TKIs. Mediterr J Hematol Infect Dis. 2014;6(1):e2014003.

70. Pan J, Quintás-Cardama A, Manshouri T, Cortes J, Kantarjian H, Verstovsek S. Sensitivity of human cells bearing oncogenic mutant kit isoforms to the novel tyrosine kinase inhibitor INNO-406. Cancer Sci. 2007;98:1223–5.

71. Weisberg E, Wright RD, Jiang J, Ray A, Moreno D, Manley PW, et al. Effects of PKC412, nilotinib, and imatinib against GIST-associated PDGFRA mutants with differential imatinib sensitivity. Gastroenterology. 2006;131:1734–42.

72. Von Bubnoff N, Gorantla SP, Thöne S, Peschel C, Duyster J. The FIP1L1-PDGFRA T674I mutation can be inhibited by the tyrosine kinase inhibitor AMN107 (nilotinib). Blood. 2006;107:4970–1.

73. Duveau DY, Hu X, Walsh MJ, Shukla S, Skoumbourdis AP, Boxer MB, et al. Synthesis and biological evaluation of analogues of the kinase inhibitor nilotinib as Abl and Kit inhibitors. Bioorganic Med Chem Lett. 2013;23:682–6.

74. Blay J-Y, von Mehren M. Nilotinib: a novel, selective tyrosine kinase inhibitor. Semin Oncol. 2011;38:S3–9. https://doi.org/10.1053/j.seminoncol.2011.01.016.

75. von Bubnoff N, Gorantla SHP, Kancha RK, Lordick F, Peschel C, Duyster J. The systemic mastocytosis-specific activating cKit mutation D816V can be inhibited by the tyrosine kinase inhibitor AMN107. Leukemia. 2005;19:1670–1.

76. Dewaele B, Wasag B, Cools J, Sciot R, Prenen H, Vandenberghe P, et al. Activity of dasatinib, a dual SRC/ABL kinase inhibitor, and IPI-504, a heat shock protein 90 inhibitor, against gastrointestinal stromal tumor-associated PDGFRAD842V mutation. Clin Cancer Res. 2008;14:5749–58.

77. Shah NP, Lee FY, Luo R, Jiang Y, Donker M, Akin C. Dasatinib (BMS-354825) inhibits KITD816V, an imatinib-resistant activating mutation that triggers

neoplastic growth in most patients with systemic mastocytosis. Blood. 2006;108:286–91.

78. Guo T, Hajdu M, Agaram NP, Shinoda H, Veach D, Clarkson BD, et al. Mechanisms of sunitinib resistance in gastrointestinal stromal tumors harboring KIT AY502-3ins mutation: an in vitro mutagenesis screen for drug resistance. Clin Cancer Res. 2009;15:6862–70.

79. Eiring AM, Deininger MW. Individualizing kinase-targeted cancer therapy: the paradigm of chronic myeloid leukemia. Genome Biol. 2014;15:461.

80. Remsing Rix LL, Rix U, Colinge J, Hantschel O, Bennett KL, Stranzl T, et al. Global target profile of the kinase inhibitor bosutinib in primary chronic myeloid leukemia cells. Leukemia. 2009;23:477–85.

81. Gozgit JM, Wong MJ, Wardwell S, Tyner JW, Loriaux MM, Mohemmad QK, et al. Potent activity of ponatinib (AP24534) in models of FLT3-driven acute myeloid leukemia and other hematologic malignancies. Mol Cancer Ther. 2011;10:1028–35. https://doi.org/10.1158/1535-7163.MCT-10-1044.

82. Lierman E, Smits S, Cools J, Dewaele B, Debiec-Rychter M, Vandenberghe P. Ponatinib is active against imatinib-resistant mutants of FIP1L1-PDGFRA and KIT, and against FGFR1-derived fusion kinases. Leukemia. 2012;26:1693–5.

83. Rix U, Remsing Rix LL, Terker AS, Fernbach NV, Hantschel O, Planyavsky M, et al. A comprehensive target selectivity survey of the BCR-ABL kinase inhibitor INNO-406 by kinase profiling and chemical proteomics in chronic myeloid leukemia cells. Leukemia. 2010;24:44–50.

84. Zabriskie MS, Eide CA, Tantravahi SK, Vellore NA, Estrada J, Nicolini FE, et al. BCR-ABL1 compound mutations combining key kinase domain positions confer clinical resistance to ponatinib in Ph chromosome-positive leukemia. Cancer Cell. 2014;26:428–42.

85. Hadzijusufovic E, Peter B, Herrmann H, Rülicke T, Cerny-Reiterer S, Schuch K, et al. NI-1: a novel canine mastocytoma model for studying drug resistance and IgER-dependent mast cell activation. Allergy. 2012;67:858–68.

86. Winter GE, Rix U, Lissat A, Stukalov A, Mullner MK, Bennett KL, et al. An integrated chemical biology approach identifies specific vulnerability of Ewing's sarcoma to combined inhibition of Aurora kinases A and B. Mol Cancer Ther. 2011;10:1846–56. https://doi.org/10.1158/1535-7163.MCT-11-0100.

87. Zhang J, Adrián FJ, Jahnke W, Cowan-Jacob SW, Li AG, Iacob RE, et al. Targeting Bcr-Abl by combining allosteric with ATP-binding-site inhibitors. Nature. 2010;463:501–6.

88. Reynolds CR, Islam SA, Sternberg MJE. EzMol: a web server wizard for the rapid visualisation and image production of protein and nucleic acid structures. J Mol Biol. 2018:1–5. https://doi.org/10.1016/j.jmb.2018.01.013.

7

Overexpression of CLC-3 is regulated by XRCC5 and is a poor prognostic biomarker for gastric cancer

Zhuoyu Gu[1,2†], Yixin Li[3†], Xiaoya Yang[2,4†], Meisheng Yu[1,2], Zhanru Chen[4], Chan Zhao[4], Lixin Chen[1*] and Liwei Wang[4*] (iD)

Abstract

Background: Recently, many potential prognostic biomarkers for gastric cancer (GC) have been identified, but the prognosis of advanced GC patients remains poor. Chloride channels are promising cancer biomarkers, and their family member chloride channel-3 (CLC-3) is involved in multiple biological behaviors. However, whether CLC-3 is a prognostic biomarker for GC patients is rarely reported. The molecular mechanisms by which CLC-3 is regulated in GC are unclear.

Methods: The expression of CLC-3 and XRCC5 in human specimens was analyzed using immunohistochemistry. The primary biological functions and pathways related to CLC-3 were enriched by RNA sequencing. A 5′-biotin-labeled DNA probe with a promoter region between − 248 and + 226 was synthesized to pull down CLC-3 promoter-binding proteins. Functional studies were detected by MTS, clone formation, wound scratch, transwell, and xenograft mice model. Mechanistic studies were investigated by streptavidin-agarose-mediated DNA pull-down, mass spectrometry, ChIP, dual-luciferase reporter assay system, Co-IP, and immunofluorescence.

Results: The results showed that CLC-3 was overexpressed in human GC tissues and that overexpression of CLC-3 was a poor prognostic biomarker for GC patients ($P = 0.012$). Furthermore, higher expression of CLC-3 was correlated with deeper tumor invasion ($P = 0.006$) and increased lymph node metastasis ($P = 0.016$), and knockdown of CLC-3 inhibited cell proliferation and migration in vitro. In addition, X-ray repair cross-complementing 5 (XRCC5) was identified as a CLC-3 promoter-binding protein, and both CLC-3 (HR 1.671; 95% CI 1.012–2.758; $P = 0.045$) and XRCC5 (HR 1.795; 95% CI 1.076–2.994; $P = 0.025$) were prognostic factors of overall survival in GC patients. The in vitro and in vivo results showed that the expression and function of CLC-3 were inhibited after XRCC5 knockdown, and the inhibition effects were rescued by CLC-3 overexpression. Meanwhile, the expression and function of CLC-3 were promoted after XRCC5 overexpression, and the promotion effects were reversed by the CLC-3 knockdown. The mechanistic study revealed that knockdown of XRCC5 suppressed the binding of XRCC5 to the CLC-3 promoter and subsequent promoter activity, thus regulating CLC-3 expression at the transcriptional level by interacting with PARP1.

Conclusions: Our findings indicate that overexpression of CLC-3 is regulated by XRCC5 and is a poor prognostic biomarker for gastric cancer. Double targeting CLC-3 and XRCC5 may provide the promising therapeutic potential for GC treatment.

Keywords: CLC-3, XRCC5, Prognosis, Biomarker, Gastric cancer

* Correspondence: tchenlixin@jnu.edu.cn; twangliwei@jnu.edu.cn
†Zhuoyu Gu, Yixin Li and Xiaoya Yang contributed equally to this work.
[1]Department of Pharmacology, Medical College, Jinan University, Guangzhou 510632, China
[4]Department of Physiology, Medical College, Jinan University, Guangzhou 510632, China
Full list of author information is available at the end of the article

Background

Gastric cancer (GC), the second leading cause of cancer-related death worldwide, is characterized by advanced clinical stages at diagnosis and poor survival rates [1, 2]. In 2012, GC accounted for 6.8% of global cancer incidence and 8.8% of cancer mortality worldwide [3]. GC development is a complicated multistep process, influenced by a *Helicobacter pylori* infection, host genetic susceptibility, and other environmental factors [4]. Achieving a detailed understanding of the molecular pathogenesis associated with GC will be critical to improving patient outcomes. Recently, many potential prognosis biomarkers for GC have been identified, including BMI1, Ezh2, and LINC00261 [5–8]. However, the prognosis of advanced GC remains poor. Therefore, the identification of further biomarkers for therapeutic purposes in GC is imperative.

Chloride channels are promising cancer biomarkers by mediating a multitude of biological functions [9]. Chloride channel-3 (CLC-3), a member of the voltage-gated chloride channel family, mainly mediates the extra- and intracellular ion homeostasis and acidification of intracellular compartments. Recent studies have revealed that CLC-3 participates in the processes of cell volume regulation, proliferation, and migration, particularly in glioma and prostate cancer cells [10–12]. Our previous studies have indicated that CLC-3 is overexpressed in nasopharyngeal carcinoma cells and plays roles in controlling cell proliferation [13]. Moreover, suppression of CLC-3 expression reduces the migration of nasopharyngeal carcinoma, hepatocellular carcinoma, and cervical carcinoma cells [14–16]. Therefore, CLC-3 may play key roles in tumor development. However, whether CLC-3 is a prognostic biomarker for GC patients is rarely reported. The molecular mechanisms by which CLC-3 is regulated in GC are unclear.

Our present study indicated that overexpression of CLC-3 was a poor prognostic marker for GC patients and that cell proliferation and migration were the primary biological functions of CLC-3 in GC cells. Moreover, XRCC5, a subunit of the Ku heterodimer protein [17, 18], was identified to be a promoter-binding protein of CLC-3. As a key mediator of DNA recombination, chemotherapy resistance, and chromosome stability maintenance [19–21], XRCC5 has elevated expression in a variety of tumors [22–24]. However, little is known about the expression of XRCC5 in GC. In this study, we showed that XRCC5 was highly expressed in GC. Importantly, the expression and function of CLC-3 were regulated by XRCC5 in vivo and in vitro, and both CLC-3 and XRCC5 were prognostic factors of overall survival in GC patients. The relative expressions of CLC-3 and XRCC5 could determine the further prognosis of GC patients.

Methods

Patient samples

Paraffin-embedded tumor tissues and adjacent normal tissues were obtained from 90 patients diagnosed with gastric adenocarcinoma between May 2007 and February 2008 at the First Affiliated Hospital of Zhengzhou University. Medical records of all patients provided information about age, gender, pathological grade, and TNM stage. The patients were followed up for 8 years. Written informed consent was obtained from each patient involved in the study, and the study was approved by the Ethics Committee of Zhengzhou University.

Cell culture and stable cell line construction

Human GC cell lines (SGC-7901, BGC-823, and AGS) and human normal gastric epithelial (GES-1) cells were obtained and authenticated from the Cell Bank of the Chinese Academy of Sciences (Shanghai, China). All cells were cultured in RPMI 1640 medium supplemented with 10% fetal bovine serum. Lentiviruses for XRCC5 knockdown (shXR-1 and shXR-2), XRCC5 overexpression (XRCC5), CLC-3 knockdown (shCLC-3), and CLC-3 overexpression (CLC-3) were purchased from GenePharma (Shanghai, China). SGC-7901 and BGC-823 cells were used to establish stable cell lines via selection with 1 μg/ml puromycin for 4 weeks. Negative control shRNA cells (sh-NC) and empty vector-transfected cells (vector) were established as controls.

Streptavidin-agarose-mediated DNA pull-down assay

A biotin-labeled double-stranded oligonucleotide probe for the − 248 to + 226 fragment of the CLC-3 promoter sequence was synthesized by Ruibiotech Co. (Beijing, China). Briefly, 1 mg of nuclear protein extract was mixed and incubated with 10 μg of probe and 100 μl of streptavidin-agarose beads (Sigma, St Louis, MO). The mixtures were then centrifuged at 800×g, resuspended in 30 μl of loading buffer, and boiled at 100 °C for 5 min. The collected samples containing the bound proteins were separated by SDS-PAGE for further silver staining or Western blot analysis.

Silver staining and mass spectrometry

After electrophoresis of the samples containing the bound proteins, the protein gel was immersed in a stationary liquid with 10% acetic acid, 50% ethanol, and 40% water at room temperature on a shaker overnight. The protein bands were visualized with a fast silver staining kit (Beyotime, Shanghai, China) and analyzed using MS by Honortech (Beijing, China).

Chromatin immunoprecipitation assay

The chromatin immunoprecipitation (ChIP) procedure was performed as illustrated in the ChIP kit (cat# 9002S,

Cell Signaling Technology, Danvers, MA). Briefly, the tested cell lines were fixed with formaldehyde, and cross-linking was performed by adding glycine. The samples were placed on ice and sonicated to separate the DNA into 100 to 1000-bp fragments. Then, they were incubated with antibodies at a dilution of 1:50 overnight, followed by incubation with protein G agarose beads at 4 °C overnight. Next, the bound DNA-protein mixtures were eluted, and cross-linking was reversed after several washes. The DNA fragments were then purified, and PCR was performed with CLC-3 primers purchased from GeneCopoeia (cat# HQP001983, Rockville, MD, USA) to amplify a 102-bp segment. The PCR products were separated on 2% agarose gels and visualized on a UV transilluminator.

Dual-luciferase reporter assay

The pGL4.13 vector was used as a positive control for the luciferase reporter system. Fragments including the CLC-3 promoter region were inserted between the HindIII and KpnI sites of the pGL4.10 luciferase vector (Promega, Madison, WI). Primer pairs were designed for the truncated promoter regions, as shown in Additional file 1: Table S1. Briefly, stable cell lines were plated in 96-well plates and transfected with luciferase plasmid. To normalize the transfection efficiency, the cells were co-transfected with the Renilla luciferase control reporter pRL-TK vector by using EndoFectin™ Max (GeneCopoeia, Inc.). Luciferase activity was detected using the Dual-Luciferase® Reporter Assay System (Promega) after 48 h.

RNA extraction and quantitative RT-PCR

Total RNA was extracted from cells using a RaPure Total RNA Micro Kit (Magen, Guangzhou, China). Endogenous cDNA was obtained by the ReverTra Ace qPCR RT Master Mix kit (Toyobo, Shanghai, China). Primers for CLC-3 (cat# HQP001983), XRCC5 (cat# HQP018568), and GAPDH (cat# HQP006940) were obtained from GeneCopoeia Inc. Finally, qRT-PCR was performed with SYBR® Green Real-time PCR Master Mix (Toyobo) in a Bio-Rad CFX96 PCR system. Relative RNA levels were calculated as the fold changes with the $2^{-\Delta\Delta CT}$ formula.

Co-immunoprecipitation (Co-IP) assay and Western blot analysis

Protein extracts were prepared and incubated with antibodies against XRCC5 or IgG for 24 h on a rotating wheel. Then, Protein A/G plus-Agarose beads (Santa Cruz, Dallas TX, USA) were added and incubated for another 24 h. After the beads were boiled, the precipitated proteins were separated by SDS-PAGE and transferred to PVDF membranes for further analysis. For Western blot (WB) analysis, equal amounts of proteins from the lysates were separated and transferred. The membranes were blocked with 5% nonfat milk for 2 h and then incubated with antibodies. The protein bands were finally detected by enhanced chemiluminescence. The density of the protein bands was quantified by ImageJ software (National Institutes of Health, Bethesda, MD) and normalized to GAPDH. Relative protein levels were calculated as the density ratios of interest protein to GAPDH. All antibodies used for WB were purchased from Cell Signaling Technology (Danvers, MA, USA).

MTS assay and clone formation assay

Cell proliferation was determined by MTS assays (Promega, Madison, WI). Different stable cell lines and stable cell lines transfected with PARP1 siRNA (GenePharma, Shanghai, China) were seeded at a density of 5000 cells per well in 96-well plates. At the time points of 24 h, 48 h, and 72 h after seeding, the cells were respectively incubated with MTS for 40 min, and the optical density (OD) was then detected with a microplate reader. For the clone formation assay, cells were seeded at a density of 500 cells per well in 6-well plates and cultured for 2 weeks. The formative colonies were then fixed with formalin and stained by crystal violet. The number of clones was counted by Image-Pro Plus 6.0 software.

Wound scratch assay and transwell assay

Cell migration ability was examined by the wound scratch assay. Briefly, cells were cultured in 6-well plates until reaching confluence and then were scratched with a 10-μl pipette tip. The gap widths at 0 h (w1) and at 36 or 48 h (w2) were measured, and the relative migration rate was calculated as (w1 − w2)/w1 × 100%. Transwell assay was performed with Boyden chambers containing 24-well transwell plates (BD, Franklin Lakes, USA). Homogeneous single-cell suspensions were added to the upper chambers coated with Matrigel. After 24 h, invaded cells on the bottom of the chambers were stained with crystal violet and counted in five random fields.

RNA sequencing

Briefly, samples (SGC-7901 cells transfected with control or CLC-3 shRNA) were used to extract total RNA for RNA-seq loading and quality control. Differential gene expression (DGE) RNA-seq was then performed, and 50-bp paired-end reads were finally produced (RiboBio, Guangzhou, China). NCBI Sequence Read Archive (SRA) sequencing data were submitted under accession number SRP135951.

In vivo tumor model

All animal experimental procedures were approved by the Animal Care and Use Committee of Jinan University. Approximately 2×10^6 cells in 100 μl of PBS were subcutaneously injected. Tumor volumes were recorded every 4 days and calculated according to the equation of volume = (width^2 × length)/2. After 4 weeks, the tumor xenografts were harvested, weighed, and processed for immunohistochemistry (IHC) staining.

Immunofluorescence and immunohistochemistry

Cells were first seeded onto coverslips in a 6-well plate. Subsequently, the cells were fixed with 4% paraformaldehyde, permeabilized with 0.5% Triton-X, and blocked with bovine serum albumin (BSA). The coverslips were then incubated with primary antibodies at a dilution of 1:200 overnight. After washing, the coverslips were incubated with secondary antibodies and stained with 4,6-diamidino-2-phenylindole (DAPI). The immunofluorescence images were captured by a confocal microscope (Olympus, Japan). For IHC staining, the paraffin-embedded sections were incubated with anti-XRCC5 and anti-CLC-3 primary antibodies at a dilution of 1:100 overnight. After washing, the sections were incubated with horseradish peroxidase-conjugated anti-goat antibodies and stained with 3,5-diaminobenzidine (DAB). The percentage of stained cells (0–100%) was multiplied by the staining intensity (0, 1, 2, or 3) to produce the final IHC scores (0–300), of which 100 or higher was considered to indicate high XRCC5 expression, and 60 or higher was considered to indicate high CLC-3 expression.

Statistical analysis

Statistical analyses were performed using SPSS statistical software. All data were presented as the mean ± SD. The significance of difference was assessed by t tests or variance analysis. Correlations between XRCC5 and CLC-3 expression were assessed using Spearman rank correlation analysis, and overall survival curves were assessed using Kaplan-Meier analysis. Multivariate cumulative survival analysis was conducted with the Cox regression model. The P values less than 0.05 were considered statistically significant.

Results

Overexpression of CLC-3 was a poor prognostic biomarker for GC patients, and CLC-3 knockdown inhibited cell proliferation and migration in vitro

To confirm whether CLC-3 was a potential cancer biomarker for GC, in this study, we first examined the expression of CLC-3 in 90 paraffin-embedded GC tumor tissues and adjacent normal tissues (ANT) by IHC analysis. Significantly, the expression of CLC-3 was higher in GC tissues than that in ANT. Moreover, CLC-3 was mainly localized to the cell membrane and cytoplasm (Fig. 1a, b). Next, we analyzed the effect of CLC-3 expression on the cumulative survival rate of these 90 GC patients. Kaplan-Meier analysis showed that high expression (IHC score ≥ 60) of CLC-3 predicted poor survival outcome, indicating that CLC-3 overexpression was a poor prognostic biomarker for GC patients ($P = 0.012$, Fig. 1c). Furthermore, we examined the relationship between the CLC-3 expression and the clinicopathological characteristics in GC patients. As shown in Table 1, higher CLC-3 expression was correlated with deeper tumor invasion ($P = 0.006$), increased lymph node metastasis ($P = 0.016$), and later clinical staging ($P = 0.015$).

We further investigated the role of CLC-3 in vitro. Basic protein expression of CLC-3 in human normal gastric epithelial cells (GES-1) and human GC cell lines (SGC-7901, BGC-823, and AGS) was detected by WB. The expression of CLC-3 was also increased in GC cell lines compared to that in normal cells (Fig. 1d). To identify the biological functions of CLC-3 in GC cells, the primary biological processes participated by CLC-3 were analyzed by RNA sequencing in SGC-7901 cells. The heatmap and volcano plot revealed that 136 and 175 genes (upregulated and downregulated, respectively) were differentially expressed after the CLC-3 knockdown. By Gene Ontology (GO) analysis of these differential genes, cell proliferation and migration were identified as the primary biological functions of CLC-3 (Fig. 1e). We then validated the effect of CLC-3 knockdown on cell proliferation and migration. Our results showed that knockdown of CLC-3 inhibited the proliferation of GC cells at different time points (Fig. 1f). Next, clone formation assay showed that knockdown of CLC-3 attenuated the clonogenicity of GC cells (Fig. 1g). Furthermore, the scratch assay and transwell assay indicated that knockdown of CLC-3 impaired the migration rate and number of invaded GC cells (Fig. 1h, i). To study the pathways related to CLC-3 in GC cells, Kyoto Encyclopedia of Genes and Genomes (KEGG) pathway enrichment was performed by RNA sequencing in SGC-7901 cells, and the PI3K/Akt signaling pathway was enriched as the primary pathway after CLC-3 knockdown (Fig. 1j). We then verified that knockdown of CLC-3 reduced the levels of key targets in the PI3K/Akt signaling pathway, which revealed that CLC-3 knockdown inhibited this pathway (Fig. 1k). Altogether, our results proved that as a prognostic biomarker for GC, CLC-3 also had important functions in vitro.

XRCC5 was identified as a CLC-3 promoter-binding protein, and both CLC-3 and XRCC5 were prognostic factors of overall survival in GC patients

To explore the molecular mechanism of CLC-3 overexpression in GC cells, we further detected the basic RNA

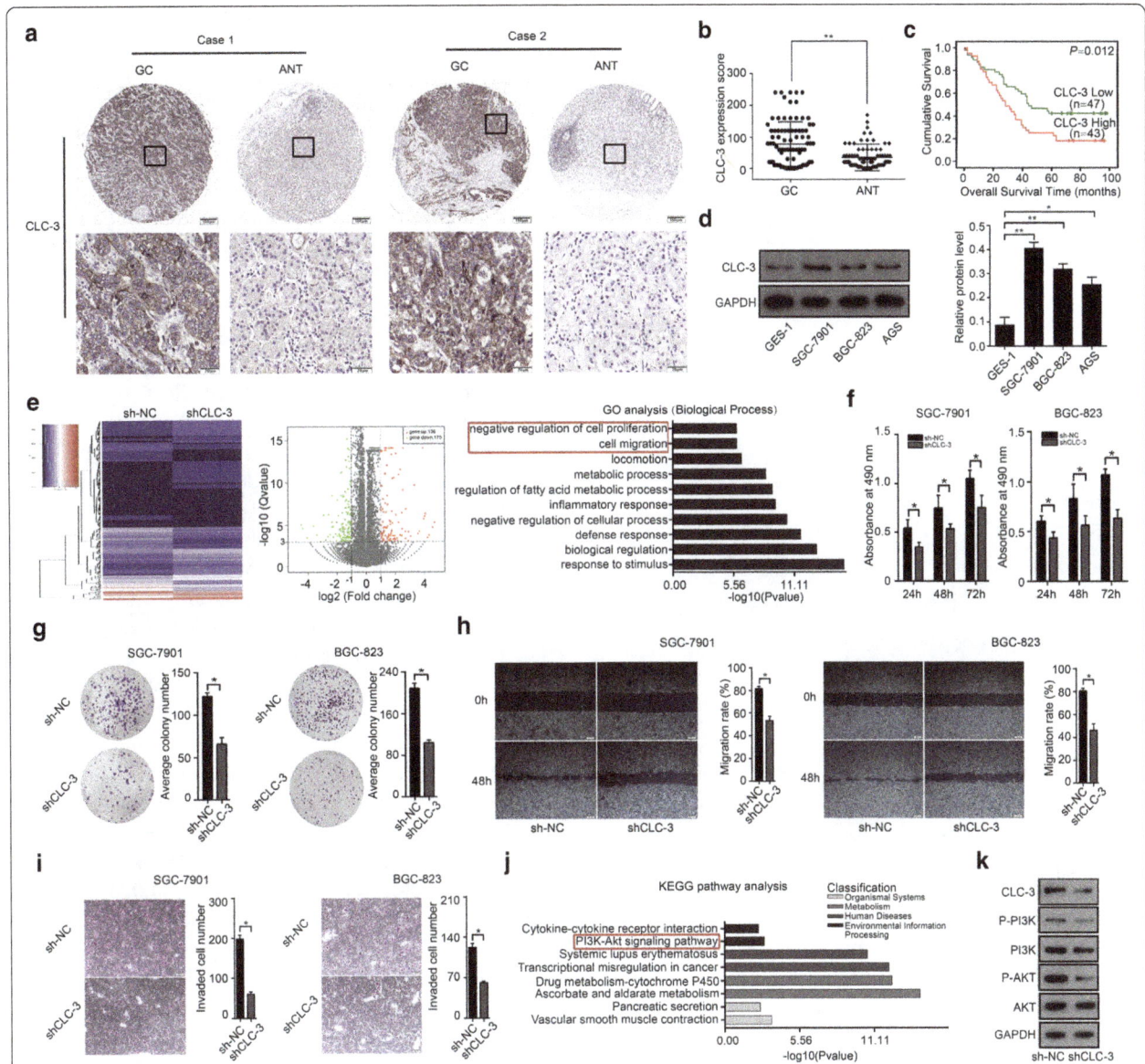

Fig. 1 Overexpression of CLC-3 was a poor prognostic biomarker for GC patients, and CLC-3 knockdown inhibited cell proliferation and migration in vitro. **a** Representative images of CLC-3 expression in GC tissues and adjacent normal tissues (ANT). **b** The expression of CLC-3 in 90 GC tissues was higher than that in ANT. **c** High expression of CLC-3 was associated with poor prognosis in GC patients. **d** The basic protein expression of CLC-3 in human normal gastric epithelial cells (GES-1) and human GC cell lines (SGC-7901, BGC-823, and AGS). **e** The heatmap and volcano plot of RNA sequencing were constructed after the CLC-3 knockdown. Cell proliferation and migration were identified as the primary biological functions of CLC-3 according to the Gene Ontology (GO) analysis. **f**, **g** Knockdown of CLC-3 inhibited the proliferation and clonogenicity of SGC-7901 and BGC-823 cells ($n=3$). **h**, **i** Knockdown of CLC-3 inhibited the migration and invasion of SGC-7901 and BGC-823 cells ($n=3$). **j** The PI3K/Akt signaling pathway was enriched according to the Kyoto Encyclopedia of Genes and Genomes (KEGG) pathway analysis of CLC-3 knockdown. **k** Knockdown of CLC-3 reduced the levels of key targets in the PI3K/Akt signaling pathway. $*P < 0.05$, $**P < 0.01$

expression of CLC-3 in the above cell lines. The RNA level of CLC-3 was also elevated in GC cells compared to that in normal cells (Fig. 2a), suggesting that the CLC-3 overexpression might be regulated by some tumor-specific factors at the transcriptional level. To study the transcriptional regulatory mechanism of CLC-3 overexpression, a series of truncated CLC-3 gene promoter fragments were amplified

by PCR and cloned into the pGL4.10-basic vector to construct dual-fluorescence reporter plasmids. The results of agarose gel electrophoresis indicated that each truncated fragment had the correct size in accordance with our designed sequence (Fig. 2b). Dual-luciferase reporter assays revealed that all reporter plasmids exhibited promoter activity in SGC-7901 cells, while the pGL4.10-CLC-3 – 248

Table 1 Correlations between CLC-3 expression and clinicopathological characteristics of GC patients

Variables	N	CLC-3		χ^2	P value
		Low expression	High expression		
Age					
≤ 70	55	29	26	0.014	0.904
> 70	35	18	17		
Gender					
Male	70	35	35	0.623	0.430
Female	20	12	8		
Pathological grade					
I/II	24	15	9	1.386	0.239
III/IV	66	32	34		
Depth of invasion					
T1/T2	11	10	1	7.517	0.006
T3/T4	79	37	42		
Lymph node metastases					
N0	23	17	6	5.826	0.016
N1/N2/N3	67	30	37		
Distant metastasis					
M0	86	45	41	0.009	0.927
M1	4	2	2		
TNM stage					
I/II	37	25	12	5.930	0.015
III/IV	53	22	31		

CLC-3 chloride channel-3, GC gastric cancer

plasmid showed higher promoter activity combined with shorter sequence length, indicating that a 5′-biotin-labeled DNA probe with a promoter region between − 248 and + 226 was optimal to pull down CLC-3 promoter-binding proteins (Fig. 2c, d).

We synthesized and incubated this probe with nuclear protein extracts to pull down potential CLC-3 promoter-binding proteins. After SDS-PAGE and silver staining, the target protein band (at almost 86 kDa) was observed, and the amount of this protein band was significantly enriched in GC cells compared with normal cells (Fig. 2e, left; red rectangle). This protein band was then excised and analyzed by MS. With the best peptide-spectrum sequence of KYAPTEAQLNAVDALIDSMSLAK, XRCC5 was identified as a candidate binding to the CLC-3 promoter (Fig. 2e, right). To ascertain the binding between XRCC5 and the CLC-3 promoter, we pulled down the nuclear protein/DNA complex in GC cells using synthesized DNA probe or nonspecific probe (NSP) and validated their binding by WB (Fig. 2f). Furthermore, ChIP assays were performed to further confirm the binding of XRCC5 protein to CLC-3 DNA. We found that XRCC5 bound the CLC-3 DNA in all cells, while the smallest

amount of binding was observed in normal cells (Fig. 2g).

We then explored the clinicopathologic significance of CLC-3 and XRCC5 in GC patients. IHC analysis revealed that XRCC5 was localized to the nucleus, and the expression of both CLC-3 and XRCC5 was higher in GC tissues than that in ANT. Moreover, by observing IHC images of the same site, we found that patients with strong XRCC5 staining tended to have strong CLC-3 staining (Fig. 2h, i). The Spearman rank correlation analysis showed that the expression of CLC-3 and XRCC5 was positively correlated ($r = 0.369$, $P < 0.001$) (Fig. 2j). Next, the Kaplan-Meier survival analysis revealed that high expression (IHC score ≥ 100) of XRCC5 predicted a poor prognosis for GC patients ($P < 0.001$, Fig. 2k). In addition, higher XRCC5 expression was correlated with deeper tumor invasion ($P = 0.036$) and later clinical staging ($P = 0.045$) (Table 2). Importantly, compared to those with low CLC-3 and high XRCC5 levels, the GC patients with high CLC-3 and low XRCC5 levels did not present a difference in overall survival ($P > 0.05$, Fig. 2l). However, patients with high expression of XRCC5 and CLC-3 had the worst prognosis ($P < 0.001$, Fig. 2m). To further check the prognostic value of CLC-3 and XRCC5, multivariate analysis was used to investigate the correlation between cumulative overall survival rates and clinicopathological characteristics. As shown in Table 3, four factors, including depth of invasion (hazard rate (HR) = 1.883; 95% CI 1.135–3.122; $P = 0.014$), TNM stage (HR = 2.349; 95% CI 1.342–4.114; $P = 0.003$), XRCC5 expression (HR = 1.795; 95% CI 1.076–2.994; $P = 0.025$), and CLC-3 expression (HR = 1.671; 95% CI 1.012–2.758; $P = 0.045$), were associated with the clinical outcomes of GC patients. Our results suggested that both CLC-3 and XRCC5 were prognostic factors of overall survival in GC patients.

The expression and function of CLC-3 were regulated by XRCC5 in vitro

To study the relationship between XRCC5 and CLC-3 in vitro, we established stable XRCC5-knockdown cell lines (SGC-7901 and BGC-823) and corresponding rescue models by transfecting lentivirus of CLC-3 overexpression. WB revealed that the expression of CLC-3 was inhibited after XRCC5 knockdown in SGC-7901 and BGC-823 cells, and the inhibition effect was rescued by CLC-3 overexpression (Fig. 3a, b). According to the primary biological functions of CLC-3, we investigated the effects of XRCC5 knockdown on cell proliferation and migration. The proliferation of GC cells was attenuated after XRCC5 knockdown, and the attenuation effect was rescued by CLC-3 overexpression (Fig. 3c, d). Furthermore, clone formation assay showed that knockdown of XRCC5 attenuated the cell clonogenicity. Similarly, the

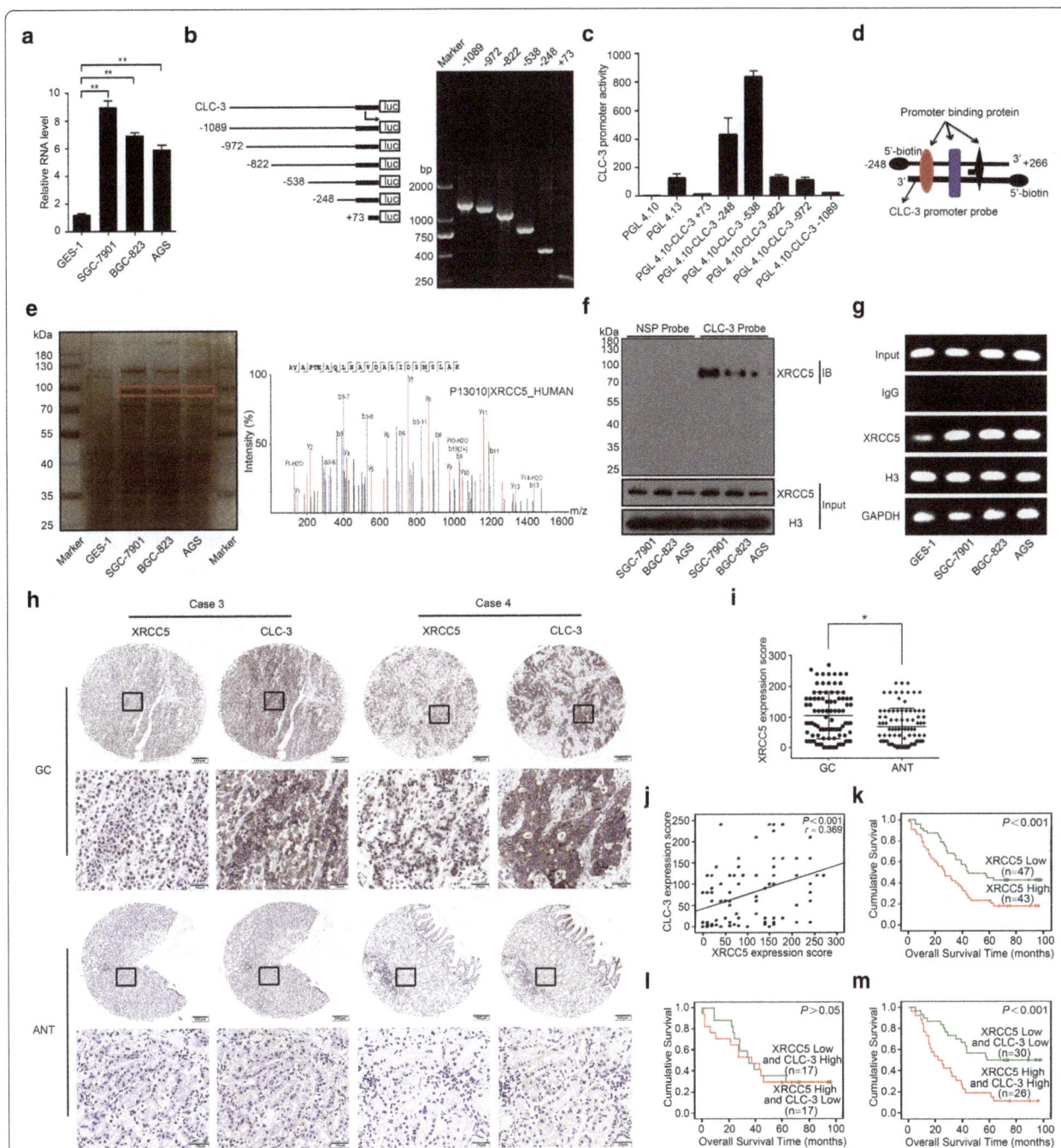

Fig. 2 XRCC5 was identified as a CLC-3 promoter-binding protein, and both CLC-3 and XRCC5 were prognostic factors of the overall survival in GC patients. **a** The basic RNA expression of CLC-3 in cell lines ($n = 3$). **b** Truncated fragments of the CLC-3 gene promoter were designed and amplified by PCR to construct dual-fluorescence reporter plasmids. **c** The promoter activity of various reporter plasmids was measured by dual-luciferase reporter assay ($n = 3$). **d** A 5′-biotin-labeled DNA probe with a promoter region between − 248 and + 226 was synthesized. **e** Potential CLC-3 promoter-binding proteins in nuclear protein extracts were pulled down using the synthesized probe. After SDS-PAGE and silver staining, the target protein band was observed (indicated with the red rectangle), which was significantly enriched in GC cells and finally analyzed by mass spectrometry. **f** Binding between XRCC5 and the CLC-3 promoter was detected by WB in the nuclear protein/DNA complex using a synthesized probe or nonspecific probe (NSP). **g** Binding of XRCC5 to the CLC-3 DNA was confirmed by ChIP assay. The PCR products were separated on 2% agarose gels. **h** Representative images of XRCC5 and CLC-3 expression in GC tissues and ANT. **i** The expression of XRCC5 in 90 GC tissues was higher than that in ANT. **j** The expression of XRCC5 and CLC-3 was positively correlated in GC tissues. **k** High expression of XRCC5 predicted a poor prognosis for GC patients. **l** There was no difference in overall survival between GC patients with high CLC-3 and low XRCC5 levels and GC patients with high XRCC5 and low CLC-3 levels. **m** GC patients with high expression of XRCC5 and CLC-3 had the worst prognosis. $*P < 0.05$, $**P < 0.01$

Table 2 Correlations between XRCC5 expression and clinicopathological characteristics of GC patients

Variables	N	XRCC5		χ^2	P value
		Low expression	High expression		
Age					
≤ 70	55	33	22	3.429	0.064
> 70	35	14	21		
Gender					
Male	70	34	36	1.683	0.195
Female	20	13	7		
Pathological grade					
I/II	24	9	15	2.843	0.092
III/IV	66	38	28		
Depth of invasion					
T1/T2	11	9	2	4.399	0.036
T3/T4	79	38	41		
Lymph node metastases					
N0	23	14	9	0.926	0.336
N1/N2/N3	67	33	34		
Distant metastasis					
M0	86	46	40	1.243	0.265
M1	4	1	3		
TNM stage					
I/II	37	24	13	4.025	0.045
III/IV	53	23	30		

XRCC5 X-ray repair cross-complementing 5, *GC* gastric cancer

attenuation effect was rescued by CLC-3 overexpression (Fig. 3e, f). Next, scratch assay and transwell assays revealed that the migration and invasion of SGC-7901 and BGC-823 cells were also inhibited after XRCC5 knockdown, and the inhibition effects were rescued by CLC-3 overexpression (Fig. 3g, h).

To further evaluate whether CLC-3 was the target of XRCC5, we established stable cell lines with XRCC5 overexpression and corresponding reverse models by transfecting lentivirus of CLC-3 knockdown. The protein expression of CLC-3 in SGC-7901 and BGC-823 cells was increased after XRCC5 overexpression, and the increase effects could be reversed by CLC-3 knockdown (Fig. 4a, b). We then found that XRCC5 overexpression promoted the cell proliferation and clonogenicity, and these promotion effects could be reversed by CLC-3 knockdown (Fig. 4c–f). Scratch and transwell assays indicated that the migration and invasion of GC cells were enhanced by XRCC5 overexpression. Similarly, these enhancement effects were reversed by CLC-3 knockdown (Fig. 4g, h). These findings confirmed that the expression and function of CLC-3 were regulated by XRCC5 in vitro.

The expression of CLC-3 was regulated at the transcriptional level by XRCC5 interacting with PARP1

The significant association between CLC-3 and XRCC5 revealed in cellular experiments and clinical outcomes led us to further examine their underlying molecular mechanisms. ChIP assays indicated that the binding of XRCC5 to the CLC-3 DNA in SGC-7901 cells was suppressed after XRCC5 knockdown (Fig. 5a). Dual-luciferase reporter assays revealed that knockdown of XRCC5 impaired the promoter activities of the pGL4.10-CLC-3 − 248 and pGL4.10-CLC-3 − 538 reporter plasmids in SGC-7901 cells (Fig. 5b). We then detected RNA expression of CLC-3 in established stable cell lines. The RNA level of CLC-3 was inhibited after XRCC5 knockdown and increased after XRCC5 overexpression, validating that the expression of CLC-3 was regulated by XRCC5 at the transcriptional level (Fig. 5c). Based on the primary related pathway of CLC-3 indicated above, we assessed whether the PI3K/Akt signaling pathway was inhibited after XRCC5 knockdown. The results demonstrated that knockdown of XRCC5 reduced the levels of key targets in the PI3K/Akt signaling

Table 3 Multivariate analysis between cumulative overall survival rates and clinicopathological characteristics of GC patients

Variables	HR (95% CI)	P value
Age, > 70 (vs. ≤ 70)	1.734 (0.650–4.628)	0.271
Gender, female (vs. male)	1.069 (0.589–1.940)	0.827
Pathological grade, III/IV (vs. I/II)	1.260 (0.661–2.401)	0.483
Depth of invasion, T3/T4 (vs. T1/T2)	1.883 (1.135–3.122)	0.014
Lymph node metastases, N1/N2/N3 (vs. N0)	2.251 (0.809–6.261)	0.120
Distant metastasis, M1 (vs. M0)	1.480 (0.815–2.687)	0.198
TNM stage, III/IV (vs. I/II)	2.349 (1.342–4.114)	0.003
XRCC5 expression, high (vs. low)	1.795 (1.076–2.994)	0.025
CLC-3 expression, high (vs. low)	1.671 (1.012–2.758)	0.045

HR hazard rate, *CI* confidence interval, *XRCC5* X-ray repair cross complementing 5, *CLC-3* chloride channel-3, *GC* gastric cancer

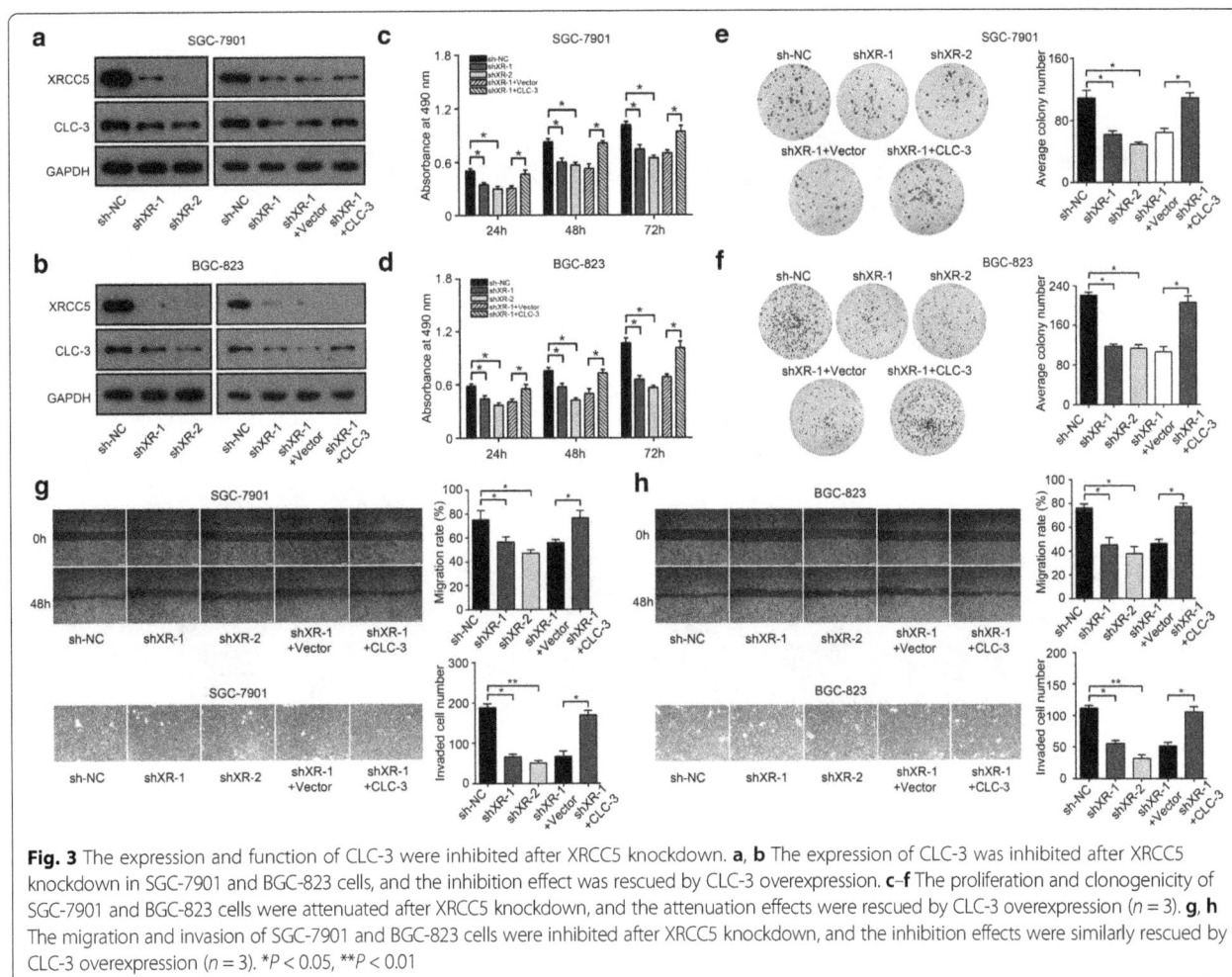

Fig. 3 The expression and function of CLC-3 were inhibited after XRCC5 knockdown. **a, b** The expression of CLC-3 was inhibited after XRCC5 knockdown in SGC-7901 and BGC-823 cells, and the inhibition effect was rescued by CLC-3 overexpression. **c-f** The proliferation and clonogenicity of SGC-7901 and BGC-823 cells were attenuated after XRCC5 knockdown, and the attenuation effects were rescued by CLC-3 overexpression ($n = 3$). **g, h** The migration and invasion of SGC-7901 and BGC-823 cells were inhibited after XRCC5 knockdown, and the inhibition effects were similarly rescued by CLC-3 overexpression ($n = 3$). *$P < 0.05$, **$P < 0.01$

pathway by downregulating CLC-3 in SGC-7901 cells (Fig. 5d).

Next, to identify the interaction partners of XRCC5 in regulating the expression of CLC-3, we performed immunoprecipitation (IP) combined with mass spectrometry (MS) in nuclear protein extracts of SGC-7901 cells with anti-XRCC5 antibodies. The MS results showed that 12 proteins were potential candidates for interaction with XRCC5, of which PARP1 was found to have the highest confidence score and coverage percentage (Fig. 5e). The best peptide-spectrum sequences of PARP1 and XRCC5 were shown in Fig. 5f, g. Next, the interaction between XRCC5 and PARP1 was confirmed by Co-IP in stable SGC-7901 cells with XRCC5 overexpression (Fig. 5h). To certify whether PARP1 also bound to the CLC-3 promoter, we pulled down the nuclear protein/DNA complex in GC cells using a CLC-3 promoter probe or NSP and validated their binding by WB (Fig. 5i). In addition, the subcellular localization of XRCC5 and PARP1 was examined by confocal microscopy analysis. The obtained images indicated that XRCC5 (green) and PARP1 (red) were both primarily expressed in the

nucleus, and the co-localization of XRCC5 and PARP1 was observed in the nucleus (yellow) (Fig. 5j). The effect of PARP1 interacting with XRCC5 on CLC-3 expression was then explored. Overexpression of XRCC5 increased the expression of CLC-3 in SGC-7901 cells, and the increase effect could be reversed by PARP1 knockdown (Fig. 5k). Functionally, the promotion effects of XRCC5 overexpression on cell proliferation and clonogenicity were also reversed by PARP1 knockdown (Fig. 5l, m). Overall, the results indicated that the expression and function of CLC-3 were regulated at the transcriptional level by XRCC5 interacting with PARP1.

The expression and function of CLC-3 were regulated by XRCC5 in vivo

The association between XRCC5 and CLC-3 was also investigated in mouse xenograft models. SGC-7901 cells were subcutaneously injected into the left flank of nude mice. Tumor volumes were measured and recorded every 4 days. After approximately 4 weeks, the tumor xenografts were harvested, weighed, and processed for IHC staining. Our observations revealed that tumor

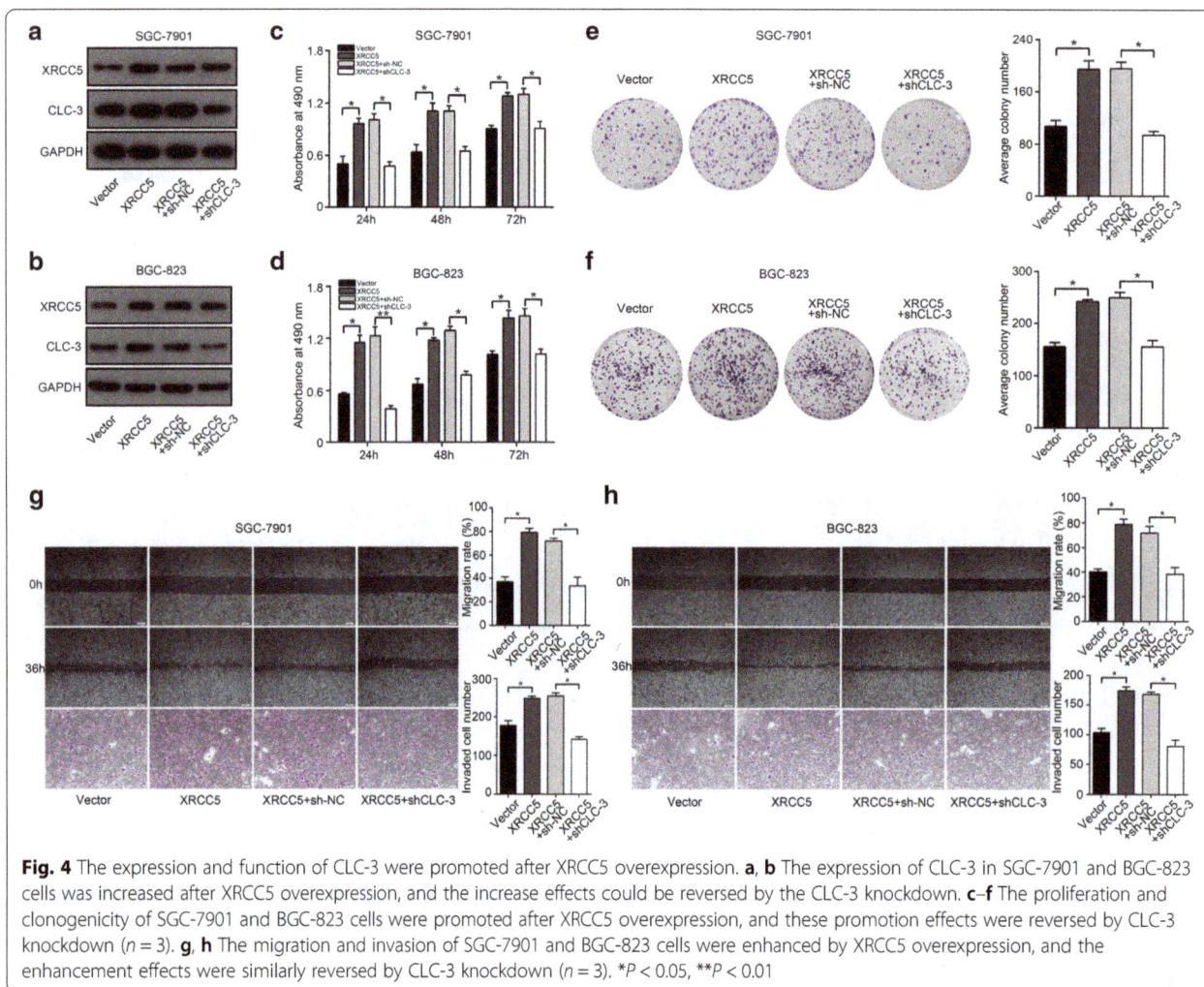

Fig. 4 The expression and function of CLC-3 were promoted after XRCC5 overexpression. **a, b** The expression of CLC-3 in SGC-7901 and BGC-823 cells was increased after XRCC5 overexpression, and the increase effects could be reversed by the CLC-3 knockdown. **c–f** The proliferation and clonogenicity of SGC-7901 and BGC-823 cells were promoted after XRCC5 overexpression, and these promotion effects were reversed by CLC-3 knockdown ($n = 3$). **g, h** The migration and invasion of SGC-7901 and BGC-823 cells were enhanced by XRCC5 overexpression, and the enhancement effects were similarly reversed by CLC-3 knockdown ($n = 3$). *$P < 0.05$, **$P < 0.01$

growth was inhibited after XRCC5 knockdown or CLC-3 knockdown. Conversely, overexpression of XRCC5 promoted tumor growth and the promotion effect could be reversed by CLC-3 knockdown (Fig. 6a–d). In addition, the expression of CLC-3 and XRCC5 in tumor tissues presented the same variation trend as tumor growth (Fig. 6e). These in vivo results were consistent with our in vitro observations and confirmed that CLC-3 could be regulated by XRCC5 in vivo.

Discussion

GC is one of the most common tumors and continues to be a serious public health problem in the clinic. To date, the prognosis of advanced GC patients remains poor. Consistently, the available targeted therapy clinical trials only target HER2 (trastuzumab) and VEGFR2 (ramucirumab) in advanced GC patients [25]. Therefore, there is a need to explore more potential biomarkers of GC for therapeutic purposes. Chloride channels are a new class of membrane proteins that are aberrantly expressed in multiple tumor types. In addition to

regulating various aspects of cancer cell behavior, chloride channels may constitute promising cancer biomarkers. However, few studies have focused on exploiting chloride channels for clinical purposes in GC. In this study, we first found that CLC-3, a member of the voltage-gated chloride channel superfamily, was overexpressed in human GC tissues and GC cell lines, suggesting a possible pivotal role of CLC-3 overexpression in GC development. Importantly, high expression of CLC-3 predicted poor prognosis in GC patients, demonstrating that overexpression of CLC-3 was a poor prognostic biomarker for GC.

CLC-3 is a crucial exchange transporter in plasma membranes and intracellular vesicles. Recently, the study of CLC-3 in cell metastasis and proliferation has attracted much attention [26–28]. Nonetheless, as a potential prognostic biomarker, the role of CLC-3 in digestive tract cancers is rarely reported, including GC. In this study, the primary biological functions of CLC-3 were identified as cell proliferation and migration, which were identical to the clinicopathological characteristics

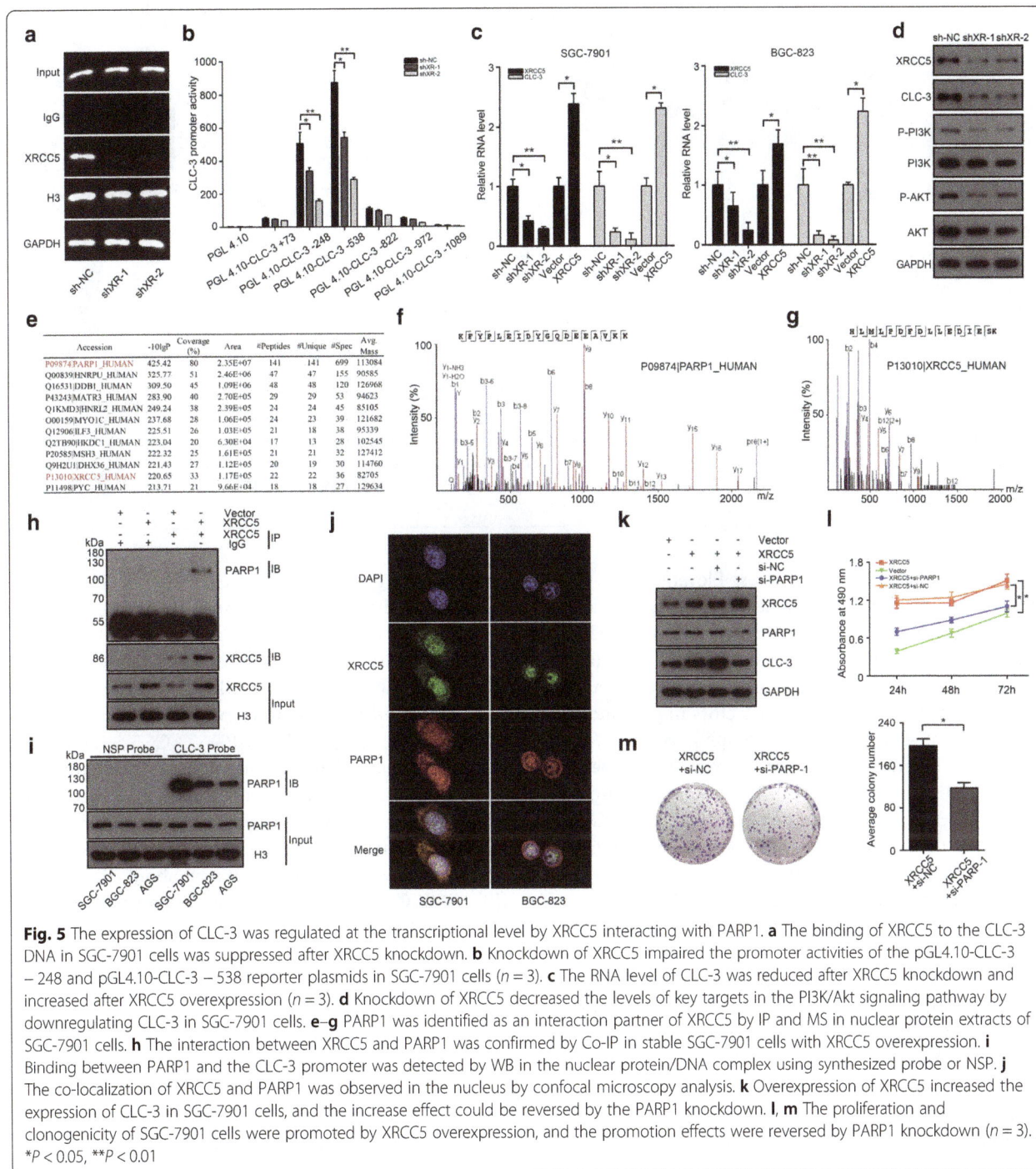

Fig. 5 The expression of CLC-3 was regulated at the transcriptional level by XRCC5 interacting with PARP1. **a** The binding of XRCC5 to the CLC-3 DNA in SGC-7901 cells was suppressed after XRCC5 knockdown. **b** Knockdown of XRCC5 impaired the promoter activities of the pGL4.10-CLC-3 − 248 and pGL4.10-CLC-3 − 538 reporter plasmids in SGC-7901 cells ($n = 3$). **c** The RNA level of CLC-3 was reduced after XRCC5 knockdown and increased after XRCC5 overexpression ($n = 3$). **d** Knockdown of XRCC5 decreased the levels of key targets in the PI3K/Akt signaling pathway by downregulating CLC-3 in SGC-7901 cells. **e–g** PARP1 was identified as an interaction partner of XRCC5 by IP and MS in nuclear protein extracts of SGC-7901 cells. **h** The interaction between XRCC5 and PARP1 was confirmed by Co-IP in stable SGC-7901 cells with XRCC5 overexpression. **i** Binding between PARP1 and the CLC-3 promoter was detected by WB in the nuclear protein/DNA complex using synthesized probe or NSP. **j** The co-localization of XRCC5 and PARP1 was observed in the nucleus by confocal microscopy analysis. **k** Overexpression of XRCC5 increased the expression of CLC-3 in SGC-7901 cells, and the increase effect could be reversed by the PARP1 knockdown. **l, m** The proliferation and clonogenicity of SGC-7901 cells were promoted by XRCC5 overexpression, and the promotion effects were reversed by PARP1 knockdown ($n = 3$). $*P < 0.05$, $**P < 0.01$

analysis of CLC-3 expression in GC patients, indicating that overexpression of CLC-3 in GC acted as a potential tumor-promoting factor by facilitating cell proliferation and migration. In addition, we found that the PI3K/Akt signaling pathway, a critical pathway mainly implicated in cell proliferation and migration [29, 30], was inhibited after the CLC-3 knockdown. This result was in accord with our previous finding indicating that the PI3K/Akt signaling pathway might be the downstream signaling pathway of CLC-3 [31]. So, we focused on the PI3K/ AKT pathway rather than other pathways, and we hypothesized that CLC-3 might regulate cell proliferation and migration via this pathway. Accordingly, as a prognostic biomarker for GC, CLC-3 also plays important roles in vitro. Investigating the molecular mechanism of CLC-3 overexpression in GC development is needed.

To further explore the molecular mechanism of CLC-3 overexpression in GC, we studied the basic RNA

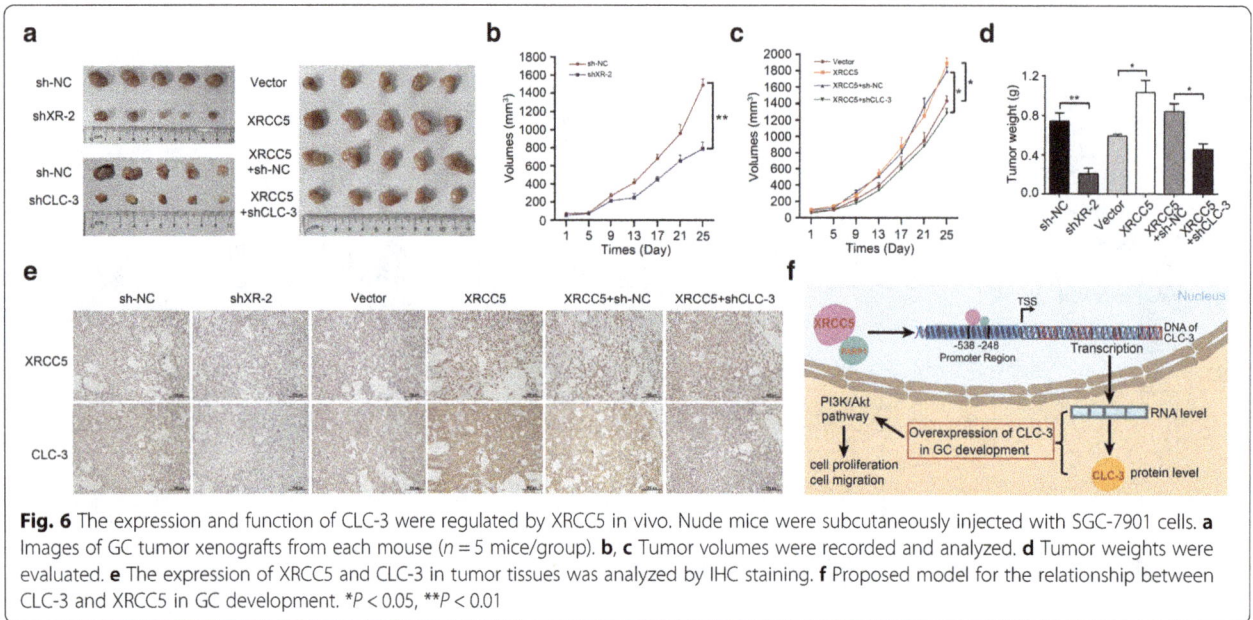

Fig. 6 The expression and function of CLC-3 were regulated by XRCC5 in vivo. Nude mice were subcutaneously injected with SGC-7901 cells. **a** Images of GC tumor xenografts from each mouse (n = 5 mice/group). **b**, **c** Tumor volumes were recorded and analyzed. **d** Tumor weights were evaluated. **e** The expression of XRCC5 and CLC-3 in tumor tissues was analyzed by IHC staining. **f** Proposed model for the relationship between CLC-3 and XRCC5 in GC development. *P < 0.05, **P < 0.01

expression of CLC-3 in cell lines. Elevated RNA level was also observed in GC cell lines, suggesting that a specific transcriptional regulatory mechanism of CLC-3 overexpression might exist in GC. With the regulatory events often occurring at gene promoters, we speculated that some tumor-specific cellular factors might bind specifically to the CLC-3 promoter to upregulate CLC-3 expression. Therefore, an optimal promoter probe was synthesized to pull down CLC-3 promoter-binding proteins [32, 33]. Our study demonstrated that XRCC5 bound the CLC-3 promoter, and increased combination was observed in GC cells, suggesting that this increased binding might be a promoting factor of CLC-3 overexpression. The novel finding of this study was the identification of XRCC5 as a CLC-3 promoter-binding protein in GC cells. To provide valuable clinical outcome prediction information, we then examined the expression of CLC-3 and XRCC5 in GC patients. Similar to most other types of tumors, the expression of XRCC5 in GC was also significantly increased [22–24]. Moreover, the expression of CLC-3 and XRCC5 presented the same variation trend, which was identified by their positive correlated expression in GC tissues. The survival analysis indicated that high expression of XRCC5 predicted poor prognosis in GC patients, prompting that XRCC5 might be a tumor-promoting factor in GC development. Importantly, the patients with high expression of XRCC5 and CLC-3 had the worst prognosis, revealing the synergistic effect of XRCC5 and CLC-3 on GC progression. Cox regression analysis further demonstrated that both CLC-3 and XRCC5 were prognostic factors of the overall survival in GC patients and that double detection of CLC-3 and XRCC5 could provide precise information

for predicting the prognosis of GC patients. These findings indicate that the expression of CLC-3 is elevated in GC tissues in response to increased XRCC5 levels, and double targeting of CLC-3 and XRCC5 may provide more useful therapeutic potential for GC treatment.

As the regulatory subunit of the DNA-dependent protein kinase complex DNA-PK, XRCC5 is associated with the development of tumors such as lung cancer, breast cancer, and bladder cancer [34–36]. Functionally, XRCC5 acts as a double-edged sword by inhibiting or promoting tumor progression in different tumor types [37, 38]. However, little is known about the role of XRCC5 in GC. Clinicopathological characteristics analysis suggested that XRCC5 might promote the proliferation and invasion of GC cells. In vitro, the primary biological functions of CLC-3 were suppressed after XRCC5 knockdown and promoted after XRCC5 overexpression, reconfirming the tumor-promoting action of XRCC5. The rescue models with CLC-3 overexpression and reverse models with CLC-3 knockdown further certified that CLC-3 was the molecular target of XRCC5. Collectively, these results indicate that the expression and function of CLC-3 are regulated by XRCC5 in vitro and that XRCC5 is a tumor-promoting factor in GC. However, XRCC5 may not be the only regulator of CLC-3, and other molecular regulators can also exist in GC cells.

The above results only illustrated that XRCC5 bound to the CLC-3 promoter in the nucleus. To further verify the molecular mechanisms underlying the interaction between CLC-3 and XRCC5, ChIP assays and luciferase assays were performed in SGC-7901 cells with XRCC5 knockdown. We proved that knockdown of XRCC5 suppressed the binding of XRCC5 to the CLC-3 DNA and impaired the promoter activity of the pGL4.10-CLC-3 – 248 and pGL4.10-CLC-3 – 538 reporter plasmids, which indicated that the potential binding site might be located between – 248 and – 538. Furthermore, the RNA level of CLC-3 was inhibited by XRCC5 knockdown and increased by XRCC5 overexpression, validating that the expression of CLC-3 was regulated by XRCC5 at the transcriptional level. Next, XRCC5 knockdown inhibited the levels of key targets in the PI3K/Akt signaling pathway by downregulating CLC-3, confirming that the observed effects of XRCC5 on proliferation and migration were reflected at the functional level of CLC-3. Previous studies have indicated that XRCC5 binds the promoter region of genes such as pS2, FAS, and COX-2, thus regulating gene transcription. The XRCC5-interacting proteins identified in these genes' promoter regions include DNA-PK, XRCC6, PARP-1, topoisomerase IIβ, PP1, and p300 [19, 20, 37]. Therefore, we tested whether XRCC5 bound to the CLC-3 promoter by interacting with other proteins. PARP1, also known as poly (ADP-ribose) polymerase 1, was discovered as a potential candidate for interaction with XRCC5 in the nucleus. Served as a transcription factor [39], PARP1 is essential for many cellular processes, including maintenance of genomic integrity, chromatin dynamics, and transcriptional regulation [40]. To ascertain whether PARP1 also bound the CLC-3 promoter, we pulled down the nuclear protein/DNA complex in GC cells using a CLC-3 promoter probe and validated their direct binding. We therefore speculated that PARP1 should also be identified in Fig. 2e. Nevertheless, the upper differential protein band (at almost 120 kDa) was not analyzed by MS. Previous studies have reported that PARP1 often forms regulatory complexes with other proteins and then regulates the expression of genes, including CCND1, CCN2, and NF-κB [41–43]. Indeed, the co-localization of XRCC5 and PARP1 was observed in the nucleus, indicating that XRCC5 and PARP1 formed a regulatory complex in the nucleus. It has been reported that PARP1 is overexpressed in GC and that PARP1 knockdown significantly attenuates the proliferation of GC cells [44, 45]. Therefore, we preliminarily explored the interaction effect of PARP1 and XRCC5 on CLC-3 expression and cell proliferation. The results indicated that the promotion effect of XRCC5 overexpression on the CLC-3 expression and cell proliferation was partly reversed by the PARP1 knockdown, which suggested that PARP1 might act as a positive regulatory factor for CLC-3 in GC cells. These findings prove that knockdown of XRCC5 suppresses the binding of XRCC5 to the CLC-3 promoter and subsequent promoter activity, thus regulating CLC-3 expression at the transcriptional level by interacting with PARP1. Currently, there

are ongoing clinical trials of many PARP1 inhibitors aimed at DNA binding and transcriptional activity [46–48], and one PARP inhibitor, olaparib, has been approved by the FDA to treat ovarian cancer patients with BRCA genes mutations [49], providing new prospects for the application of this inhibitor in future studies.

The relationship between CLC-3 and XRCC5 was also investigated in mouse xenograft models. The results were consistent with our in vitro data and showed that CLC-3 could be regulated by XRCC5 in vivo. Here, we propose a model for the relationship between CLC-3 and XRCC5 in GC development (Fig. 6f). Overexpression of CLC-3 is a poor prognostic biomarker for GC, and CLC-3 may regulate cell proliferation and migration via the PI3K/AKT signaling pathway. The regulatory mechanism of CLC-3 overexpression in GC is that XRCC5 binds the CLC-3 promoter region and affects subsequent promoter activity, thus regulating CLC-3 expression at the transcriptional level by interacting with PARP1.

Conclusions

In summary, this study has illustrated that overexpression of CLC-3 is regulated by XRCC5 and is a poor prognostic biomarker for gastric cancer. Double targeting CLC-3 and XRCC5 may provide promising therapeutic potential for GC treatment.

Additional file

Additional file 1: Table S1. The truncated promoter regions of CLC-3 were designed with primer pairs as follows. (DOCX 29 kb)

Abbreviations
ANT: Adjacent normal tissues; BSA: Bovine serum albumin; cDNA: Complementary DNA; ChIP: Chromatin immunoprecipitation; CI: Confidence interval; CLC-3: Chloride channel-3; Co-IP: Co-immunoprecipitation; DAB: 3,5-Diaminobenzidine; DAPI: 4,6-Diamidino-2-phenylindole; DGE: Differential gene expression; DNA-PK: DNA-dependent protein kinase; FBS: Fetal bovine serum; GC: Gastric cancer; GO: Gene Ontology; HR: Hazard rate; IF: Immunofluorescence; IHC: Immunohistochemistry; IP: Immunoprecipitation; KEGG: Kyoto Encyclopedia of Genes and Genomes; MS: Mass spectrometry; MTS: 3-(4,5-Dimethylthiazol-2-yl)-5-(3-carboxymethoxyphenyl)-2-(4-sulfophenyl)-2H-tetrazolium; NSP: Nonspecific probe; OD: Optical density; PAGE: Polyacrylamide gel electrophoresis; PARP1: Poly (ADP-ribose) polymerase 1; PBS: Phosphate-buffered solution; PCR: Polymerase chain reaction; PVDF: Polyvinylidene fluoride; qRT-PCR: Quantitative real-time polymerase chain reaction; RPMI: Roswell Park Memorial Institute; SDS: Sodium dodecyl sulfate; SRA: Sequence Read Archive; WB: Western blot; XRCC5: X-ray repair cross-complementing 5

Funding
This work was supported by the funds from the National Natural Science Foundation of China (81272223, 81273539), the Ministry of Education of China (201244401110009), the Natural Science Foundation of Guangdong Province (2016A030313495), and the Science and Technology Programs of Guangdong (2017A050501021, 2013B051000059).

Authors' contributions
ZG and YL conceived and designed the study. YL collected GC samples and clinical information. ZG, YL, and XY performed the experiments and acquired the result data. MY, ZC, and CZ helped to perform the partial experiments and review the statistical analysis. ZG and YL drafted the manuscript. LC and LW critically revised the manuscript and supervised the study. All authors read and approved the final manuscript.

Consent for publication
Not applicable

Competing interests
The authors declare that they have no competing interests.

Author details
[1]Department of Pharmacology, Medical College, Jinan University, Guangzhou 510632, China. [2]Department of Pathophysiology, Medical College, Jinan University, Guangzhou, China. [3]Department of Clinical Oncology, The First Affiliated Hospital, Zhengzhou University, Zhengzhou, China. [4]Department of Physiology, Medical College, Jinan University, Guangzhou 510632, China.

References
1. Van Cutsem E, Sagaert X, Topal B, Haustermans K, Prenen H. Gastric cancer. Lancet. 2016;388:2654–64.
2. Badgwell B, Das P, Ajani J. Treatment of localized gastric and gastroesophageal adenocarcinoma: the role of accurate staging and preoperative therapy. J Hematol Oncol. 2017;10:149.
3. Ferlay J, Soerjomataram I, Dikshit R, Eser S, Mathers C, Rebelo M, Parkin DM, Forman D, Bray F. Cancer incidence and mortality worldwide: sources, methods and major patterns in GLOBOCAN 2012. Int J Cancer. 2015;136: E359–86.
4. Zheng L, Wang L, Ajani J, Xie K. Molecular basis of gastric cancer development and progression. Gastric Cancer. 2004;7:61–77.
5. Zhang XW, Sheng YP, Li Q, Qin W, Lu YW, Cheng YF, Liu BY, Zhang FC, Li J, Dimri GP, Guo WJ. BMI1 and Mel-18 oppositely regulate carcinogenesis and progression of gastric cancer. Mol Cancer. 2010;9:40.
6. Wang X, Wang C, Zhang X, Hua R, Gan L, Huang M, Zhao L, Ni S, Guo W. Bmi-1 regulates stem cell-like properties of gastric cancer cells via modulating miRNAs. J Hematol Oncol. 2016;9:90.
7. Gan L, Xu M, Hua R, Tan C, Zhang J, Gong Y, Wu Z, Weng W, Sheng W, Guo W. The polycomb group protein EZH2 induces epithelial-mesenchymal transition and pluripotent phenotype of gastric cancer cells by binding to PTEN promoter. J Hematol Oncol. 2018;11:9.
8. Fan Y, Wang YF, Su HF, Fang N, Zou C, Li WF, Fei ZH. Decreased expression of the long noncoding RNA LINC00261 indicate poor prognosis in gastric cancer and suppress gastric cancer metastasis by affecting the epithelial-mesenchymal transition. J Hematol Oncol. 2016;9:57.
9. Jentsch TJ, Pusch M. CLC chloride channels and transporters: structure, function, physiology, and disease. Physiol Rev. 2018;98:1493–590.
10. Habela CW, Olsen ML, Sontheimer H. ClC3 is a critical regulator of the cell cycle in normal and malignant glial cells. J Neurosci. 2008;28:9205–17.
11. Cuddapah VA, Turner KL, Seifert S, Sontheimer H. Bradykinin-induced chemotaxis of human gliomas requires the activation of KCa3.1 and ClC-3. J Neurosci. 2013;33:1427–40.
12. Lemonnier L, Shuba Y, Crepin A, Roudbaraki M, Slomianny C, Mauroy B, Nilius B, Prevarskaya N, Skryma R. Bcl-2-dependent modulation of swelling-activated Cl⁻ current and ClC-3 expression in human prostate cancer epithelial cells. Cancer Res. 2004;64:4841–8.
13. Zhu L, Yang H, Zuo W, Yang L, Zhang H, Ye W, Mao J, Chen L, Wang L. Differential expression and roles of volume-activated chloride channels in control of growth of normal and cancerous nasopharyngeal epithelial cells. Biochem Pharmacol. 2012;83:324–34.
14. Mao J, Chen L, Xu B, Wang L, Li H, Guo J, Li W, Nie S, Jacob TJ, Wang L. Suppression of ClC-3 channel expression reduces migration of nasopharyngeal carcinoma cells. Biochem Pharmacol. 2008;75:1706–16.
15. Mao J, Yuan J, Wang L, Zhang H, Jin X, Zhu J, Li H, Xu B, Chen L. Tamoxifen inhibits migration of estrogen receptor-negative hepatocellular carcinoma cells by blocking the swelling-activated chloride current. J Cell Physiol. 2013; 228:991–1001.
16. Mao J, Chen L, Xu B, Wang L, Wang W, Li M, Zheng M, Li H, Guo J, Li W, et al. Volume-activated chloride channels contribute to cell-cycle-dependent regulation of HeLa cell migration. Biochem Pharmacol. 2009;77: 159–68.
17. Taccioli GE, Gottlieb TM, Blunt T, Priestley A, Demengeot J, Mizuta R, Lehmann AR, Alt FW, Jackson SP, Jeggo PA. Ku80: product of the XRCC5 gene and its role in DNA repair and V(D)J recombination. Science. 1994;265: 1442–5.
18. Gottlieb TM, Jackson SP. The DNA-dependent protein kinase: requirement for DNA ends and association with Ku antigen. Cell. 1993;72:131–42.
19. Ju BG, Lunyak VV, Perissi V, Garcia-Bassets I, Rose DW, Glass CK, Rosenfeld MG. A topoisomerase IIbeta-mediated dsDNA break required for regulated transcription. Science. 2006;312:1798–802.
20. Wong RH, Chang I, Hudak CS, Hyun S, Kwan HY, Sul HS. A role of DNA-PK for the metabolic gene regulation in response to insulin. Cell. 2009;136: 1056–72.
21. Trinh BQ, Ko SY, Barengo N, Lin SY, Naora H. Dual functions of the homeoprotein DLX4 in modulating responsiveness of tumor cells to topoisomerase II-targeting drugs. Cancer Res. 2013;73:1000–10.
22. Moeller BJ, Yordy JS, Williams MD, Giri U, Raju U, Molkentine DP, Byers LA, Heymach JV, Story MD, Lee JJ, et al. DNA repair biomarker profiling of head and neck cancer: Ku80 expression predicts locoregional failure and death following radiotherapy. Clin Cancer Res. 2011;17:2035–43.
23. Grabsch H, Dattani M, Barker L, Maughan N, Maude K, Hansen O, Gabbert HE, Quirke P, Mueller W. Expression of DNA double-strand break repair proteins ATM and BRCA1 predicts survival in colorectal cancer. Clin Cancer Res. 2006;12:1494–500.
24. Ma Q, Li P, Xu M, Yin J, Su Z, Li W, Zhang J. Ku80 is highly expressed in lung adenocarcinoma and promotes cisplatin resistance. J Exp Clin Cancer Res. 2012;31:99.
25. Tan P, Yeoh KG. Genetics and molecular pathogenesis of gastric adenocarcinoma. Gastroenterology. 2015;149:1153–62. e1153
26. Guan YT, Huang YQ, Wu JB, Deng ZQ, Wang Y, Lai ZY, Wang HB, Sun XX, Zhu YL, Du MM, et al. Overexpression of chloride channel-3 is associated with the increased migration and invasion ability of ectopic endometrial cells from patients with endometriosis. Hum Reprod. 2016;31:986–98.
27. Qin C, He B, Dai W, Lin Z, Zhang H, Wang X, Wang J, Zhang X, Wang G, Yin L, Zhang Q. The impact of a chlorotoxin-modified liposome system on receptor MMP-2 and the receptor-associated protein ClC-3. Biomaterials. 2014;35:5908–20.
28. Zeng JW, Wang XG, Ma MM, Lv XF, Liu J, Zhou JG, Guan YY. Integrin beta3 mediates cerebrovascular remodelling through Src/ClC-3 volume-regulated Cl(-) channel signalling pathway. Br J Pharmacol. 2014;171: 3158–70.
29. Hennessy BT, Smith DL, Ram PT, Lu Y, Mills GB. Exploiting the PI3K/AKT pathway for cancer drug discovery. Nat Rev Drug Discov. 2005;4:988–1004.
30. Fu QF, Liu Y, Fan Y, Hua SN, Qu HY, Dong SW, Li RL, Zhao MY, Zhen Y, Yu XL, et al. Alpha-enolase promotes cell glycolysis, growth, migration, and invasion in non-small cell lung cancer through FAK-mediated PI3K/AKT pathway. J Hematol Oncol. 2015;8:22.
31. Liu J, Zhang D, Li Y, Chen W, Ruan Z, Deng L, Wang L, Tian H, Yiu A, Fan C, et al. Discovery of bufadienolides as a novel class of ClC-3 chloride channel activators with antitumor activities. J Med Chem. 2013;56:5734–43.

32. Liu T, Li W, Lu W, Chen M, Luo M, Zhang C, Li Y, Qin G, Shi D, Xiao B, et al. RBFOX3 promotes tumor growth and progression via hTERT signaling and predicts a poor prognosis in hepatocellular carcinoma. Theranostics. 2017;7: 3138–54.

33. Huang R, Chen Z, He L, He N, Xi Z, Li Z, Deng Y, Zeng X. Mass spectrometry-assisted gel-based proteomics in cancer biomarker discovery: approaches and application. Theranostics. 2017;7:3559–72.

34. Lee MN, Tseng RC, Hsu HS, Chen JY, Tzao C, Ho WL, Wang YC. Epigenetic inactivation of the chromosomal stability control genes BRCA1, BRCA2, and XRCC5 in non-small cell lung cancer. Clin Cancer Res. 2007;13:832–8.

35. Pucci S, Mazzarelli P, Rabitti C, Giai M, Gallucci M, Flammia G, Alcini A, Altomare V, Fazio VM. Tumor specific modulation of KU70/80 DNA binding activity in breast and bladder human tumor biopsies. Oncogene. 2001;20: 739–47.

36. Wang S, Wang M, Yin S, Fu G, Li C, Chen R, Li A, Zhou J, Zhang Z, Liu Q. A novel variable number of tandem repeats (VNTR) polymorphism containing Sp1 binding elements in the promoter of XRCC5 is a risk factor for human bladder cancer. Mutat Res. 2008;638:26–36.

37. Zhang Z, Zheng F, Yu Z, Hao J, Chen M, Yu W, Guo W, Chen Y, Huang W, Duan Z, Deng W. XRCC5 cooperates with p300 to promote cyclooxygenase-2 expression and tumor growth in colon cancers. PLoS One. 2017;12: e0186900.

38. Wei S, Xiong M, Zhan DQ, Liang BY, Wang YY, Gutmann DH, Huang ZY, Chen XP. Ku80 functions as a tumor suppressor in hepatocellular carcinoma by inducing S-phase arrest through a p53-dependent pathway. Carcinogenesis. 2012;33:538–47.

39. Forrest AR, Kawaji H, Rehli M, Baillie JK, de Hoon MJ, Haberle V, Lassmann T, Kulakovskiy IV, Lizio M, Itoh M, et al. A promoter-level mammalian expression atlas. Nature. 2014;507:462–70.

40. Schiewer MJ, Knudsen KE. Transcriptional roles of PARP1 in cancer. Mol Cancer Res. 2014;12:1069–80.

41. Shan L, Li X, Liu L, Ding X, Wang Q, Zheng Y, Duan Y, Xuan C, Wang Y, Yang F, et al. GATA3 cooperates with PARP1 to regulate CCND1 transcription through modulating histone H1 incorporation. Oncogene. 2014;33:3205–16.

42. Okada H, Inoue T, Kikuta T, Kato N, Kanno Y, Hirosawa N, Sakamoto Y, Sugaya T, Suzuki H. Poly(ADP-ribose) polymerase-1 enhances transcription of the profibrotic CCN2 gene. J Am Soc Nephrol. 2008;19:933–42.

43. Hassa PO, Haenni SS, Buerki C, Meier NI, Lane WS, Owen H, Gersbach M, Imhof R, Hottiger MO. Acetylation of poly(ADP-ribose) polymerase-1 by p300/CREB-binding protein regulates coactivation of NF-kappaB-dependent transcription. J Biol Chem. 2005;280:40450–64.

44. Park SH, Jang KY, Kim MJ, Yoon S, Jo Y, Kwon SM, Kim KM, Kwon KS, Kim CY, Woo HG. Tumor suppressive effect of PARP1 and FOXO3A in gastric cancers and its clinical implications. Oncotarget. 2015;6:44819–31.

45. Liu Y, Zhang Y, Zhao Y, Gao D, Xing J, Liu H. High PARP-1 expression is associated with tumor invasion and poor prognosis in gastric cancer. Oncol Lett. 2016;12:3825–35.

46. Hu X, Huang W, Fan M. Emerging therapies for breast cancer. J Hematol Oncol. 2017;10:98.

47. Dholaria B, Hammond W, Shreders A, Lou Y. Emerging therapeutic agents for lung cancer. J Hematol Oncol. 2016;9:138.

48. Laroche A, Chaire V, Le Loarer F, Algeo MP, Rey C, Tran K, Lucchesi C, Italiano A. Activity of trabectedin and the PARP inhibitor rucaparib in soft-tissue sarcomas. J Hematol Oncol. 2017;10:84.

49. Du Y, Yamaguchi H, Wei Y, Hsu JL, Wang HL, Hsu YH, Lin WC, Yu WH, Leonard PG, GRt L, et al. Blocking c-Met-mediated PARP1 phosphorylation enhances anti-tumor effects of PARP inhibitors. Nat Med. 2016;22:194–201.

8

Emerging roles of long non-coding RNAs in tumor metabolism

Hui Sun[1], Zhaohui Huang[2], Weiqi Sheng[1*] and Mi-die Xu[1,3*]

Abstract

Compared with normal cells, tumor cells display distinct metabolic characteristics. Long non-coding RNAs (lncRNAs), a large class of regulatory RNA molecules with limited or no protein-coding capacity, play key roles in tumorigenesis and progression. Recent advances have revealed that lncRNAs play a vital role in cell metabolism by regulating the reprogramming of the metabolic pathways in cancer cells. LncRNAs could regulate various metabolic enzymes that integrate cell malignant transformation and metabolic reprogramming. In addition to the known functions of lncRNAs in regulating glycolysis and glucose homeostasis, recent studies also implicate lncRNAs in amino acid and lipid metabolism. These observations reveal the high complexity of the malignant metabolism. Elucidating the metabolic-related functions of lncRNAs will provide a better understanding of the regulatory mechanisms of metabolism and thus may provide insights for the clinical development of cancer diagnostics, prognostics and therapeutics.

Keywords: lncRNAs, Tumor, Metabolism, Reprogramming, Dysregulation

Background

Metabolism is the set of life-sustaining chemical transformations within the cells of organisms. Most of the structures that make up living organisms are made from three basic classes of molecule: carbohydrates, lipids, and amino acids. The metabolic pathways in the human body focus either on making these molecules during the construction of cells and tissues or on breaking them down by digestion and using them as a source of energy. Malignancy is a disease characterized by the evasion of cell proliferation checkpoints. In general, tumor cells metabolize glucose, glutamine, and fatty acids (FAs) at much higher rates than their normal counterparts. The metabolic ecology of tumors is complex, and tumor cells undergo fundamental changes in metabolic pathways. Multiple molecular mechanisms converge to alter the overall cell metabolism and to provide support for the three basic needs of proliferating cells: rapid ATP generation to maintain energy status; increased biosynthesis of macromolecules; and strict maintenance of appropriate redox status [1]. To satisfy these needs, cancer cells alter the metabolism of the four major macromolecules, carbohydrates, proteins, lipids,

and nucleic acids. A number of similar alterations have also been observed in normal cells that are rapidly proliferating in response to pathophysiological growth signals [2, 3].

Normal cells produce energy primarily through mitochondrial oxidative phosphorylation, which is the metabolic pathway in which cells use enzymes to oxidize organic compounds including carbohydrates, lipids, and amino acids, thereby releasing energy for the production of adenosine triphosphate (ATP) [2]. Tumor cells can satisfy the needs of their rapid and unrestrained proliferation by a high rate of glycolysis followed by lactic acid fermentation even in the presence of abundant oxygen. This process is called aerobic glycolysis, also known as the Warburg effect [4]. Aerobic glycolysis was first recognized in the 1920s by Otto Warburg, who found that cancer tissues metabolized glucose to lactate through glycolysis at an increased rate, even under normal oxygen concentrations [5, 6]. The Warburg effect has been observed in different types of tumors and has been widely accepted as a hallmark of altered metabolism in cancer cells [7]. However, these alterations are not specific to tumors, because similar changes have also been observed in rapidly proliferating normal cells [2, 3, 8].

Although glucose metabolism is important for cell proliferation, it has recently been recognized that other nutrients, such as amino acids and lipids, also significantly contribute to cell proliferation [9, 10]. "Glutamine metabolism"

---

* Correspondence: shengweiqi2006@163.com; xumd27202003@163.com;
12111230022@fudan.edu.cn
[1]Department of Pathology, Fudan University Shanghai Cancer Center,
Shanghai 200032, China
Full list of author information is available at the end of the article

(i.e., accelerated glutamine intake and glutaminolysis in tumor cells) is another important energy metabolic mode of tumor cells in addition to the Warburg effect [11–14]. Like glucose, glutamine is anaplerotic, meaning that it provides energetic precursors such as oxaloacetate for the Krebs Cycle (also called the tricarboxylic acid cycle, TCA). Glycolysis and glutaminolysis increase carbon flux inside the cell, resulting in the accumulation of the Krebs cycle precursor intermediate to activate another metabolic pathway—the pentose phosphate pathway [15], which generates NADPH, reducing glutathione and enhancing the amelioration of oxidative stress. The pentose phosphate pathway also produces ribose-5-phosphate, which is essential for the biosynthesis of nucleic acids. While normal cells obtain most FAs from circulating lipids, tumor cells show increased dependence on endogenous FA synthesis to satisfy their rapacious metabolic needs [16]. Under hypoxic conditions, when glucose metabolism in the tumor is blocked, the glutamine metabolism can supply the necessary energy for tumor cell survival. In addition, tumor cells could take more acetic acid from the outside environment to supplement the acetyl-CoA supply in cells and further feed the FA synthesis pathway to promote tumor growth.

The implications of the Warburg effect have been further extended in recent years as cumulative evidence confirmed that the mode of metabolism during tumorigenesis undergoes dramatic changes involving glycolysis, the Krebs cycle, oxidative phosphorylation, amino acid metabolism, FA metabolism, and nucleic acid metabolism, among many other aspects. This phenomenon is called metabolic reprogramming. Malignant transformation involves excessive glucose uptake, lactate excretion, aerobic glycolysis, glutamine, and lipid metabolism, all of which allow cancer cells to survive in adverse microenvironments [17]. The metabolic profiles of tumors with the same genetic alterations show differences depending on the origin of the tissue, suggesting that the tissue microenvironment may affect the metabolic activity of cancer cells [18]. Elucidating the mechanism of cell metabolism reprogramming and its relationship with the occurrence and development of the tumor and developing methods for the intervention and correction of abnormal cell metabolism are promising new ideas for the diagnosis, prevention, and treatment of tumors.

Long non-coding RNAs (lncRNAs) are defined as mRNA-like transcripts longer than 200 nucleotides that have little or no protein-coding potential [19–21]. LncRNAs were previously regarded as "junk products" of transcription and were neglected, but recently, many lncRNAs have been identified as regulators of tumorigenesis and progression via a series of cellular processes, including cell proliferation [22, 23], apoptosis [24, 25], metastasis [26], and differentiation [27] at the transcriptional and posttranscriptional levels [28].

LncRNAs are extensively dysregulated in human malignancies and control different aspects of cellular energy metabolism, including glucose metabolism [29, 30], plasma lipid homeostasis [31], and glutamine metabolism [32] (Fig. 1), and multiple altered metabolic pathways in cancers are tightly regulated by lncRNAs [33, 34] (Figs. 2 and 3). In this review, we discuss the regulatory roles of lncRNAs in the essential metabolic rearrangement and the pathways affected in cancer.

LncRNAs and metabolic reprogramming
LncRNAs and glycometabolism

Malignant cells are known for accelerated nutrient and energy metabolism and increased glucose metabolism and uptake. In eukaryotic cells, glucose transport consists of two different types of membrane-related carrier proteins, namely, Na^+-glucose linked transporters (SGLTs) and glucose transporters (GLUTs) [35]. GLUTs play a crucial role in glucose metabolism in transformed cells [36, 37]. A number of lncRNAs can regulate glycolytic steps by binding GLUTs. A novel large antisense non-coding RNA (named ANRIL) spans a 126.3 kb region and transcribes as a 3.8 kb lncRNA in the antisense orientation of the INK4B-ARF-INK4A gene cluster [16, 38, 39]. ANRIL is upregulated in nasopharyngeal carcinoma (NPC). By activating the AKT/mTOR signal, ANRIL upregulates GLUT1 and LDHA expression, thus increasing glucose uptake and promoting cancer progression in NPC cells [40]. Adenosine monophosphate-activated protein kinase (AMPK) is a critical sensor of cellular energy status in eukaryotic cells, and activated AMPK functions to promote catabolic processes (such as glycolysis, FA oxidation, and autophagy) and repress anabolic processes (such as lipid, protein, and sterol synthesis), resulting in restoration of the energy balance [41]. As anabolic processes are often required to support tumor survival and growth, the AMPK signaling pathway plays tumor-suppressive roles in many types of cancers. Currently, a glucose starvation-induced lncRNA called NBR2 (the neighbor of BRCA1 gene 2) was found to be induced in cancer cells by the LKB1–AMPK pathway under energy stress conditions [42]. Intriguingly, NBR2 can in turn interact with the kinase domain of AMPKα and promote AMPK kinase activity, thus forming a feed-forward loop to potentiate AMPK activation upon glucose starvation [34]. However, under the energy stress imposed by phenformin treatment, NBR2 promotes glucose uptake by upregulating GLUT1 expression but not by affecting phenformin-induced AMPK activation [43]. Thus, NBR2 may promote cancer cell glucose uptake by participating in alterable biological processes in response to different intracellular environments. GLUT4 is directly associated with carbohydrate metabolism. It translocates to the plasma membrane and facilitates the intracellular transport of

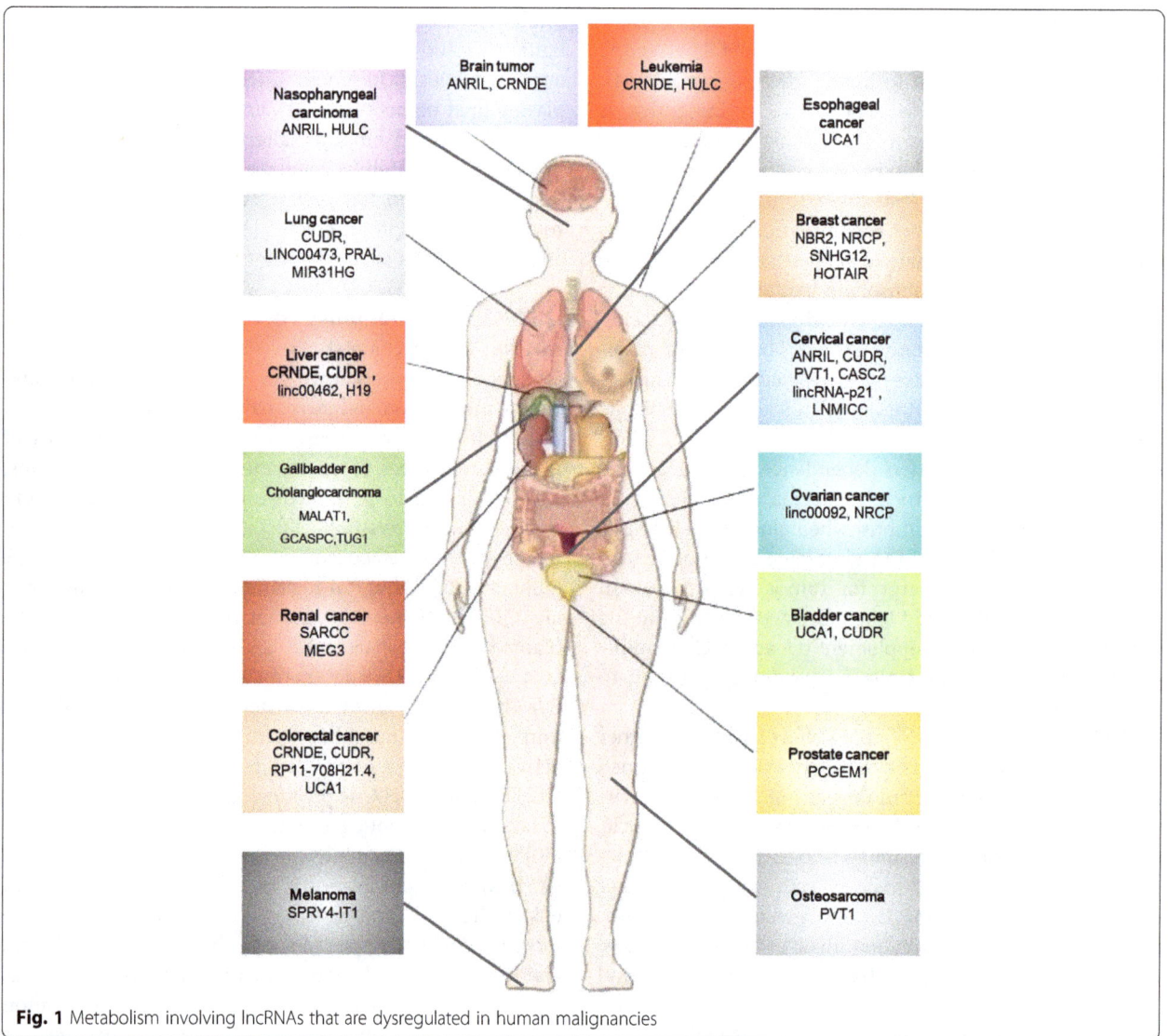

Fig. 1 Metabolism involving lncRNAs that are dysregulated in human malignancies

glucose under insulin stimulation [44]. Ellis et al. found that the lncRNA CRNDE, which is upregulated in colorectal tumors, whereas little to none is expressed in the normal colorectal epithelium [45], can positively regulate GLUT4 transcription and glucose intake [30].

In addition to binding to glycolysis transporters, lncRNAs can also regulate glycolytic steps by binding to key enzymes (Fig. 2). The glycolytic enzyme 6-phosphofructo-2-kinase/fructose-2,6-bisphosphatase 2 (PFKFB2) acts as a functional homodimer that catalyzes both the synthesis and hydrolysis of fructose-2,6-bisphosphate (Fru-2,6-P2). By directly binding with PFKFB2, linc00092 promotes ovarian cancer metastasis by altering glycolysis and sustaining the local supportive function of cancer-associated fibroblasts (CAFs) one of the most abundant cell components in the tumor microenvironment, which promotes carcinogenesis and cancer progression in different cancer cell types [46]. miR-17-3p belongs to the polycistronic miR-17-92 cluster,

which could associate with c-Myc, a well-studied oncogenic transcription factor showing pivotal promoting effects on cellular glycolysis [47]. miR-17-3p, which targets GCASPC (gallbladder cancer-associated suppressor of pyruvate carboxylase), can suppress pyruvate carboxylase-dependent cell proliferation in gallbladder cancer by binding and destabilizing the pyruvate carboxylase (PC) protein [48]. NRCP (lncRNA ceruloplasmin) can function as an intermediary molecule by connecting STAT1 to RNA polymerase II, which leads to upregulation of the key glycolysis enzyme glucose-6-phosphate isomerase (GP6I) and thus promotes glycolysis and cancer progression [49]. Pyruvate kinase M2 (PKM2) is essential for glucose metabolism, cell proliferation, cell migration, and tumor angiogenesis because dimeric PKM2 diverts glucose metabolism towards anabolism through aerobic glycolysis [50, 51]. The lncRNA CUDR is well known to be involved in tumorigenesis. Acting as a sponge cushion

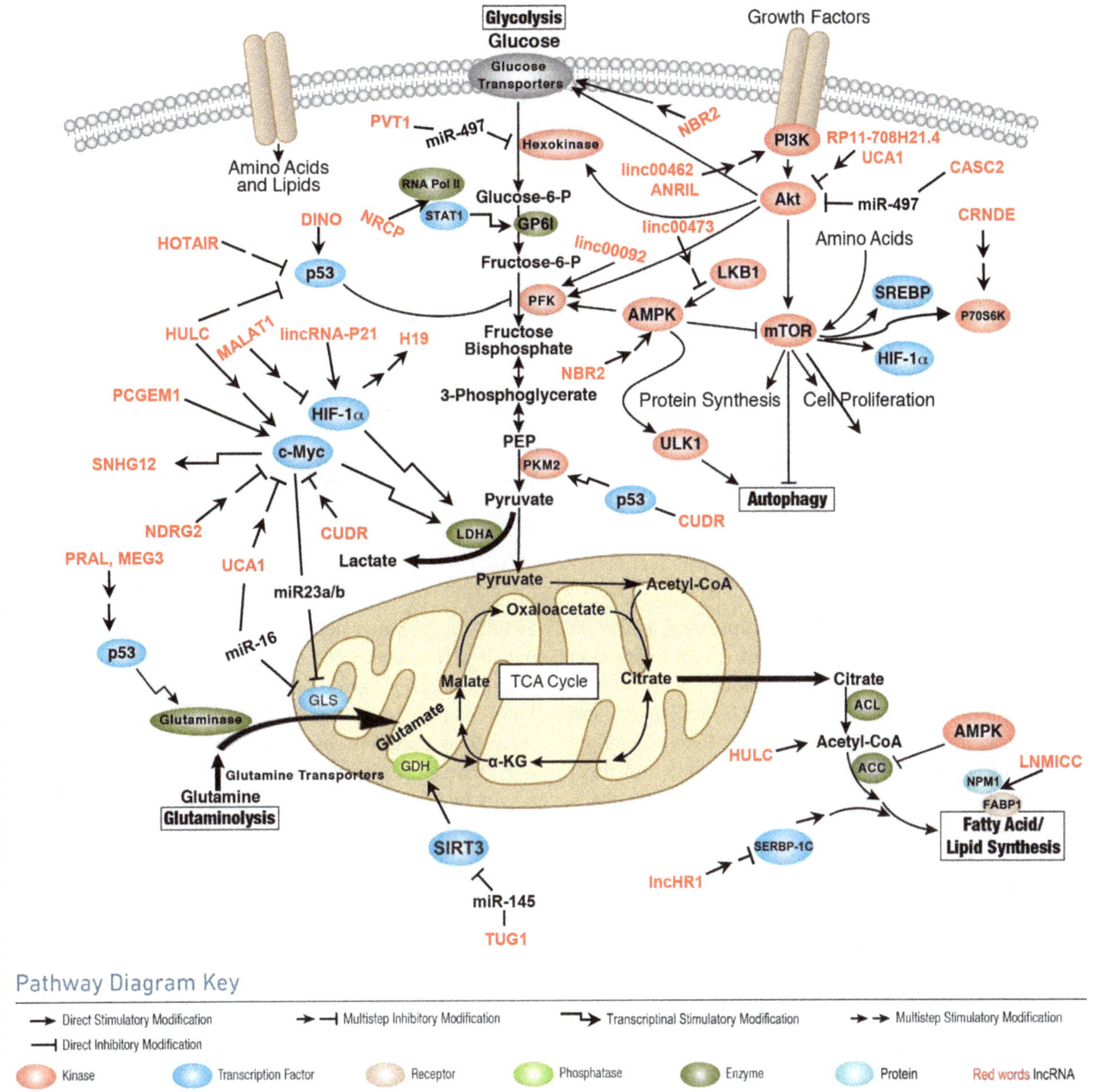

Fig. 2 LncRNAs regulate metabolic rearrangement by targeting metabolism-related signals

linking SET1A and pRB1, CUDR increases the expression of HULC, β-catenin, TERT, and c-Myc in human liver cancer stem cells, thus initiating stem cell malignant transformation [52–54] in a metabolic paradigm; however, CUDR can form a complex with p53 to promote hepatocarcinogenesis by transcriptionally activating PKM2 [55]. Our recent work revealed that FEZF1-AS1 enhances glycolysis through binding and increasing the stability of PKM2 in CRC cells [56]. Hexokinase catalyzes the first irreversible step of glucose metabolism, thereby producing glucose-6-phosphate through the ATP-dependent phosphorylation of glucose [57]. In bladder carcinoma, lncRNA

UCA1 is overexpressed and promotes glycolysis by upregulating hexokinase 2 (HK2), which promotes aerobic glycolysis and acts as the key indicator of the Warburg effect [58, 59]. LncRNA PVT1 promotes glucose metabolism in osteosarcoma by inhibiting miR-497/HK2 signaling through a competing endogenous RNA (ceRNA) mechanism [60].

The let-7/Lin28 pathway plays a central role in mammalian glucose metabolism [61]. Lin28 promotes malignancy by blocking the biogenesis of tumor-suppressive let-7 and by derepressing the expression of oncogenic lncRNA—H19 [62]. Moreover, H19 can act as a ceRNA to

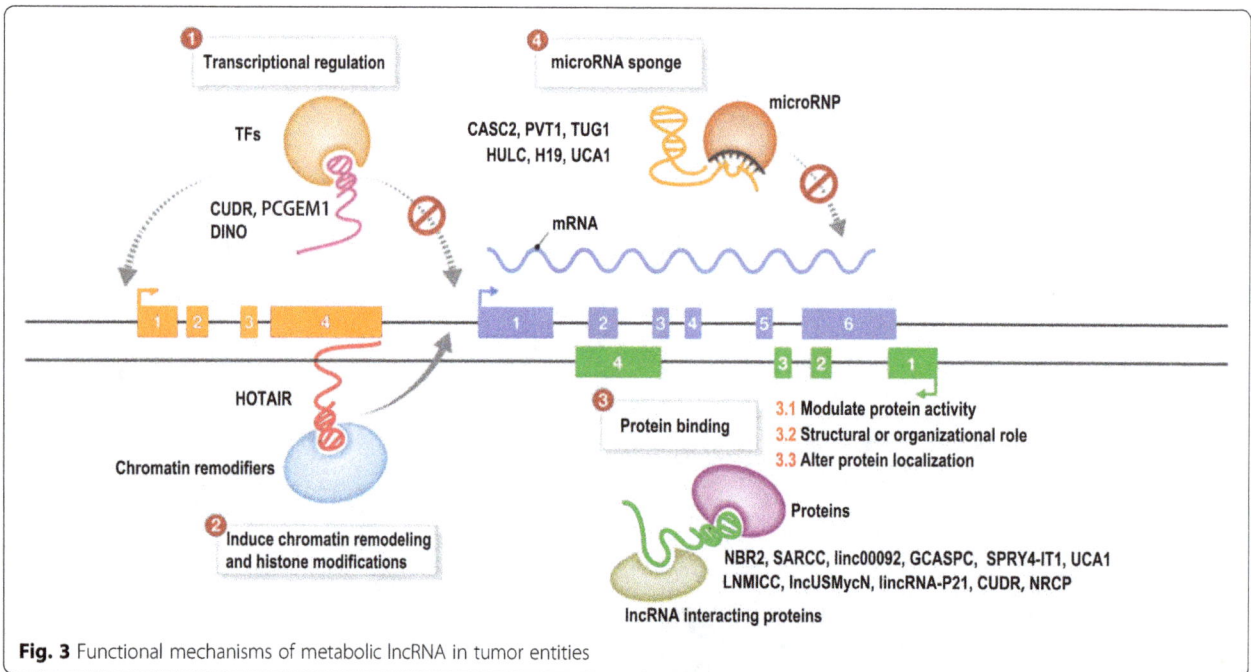

Fig. 3 Functional mechanisms of metabolic lncRNA in tumor entities

sponge let-7 and upregulates Lin28 expression in breast cancer cells; in turn, this induction of Lin28 expression further restricts let-7 function [62]. In addition, by directly binding to let-7, H19 can decrease let-7 availability and suppress the insulin pathway [63, 64]. Taken together, these findings suggest that H19, let-7, and Lin28 may form a glucose metabolism-related double-negative feedback loop in breast cancer cells.

LncRNA and lipid metabolism

Lipids are a class of water-insoluble molecules that include triglycerides, phospholipids, sterols, and sphingolipids. The main structural components of biological membranes include phospholipids, sterols, and sphingolipids, whereas triglycerides provide energy storage. Lipids not only play a pivotal role in metabolic processes but also act as signaling molecules [65]. Similar to glucose metabolism, aberrant alterations in lipid metabolism have also been observed in cancer cells [66]. Regardless of the concentration of extracellular lipids, the main synthetic pathway of FAs is de novo synthesis. Instead of increase glucose uptake, certain tumor cells could utilize increase lipid oxidation as their main energy source. For example, malignant prostate cells are characterized by a low rate of glucose uptake but a high FA intake [67].

As master regulators of hepatic lipid homeostasis, sterol regulatory element binding proteins (SREBPs) play extensive roles in lipid metabolism. Mammals have three SREBPs (-1a, -1c, and -2), of which SREBP-1a and SREBP-1c preferentially activate the genes for FA synthesis, and SREBP-2 activates the cholesterol synthesis genes [68]. LncHR1 was found to decrease lipid metabolism by repressing the SREBP-1c promoter activity and FA synthase (FAS), resulting in decreased accumulation of oleic acid-induced hepatic cell triglyceride (TG) and lipid droplet (LD) in the Huh7 human hepatoma cell line [69]. FA-binding proteins (FABP), as indispensable carriers of FA uptake and transport, have been proven to be critical central regulators of FA metabolism [70]. FABP5 is a member of the FABP family and exhibits high-affinity binding to long-chain FAs. LncRNA LNMICC can recruit the nuclear factor NPM1 to the promoter of FABP5, thus reprogramming FA metabolism and promoting lymph node metastasis in cervical cancer [71].

Acyl-CoA synthase long-chain (ACSL) family members catalyze the initial step in cellular long-chain FA metabolism in mammals; ACSL1, one of the major isoforms of the ACSL family, can increase the uptake of FAs in hepatoma cells and can be regulated by the transcriptional factor PPARα [72–74]. HULC is the first lncRNA found to be specifically overexpressed in hepatocellular carcinoma (HCC) [75]. In hepatoma cells, HULC suppresses miR-9 targeting PPARα silencing by eliciting the methylation of CpG islands in the miR-9 promoter, and PPARα activates ACSL1 transcription. In this case, HULC stimulates the accumulation of intracellular triglycerides and cholesterol through the miR-9/PPARα/ACSL1 signaling pathway in hepatoma cells [76].

Fatty liver is an early manifestation of various liver toxicities and is not directly related to the occurrence of primary liver cancer. However, some of the etiologies of fatty liver, such as alcohol, malnutrition, drugs, and toxic damage, are pathogens of both fatty liver disease and liver cancer; therefore, fatty liver and hepatic cancer are often intertwined and share a common molecular regulatory mechanism. LncRNA has been potentially implicated in adipogenesis. Peroxisome proliferator-activated receptor-γ (PPARγ) is a master transcriptional regulator of adipogenesis. Insulin influences adipocyte differentiation through the regulation of MAPKs, including ERK1/2 (p44/p42), p38 and c-Jun amino-terminal kinase (JNK), each of which can regulate adipogenesis [77]. LncRNA-SRA (steroid receptor RNA) functions as an RNA coactivator for nonsteroid nuclear receptors and contributes to adipogenesis and insulin sensitivity via regulating PPARγ and P38/JNK phosphorylation [77, 78], and SRA knockout downregulates the size of adipocytes and improves glucose tolerance by protecting against high-fat diet-induced obesity and fatty liver [79]. We speculated that the SRA-PPARγ-P38/JNK pathway may also be implicated in HCC-related lipid metabolism rearrangement.

Lipin 2 is an enzyme that converts phosphatidate to diacylglycerol (DAG), and diacylglycerol O-acyltransferase 2 (DGAT2) is an enzyme involved in the conversion of DAG to triacylglycerol. LncRNA SPRY4-IT1 expression is low in normal human melanocytes but elevated in melanoma cells. By directly binding with lipin 2, SPRY4-IT1 downregulates the expression of DGAT2, acyl carnitine, fatty acyl chains, and triacylglycerol, thereby leading to cellular lipotoxicity and functioning as an oncogene in human melanoma cells, which provides novel insight into the mechanisms by which extranuclear processing of lncRNAs contributes to lipid metabolism [80].

LncRNA and amino acid metabolism

In addition to the rearrangement of glucose metabolism, tumor cells also exhibit accelerated glutamine intake and glutaminolysis. Recent work has shown that TUG1 increased glutamine metabolism and increased tumorigenic potential by functioning as an endogenous competing RNA (ceRNA), antagonizing miR-145 and indirectly upregulating sirtuin 3 (Sirt3) and glutamate dehydrogenase (GDH) expression, which provides evidence for its pivotal role in intrahepatic cholangiocarcinoma (ICC) [81]. Reactive oxygen species (ROS), as by-products of cell metabolism, can induce genetic and epigenetic alterations in human carcinogenesis [82]. Tumor cells depend for their survival not only on glycolysis but also on glutamine metabolism [11–13]. For instance, glutamine metabolism plays a key role in maintaining redox balance and ROS levels in tumor cells [83], and glutamine can be converted to glutamate, a precursor of glutathione, by glutaminase 2 (GLS2, a GLS enzyme catalyzing the conversion of glutamine to glutamate) during ROS-induced stress [84].

The c-Myc family are pivotal glutamine metabolism regulators that regulate the intracellular transposition of glutamate and promote the conversion of glutamine to glutamate [17, 85]. In colorectal cancer, by suppressing the expression of β-catenin and thereby decreasing c-Myc expression, the lncRNA N-Myc downstream-regulated gene 2 (NDRG2) could inhibit glycolysis, glutaminolysis, and thus cancer growth [86]. Previous data showed that UCA1 plays a tumor suppressor role by reducing the expression level of c-Myc in esophageal squamous cell carcinoma [87]. Moreover, in bladder cancer cells, by acting as a miR-16 sponge and upregulating the expression of miR-16 targeting GLS2, UCA1 contributes to glutamine metabolism and represses ROS formation in bladder cancer [32]. These reports reveal that UCA1 may implement its role in glutamine metabolism by multiple mechanisms.

Functions of lncRNA and mitochondria

In eukaryotic cells, mitochondria are critical hubs for the integration of several key metabolic processes (Fig. 2). To maintain homeostasis, the genome produces specific lncRNA nucleic acids and proteins to coordinate the intense cross-talk between the mitochondria and the nucleus. Currently, the concept of regulation driven by lncRNAs is extending from the nuclear and cytosolic compartments to the mitochondria. Based on the discoveries that (i) the mitochondrial genome can encode lncRNAs [88, 89] and (ii) lncRNAs may be transcribed in the nucleus but reside in the mitochondria [90–92], a role for mitochondrial lncRNAs in the regulation of mitochondrial functions was suggested.

The first reported human mitochondrial-encoded long noncoding RNAs are SncmtRNA, a long chimeric transcript containing an inverted repeat (IR) of 820 nt covalently bound to the 5′ terminus of the mitochondrial 16S ribosomal RNA, and its two antisense transcripts (ASncmtRNA-1 and ASncmtRNA-2). All three lncRNAs are exported from the mitochondria to the nucleus and can be expressed both in normal proliferating cells and in tumor cells. Notably, both antisense transcripts are universally downregulated in cancer cells [88]. ASncmtRNA knockdown induces tumor cell apoptosis by inhibiting the expression of survivin, a member of the inhibitor of apoptosis (IAP) family, suggesting that ASncmtRNAs may take part in mitochondrial retrograde signaling [93]. In addition, although little is known regarding their potential function, several mitochondrial-encoded lncRNAs have been identified [89, 94] and could provide a new paradigm for understanding mitochondrial function.

Evidence is now emerging that several nuclear-encoded lncRNAs can execute regulatory roles in mitochondria. The lncRNA SAMMSON is predominantly localized to the cytoplasm of human melanoblasts and melanoma cells [91]. SAMMSON depletion in melanoma cells decreases the mitochondrial targeting of p32, a mitoribosome assembly and mitochondrial protein synthesis regulator, and attenuates mitochondrial protein synthesis [95], which ultimately triggers cell apoptosis. ARL2 is present in the inner membrane space of mitochondria and is an activator of ATP/ADP transporters. UCA1 can act as a competing endogenous RNA (ceRNA) and contributes to ARL2-induced mitochondrial activity by inhibiting miR-195-5p in bladder cancer [96]. The peroxisome proliferator-activated receptor γ (PPARγ) coactivator α (PGC-1α) is encoded by Ppargc1a and is a well-characterized transcriptional coactivator that plays an integral role in maintaining energy homeostasis and mitochondrial biogenesis in response to a myriad of nutrient and hormonal signals [97]. PGC-1α enhances its own transcription via an autoregulatory loop [98]. By binding directly to an R/S-rich region of the CTD of PGC-1α, the lncRNA TUG1 recruits PGC-1α protein to the Ppargc1a promoter, which enhances PGC-1α expression, leading to increased mitochondrial content, enhanced mitochondrial respiration, increased cellular ATP levels, and reduced mitochondrial ROS [99]. Bcl2 plays a key role in the mitochondrial pathway and regulates cell death by controlling the permeability of the mitochondrial membrane [100]. Tumor-suppressive MEG3 can induce the apoptosis of renal cell carcinoma cells by downregulating Bcl2 expression and thereby stimulating the mitochondrial pathway [101]; similarly, blockage of oncogenic HOTAIR induces mitochondrial calcium uptake 1 (MICU1)-dependent cell death and changes mitochondrial membrane potential by regulating mitochondrial related cell death pathway (Bcl-2, BAX, caspase-3, cleaved caspase-3, cytochrome c) [102]. LncRNA NDRG2 prevents p53 from entering the nucleus and promotes the accumulation of P53 in the mitochondria by increasing the half-life of Bad, thus promoting apoptosis in a p53-dependent manner in breast cancer cells [103]. Considering these pieces of evidence, we concluded that lncRNAs are required for mitochondrial bioenergetics and thus for the maintenance of mitochondrial energy homeostasis.

LncRNA regulation of metabolic signaling

LncRNAs play pivotal regulatory roles in human malignancy-related metabolic reprogramming. Accordingly, the interrelation between dysregulated lncRNAs and metabolism-related factors and signaling pathways contributes greatly to the metabolic abnormalities of cancer cells, thereby promoting carcinogenesis and tumor progression (Table 1 and Figs. 2 and 3).

HIF1 and MYC

Hypoxia-inducible factor (HIF) complexes are transcription factors that regulate cellular gene expression in anoxic conditions. HIF1α and HIF2α are stable in anoxic environments and form heterodimers with HIF1β, which enhances the glycolytic capacity of cells by activating genes that

encode transporters and most glycolytic enzymes and by reinforcing the glycolytic phenotype, through the activation of pyruvate dehydrogenase kinases (PDKs), to reduce the flow of pyruvate into the TCA cycle [1, 104]. HIF1α usually contributes to metabolic transformation in cooperation with lncRNAs. LnRNA H19 is induced by HIF1α upon oxygen deprivation in tumor cells [105]; however, H19 was efficiently repressed when HIF1-α transcriptional activity was inhibited by P53, demonstrating an important role of the p53-HIF1α-H19 pathway in hypoxia [106]. Under arsenite exposure, MALAT1, a hypoxia-inducible lncRNA, influences HIF1α protein levels via blocking HIF1α hydroxylation. In this scenario, MALAT1 disrupts HIF1α-von Hippel-Lindau (VHL) interaction and HIF1α stabilization and increases the expression of glycolytic enzymes, such as HK2 and GLUT4, thereby promoting arsenite-induced glycolysis in human hepatic cells [107]. LincRNA-p21 is a hypoxia-responsive lncRNA and can be specifically upregulated by HIF-1α under hypoxic conditions. Intriguingly, hypoxia/HIF-1a-induced lincRNA-p21 is able in turn to bind to HIF-1α and VHL and thus disrupt the VHL-HIF-1α interaction, resulting in disassociation and thereby attenuating VHL-mediated HIF-1α ubiquitination and stabilizing HIF-1α; in turn, HIF-1α increases the expression of HIF-1α responsive genes, such as those encoding the glycolytic enzymes GLUT1 and LDAH, which increases glycolysis and thus suppresses tumorigenicity [108]. The positive feedback loop between HIF-1a and lincRNA-p21 promoting glycolysis under hypoxia provides a new mechanical paradigm for the Warburg effect in human malignancies.

Myc is a canonical oncogene family that includes c-Myc, n-Myc, and l-Myc. c-Myc has been reported to promote increased aerobic glycolysis through the constitutive elevation of PFK and LDHA as well as through the expression of enzymes involved in nucleotide and amino acid metabolism [84, 85, 109]. In addition, Myc regulates glutamine metabolism and mitochondrial function by activating genes involved in mitochondrial biogenesis [17, 85]. In prostate cancer, Myc regulates glutamine metabolism by regulating the levels of SLC1A4 and SLC1A5 [110]. Prostate cancer gene expression marker 1 (PCGEM1) is an androgen-induced prostate-specific lncRNA whose overexpression is highly related to prostate cancer [111]. PCGEM1 mediates gene regulation partly through activated AR but predominantly through activated c-Myc: PCGEM1 directly binds c-Myc, promotes the chromatin recruitment of c-Myc, and enhances its transactivation activity, then increases the activity of glucose-6-phosphate dehydrogenase (G6PD), a rate-limiting enzyme of the pentose pathway, to shunt the carbon flow from glucose to ribose-5-phosphate; NADPH is generated for redox homeostasis and then participates in multiple metabolic pathways, including glucose and glutamine

Table 1 LncRNAs deregulated in cancer through targeting the signals of metabolism

LncRNA	Location	Target	Up/down	Disease
HIF1 and MYC				
H19	Chr 11p15.5	HIF1A	Up	HCC [105]
SNHG12	/	C-MYC	Up	Breast cancer [113]
SARCC	/	AR	Down	RCC [115]
PCGEM1	Chr 2q32	C-MYC	Up	Prostatic cancer [111]
P53				
HULC	Chr 6p24.3	P53	Up	NPC [123]
HOTAIR	Chr 12	P53	Up	Breast cancer [124]
PRAL	Chr 17p13.1	P53	Down	Lung cancer [125]
PI3K/AKT/MTOR				
RP11-708H21.4	Chr 17q21	MTOR	Down	CRC [138]
UCA1	Chr 19	MTOR/STAT3	Up	CRC [63, 122]
linc00462	/	PI3/AKT	Down	HCC [139]
MALAT1	Chr 11q13	PI3/AKT	Down	Cholangiocarcinoma [177]
CASC2	Chr 10q26	PTEN	Down	CESC [7]
HULC	Chr 6p24.3	PI3/AKT	Up	Myeloid leukemia [135]
ANRIL	Chr 9q21	AKT	Up	NPC, glioma, CESC [33, 40]
AMP-activated protein kinase				
LINC00473	Chr 6q27	LKB1	Up	Lung cancer [143]
NBR2	Chr 17q21	AMPK	Down	Breast cancer [34, 42]

Chr chromosome, *HCC* hepatocellular carcinoma, *NPC* nasopharyngeal carcinoma, *RCC* renal cell carcinoma, *CESC* cervical cancer

metabolism, the pentose phosphate pathway, nucleotide and FA biosynthesis, and the TCA cycle [111, 112]. The c-Myc-induced lncRNA SNHG12 is upregulated in triple-negative breast cancer, indicating that SNHG12 may potentially be a downstream regulator of c-Myc-regulated metabolic abnormalities [113]. Another Myc oncoprotein, N-Myc, is upregulated by lncUSMycN, leading to neuroblastoma cell proliferation via binding to the RNA-binding protein NonO [114].

In combination with the oncogenic transcription factor HIF, Myc activates the glycolytic enzymes PDK1 and LDH. As the substrate recognition module of the ubiquitin ligase complex, the VHL tumor suppressor protein (pVHL) can participate in proteasomal degradation by targeting the alpha subunits of the heterodimeric HIF transcription factor [115]. Inactivation of pVHL is a common event in clear cell renal carcinoma (ccRCC). Under hypoxic conditions, lncRNA-SARCC can physically bind and destabilize AR protein to suppress the VHL-mutant, yet it promotes wild-type RCC cell proliferation by modulating the AR/HIF-2α/c-Myc axis [116].

TP53

The transcription factor p53 is a tumor suppressor that is downregulated in most human malignancies [117]. P53 enhances the expression of HK, TIGAR (TP53-inducible glycolysis and apoptosis regulator), PTEN, and SCO2 [118–121]. SCO2 enhances TCA, PTEN decreases the PI3K signal, and TIGAR suppresses the glycolytic activator Fru-2,6-P2. Various p53-related lncRNAs are reported to participate in tumorigenesis. For example, the lncRNA DINO (damage-induced noncoding) directly binds and stabilizes p53 protein, resulting in enhanced p53 activity [122]. MEG3 plays a tumor-suppressive role by both p53-independent and p53-dependent pathways. MEG3-activated p53 can transcriptionally activate the expression of the growth differentiation factor 15 (GDF15), thus inhibiting cell proliferation. HULC suppresses the activity of p53 and p21 to promote cell growth in nasopharyngeal carcinoma (NPC) [123]. The knockdown of oncogenic HOTAIR increases the level of p53 expression in breast cancer and thereby markedly decreases the proliferation, migration, and invasion ability of MCF-7 cells [124]. P53 was found to be downregulated in lung cancer and to be related to the tumor-suppressive lncRNA PRAL [125]. The lncRNA MIR31HG downregulates p53, promotes cell proliferation, and decreases apoptosis in non-small cell lung cancer by activating the EGFR/PI3K/AKT pathway [126]. All these findings powerfully demonstrated that lncRNAs act as regulators of p53 or its downstream effectors. Thus, the aforementioned lncRNAs likely play their role in tumor metabolism by regulating p53, and further studies are needed to clarify these specific linkages.

The PI3K/AKT/mTOR pathway

The AKT/mTOR signaling pathway plays a pivotal role in various physiological and pathological processes, including tumorigenesis [127]. As a crucial downstream target of P13K, AKT can stimulate aerobic glycolysis by upregulating glucose transporters and glycolytic enzymes, such as hexokinase-II [128–130]. As indicated by recent studies, UCA1 activates mTOR by upregulating HK2 and increases glycolysis through both the activation of STAT3 and the repression of miR-143, thereby revealing a novel glucose metabolism regulatory pathway, UCA1-mTOR-STAT3/miR-143/HK2, in bladder cancer cells [131, 132]. Interestingly, mTOR can also be activated by CUDR, thus regulating HK2 expression through the activation of STAT3 and the repression of miR-143 [133].

Several lncRNAs have been implicated to function in the PI3K/AKT/mTOR pathway as ceRNAs. Cancer susceptibility candidate 2 (CASC2) upregulates PTEN expression and downregulates p-AKT expression by competitively binding to miR-21, thus promoting the chemosensitivity of cervical cancer cells to cisplatin [134]. HULC upregulates c-Myc and Bcl-2 by sequestering miR-200a-3p, thus activating the PI3K/AKT signaling pathway and promoting cell proliferation [135].

In addition, although the direct regulatory targets have not been elucidated, many lncRNAs have also been found to be involved in the PI3K/AKT/mTOR pathway. CRNDE promotes glioma cell growth and invasion through phosphorylation of the P70S6K-mediated mTOR pathway [136]. As mentioned above, CRNDE can increase GLUT4 transcription and contribute to glucose intake. Therefore, it is possible that CRNDE upregulates the expression of GLUT4 to promote glucose metabolism via the AKT/mTOR signaling pathway. UCA1 regulates the cell cycle via affecting CREB expression and activity through a PI3K-AKT-dependent pathway [137]. Previous data showed that ANRIL can enhance NPC progression by contributing to the expression of GLUT1 and LDHA in NPC cells [40]. The mechanism underlying the ANRIL-dependent enhancement of NPC progression may involve the ANRIL-induced phosphorylation of Akt and thus activate the mTOR pathway, which further upregulates the expression of GLUT1 and LDHA and thus promotes NPC development [138]. The lncRNA RP11-708H21.4, located in the 17q21 gene desert region, is downregulated in colorectal cancer and could regulate CyclinD1 and p27 expression by inactivating AKT/mTOR signaling, thus inhibiting tumorigenesis [139]. Linc00462 is downregulated in hepatocellular carcinoma and contributes to the inactivation of P13K/AKT signaling, thus mediating carcinogenic activity [140]. Whether RP11-708H21.4 and linc00462 participate in metabolic transformation via modulating AKT/mTOR signaling needs further comprehensive investigation.

The AMP-activated protein kinase pathway

AMP-activated protein kinase (AMPK) is a key sensor of cellular energy, and tumor cells downregulate AMPK in order to evade restraining influences on growth and biosynthesis [141]. As a critical metabolic checkpoint, defective AMPK signaling leads to increased cell proliferation and decreased autophagy under conditions of energy stress [142]. Many types of cancer cells show AMPK signal loss, which may lead to their glycolytic phenotype [1, 141]. The tumor suppressor LKB1 is a major upstream regulator of kinases when intracellular levels of ATP are low; as such, LKB1 phosphorylates and activates AMPK, resulting in the downregulation of ATP-consuming processes and the upregulation of ATP production in the presence of AMP [143]. AMPK is activated in response to an increased AMP/ATP ratio, which causes cells to shift to an oxidative metabolic phenotype and inhibit cell proliferation. The growth-promoting role of linc00473 in lung cancer has been shown to be related to the function loss of LKB1 [144], and the lncRNA NBR2 is downregulated in breast cancer under energy stress. NBR2 executes its regulatory role by forming a feed-forward loop to potentiate AMPK activation upon glucose starvation [34]. Thus, the linc00473, NBR2, and LKB1/AMPK axis may play a pivotal role in cancer cells by regulating metabolic rearrangement.

miRNA in cancer metabolism

miRNAs are endogenous small non-coding RNAs, 18 to 25 nt in length, that regulate gene expression [145]. Recent studies have shown that miRNAs control different aspects of energy metabolism including glucose transport and metabolism, cholesterol and lipid homeostasis, insulin production and signaling, and amino acid biogenesis [146]. The involvement of miRNAs in carcinogenesis has been well documented for almost a decade. miRNAs mediate the fine-tuning of genes involved directly or indirectly in cancer metabolism. We list the metabolic lncRNAs and miRNAs involved in regulating cancer metabolism in Table 2 [30, 33, 34, 40, 43, 48, 60, 62, 69, 71, 77–79, 81, 136, 147–162]. Obviously, both miRNAs and lncRNAs are currently known to regulate metabolic rearrangement based on various signaling pathways, as mentioned above. However, miRNAs function only at the post-transcriptional level, whereas lncRNAs exhibit great mechanical diversification, even interacting with miRNAs in cancer metabolism (Fig. 3). Studies on the roles and the underlying mechanisms of lncRNAs in metabolic rearrangement can improve the understanding of the regulatory networks of miRNAs in cancer.

LncRNAs and autophagy in cancer metabolism

Autophagy is an evolutionarily conserved catabolic process involving the formation of autophagosome vacuoles that

Table 2 LncRNAs and miRNAs involved in regulating tumor metabolism

Gene	Target	Signaling	Potential functions and indication	Ref.
lncRNA and glucose metabolism				
ANRIL	GLUT1 and LDHA	PI3/AKT/mTOR	Increase glucose uptake, prognosis	[33, 40]
NBR2	GLUT1	LKB1/AMPK	Decrease glucose uptake, increases autophagy, prognosis	[34]
CRNDE	GLUT4	PI3/AKT/mTOR	Increases glucose uptake	[30, 136]
GCASPC	miR-17-3P	HIF1/MYC	Decrease pyruvate carboxylase, prognosis	[48]
NRCP	STAT1	Not mentioned	Increase glycolysis, prognosis	[49]
PVT1	HK2	miR-497/HK2 axis	Increase glucose metabolism, prognosis	[60]
H19	let-7	HIF1/MYC	Increase insulin sensitivity, enhance glucose tolerance, prognosis	[62]
MALAT1		HIF1/MYC	Increase glycolysis	[146]
microRNA and glucose metabolism				
miR-195-5p	GLUT3	LKB1/AMPK	Decrease glucose uptake	[148]
miR-210	GPD1L	HIF1/MYC	Decrease glycolysis, prognosis	[149, 150]
miR-223	c-MYC	HIF1/MYC	Increase glucose uptake, prognosis	[151]
miR-143	HK2	PI3K/AKT/mTOR	Decrease glucose metabolism	[147]
miR-21	PTEN	PI3K/AKT/mTOR	Increase glucose metabolism, prognosis	[152]
miR-326	PKM2	LKB1/AMPK	Decrease glycolysis	[153]
miR-451	CAB39	LKB1/AMPK	Increase glucose metabolism, prognosis	[156]
miR-29	MCT1	P53, PI3K/AKT/mTOR	Caused insulin resistance, prognosis	[154, 155]
LncRNA and lipid metabolism				
LncHR1	SREBP-1c and FAS	PI3K/AKT/mTOR	Decrease lipid metabolism	[69]
LNMICC	miR-190	miR-190/LNMICC/FABP5 axis	Increase fatty acid metabolism, prognosis	[71]
SRA	Not mentioned	AKT/FOXO1 axis	Decrease adipogenesis and glucose uptake	[77]
HULC	miR-9	miR-9/PPARγ/ACSL1 axis	Increase the deregulation of lipid metabolism	[76]
miRNA and lipid metabolism				
miR-122	CyclinB1	P53	Increase cholesterol synthesis and lipogenesis	[157]
lncRNA and glutamine metabolism				
TUG1	miR-145	Sirt3/GDH axis	Increase glutamine metabolism, prognosis	[81]
UCA1	miR-16	PI3/AKT/mTOR	Increase glutamine metabolism	[160]
miRNA and glutamine metabolism				
miR-23b	c-MYC	HIF1/MYC	Increase the biosynthesis of proline from glutamine	[161]

engulf cellular macromolecules and dysregulated organelles, leading to their breakdown after fusion with lysosomes [163]. Much as autophagy promotes survival during starvation, cancer cells can use autophagy-mediated recycling to maintain mitochondrial function and energy homeostasis to meet the elevated metabolic demands of growth and proliferation. LncRNAs are also pivotal regulators in cancer cell autophagy. A lncRNA named lung cancer progression-association transcript 1 (LCPAT1) was shown to bind to RCC2, which upregulates autophagy and promotes lung cancer progression [164]. The lncRNA DICER1-AS1 was significantly upregulated in osteosarcoma cells. DICER1-AS1 promotes tumor proliferation, invasion, and autophagy via the miR-30b/ATG5 axis in osteosarcoma cells [165].

Cancer cells tend to constitutively activate autophagy via metabolic reprogramming [166, 167], and autophagy is also a pivotal biological process implicated in metabolic reprogramming (Fig. 2), suggesting that metabolic reprogramming and autophagy are often intertwined. Some lncRNAs have been implicated in tumor autophagy because they regulate common molecular regulatory mechanisms for both metabolic reprogramming and autophagy, such as AKT and AMPK/mTOR signaling [142, 168]. For example, linc00470 binds to FUS and AKT to form a ternary complex, anchoring FUS in the cytoplasm to increase AKT activity, which was found to inhibit the ubiquitination of HK1, affect glycolysis, and inhibit autophagy in glioblastoma cells [169]. The aforementioned metabolic lncRNAs NBR2 and ANRIL can also influence cellular autophagy by interacting with the AMPK/mTOR pathway [170, 171]. Thus, we speculated that in the process of the regulation of tumorigenesis and development by lncRNAs, metabolism and autophagy influence and promote each other to form a complex network in tumor cells. However, if specific lncRNAs regulate both autophagy and metabolism, which pathway is the predominant regulatory process in specific tumors is currently not fully clarified.

Therapeutic potential of metabolism-related lncRNAs

Previous investigations detailing the mechanism(s) of lncRNA function in metabolic rearrangement demonstrate the potential applications of lncRNAs in novel antitumor therapies. LncRNAs are strongly associated with metabolic processes in cancer because they regulate key signaling or regulatory factors; moreover, certain lncRNAs can function as driving factors for highly tissue-specific cancer phenotypes. Thus, the rationale for using lncRNAs in metabolism is clear. Studies have reported that metformin inhibits aerobic glycolysis in cancer cells by regulating UCA1, which in turn modulates the mTOR-STAT3-HK2 pathway [172]. The upregulation of lncRNA RP11-708H21.4 inhibits migration and invasion, induces apoptosis, and enhances 5-FU sensitivity in CRC cells by inactivating mTOR signaling [139]. FA synthase (FASN) is a key lipogenic enzyme that catalyzes the terminal steps in the de novo biogenesis of FAs during cancer pathogenesis [66]. The lncRNA PVT1 has been reported to be overexpressed in osteosarcoma and to promote migration and invasion through regulating the miR-195/FASN pathway [60]. Silencing PVT1 expression restores the miR-195-mediated inhibition of FNSN, resulting in decreased tumor proliferation, migration and invasion. Therefore, PVT1 may be used as a lipid therapeutic target for the treatment of osteosarcoma. All these findings support lncRNAs as promising therapeutic targets for cancer.

We should adapt the strategies for tumor screening, diagnosis, and especially therapeutic regimens to address the metabolic reprogramming characteristics of tumors. Tumor nutritional and metabolic regulation therapies could become the main battlefield of tumor treatment. Tumor cells are characterized by high metabolic fitness and can automatically switch to other pathways when one metabolic pathway meets any obstacle, in order to avoid stress damage. Therefore, tumor metabolic regulation therapeutic regimens should be designed to sever or control multiple metabolic pathways simultaneously. Conspicuously, lncRNAs can interact with multiple molecules and/or signaling pathways (e.g., HULC with C-Myc and p53); they participate in diverse physiological and pathological processes by acting as transcriptional, post-transcriptional, or epigenetic regulators (e.g., UCA1

with HK2, C-Myc, miR-143 and miR-16); and they can target multiple metabolic processes (e.g., UCA1 in glycolysis and glutaminolysis) in a tumor simultaneously, which undoubtedly will illuminate the development and selection of therapeutic targets to prevent tumorigenesis and progression.

However, the development of lncRNA-based therapies is complicated by several common challenges in RNA therapeutics, such as the lack of reliable delivery methods and optimal dosage regimes as well as undetermined side effects. Although lncRNAs act as modulators of various human malignancies, the mechanism by which lncRNAs regulate metabolism remains largely uncharacterized. Further research will hopefully enhance the understanding of the regulatory network of cancer metabolism and provide potential targets for the development of cancer therapeutic strategies. Nevertheless, although it may currently be premature to expect lncRNA-targeted therapy to correct metabolism, the rapid development of the mechanistic modeling of lncRNA function and metabolic signaling in recent years will undoubtedly stimulate research in the field of ideal therapeutics for tumor patients with metabolic disorders in the near future.

Conclusion

LncRNAs are well known to be able to regulate gene expression through diverse mechanisms [173]. Although the mechanisms of most lncRNAs have not been fully characterized, an elegant framework for categorizing the emerging roles of lncRNAs was recently proposed as follows: the signal archetype, a molecular signal or indicator of transcriptional activity; the decoy archetype, which binds with other regulatory RNAs or proteins to attenuate regulation; the guide archetype, which directs the localization of chromatin-modifying complex (es) and other nuclear protein (s) to specific targets to exert their effects; and the scaffold archetype, an adaptor to bring two or more RNAs and/or proteins into discrete complexes [174]. In Fig. 3, we provide an overview of currently clearly defined metabolic lncRNA function mechanisms in human tumor entities. The small number of characterized human lncRNAs have been associated with a spectrum of biological processes including transcriptional interference, the induction of chromatin remodeling and histone modifications, service as structural components, protein binding to modulate protein activity or alter protein localization, and even service as miRNA sponges. However, additional functions and detailed signaling pathways of lncRNAs remain to be clarified.

Without question, the dysregulation of lncRNAs affects multiple metabolic processes and plays a critical role in tumorigenesis and progression. Despite cumulative studies investigating the altered expression profiles of lncRNAs during metabolic rearrangement in cancer, the roles and molecular characteristics of these lncRNAs remain largely unexplored. The expression pattern and role of one lncRNA may be significantly different in different metabolic processes due to the complicated structures, specific temporal and spatial expression patterns, and tissue-specific expression of lncRNAs. Therefore, to attain a comprehensive understanding of the role of lncRNAs during tumor development, in addition to elucidating the expression patterns and functions of lncRNAs in metabolic rearrangement, further studies should also focus on structural and mechanistic characterizations. Thus far, the elucidation of the molecular mechanism underlying the Warburg effect has been of great interest in efforts to simulate tumor metabolism and to select target combinations for possible therapeutic interventions. Due to the development of software procedures, PET-CT is currently used as a clinical method for detecting cancer glucose metabolism. Metabolic tumor volume (MTV) and total lesion glycolysis (TLG) on F-18 FDG PET/CT (positron emission tomography/computed tomography) may be useful quantitative parameters for prognostic evaluation [175, 176]. However, other aspects of carbohydrate, lipid, and amino acid metabolism are rarely involved in the clinical detection and diagnosis of human malignancies. Despite decades of research, the poor understanding of tumor metabolism can clearly be attributed to the limitations of current research methods. Therefore, more comprehensive analytical strategies are desired for the study of metabolic disorders and the determination of the advantages of new strategies in different cancer diagnoses. The systematic identification and annotation of metabolism-specific lncRNA signatures and their expression patterns in tumors shows great promise for the development of accurate, noninvasive diagnostic and prognostic biomarkers. The successful development of lncRNA biotechnology and metabonomics may ultimately translate our understanding of the function of lncRNAs in cancer into a strategy for the diagnosis and treatment of cancer.

In conclusion, lncRNAs have been identified as major participants in the complex metabolic gene regulatory networks and have been found to be involved in many aspects of human malignancies. LncRNAs are crucial regulators of cell metabolism, which reinforces the importance of complementing regulatory models with the functions of lncRNAs in malignancies.

Abbreviations
ACSL: Acyl-CoA synthase long-chain; AMPK: AMP-activated protein kinase; ANRIL: A novel large antisense noncoding RNA; ARL2: ADP-ribosylation factor-like 2; CAFs: Cancer-associated fibroblasts; CASC2: Cancer susceptibility candidate 2; ccRCC: Clear cell renal carcinoma; ceRNA: Competing endogenous RNA; CRNDE: Colorectal neoplasia differentially expressed; DDP: Cisplatin; DINO: Damage-induced noncoding; FA: Fatty acid; FABP: Fatty acid-binding proteins; FAS: Fatty acid synthase; FASN: Fatty acid synthase; Fru-2,6-P2: Fructose-2,6-bisphosphate; GCASPC: Gallbladder cancer-associated suppressor of pyruvate carboxylase; GDF15: Growth differentiation factor 15; GDH: Glutamate dehydrogenase; GLS2: Glutaminase 2; GLUTs: Glucose transporters; H3K9me1: One methylation of histone H3 on the ninth lysine; HCC: Hepatocellular carcinoma; HIF: Hypoxia-inducible factor; HK2: Hexokinase 2; ICC: Cholangiocarcinoma; LD: Lipid droplet; LDH: Lactate dehydrogenase; lncRNAs: Long noncoding RNAs; MICU1: Mitochondrial calcium uptake 1; MTV: Metabolic tumor volume; NBR2: The neighbor of BRCA1 gene 2; NDRG2: N-Myc downstream regulated gene 2; NPC: Nasopharyngeal carcinoma; NRCP: lncRNA ceruloplasmin; PC: Pyruvate carboxylase; PCGEM1: Prostate cancer gene expression marker 1; PDKs: Pyruvate dehydrogenase kinases; PFKFB2: 6-Phosphofructo-2-kinase/fructose-2,6-biphosphatase 2; PGC-1α: Peroxisome proliferator-activated receptor γ coactivator α; PKM2: Pyruvate kinase M2; PPAR: Peroxisome proliferator-activated receptor; ROS: Reactive oxygen species; RXRA: Retinoid X receptor alpha; SGLTs: Na$^+$-glucose linked transporters; Sirt3: Sirtuin 3; SRA: Steroid receptor RNA; SREBs: Sterol regulatory element binding proteins; TCA: Tricarboxylic acid cycle; TERT: Telomerase reverse transcriptase; TG: Triglyceride; TIGAR: TP53-inducible glycolysis and apoptosis regulator; TLG: Total lesion glycolysis; VHL: Von Hippel-Lindau

Acknowledgements
We thank Hu [173] and Cell signaling Technology, Inc. (U.S.A), for providing us materials for figure preparation.

Funding
This study was supported by the grant from the National Natural Science Foundation of China (81602078, 81672328 and 81272299), Natural Science Foundation of Jiangsu Province (BK20150004), Fundamental Research Funds for the Central Universities (NOJUSRP51619B and JUSRP51710A), and Natural Science Foundation of Shanghai (No.17ZR1406500).

Authors' contributions
HS performed the study and drafted the manuscript. ZHH performed the study and revised the manuscript. MDX and WQS supervised the study and revised the manuscript. All authors read and approved the final manuscript.

Consent for publication
Not applicable

Competing interests
The authors declare that they have no competing interests.

Author details
[1]Department of Pathology, Fudan University Shanghai Cancer Center, Shanghai 200032, China. [2]Wuxi Cancer Institute, Affiliated Hospital of Jiangnan University, Wuxi, Jiangsu, China. [3]Department of Pathology, Tissue bank, Fudan University Shanghai Cancer Center, Shanghai 200032, China.

References
1. Cairns RA, Harris IS, Mak TW. Regulation of cancer cell metabolism. Nat RevCancer. 2011;11(2):85–95.
2. Vander Heiden MG, Cantley LC, Thompson CB. Understanding the Warburg effect: the metabolic requirements of cell proliferation. Science (New York, NY). 2009;324(5930):1029–33.
3. Newsholme EA, Crabtree B, MSM A. The role of high rates of glycolysis and glutamine utilization in rapidly dividing cells. Bioscience. 1985;5:393–400.

4. Koppenol WH, Bounds PL, Dang CV. Otto Warburg's contributions to current concepts of cancer metabolism. Nat Rev Cancer. 2011;11(5):325–37.

5. Warburg O, Wind F, Negelein E. The metabolism of tumors in the body. General Physiology. 1926;8(6):519–30.

6. Warburg O, Posener K, Negelein E. Uber den Stoffwechsol der Carcinomzelle. Eingegangen. 1924;6:310–44.

7. Li L, Kang L, Zhao W, Feng Y, Liu W, Wang T, et al. miR-30a-5p suppresses breast tumor growth and metastasis through inhibition of LDHA-mediated Warburg effect. Cancer Lett. 2017;400:89–98.

8. Chen Z, Liu M, Li L, Chen L. Involvement of the Warburg effect in non-tumor diseases processes. J Cell Physiol. 2018;233(4):2839–49.

9. Knowles LM, Smith JW. Genome-wide changes accompanying knockdown of fatty acid synthase in breast cancer. BMC Genomics. 2007;8:168.

10. DeBerardinis RJ, Cheng T. Q's next: the diverse functions of glutamine in metabolism, cell biology and cancer. Oncogene. 2010;29(3):313–24.

11. Hensley CT, Wasti AT, DeBerardinis RJ. Glutamine and cancer: cell biology, physiology, and clinical opportunities. J Clin Invest. 2013;123(9):3678–84.

12. Wise DR, Thompson CB. Glutamine addiction: a new therapeutic target in cancer. Trends Biochem Sci. 2010;35(8):427–33.

13. Rajagopalan KN, DeBerardinis RJ. Role of glutamine in cancer: therapeutic and imaging implications. J Nucl Med. 2011;52(7):1005–8.

14. Yang L, Venneti S, Nagrath D. Glutaminolysis: a hallmark of cancer metabolism. Annu Rev Biomed Eng. 2017;19:163–94.

15. Lamonte G, Tang X, Chen JL, Wu J, Ding CK, Keenan MM, et al. Acidosis induces reprogramming of cellular metabolism to mitigate oxidative stress. Cancer Metab. 2013;1(1):23.

16. Cunnington MS, Santibanez Koref M, Mayosi BM, Burn J, Keavney B. Chromosome 9p21 SNPs associated with multiple disease phenotypes correlate with ANRIL expression. PLoS Genet. 2010;6(4):e1000899.

17. Jones RG, Thompson CB. Tumor suppressors and cell metabolism: a recipe for cancer growth. Genes Dev. 2009;23(5):537–48.

18. Yuneva MO, Fan TW, Allen TD, Higashi RM, Ferraris DV, Tsukamoto T, et al. The metabolic profile of tumors depends on both the responsible genetic lesion and tissue type. Cell Metab. 2012;15(2):157–70.

19. Fatica A, Bozzoni I. Long non-coding RNAs: new players in cell differentiation and development. Nat Rev Genet. 2014;15(1):7–21.

20. Rinn JL, Chang HY. Genome regulation by long noncoding RNAs. Annu Rev Biochem. 2012;81:145–66.

21. Perkel JM. Visiting "Noncodarnia". BioTechniques. 2016;54:301–4.

22. Wang ZH, Guo XQ, Zhang QS, Zhang JL, Duan YL, Li GF, et al. Long non-coding RNA CCAT1 promotes glioma cell proliferation via inhibiting microRNA-410. Biochem Biophys Res Commun. 2016;480(4):715–20.

23. Bian Z, Jin L, Zhang J, Yin Y, Quan C, Hu Y, et al. LncRNA-UCA1 enhances cell proliferation and 5-fluorouracil resistance in colorectal cancer by inhibiting miR-204-5p. Sci Rep. 2016;6:23892.

24. Pauli A, Rinn JL, Schier AF. Non-coding RNAs as regulators of embryogenesis. Nat Rev Genet. 2011;12(2):136–49.

25. Yang SZ, Xu F, Zhou T, Zhao X, McDonald JM, Chen Y. The long non-coding RNA HOTAIR enhances pancreatic cancer resistance to TNF-related apoptosis-inducing ligand. J Biol Chem. 2017;292(25):10390–7.

26. Cao MX, Jiang YP, Tang YL, Liang XH. The crosstalk between lncRNA and microRNA in cancer metastasis: orchestrating the epithelial-mesenchymal plasticity. Oncotarget. 2016;8:12472–83.

27. Rinn JL, Kertesz M, Wang JK, Squazzo SL, Xu X, Brugmann SA, et al. Functional demarcation of active and silent chromatin domains in human HOX loci by non-coding RNAs. Cell. 2007;129(7):1311–23.

28. Li H, Ma SQ, Huang J, Chen XP, Zhou HH. Roles of long noncoding RNAs in colorectal cancer metastasis. Oncotarget. 2017;8(24):39859–76.

29. Zhu X, Wu YB, Zhou J, Kang DM. Upregulation of lncRNA MEG3 promotes hepatic insulin resistance via increasing FoxO1 expression. Biochem Biophys Res Commun. 2016;469(2):319–25.

30. Ellis BC, Graham LD, Molloy PL. CRNDE, a long non-coding RNA responsive to insulin/IGF signaling, regulates genes involved in central metabolism. Biochim Biophys Acta. 2014;1843(2):372–86.

31. Zhao XY, Lin JD. Long noncoding RNAs: a new regulatory code in metabolic control. Trends Biochem Sci. 2015;40(10):586–96.

32. Li HJ, Li X, Pang H, Pan JJ, Xie XJ, Chen W. Long non-coding RNA UCA1 promotes glutamine metabolism by targeting miR-16 in human bladder cancer. Jpn J Clin Oncol. 2015;45(11):1055–63.

33. Zhang D, Sun G, Zhang H, Tian J, Li Y. Long non-coding RNA ANRIL indicates a poor prognosis of cervical cancer and promotes carcinogenesis via PI3K/Akt pathways. Biomed Pharmacother. 2017;85:511–6.

34. Liu X, Xiao ZD, Han L, Zhang J, Lee SW, Wang W, et al. LncRNA NBR2 engages a metabolic checkpoint by regulating AMPK under energy stress. Nat Cell Biol. 2016;18(4):431–42.

35. Balon TW. SGLT and GLUT: are they teammates? Focus on "mouse SGLT3a generates proton-activated currents but does not transport sugar". Am J Physiol Cell Physiol. 2012;302(8):C1071–2.

36. Thorens B, Mueckler M. Glucose transporters in the 21st century. Am J Physiol Endocrinol Metab. 2010;298(2):E141–5.

37. Hatanaka M. Transport of sugars in tumor cell membranes. Biochim Biophys Acta. 1974;355(1):77–104.

38. Tano K, Akimitsu N. Long non-coding RNAs in cancer progression. Front Genet. 2012;3:219.

39. Pasmant E, Laurendeau I, Heron D, Vidaud M, Vidaud D, Bieche I. Characterization of a germ-line deletion, including the entire INK4/ARF locus, in a melanoma-neural system tumor family: identification of ANRIL, an antisense noncoding RNA whose expression coclusters with ARF. Cancer Res. 2007;67(8):3963–9.

40. Zou ZW, Ma C, Medoro L. LncRNA ANRIL is up-regulated in nasopharyngeal carcinoma and promotes the cancer progression via increasing proliferation, reprograming cell glucose metabolism and inducing side- population stem-like cancer cells. Oncotarget. 2016;7:38.

41. Hardie DG, Ross FA, Hawley SA. AMPK: a nutrient and energy sensor that maintains energy homeostasis. Nat Rev Mol Cell Biol. 2012;13(4):251–62.

42. Xiao ZD, Liu X, Zhuang L, Gan B. NBR2: a former junk gene emerges as a key player in tumor suppression. Mol Cell Oncol. 2016;3(4):e1187322.

43. Liu X, Gan B. lncRNA NBR2 modulates cancer cell sensitivity to phenformin through GLUT1. Cell cycle (Georgetown, Tex). 2016;15:3471–81.

44. Chang L, Chiang SH, Saltiel AR. Insulin signaling and the regulation of glucose transport. Mol Med. 2004;10(7–12):65–71.

45. Graham LD, Pedersen SK, Brown GS, Ho T, Kassir Z, Moynihan AT, et al. Colorectal neoplasia differentially expressed (CRNDE), a novel gene with elevated expression in colorectal adenomas and adenocarcinomas. Genes Cancer. 2011;2(8):829–40.

46. Zhao L, Ji G, Le X, Wang C, Xu L, Feng M, et al. Long noncoding RNA LINC00092 acts in cancer-associated fibroblasts to drive glycolysis and progression of ovarian cancer. Cancer Res. 2017;77(6):1369–82.

47. Sand M, Hessam S, Amur S, Skrygan M, Bromba M, Stockfleth E, et al. Expression of oncogenic miR-17-92 and tumor suppressive miR-143-145 clusters in basal cell carcinoma and cutaneous squamous cell carcinoma. J Dermatol Sci. 2017;86(2):142–8.

48. Ma MZ, Zhang Y, Weng MZ, Wang SH, Hu Y, Hou ZY, et al. Long noncoding RNA GCASPC, a target of miR-17-3p, negatively regulates pyruvate carboxylase-dependent cell proliferation in gallbladder cancer. Cancer Res. 2016;76(18):5361–71.

49. Rupaimoole R, Lee J, Haemmerle M, Ling H, Previs RA, Pradeep S, et al. Long noncoding RNA ceruloplasmin promotes cancer growth by altering glycolysis. Cell Rep. 2015;13(11):2395–402.

50. Li L, Zhang Y, Qiao J, Yang JJ, Liu ZR. Pyruvate kinase M2 in blood circulation facilitates tumor growth by promoting angiogenesis. J Biol Chem. 2014;289(37):25812–21.

51. Wong N, Ojo D, Yan J, Tang D. PKM2 contributes to cancer metabolism. Cancer Lett. 2015;356(2 Pt A):184–91.

52. Gui X, Li H, Li T, Pu H, Lu D. Long noncoding RNA CUDR regulates HULC and beta-catenin to govern human liver stem cell malignant differentiation. Mol Ther. 2015;23(12):1843–53.

53. Li T, Zheng Q, An J, Wu M, Li H, Gui X, et al. SET1A cooperates with CUDR to promote liver cancer growth and hepatocyte-like stem cell malignant transformation epigenetically. Mol Ther. 2016;24(2):261–75.

54. Hu P, Zheng QD, Li HY, Wu MY, An JH, et al. CUDR promotes liver cancer stem cell growth through upregulating TERT and C-Myc. Oncotarget. 2015;6:40775–98.

55. Wu MY, Zheng QD, An JH, et al. Double mutant P53 (N340Q/L344R) promotes hepatocarcino- genesis through upregulation of Pim1 mediated by PKM2 and LncRNA CUDR. Oncotarget. 2016;7:66525–39.

56. Bian Z, Zhang J, Li M, Feng Y, Wang X, Zhang J, et al. LncRNA-FEZF1-AS1 promotes tumor proliferation and metastasis in colorectal cancer by regulating PKM2 signaling. Clin Cancer Res. 2018.

57. Robey RB, Hay N. Mitochondrial hexokinases, novel mediators of the antiapoptotic effects of growth factors and Akt. Oncogene. 2006;25(34):4683–96.

58. Mathupala SP, Ko YH, Pedersen PL. Hexokinase-2 bound to mitochondria: cancer's stygian link to the "Warburg Effect" and a pivotal target for effective therapy. Semin Cancer Biol. 2009;19(1):17–24.

59. Li Z, Li X, Wu S, Xue M, Chen W. Long non-coding RNA UCA1 promotes glycolysis by upregulating hexokinase 2 through the mTOR-STAT3/microRNA143 pathway. Cancer Sci. 2014;105(8):951–5.

60. Song J, Wu X, Liu F, Li M, Sun Y, Wang Y, et al. Long non-coding RNA PVT1 promotes glycolysis and tumor progression by regulating miR-497/HK2 axis in osteosarcoma. Biochem Biophys Res Commun. 2017;490(2):217–24.

61. Pérez LM, Bernal A, Martín NS, et al. Metabolic rescue of obese adipose-derived stem cells by Lin28/Let7 pathway. Diabetes. 2013;62:2368–79.

62. Peng F, Li TT, Wang KL, Xiao GQ, Wang JH, Zhao HD, et al. H19/let-7/LIN28 reciprocal negative regulatory circuit promotes breast cancer stem cell maintenance. Cell Death Dis. 2017;8(1):e2569.

63. Gao Y, Wu F, Zhou J, Yan L, Jurczak MJ, Lee HY, et al. The H19/let-7 double-negative feedback loop contributes to glucose metabolism in muscle cells. Nucleic Acids Res. 2014;42(22):13799–811.

64. Kallen AN, Zhou XB, Xu J, Qiao C, Ma J, Yan L, et al. The imprinted H19 lncRNA antagonizes let-7 microRNAs. Mol Cell. 2013;52(1):101–12.

65. Santos CR, Schulze A. Lipid metabolism in cancer. FEBS J. 2012;279(15):2610–23.

66. Menendez JA, Lupu R. Fatty acid synthase and the lipogenic phenotype in cancer pathogenesis. Nat Rev Cancer. 2007;7(10):763–77.

67. Liu Y, Zuckier LS, Ghesani NV. Dominant uptake of fatty acid over glucose by prostate cells: a potential new diagnostic and therapeutic approach. Anticancer Res. 2010;30(2):369–74.

68. Rawson RB. Control of lipid metabolism by regulated intramembrane proteolysis of sterol regulatory element binding proteins (SREBPs). Biochem Soc. 2003;70:221–31.

69. Li D, Cheng M, Niu Y, Chi X, Liu X, Fan J, et al. Identification of a novel human long non-coding RNA that regulates hepatic lipid metabolism by inhibiting SREBP-1c. Int J Biol Sci. 2017;13(3):349–57.

70. Storch J, Thumser AE. Tissue-specific functions in the fatty acid-binding protein family. J Biol Chem. 2010;285(43):32679–83.

71. Shang C, Wang W, Liao Y, Chen Y, Liu T, Du Q, et al. LNMICC promotes nodal metastasis of cervical cancer by reprogramming fatty acid metabolism. Cancer Res. 2018;78(4):877–90.

72. Mashek DGBK, Coleman RA, Berger J, Bernlohr DA, Black P, et al. Revised nomenclature for the mammalian long-chain acyl-CoA synthetase gene family. J Lipid Res. 2004;45:1958–61.

73. Phillips CMGL, Bertrais S, Field MR, Cupples LA, Ordovas JM, et al. Gene-nutrient interactions with dietary fat modulate the association between genetic variation of the ACSL1 gene and metabolic syndrome. J Lipid Res. 2010;51:1973–800.

74. Ong KT, Mashek M, Bu SY, Greenberg AS, Mashek DG. Adipose triglyc- eride lipase is a major hepatic lipase that regulates triacylglycerol turnover and fatty acid signaling and partitioning. Hepatology. 2011;53:116–26.

75. Panzitt K, Tschernatsch MM, Guelly C, Moustafa T, Stradner M, Strohmaier HM, et al. Characterization of HULC, a novel gene with striking up-regulation in hepatocellular carcinoma, as noncoding RNA. Gastroenterology. 2007;132(1):330–42.

76. Cui M, Xiao Z, Wang Y, Zheng M, Song T, Cai X, et al. Long noncoding RNA HULC modulates abnormal lipid metabolism in hepatoma cells through an miR-9-mediated RXRA signaling pathway. Cancer Res. 2015;75(5):846–57.

77. Liu S, Xu R, Gerin I, Cawthorn WP, Macdougald OA, Chen XW, et al. SRA regulates adipogenesis by modulating p38/JNK phosphorylation and stimulating insulin receptor gene expression and downstream signaling. PLoS One. 2014;9(4):e95416.

78. Xu B, Gerin I, Miao H, Vu-Phan D, Johnson CN, Xu R, et al. Multiple roles for the non-coding RNA SRA in regulation of adipogenesis and insulin sensitivity. PLoS One. 2010;5(12):e14199.

79. Liu S, Sheng L, Miao H, Saunders TL, MacDougald OA, Koenig RJ, et al. SRA gene knockout protects against diet-induced obesity and improves glucose tolerance. J Biol Chem. 2014;289(19):13000–9.

80. Mazar J, Zhao W, Khalil AM, Lee B, et al. The functional characterization of long noncoding RNA SPRY4- IT1 in human melanoma cells. Oncotarget. 2014;5:8959–69.

81. Zeng B, Ye HL, Chen JM, Cheng D, Cai CF, et al. LncRNA TUG1 sponges miR-145 to promote cancer progression and regulate glutamine metabolism via Sirt3/GDH axis. Oncotarget. 2017;8:113650–61.

82. Ziech D, Franco R, Pappa A, Panayiotidis MI. Reactive oxygen species (ROS)--induced genetic and epigenetic alterations in human carcinogenesis. Mutat Res. 2011;711(1–2):167–73.

83. Shanware NP, Mullen AR, DeBerardinis RJ, Abraham RT. Glutamine: pleiotropic roles in tumor growth and stress resistance. J Mol Med (Berl). 2011;89(3):229–36.

84. Hu W, Zhang C, Wu R, Sun Y, Levine A, Feng Z. Glutaminase 2, a novel p53 target gene regulating energy metabolism and antioxidant function. Proc Natl Acad Sci U S A. 2010;107(16):7455–60.

85. Wise DR, DeBerardinisb RJ, Mancuso A, et al. Myc regulates a transcriptional program that stimulates mitochondrial glutaminolysis and leads to glutamine addiction. PNAS. 2008;105:18782–7.

86. Xu XY, Li JY, Sun X, et al. Tumor suppressor NDRG2 inhibits glycolysis and glutaminolysis in colorectal cancer cells by repressing c-Myc expression. Oncotarget. 2015;6:26161–76.

87. Wang X, Gao Z, Liao J, Shang M, Li X, Yin L, et al. lncRNA UCA1 inhibits esophageal squamous-cell carcinoma growth by regulating the Wnt signaling pathway. J Toxicol Environ Health A. 2016;79(9–10):407–18.

88. Burzio VA, Villota C, Villegas J, Landerer E, Boccardo E, Villa LL, et al. Expression of a family of noncoding mitochondrial RNAs distinguishes normal from cancer cells. Proc Natl Acad Sci U S A. 2009;106(23):9430–4.

89. Rackham O, Shearwood AM, Mercer TR, Davies SM, Mattick JS, Filipovska A. Long noncoding RNAs are generated from the mitochondrial genome and regulated by nuclear-encoded proteins. RNA (New York, NY). 2011;17(12):2085–93.

90. Mercer TR, Neph S, Dinger ME, Crawford J, Smith MA, Shearwood AM, et al. The human mitochondrial transcriptome. Cell. 2011;146(4):645–58.

91. Leucci E, Vendramin R, Spinazzi M, Laurette P, Fiers M, Wouters J, et al. Melanoma addiction to the long non-coding RNA SAMMSON. Nature. 2016;531(7595):518–22.

92. Noh JH, Kim KM, Abdelmohsen K, Yoon JH, Panda AC, Munk R, et al. HuR and GRSF1 modulate the nuclear export and mitochondrial localization of the lncRNA RMRP. Genes Dev. 2016;30(10):1224–39.

93. Vidaurre S, Fitzpatrick C, Burzio VA, Briones M, Villota C, Villegas J, et al. Down-regulation of the antisense mitochondrial non-coding RNAs (ncRNAs) is a unique vulnerability of cancer cells and a potential target for cancer therapy. J Biol Chem. 2014;289(39):27182–98.

94. Kumarswamy R, Bauters C, Volkmann I, Maury F, Fetisch J, Holzmann A, et al. Circulating long noncoding RNA, LIPCAR, predicts survival in patients with heart failure. Circ Res. 2014;114(10):1569–75.

95. Fogal V, Richardson AD, Karmali PP, Scheffler IE, Smith JW, Ruoslahti E. Mitochondrial p32 protein is a critical regulator of tumor metabolism via maintenance of oxidative phosphorylation. Mol Cell Biol. 2010;30(6):1303–18.

96. Li HJ, Sun XM, Li ZK, Yin QW, Pang H, Pan JJ, et al. LncRNA UCA1 promotes mitochondrial function of bladder cancer via the MiR-195/ARL2 signaling pathway. Cell Physiol Biochem. 2017;43(6):2548–61.

97. Handschin C, Spiegelman BM. Peroxisome proliferator-activated receptor gamma coactivator 1 coactivators, energy homeostasis, and metabolism. Endocr Rev. 2006;27(7):728–35.

98. Handschin C, Rhee J, Lin J, Tarr PT, Spiegelman BM. An autoregulatory loop controls peroxisome proliferator-activated receptor gamma coactivator 1alpha expression in muscle. Proc Natl Acad Sci US A. 2003;100(12):7111–6.

99. Long J, Badal SS, Ye Z, Wang Y, Ayanga BA, Galvan DL, et al. Long noncoding RNA Tug1 regulates mitochondrial bioenergetics in diabetic nephropathy. J Clin Invest. 2016;126(11):4205–18.

100. Shimizu SNM, Tsujimoto Y. Bcl-2 family proteins regulate the release of apoptogenic cytochrome c by the mitochondrial channel VDAC. Nature. 1999;399:483–7.

101. MiaoW T, Gang L. long non-coding RNA MEG3 induces renal cell carcinoma cells apoptosis by activating the mitochondrial pathway J Huazhoung Univ sci Technol 2015;35:541–545.

102. Kong LZX, Wu Y. Targeting HOTAIR induces mitochondria related apoptosis and inhibits tumor growth in head and neck aquamous cell carcinoma in vitro and invivo. Curr Mol Med. 2015;15:952–60.

103. Wei YF, Yu ST, Zhang YP, et al. NDRG2 promotes adriamycin sensitivity through a Bad/p53 complex at the mitochondria in breast cancer. Oncotarget. 2017;8:29038–47.

104. Bertout JA, Patel SA, Simon MC. The impact of O2 availability on human cancer. Nat Rev Cancer. 2008;8:967–75.

105. Matouk IJ, Mezan S, Mizrahi A, Ohana P, Abu-Lail R, Fellig Y, et al. The oncofetal H19 RNA connection: hypoxia, p53 and cancer. Biochim Biophys Acta. 2010;1803(4):443–51.

106. Shi J, Dong B, Cao J, Mao Y, Guan W, et al. Long non-coding RNA in glioma: signaling pathways. Oncotarget. 2017;8:27582–92.

107. Luo F, Liu X, Ling M, Lu L, Shi L, Lu X, et al. The lncRNA MALAT1, acting through HIF-1alpha stabilization, enhances arsenite-induced glycolysis in human hepatic L-02 cells. Biochim Biophys Acta. 2016;1862(9):1685–95.

108. Yang F, Zhang H, Mei Y, Wu M. Reciprocal regulation of HIF-1alpha and lincRNA-p21 modulates the Warburg effect. Mol Cell. 2014;53(1):88–100.

109. Osthus RC, Shim H, Kim S, Li Q, Reddy R, Mukherjee M, et al. Deregulation of glucose transporter 1 and glycolytic gene expression by c-Myc. J Biol Chem. 2000;275(29):21797–800.

110. White MA, Lin C, Rajapakshe K, Dong J, Shi Y, Tsouko E, et al. Glutamine transporters are targets of multiple oncogenic signaling pathways in prostate cancer. Mol Cancer Res. 2017;15(8):1017–28.

111. Hung CL, Wang LY, Yu YL, Chen HW, Srivastava S, Petrovics G, et al. A long noncoding RNA connects c-Myc to tumor metabolism. Proc Natl Acad Sci U S A. 2014;111(52):18697–702.

112. Srikantan V, Zou Z, Petrovics G, Xu L, Augustus M, et al. PCGEM1, a prostate-specific gene, is overexpressed in prostate cancer. NPNAS. 2000;97:12216–21.

113. Wang O, Yang F, Liu Y, Lv L, Ma R, et al. C-MYC-induced upregulation of lncRNA SNHG12 regulates cell proliferation, apoptosis and migration in triple-negative breast cancer. Am J Transl Res. 2017;9:533–45.

114. Liu PY, Atmadibrata B, Mondal S, Tee AE, Liu T. NCYM is upregulated by lncUSMycN and modulates N-Myc expression. Int J Oncol. 2016;49(6):2464–70.

115. Shen C, Jr WGK. The VHL/HIF axis in clear cell renal carcinoma. Semin Cancer Biol. 2013;23:18–25.

116. Zhai W, Sun Y, Jiang M, Wang M, Gasiewicz TA, Zheng J, et al. Differential regulation of LncRNA-SARCC suppresses VHL-mutant RCC cell proliferation yet promotes VHL-normal RCC cell proliferation via modulating androgen receptor/HIF-2alpha/C-MYC axis under hypoxia. Oncogene. 2016;35(37):4866–80.

117. Miyamoto T, Lo PHY, Saichi N, Ueda K. Argininosuccinate synthase 1 is an intrinsic Akt repressor transactivated by p53. Mol Biol. 2017;3(5):e1603204.

118. Mathupala SP, Heese C, Pedersen PL. Glucose catabolism in cancer cells. J Biol Chem. 1997;272:22776–80.

119. Bensaad K, Tsuruta A, Selak MA, Vidal MN, Nakano K, Bartrons R, et al. TIGAR, a p53-inducible regulator of glycolysis and apoptosis. Cell. 2006;126(1):107–20.

120. Stambolic V, MacPherson D, Sas D, Lin Y, et al. Regulation of PTEN transcription by p53. Mol Cell. 2001;8:317–25.

121. Matoba S, Kang JG, Patino WD, et al. P53 regulates mitochondrial respiration. Science (New York, NY). 2006;312:1650–3.

122. Schmitt AM, Garcia JT, Hung T, Flynn RA, Shen Y, Qu K, et al. An inducible long noncoding RNA amplifies DNA damage signaling. Nat Genet. 2016;48(11):1370–6.

123. Jiang X, Liu W. Long noncoding RNA highly upregulated in liver cancer activates p53-p21 pathway and promotes nasopharyngeal carcinoma cell growth. DNA Cell Biol. 2017;36(7):596.

124. Yu Y, Lv F, Liang D, Yang Q, Zhang B, Lin H, et al. HOTAIR may regulate proliferation, apoptosis, migration and invasion of MCF-7 cells through regulating the P53/Akt/JNK signaling pathway. Biomed Pharmacother. 2017;90:555–61.

125. Su P, Wang F, Qi B, Wang T, Zhang S. P53 regulation-association long non-coding RNA (LncRNA PRAL) inhibits cell proliferation by regulation of P53 in human lung cancer. Med Sci Monit. 2017;23:1751–8.

126. Wang B, Jiang H, Wang L, Chen X, Wu K, Zhang S, et al. Increased MIR31HG lncRNA expression increases gefitinib resistance in non-small cell lung cancer cell lines through the EGFR/PI3K/AKT signaling pathway. Oncol Lett. 2017;13(5):3494–500.

127. Bauer TM, Patel MR, Infante JR. Targeting PI3 kinase in cancer. Pharmacol Ther. 2015;146:53–60.

128. Elstrom RL, Bauer DE, Buzzai M, et al. Akt stimulates aerobic glycolysis in cancer cells. Cancer Res. 2004;64:3892–9.

129. Miyamoto S, Murphy AN, Brown JH. Akt mediates mitochondrial protection in cardiomyocytes through phosphorylation of mitochondrial hexokinase-II. Cell Death Differ. 2008;15(3):521–9.

130. Vivanco I, Sawyers CL. The phosphatidylinositol 3-Kinase AKT pathway in human cancer. Nat Rev Cancer. 2002;2(7):489–501.

131. Li Y, Lin X, Zhao X, Xie J, JunNan W, Sun T, et al. Ozone (O3) elicits neurotoxicity in spinal cord neurons (SCNs) by inducing ER ca(2+) release and activating the CaMKII/MAPK signaling pathway. Toxicol Appl Pharmacol. 2014;280(3):493–501.

132. Yang C, Li X, Wang Y, Zhao L, Chen W. Long non-coding RNA UCA1 regulated cell cycle distribution via CREB through PI3-K dependent pathway in bladder cancer cells. Gene. 2012;496(1):8–16.

133. Zheng Q, Lin Z, Li X, Xin X, Wu M, An J, et al. Inflammatory cytokine IL6 cooperates with CUDR to aggravate hepatocyte-like stem cells malignant transformation through NF-kappaB signaling. Sci Rep. 2016;6:36843.

134. Feng Y, Zou W, Hu C, Li G, Zhou S, He Y, et al. Modulation of CASC2/miR-21/PTEN pathway sensitizes cervical cancer to cisplatin. Arch Biochem Biophys. 2017;623-624:20–30.

135. Lu Y, Li Y, Chai X, Kang Q, Zhao P, Xiong J, et al. Long noncoding RNA HULC promotes cell proliferation by regulating PI3K/AKT signaling pathway in chronic myeloid leukemia. Gene. 2017;607:41–6.

136. Wang Y, Wang Y, Li J, Zhang Y, Yin H, Han B. CRNDE, a long-noncoding RNA, promotes glioma cell growth and invasion through mTOR signaling. Cancer Lett. 2015;367(2):122–8.

137. Chen YX, Yu W, Le Z, Wei C. Long non-coding RNA UCA1 regulated cell cycle distribution via CREB through PI3-K dependent pathway in bladder carcinoma cells. Gene. 2012;496:8–16.

138. Sun LC, Jiang CH, Xu CJ, et al. Down-regulation of long non-coding RNA RP11-708H21.4 is associated with poor prognosis for colorectal cancer and promotes tumorigenesis through regulating AKT/mTOR pathway. Oncotarget. 2017;8:27929–42.

139. Gong J, Qi X, Zhang Y, Yu Y, Lin X, Li H, et al. Long noncoding RNA linc00462 promotes hepatocellular carcinoma progression. Biomed Pharmacother. 2017;93:40–7.

140. Hardie DG. AMP-activated protein kinase: an energy sensor that regulates all aspects of cell function. Genes Dev. 2011;25(18):1895–908.

141. Kim J, Kundu M, Viollet B, Guan KL. AMPK and mTOR regulate autophagy through direct phosphorylation of Ulk1. Nat Cell Biol. 2011;13(2):132–41.

142. Hezel AF, Bardeesy N. LKB1; linking cell structure and tumor suppression. Oncogene. 2008;27(55):6908–19.

143. Chen Z, Li JL, Lin S, Cao C, Gimbrone NT, Yang R, et al. cAMP/CREB-regulated LINC00473 marks LKB1-inactivated lung cancer and mediates tumor growth. J Clin Invest. 2016;126(6):2267–79.

144. Yanaihara N, Harris CC. MicroRNA involvement in human cancers. Clin Chem. 2013;59(12):1811–2.

145. Kasomva K, Sen A, Paulraj MG, et al. Roles of microRNA on cancer cell metabolism. J Transl Med. 2012;10:228.

146. Luo FLX, Ling M, Lu L, Shi L, Lu X, et al. The lncRNA MALAT1, acting through HIF-1alpha stabilization, enhances arsenite-induced glycolysis in human hepatic L-02 cells. Biochim Biophys Acta. 1862;2016:1865–95.

147. Peschiaroli A, Giacobbe A, Formosa A, Markert EK, Bongiorno-Borbone L, Levine AJ, et al. miR-143 regulates hexokinase 2 expression in cancer cells. Oncogene. 2013;32(6):797–802.

148. Fei X, Qi M, Wu B, Song Y, Wang Y, Li T. MicroRNA-195-5p suppresses glucose uptake and proliferation of human bladder cancer T24 cells by regulating GLUT3 expression. FEBS Lett. 2012;586(4):392–7.

149. Hong L, Yang J, Han Y, Lu Q, Cao J, Syed L. High expression of miR-210 predicts poor survival in patients with breast cancer: a meta-analysis. Gene. 2012;507(2):135–8.

150. Kelly TJ, Souza AL, Clish CB, Puigserver P. A hypoxia-induced positive feedback loop promotes hypoxia-inducible factor 1alpha stability through miR-210 suppression of glycerol-3-phosphate dehydrogenase 1-like. Mol Cell Biol. 2011;31(13):2696–706.

151. Earle JS, Luthra R, Romans A, Abraham R, Ensor J, Yao H, et al. Association of microRNA expression with microsatellite instability status in colorectal adenocarcinoma. J Mol Diagn. 2010;12(4):433–40.

152. MengF H, Janek HW. MicroRNA-21 regulates expression of the PTEN tumor suppressor gene in human hepatocellular cancer. Gastroenterology. 2007;133:647–58.

153. Kefas B, Comeau L, Erdle N, Montgomery E, Amos S, Purow B. Pyruvate kinase M2 is a target of the tumor-suppressive microRNA-326 and regulates the survival of glioma cells. Neuro-Oncology. 2010;12(11):1102–12.

154. Park SY, Lee JH, Ha M, Nam JW, Kim VN. miR-29 miRNAs activate p53 by targeting p85 alpha and CDC42. Nat Struct Mol Biol. 2009;16(1):23–9.

155. Pandey AK, Verma G, Vig S, Srivastava S, Srivastava AK, Datta M. miR-29a levels are elevated in the db/db mice liver and its overexpression leads to attenuation of insulin action on PEPCK gene expression in HepG2 cells. Mol Cell Endocrinol. 2011;332(1–2):125–33.

156. Godlewski J, Nowicki MO, Bronisz A, Nuovo G, Palatini J, De Lay M, et al. MicroRNA-451 regulates LKB1/AMPK signaling and allows adaptation to metabolic stress in glioma cells. Mol Cell. 2010;37(5):620–32.

157. Fornari F, Gramantieri L, Giovannini C, Veronese A, Ferracin M, Sabbioni S, et al. MiR-122/cyclin G1 interaction modulates p53 activity and affects

doxorubicin sensitivity of human hepatocarcinoma cells. Cancer Res. 2009;69(14):5761–7.

158. Lynn FC. Meta-regulation: microRNA regulation of glucose and lipid metabolism. Trends Endocrinol Metab. 2009;20(9):452–9.

159. Cheung O, Puri P, Eicken C, Contos MJ, Mirshahi F, Maher JW, et al. Nonalcoholic steatohepatitis is associated with altered hepatic MicroRNA expression. Hepatology. 2008;48(6):1810–20.

160. Jin LH, Xu L, Pang H, Pan JJ, Xie XJ, Chen W. Long non-coding RNA UCA1 promotes glutamine metabolism by targeting miR-16 in human bladder cancer. Jpn J Clin Oncol. 2015;45:1055–63.

161. Liu W, Le A, Hancock C, Lane AN, Dang CV, Fan TW, et al. Reprogramming of proline and glutamine metabolism contributes to the proliferative and metabolic responses regulated by oncogenic transcription factor c-MYC. Proc Natl Acad Sci U S A. 2012;109(23):8983–8.

162. Yoshida GJ. Therapeutic strategies of drug repositioning targeting autophagy to induce cancer cell death: from pathophysiology to treatment. J Hematol Oncol. 2017;10(1):67.

163. Lin H, Zhang X, Feng N, Wang R, Zhang W, Deng X, et al. LncRNA LCPAT1 mediates smoking/particulate matter 2.5-induced cell autophagy and epithelial-mesenchymal transition in lung cancer cells via RCC2. Cell Physiol Biochem. 2018;47(3):1244–58.

164. Gu Z, Hou Z, Zheng L, Wang X, Wu L, Zhang C. LncRNA DICER1-AS1 promotes the proliferation, invasion and autophagy of osteosarcoma cells via miR-30b/ATG5. Biomed Pharmacother. 2018;104:110–8.

165. Phan LM, Yeung SC, Lee MH. Cancer metabolic reprogramming: importance, main features, and potentials for precise targeted anti-cancer therapies. Cancer Biol Med. 2014;11(1):1–19.

166. Ward PS, Thompson CB. Metabolic reprogramming: a cancer hallmark even Warburg did not anticipate. Cancer Cell. 2012;21(3):297–308.

167. Wang RC, Wei Y, An Z, Zou Z, Xiao G, Bhagat G, et al. Akt-mediated regulation of autophagy and tumorigenesis through Beclin 1 phosphorylation. Science (New York, NY). 2012;338(6109):956–9.

168. Liu C, Zhang Y, She X, Fan L, Li P, Feng J, et al. A cytoplasmic long noncoding RNA LINC00470 as a new AKT activator to mediate glioblastoma cell autophagy. J Hematol Oncol. 2018;11(1):77.

169. Kang YH, Kim D, Jin EJ. Down-regulation of phospholipase D stimulates death of lung cancer cells involving up-regulation of the long ncRNA ANRIL. Anticancer Res. 2015;35:2795–804.

170. Liu YM, Ma JH, Zeng QL, Lv J, Xie XH, Pan YJ, et al. MiR-19a affects hepatocyte autophagy via regulating lncRNA NBR2 and AMPK/PPARalpha in D-GalN/lipopolysaccharide-stimulated hepatocytes. J Cell Biochem. 2018; 119(1):358–65.

171. Li T, Sun XZ, Jiang XH. UCA1 involved in the metformin- regulated bladder cancer cell proliferation and glycolysis. Tumor Biol. 2017;39(6):1010428317710823.

172. Zhou Q, Chen FL, JI Z. Long non-coding RNA PVT1 promotes osteosarcoma development by acting as a molecular sponge to regulate miR-195. Oncotarget. 2016;7(50):82620–33.

173. Hu W, Alvarez-Dominguez JR, Lodish HF. Regulation of mammalian cell differentiation by long non-coding RNAs. EMBO Rep. 2012;13(11):971–83.

174. Li X, Wu Z, Fu X, Han W. lncRNAs: insights into their function and mechanics in underlying disorders. Mutat Res Rev Mutat Res. 2014;762:1–21.

175. Liu FY, Chao A, Lai CH, Chou HH, Yen TC. Metabolic tumor volume by 18F-FDG PET/CT is prognostic for stage IVB endometrial carcinoma. Gynecol Oncol. 2012;125(3):566–71.

176. Arslan N, Tuncel M, Kuzhan O, Alagoz E, Budakoglu B, Ozet A, et al. Evaluation of outcome prediction and disease extension by quantitative 2-deoxy-2-[18F] fluoro-D-glucose with positron emission tomography in patients with small cell lung cancer. Ann Nucl Med. 2011;25(6):406–13.

177. Wang C, Mao ZP, Wang L, Wu GH, Zhang FH, Wang DY, et al. Long non-coding RNA MALAT1 promotes cholangiocarcinoma cell proliferation and invasion by activating PI3K/Akt pathway. Neoplasma. 2017;64(5):725–31.

9

Anlotinib: a novel multi-targeting tyrosine kinase inhibitor in clinical development

Guoshuang Shen[1†], Fangchao Zheng[1,2†], Dengfeng Ren[1†], Feng Du[3], Qiuxia Dong[4], Ziyi Wang[1], Fuxing Zhao[1], Raees Ahmad[1] and Jiuda Zhao[1*]

Abstract

Anlotinib is a new, orally administered tyrosine kinase inhibitor that targets vascular endothelial growth factor receptor (VEGFR), fibroblast growth factor receptor (FGFR), platelet-derived growth factor receptors (PDGFR), and c-kit. Compared to the effect of placebo, it improved both progression-free survival (PFS) and overall survival (OS) in a phase III trial in patients with advanced non-small-cell lung cancer (NSCLC), despite progression of the cancer after two lines of prior treatments. Recently, the China Food and Drug Administration (CFDA) approved single agent anlotinib as a third-line treatment for patients with advanced NSCLC. Moreover, a randomized phase IIB trial demonstrated that anlotinib significantly prolonged the median PFS in patients with advanced soft tissue sarcoma (STS). Anlotinib also showed promising efficacy in patients with advanced medullary thyroid carcinoma and metastatic renal cell carcinoma (mRCC). The tolerability profile of anlotinib is similar to that of other tyrosine kinase inhibitors that target VEGFR and other tyrosine kinase-mediated pathways; however, anlotinib has a significantly lower incidence of grade 3 or higher side effects compared to that of sunitinib. We review the rationale, clinical evidence, and future perspectives of anlotinib for the treatment of multiple cancers.

Keywords: Anlotinib, Tyrosine kinase inhibitor, VEGFR, NSCLC, STS

Background

Receptor tyrosine kinases (RTKs) are transmembrane glycoproteins that communicate with cellular growth factors and extracellular ligands. They play important roles in intracellular tyrosine phosphorylation and intracellular signaling. RTK activation mediates many vital physiological processes including cell proliferation, cell growth, cell migration, cell differentiation, and apoptosis. In addition, RTKs have been implicated in a variety of pathological conditions, including cancer, metabolic and autoimmune disorders, infectious diseases, and neurodegenerative disorders.

RTK activity is regulated by protein tyrosine kinases (PTKs) and protein tyrosine phosphatases (PTPs) [1]. Normal tissues show no or low activity and expression of most oncogenic RTKs, while many malignant cells show hyperactive RTKs or upregulated oncogenic RTK

levels [2, 3]. Downregulation of PTK activity can attenuate tumor cell growth, angiogenesis, and anti-apoptotic effects [4].

To date, targeted RTK inhibitors have been successfully utilized in the treatment of several cancer types [5]. Most of these inhibitors are multi-targeting drugs such as imatinib, sorafenib, sunitinib, and pazopanib, which achieve therapeutic efficacy in some tumors. For example, sorafenib inhibits multiple targets including the vascular endothelial growth factor (VEGF) receptors, VEGFR-1, VEGFR-2, and VEGFR-3, as well as Raf serine/threonine kinases and platelet-derived growth factor receptor (PDGFR)-β [5, 6]. Sunitinib can inhibit VEGFR types 1 and 2 (i.e., FLT1 and FLK1/KDR, respectively), PDGFR-α, PDGFR-β, the stem cell factor receptor c-KIT, as well as FLT3 and RET kinases [7]. In patients with renal cell carcinoma (RCC), sorafenib can significantly improve progression-free survival (PFS) from 2.8 to 5.6 months compared to that of placebo [8] and sunitinib can increase PFS from 5.0 to 11.0 months compared to that of interferon (IFN) [9]. Regorafenib can inhibit the activity of both angiogenic (VEGFR1,

* Correspondence: jiudazhao@126.com
†Guoshuang Shen, Fangchao Zheng and Dengfeng Ren contributed equally to this work.
[1]Affiliated Hospital of Qinghai University, Affiliated Cancer Hospital of Qinghai University, Xining 810000, China
Full list of author information is available at the end of the article

VEGFR2, VEGFR3, TIE2), stromal (PDGFR, FGFR), and oncogenic (KIT, RET, RAF-1, BRAF, BRAF^{V600E}) receptor tyrosine kinases, as well as the activity of Abl. It also significantly prolongs both overall survival (OS) and PFS in patients with refractory metastatic colorectal cancer [10, 11]. Pazopanib targets several RTKs, including VEGFR-1, VEGFR-2, VEGFR-3, and PDGFR-α. Compared with that of placebo, pazopanib showed significant prolongation of PFS in patients with advanced nonadipocytic soft tissue sarcoma (STS) (1.6 months versus 4.6 months) [12].

Nevertheless, considering the unsatisfactory efficacies and limitations of current therapies for the different stages of many cancers, there is still a need to develop innovative, more effective, and safer anticancer drugs. For example, there is currently no standard third-line treatment for advanced non-small-cell lung cancer (NSCLC). Moreover, although several targeted drugs, including olaratumab, pazopanib, sunitinib, and everolimus, are efficacious for STS according to the National Comprehensive Cancer Network (NCCN) and European guidelines [13, 14], the current targeted-therapy drugs for non-gastrointestinal stromal tissue (GIST) STS are still limited. Indeed, pazopanib is the only small-molecule tyrosine kinase inhibitor (TKI) approved by the Food and Drug Administration (FDA) as a second-line non-GIST STS treatment. In addition, no standard treatment is available to date in China for patients with STS who progressed after first-line chemotherapy [15]. For these reasons, multi-targeting RTK inhibitors are one of the most popular and important drug classes being studied, and they may play a significant role in the treatment of cancers.

Anlotinib: a novel inhibitor that targets multiple RTKs

Anlotinib (1-[[4-(4-fluoro-2-methyl-1H-indol-5-yloxy)-6-methoxyquinolin-7-yl]oxy] methyl]cyclopropanamine dihydrochloride) is a newly developed oral small-molecule RTK inhibitor that targets VEGFR1, VEGFR2/KDR, VEGFR3, c-Kit, PDGFR-α, and the fibroblast growth factor receptors (FGFR1, FGFR2, and FGFR3). Further, it can inhibit both tumor angiogenesis and tumor cell proliferation [16, 17] (Fig. 1). Anlotinib can inhibit more targets than other RTK inhibitors can, including sorafenib, sunitinib, and pazopanib. The various targets of anlotinib and other RTK inhibitors are summarized in Table 1. Anlotinib was developed by Chia-tai Tianqing Pharmaceutical Co., Ltd. in China.

Preclinical studies have shown that anlotinib inhibits cell migration and the formation of capillary-like tubes induced by VEGF/PDGF-BB/FGF-2 in endothelial cells. Furthermore, anlotinib significantly suppressed VEGF/PDGF-BB/FGF-2-induced angiogenesis in vitro and in vivo. Research into possible mechanisms indicated that anlotinib inhibits the activation of VEGFR2, PDGFRβ, and FGFR1, as

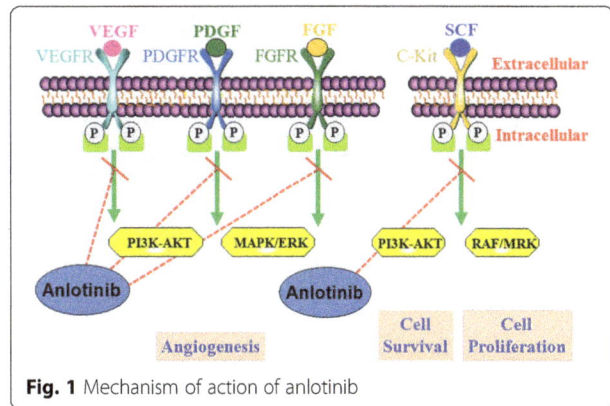

Fig. 1 Mechanism of action of anlotinib

well as downstream ERK signaling. The anti-angiogenic activity of anlotinib is stronger than that of three other anti-angiogenesis drugs, including sunitinib, sorafenib, and nintedanib [18]. Another study revealed that anlotinib binds to the ATP-binding pocket of VEGFR2 tyrosine kinase and inhibits VEGFR2 with high selectivity (IC$_{50}$ <1 nmol/L), thereby inhibiting VEGF-stimulated proliferation of human umbilical vein endothelial cells (HUVECs). Moreover, anlotinib suppressed HUVEC migration, tube formation, and microvessel growth in vitro and reduced vascular density in vivo. Anlotinib had broader and better antitumor efficacy than did sunitinib in vivo [16]. In cell lines expressing mutated FGFR2 protein, anlotinib decreased the number of cells. Nevertheless, similar to that of other oral RTK inhibitors, the combined treatment of anlotinib with carboplatin and paclitaxel did not appear to be more efficacious than anlotinib alone [19].

Anlotinib dosing and pharmacokinetics

The pharmacokinetic properties of anlotinib have been estimated in studies on animals and patients with advanced solid tumors [20–22].

The results of pharmacokinetic and disposition investigations in rats and dogs showed that anlotinib had good membrane permeability and was absorbed quickly. The oral bioavailability of anlotinib was 28–58% and 41–77% in rats and dogs, respectively. The biotransformation of anlotinib showed a significant difference between species, with a terminal half-life of 22.8 ± 11.0 h in dogs and 5.1 ± 1.6 h in rats. The difference appeared to be related to differences in total plasma clearance (rats, 5.35 ± 1.31 L/h/kg; dogs, 0.40 ± 0.06 L/h/kg). Anlotinib had large apparent volumes of distribution in rats (27.6 ± 3.1 L/kg) and dogs (6.6 ± 2.5 L/kg). It was highly bound to plasma in all species, including rat (97%), dog (96%), and human (93%). In human plasma, anlotinib was bound mainly to albumin and lipoproteins. The levels of anlotinib in the tissues of rats and tumor-bearing mice were significantly higher than the corresponding level in the plasma [20].

Table 1 The different targets between anlotinib and other RTK inhibitors

	VEGFR			PDGFR		FGFR				Others
	1	2	3	α	β	1	2	3	4	
Sorafenib	+	+	+	−	+	−	−	−	−	RET (+), c-KIT(+), FLT3(+)
Sunitinib	+	+	+	+	+	−	−	−	−	FLT3(+), c-KIT(+), RET(+), CSF1R(+)
Axitinib	+	+	+	−	−	−	−	−	−	−
Vatalanib	+	+	+	−	+	−	−	−	−	c-KIT(+)
Nintedanib	+	+	+	+	+	+	+	+	−	FLT3(+), Src(+)
Pazopanib	+	+	+	+	+	+	−	−	−	c-KIT(+)
Anlotinib	+	+	+	+	+	+	+	+	+	c-KIT(+)

+ = target, − = no target

In vitro, anlotinib could be metabolized by various human cytochrome P450 isoforms; CYP3A4 and CYP3A5 were mainly responsible. This suggests that circulating anlotinib levels are easily influenced by hepatic drugs that alter the function of P450 enzymes [20]. In vivo, anlotinib exerted a significant effect on the induction of CYP2D1 and CYP3A1/2, while it did not have a significant effect on CYP1A2, CYP2D2, or CYP2C6 after oral administration in rats. Caution, therefore, is warranted when anlotinib is administered with other drugs that are metabolized by CYP2D1 and CYP3A1/2 [23].

There have been two phase I clinical trials investigating the pharmacokinetic properties of anlotinib. In a phase I clinical study in China, the plasma concentration of anlotinib increased significantly 1 h after dosing in most patients, confirming that anlotinib was rapidly absorbed from the intestines. The peak plasma concentration (C_{max}) and area under the concentration-time curve to 120 h post-dose ($AUC_{0-120\ h}$) of anlotinib both increased with increasing doses from 5 to 16 mg anlotinib/person, while the dose proportionality was indeterminate [21]. After a dose of 16 mg anlotinib/person, the mean C_{max} of anlotinib was 10.5 ± 2.9 ng/mL. The time taken to achieve C_{max} (T_{max}) and the elimination half-life ($t_{1/2}$) of anlotinib were 4–11 h and 96 ± 17 h following dosing, respectively [21]. Anlotinib has a significantly longer $t_{1/2}$ in patients than do most tyrosine kinase inhibitors that have been used clinically to date (i.e., 3–60 h) [24]. This extremely long $t_{1/2}$ leads to a significant accumulation of plasma anlotinib over time, with a mean accumulation ratio (Rac) of 12 ± 7. A 2-week subchronic dosing regimen resulted in the continuous elevation of plasma anlotinib concentration, with the maximum achieved on day 14. Thereafter, the plasma level of anlotinib decreased over a 7-day washout period. Based on the above data and toxicity profile (see toxicity section below), this phase I study recommended a dosing regimen in future studies of 12 mg daily for 2 weeks, followed by a 1-week break [21].

In another phase I study performed in a Caucasian population, the average T_{max} and C_{max} after a single 12-mg dose of anlotinib were 10 (4–24) h and 9.60 (8.47–11.50) ng/mL, respectively, which were very similar to the values found in the Chinese patients. Following multiple, continuous doses of anlotinib, the average T_{max} and C_{max} were 360 h and 63.80 (52.90–80.30) ng/mL, respectively. The authors of this phase I study also suggested a dosing regimen of 12 mg daily, 2 weeks on/1 week off for phase II studies [22].

Therapeutic efficacy of anlotinib
Advanced NSCLC

NSCLC is one of the most common diseases used to study the efficacy and safety of anlotinib. As no standard third-line treatment is available for patients with advanced NSCLC, anlotinib has mainly been investigated in this population to date.

A randomized, double-blind, multicenter, placebo-#controlled phase II clinical trial was conducted to estimate the safety and efficacy of anlotinib monotherapy for refractory NSCLC in patients who had failed at least two types of systemic chemotherapy or experienced drug intolerance, revealing the roles of anlotinib as a third-line therapy or beyond in previously treated NSCLC [25]. Overall, 117 patients were enrolled and randomized 1:1 to receive anlotinib (12 mg per day, per os; days 1–14; 21 days per cycle) or placebo. Patients receiving anlotinib had longer PFS than patients receiving placebo (4.8 vs 1.2 months; hazard ratio (HR) = 0.32; 95% confidence interval (CI), 0.20–0.51; $P < 0.0001$). Moreover, the overall response rate (ORR) in the anlotinib group was greater than that in the placebo group (10.0%; 95% CI 2.4–17.6% vs 0%; 95% CI 0–6.27%; $P = 0.028$). Notably, anlotinib treatment benefited all subgroups independent of age, sex, smoking history, stage, efficacy of previous treatments, and histology, except the subgroup with three or fewer metastases. In addition, the OS was longer in the anlotinib group than in the control group, although the difference was not statistically significant (9.3 vs 6.3 months; HR = 0.32; 95% CI

0.51–1.18; $P = 0.2316$). The failure in obtaining a statistically significant difference in the OS might be related to the small sample size.

ALTER-0303 was a randomized, double-blind, placebo-controlled, multicenter, phase III trial that compared the efficacy and safety of anlotinib with that of placebo in patients with advanced NSCLC who progressed after at least two lines of prior treatments [26]. A total of 437 patients were randomized 2:1 to receive either oral anlotinib or placebo (12 mg QD from days 1 to 14 of a 21-day cycle). Treatment continued until tumor progression or discontinuation due to toxicity. Patients with epidermal growth factor receptor (EGFR) mutations or anaplastic lymphoma kinase (ALK) translocations who were enrolled in the study must have had treatment failure with prior targeted therapies. The results showed that anlotinib was more effective than placebo in third-line treatment of patients with advanced NSCLC. Improvements in the ORR and disease control rate (DCR) were seen in the anlotinib group compared with that of the placebo group (ORR 9.18% vs 0.7%, $P < 0.0001$; DCR 80.95% vs 37.06%, $P < 0.0001$). In addition, anlotinib significantly prolonged median PFS and OS compared with the placebo values (PFS 5.37 vs 1.40 months: HR = 0.28, 95% CI 0.19–0.31, $P < 0.0001$; OS 9.63 vs 6.30 months: HR = 0.68, 95% CI 0.54–0.87, $P < 0.0001$).

An exploratory subgroup analysis of the ALTER0303 trial showed that anlotinib significantly improved PFS and OS in patients with both sensitive EGFR mutations and wild-type EGFR. The PFS and OS in patients with sensitive EGFR mutations receiving anlotinib and placebo were 5.57 months and 0.83 months (PFS, HR = 0.15, 95% CI 0.09–0.24, $P < 0.0001$), respectively, and 10.70 months and 6.27 months (OS, HR = 0.59, 95% CI 0.37–0.93, $P = 0.0227$), respectively. Furthermore, the PFS and OS in patients with wild-type EGFR receiving anlotinib and placebo were 5.37 months and 1.57 months (PFS, HR = 0.29, 95% CI 0.22–0.39, $P < 0.0001$), respectively, and 8.87 months and 6.47 months (OS, HR = 0.73, 95% CI 0.55–0.97, $P = 0.0282$), respectively [27]. More recently, the study investigators reported that anlotinib led to a greater improvement in OS time in patients with sensitive EGFR mutations than in those with wild-type EGFR (10.70 vs 8.87, HR = 0.685, 95% CI 0.50–0.95, $P = 0.0204$) [28]. Other studies have shown that anlotinib increases survival in patients with adenocarcinomas or squamous cell carcinomas [29] and in elderly patients (over 70 years) [30]. The PFS and OS benefit from anlotinib was also independent of any previous therapeutic strategy, including conventional platinum-based chemotherapy or TKIs (gefitinib, erlotinib, and icotinib) [31].

Based on the results of ALTER-0303, anlotinib was approved by the China Food and Drug Administration (CFDA) for third-line treatment or beyond in advanced NSCLC on May 8, 2018, in China [32]. Moreover, anlotinib is recommended in the Chinese Society of Clinical Oncology Guidelines for the Diagnosis and Treatment of Primary Lung Cancer (2018 Edition) for the same indication [33].

Advanced STS

In recent years, an increasing number of targeted drugs have demonstrated good clinical efficacy in patients with certain histological types of advanced STS. These agents include multi-targeted kinase inhibitors, such as pazopanib, imatinib, sunitinib, and sorafenib; ALK inhibitors, such as crizotinib and ceritinib; anti-PDGFRs, such as the anti-PDGFRα monoclonal antibody olaratumab; and anti-angiogenic drugs, such as bevacizumab [12, 34–41]. However, pazopanib is the only small molecule TKI approved by the FDA for second-line STS treatment to date.

Considering that anlotinib induced tumors to shrink in soft tissue sarcomas in a phase I study, a multicenter, single-arm, phase II study subsequently explored anlotinib activity in patients with advanced STS who had failed previous conventional treatments [42]. The enrolled patients had malignant fibrous histiocytoma (MFH), liposarcoma, leiomyosarcoma (LMS), synovial sarcoma (SS), or other sarcomas, but not rhabdomyosarcoma (RMS), chondrosarcoma, or GIST STS. Among the 166 patients included, the progression-free rate at week 12 (PFR_{12w}) was 57.23%, median PFS was 5.63 months, and the ORR was 11.45%. Overall, anlotinib demonstrated better clinical benefits in many pathological types of STS. Specifically, alveolar soft part sarcoma (ASPS) showed a high PFR_{12w} (76.92%), similar to the efficacy of sunitinib toward ASPS [43].

The study team further conducted a phase IIB study to demonstrate the role of anlotinib in advanced STS. Overall, 233 patients who were treatment-intolerant or progressed on anthracycline-based chemotherapy were enrolled. The included pathological subtypes were SS, ASPS, LMS, and others; participants with each type were randomized 2:1 to receive anlotinib or placebo. The ORR and DCR in the anlotinib group were significantly higher than those in the control group (ORR 10.13% vs 1.33%, $P = 0.0145$; DCR 55.7% vs 22.67%, $P < 0.0001$). Additionally, anlotinib treatment significantly improved the median PFS relative to the control (6.27 months, 95% CI 4.30–8.40 vs 1.47 months, 95% CI 1.43–1.57, HR = 0.33, $P < 0.0001$). The pathological subtype with the greatest increase in survival was ASPS, whose median PFS was 18.23 months in the anlotinib group compared with 3 months in the control group (HR = 0.14, $P < 0.0001$). This trial further confirmed the efficacy and safety of anlotinib in advanced STS [44].

The results of these two clinical studies were presented in the oral report section at the American

Society of Clinical Oncology (ASCO) annual meeting due to the excellent therapeutic efficacy of anlotinib in STS. It is likely that anlotinib will be approved to treat STS in China in the future.

Metastatic renal cell carcinoma
More recently, a number of targeted treatments have become widely used as first- and second-line treatments in patients with metastatic renal cell carcinoma (mRCC). Multi-targeting kinase inhibitors, including pazopanib, sunitinib, sorafenib, cabozantinib, axitinib, and lenvatinib, were all efficacious in these patients [8, 9, 45–49].

Two phase II clinical trials have also assessed anlotinib efficacy in the treatment of mRCC. Sequential treatment with targeted therapies is effective and has been the current standard of care for patients with mRCC who failed a previous therapy. A multicenter, single-arm, phase II trial enrolled 43 patients who progressed while on, or were intolerant to, sorafenib or sunitinib. The median PFS in the whole group and in patients who had progressed while being treated with a TKI was 11.8 and 8.5 months, respectively. In intention-to-treat (ITT) patients, the ORR and 6-week DCR were 19.1% (95% CI 8.60–34.12) and 90.5% (95% CI 77.4–97.3%), respectively. Anlotinib was preliminarily shown to have promising efficacy with a favorable toxicity profile for patients with mRCC who failed sorafenib or sunitinib treatment [50].

The same authors also conducted a multicenter randomized phase II trial to compare the efficacies and safeties of anlotinib and sunitinib as first-line treatments in patients with mRCC. One-hundred and thirty-three patients (93 with anlotinib, 40 with sunitinib) were enrolled. The results showed that the anlotinib and sunitinib groups had similar PFS (11.3 vs 11.0 months, $P = 0.30$), ORR (24.4% vs 23.3%), and 6-week DCR (97.8% vs 93.0%, $P = 0.33$). More importantly, the incidence of over-grade 3 side effects was lower in the anlotinib group than in the sunitinib group (28.9% vs 55.8%, $P = 0.0039$), particularly for grade 3 or 4 thrombocytopenia (0 vs 11.6%, $P = 0.003$) and neutropenia (0.0 vs 9.3%, $P = 0.009$). These results support the hypothesis that anlotinib has a similar efficacy, but milder side effects, to that of sunitinib in patients with mRCC [51].

Advanced medullary thyroid cancer
The kinases RET and VEGFR2 are the main targets of agents used in patients with advanced medullary thyroid cancer (MTC). Several multi-targeting kinase inhibitors, such as sorafenib, sunitinib, cabozantinib, vandetanib, and pazopanib, have shown promise in patients with differentiated and advanced MTC [52–56].

A single-arm, multicenter phase II trial estimated the efficacy and safety of anlotinib in advanced MTC. The trial enrolled 58 patients with advanced or relapsed MTC, who could not receive radical surgery, and treated them with anlotinib. The average PFS was 12.8 months (median PFS not reached), the overall ORR was 48.28% (full analysis set, FAS), and the DCR at weeks 24 and 48 was 92.16% and 84.53%, respectively. These results indicate that anlotinib has the potential to treat advanced MTC [57].

The existing clinical trial treatment efficiency data of anlotinib are summarized in Table 2. In addition, a phase III trial of anlotinib in treating metastatic colorectal cancer is completed and the results will be released in the near future.

Anlotinib tolerability
Once-daily anlotinib 12 mg, administered as 2 weeks on/1 week off, was the suggested regimen from a phase I study. This dosage and administration schedule was used in all subsequent phase II–III trials.

All adverse events (AEs) appeared to be manageable in the phase I trial. The most common AEs with over 30% incidence were hand-foot skin reaction (53%), hypertension (34%), proteinuria (67%), triglyceride elevation (62%), total cholesterol elevation (62%), hypothyroidism (57%), alanine aminotransferase (ALT) elevation (48%), aspartate transaminase (AST) elevation (43%), total bilirubin elevation (38%), serum amylase (43%), myocardial enzymes abnormal (38%), leucopenia (33%), and neutropenia (33%) [21]. The overall incidence of any AE with anlotinib was 100%, while 29% of patients reported grade 3/4 AEs, including hand-foot skin reaction (5%), hypertension (10%), triglyceride elevation (10%), and lipase elevation (5%) (Fig. 2) [21]. As the authors indicated, it is noteworthy that anlotinib appeared to cause less and milder diarrhea than did other oral anti-VEGFR TKIs [58–60]. However, it also should be noted that patients receiving anlotinib treatment had a high occurrence of triglyceride and cholesterol elevation. Although these effects did not induce noticeable symptoms, the authors suggested that patients taking anlotinib undergo regular monitoring, particularly considering that some of the listed AEs are related to arterial thromboembolic events; such events were significantly more common in patients treated with anti-VEGFR TKIs, however [61].

Anlotinib had a similar toxicity in another phase I trial and a manageable AE profile in phase II–III trials. Among 58 patients with advanced MTC who received anlotinib treatment in a phase II study, 20.7% required a dose adjustment to 10 mg daily in a 2 weeks on/1 week off schedule because of grade III/IV AEs [57]. It is noteworthy that 5 of 166 patients (3.01%) with advanced STS treated with anlotinib experienced grade III/IV pneumothorax [42]. Additionally, in patients with mRCC, anlotinib induced significantly fewer cases of grade 3/4 side effects, especially thrombocytopenia and

Table 2 Summary of clinical efficacy results evaluating anlotinib in patients with cancer

Cancer type	Phase	Number of patients	ORR, % (anlotinib group).	ORR, % (control group).	PFS (median, months, anlotinib group).	PFS (median, months, control group).	OS (median, months, anlotinib group).	OS (median, months, control group).	Author	Ref
Advanced NSCLC	II (randomized control)	117	10.0	0.00	4.8	1.2	9.30	6.30	Han B	[25]
Advanced NSCLC	III	437	9.18	0.7	5.37	1.40	9.63	6.30	Han B	[26]
Advanced STS	II (single-arm)	166	11.45	/	5.63	/	NA	/	Chi Y	[42]
Advanced STS	IIB (randomized control)	233	10.13	1.33	6.27	1.47	NA	NA	Chi Y	[44]
mRCC	II (single-arm)	43	19.1	/	11.8 (whole group);8.5 (progressed on a TKI group)	/	NA	NA	Zhou A P	[50]
mRCC	II (randomized control)	133	24.4	23.3	11.3	11.0	NA	NA	Zhou AP	[51]
Advanced MTC	II (single-arm)	58	48.28	/	12.8	/	NA	/	Sun Y	[57]

NSCLC non-small-cell lung cancer, ORR overall response rate, PFS progression-free survival, OS overall survival, NA data not available, STS soft tissues sarcoma, mRCC metastatic renal cell carcinoma, TKI tyrosine kinase inhibitor, MTC medullary thyroid cancer

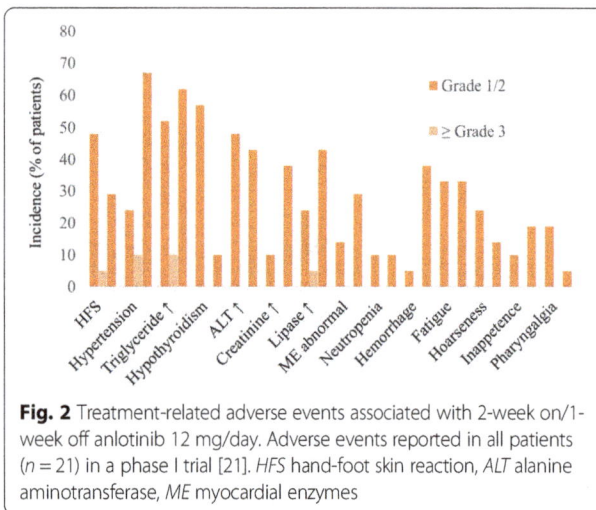

Fig. 2 Treatment-related adverse events associated with 2-week on/1-week off anlotinib 12 mg/day. Adverse events reported in all patients (n = 21) in a phase I trial [21]. *HFS* hand-foot skin reaction, *ALT* alanine aminotransferase, *ME* myocardial enzymes

neutropenia, than sunitinib did, but caused a greater incidence of hypercholesterolemia [51]. In a phase III trial, grade 3 or higher AEs, including dermal toxicity (3.74%) and hypertriglyceridemia (3.06%), were reported in patients with refractory advanced NSCLC administered anlotinib as a third-line treatment. However, there were no treatment-related deaths [26]. More recently in a phase II trial, additional grade 3 or higher AEs, including hyponatremia (3.16%) and neutrophil count reduction (3.16%), were observed in patients with metastatic STS receiving anlotinib treatment [44].

Biomarkers

Appropriate biomarkers can accurately predict and monitor early efficacy and indicate emerging resistance to anlotinib. Fortunately, several clinical trials have identified circulating biomarkers that predict anlotinib activity, specifically activated circulating endothelial cells (aCECs) and EGFR-sensitizing mutations or T790M mutation.

In the ALTER0303 trial, aCECs were measured in 49 patients receiving anlotinib and 30 patients receiving placebo. There were no statistically significant differences in baseline characteristics between the groups. Using a cutoff of 1 for the ratio of the minimal aCEC numbers at every time point to baseline (aCEC min/baseline), the 49 patients receiving anlotinib were subdivided into two groups. The median PFS of the aCEC min/baseline < 1 group (35 patients) was longer than that of the aCEC min/baseline > 1 group (14 patients) (193 vs 124 days, HR = 0.439, 95% CI 0.211–0.912, P = 0.023). However, there was no significant relationship between PFS and the number of aCEC min/baseline in patients receiving placebo. Therefore, aCECs are a potential biomarker for PFS during anlotinib treatment [62].

The ALTER0303 trial also estimated whether circulating tumor DNA (ctDNA) levels can predict the efficacy

of anlotinib treatment in patients with advanced NSCLC. Overall, 92 blood samples were analyzed through capture-based targeted ultradeep sequencing. The results revealed that 58% (53/92) had driver mutations. The maximum mutation allele frequency (MAF) at baseline had a reciprocal effect on PFS (HR = 0.612, 95% CI 0.402–0.932, P = 0.006). Moreover, there was no correlation between sensitizing EGFR mutations and PFS in 27 patients (5.53 vs 5.53 months, HR = 1.16, 95% CI 0.73–1.85, P = 0.495). Similarly, the EGFR T790M mutation did not reflect the treatment effectiveness of anlotinib in 17 patients with advanced NSCLC (5.53 vs 5.53 months, HR = 1.35, 95% CI 0.75–2.41, P = 0.253). Considering the possibility of bias found in small samples, an ongoing, larger scale analysis is needed to reaffirm these conclusions [63].

Ongoing clinical trials

Clinical trials have been conducted to estimate the efficacy and side effects of anlotinib in several advanced solid tumors, including sarcomas, hepatocellular carcinoma, thyroid carcinoma, esophageal squamous cell carcinoma, gastroenteropancreatic neuroendocrine tumor G3, colorectal cancer, gastric cancer, mRCC, small cell lung cancer, and NSCLC (Table 3).

Several ongoing trials are attempting to clarify the roles of anlotinib in STS, particularly the activity of anlotinib in several STS subtypes, such as Ewing sarcoma, ASPS, leiomyosarcoma, and synovial sarcoma. It is noteworthy that most of these are phase III studies due to the rare incidence of STS. Further, several trials are attempting to determine the efficacy of anlotinib in gastrointestinal tumors. Considering the very limited number of multi-targeting RTK inhibitors that have shown efficacy in esophageal squamous cell carcinoma and gastric cancer to date, it is important to fully understand the potential role of anlotinib treatment in these tumors. Moreover, phase I trials in neuroendocrine cancer, for which there are no ideal targeted drugs, have shown evidence of anlotinib treatment efficacy; clinical trials have also been designed to evaluate the efficacy of anlotinib treatment in gastroenteropancreatic neuroendocrine tumor G3 and small cell lung cancers.

Future perspectives

Anlotinib has exceptional efficacy and acceptable toxicity for the treatment of advanced NSCLC and STS. Anlotinib received its first approval on May 8, 2018, for patients with advanced NSCLC who have progressed after at least two lines of prior treatments in China. In the near future, it is very likely that anlotinib will also be approved in China to treat patients with STS who failed previous conventional treatments. Anlotinib also has

Table 3 Current anlotinib clinical trials for multiple cancers

Regimen	Study type	Enrollment	Population
Anlotinib and irinotecan	Phase III	Recruiting	Advanced Ewing sarcoma
Anlotinib	Phase II/III	Not recruiting	Advanced soft tissue sarcoma
Anlotinib	Phase II	Unknown status	Soft tissue sarcoma
Anlotinib	Phase III	Recruiting	Metastatic or advanced alveolar soft part sarcoma, leiomyosarcoma and synovial sarcoma
Anlotinib	Phase II	Recruiting	Hepatocellular carcinoma
Anlotinib	Phase II/III	Recruiting	Medullary thyroid carcinoma
Anlotinib	Phase II/III	Recruiting	Differentiated thyroid cancer
Anlotinib	Phase II	Not recruiting	Advanced renal cell carcinoma
Anlotinib	Phase II	Recruiting	Esophageal squamous cell carcinoma
Anlotinib plus irinotecan	Phase II	Not recruiting	Esophageal squamous cell carcinoma
Anlotinib	Phase II	Recruiting	Gastroenteropancreatic neuroendocrine tumor G3
Anlotinib	Phase II	Not recruiting	Colorectal cancer
Anlotinib	Phase II	Recruiting	Small cell lung cancer
Anlotinib	Phase II/III	Recruiting	Gastric cancer
Anti-angiogenesis plus EGFR-TKI	Phase II	Not recruiting	Non-squamous non-small cell lung cancer

EGFR epidermal growth factor receptor, *TKI* tyrosine kinase inhibitor

potential as a new treatment for other solid tumors, such as mRCC and thyroid carcinoma.

Although anlotinib showed activity against several cancers, there are still some questions that require further investigation and solutions prior to its general use. First, predictive biomarkers should be further investigated to help select optimal patients for anlotinib treatment. Although some biomarkers appeared to define patients who are most likely to benefit from anlotinib treatment, the overall number of predictive biomarkers is insufficient. Moreover, the current potential biomarkers were identified from one clinical trial that used a limited number of samples from NSCLC patients. Predictive biomarkers for other cancer types remain elusive. Future trials should further investigate the optimal indications for patients likely to benefit from anlotinib.

Second, an estimate of the efficacy of anlotinib in other tumors and the appropriate schedule of anlotinib when combined with other treatments is still needed. Whether anlotinib can be expanded to the treatment of other cancers or as a first-line drug, particularly in some subtypes of STS, also requires further study. Generally, multi-targeting RTK inhibitors, such as sunitinib, sorafenib, and regorafenib, can be used to treat multiple cancers. As a novel agent, anlotinib is assumed to be effective only in limited cancer types while studies on other tumors are still ongoing. It is expected that anlotinib will show efficacy against other tumors. Therefore, more high-quality, randomized trials should be conducted to define its therapeutic efficacy in

other diseases. Additionally, it is likely that anlotinib will perform different treatment roles in different cancer types. Thus, the optimal anlotinib treatment regimen for these cancers needs further evaluation.

Moreover, when the anti-angiogenesis drug ramucirumab is combined with chemotherapy, a synergistic effect is seen [64, 65]. Indeed, some targeted therapies can also modulate the host immune response and, therefore, may further improve clinical outcomes when combined with immunotherapies. Nevertheless, most studies to date have only examined anlotinib monotherapy treatments [66, 67]. Thus, future studies are needed to evaluate the combination of anlotinib and other therapies. Considering the strong efficacy of anlotinib in ASPS, further study is needed to estimate whether anlotinib could be administered as a first-line treatment in these patients.

Third, the long-term toxicity profile of anlotinib remains unclear and requires further study. A phase II and phase III trial found several new ≥ 3 grade AEs, including dermal toxicity, hypertriglyceridemia, hyponatremia, and neutrophil count reduction, which were not reported in previous clinical trials [31, 44]. Thus, with the increasing number of anlotinib studies, potential long-term toxicity should be clarified.

Last, we know nearly nothing about tumor resistance to anlotinib and its possible mechanisms, as studies of anlotinib were just started in recent years. However, the knowledge of how to assess and reverse resistance to anlotinib is an important issue. Future trials should also develop personalized therapy strategies to conquer resistance.

Conclusions

As a novel multi-targeting RTK inhibitor, anlotinib shows substantial antitumor activity against VEGFR1, VEGFR2/KDR, and VEGFR3, and lesser activity against c-kit, PDGFRα, FGFR1, FGFR2, and FGFR3. It is the first drug approved in China as a third-line treatment for patients with advanced NSCLC. With the development of future studies and accumulation of clinical experience, it is hopeful that anlotinib will be used in the treatment of other cancers, especially STS. In addition, anlotinib is well-tolerated and most AEs are manageable or reversible by medical intervention. Anlotinib has fewer or milder side effects compared to those of other anti-VEGFR TKIs, particularly the thrombocytopenia and neutropenia found with sunitinib. Thus, anlotinib is likely to become a new multi-targeting RTK inhibitor that is efficacious against multiple cancers.

Abbreviations

aCECs: activated circulating endothelial cells; AE: Adverse event; ASPS: Alveolar soft part sarcoma; CFDA: China Food and Drug Administration; CI: Confidence interval; DCR: Disease control rate; EGFR: Epidermal growth factor receptor; FGFR: Fibroblast growth factor receptor; HR: Hazard ratio; mRCC: metastatic renal cell carcinoma; MTC: Medullary thyroid cancer; NSCLC: Non-small-cell lung cancer; ORR: Overall response rate; OS: Overall survival; PDGFR: Platelet-derived growth factor receptors; PFS: Progression-free survival; RTK: Receptor tyrosine kinase; STS: Soft tissue sarcoma; TKI: Tyrosine kinase inhibitor; VEGFR: Vascular endothelial growth factor receptor

Funding

This work was supported by grants from the Thousand Talents of Program of High-end Innovation of Qinghai Province in China (for Dr. Jiuda Zhao and Dr. Guoshuang Shen) and Clinical Oncology Medicine Research Center of Qinghai Province (2018-SF-113).

Authors' contributions

GS, FZhe, DR, and JZ conceived of the study and drafted the manuscript. FD, QD, ZW, FZha, and RA participated in its coordination and modification. All authors read and approved the final manuscript.

Consent for publication

Not applicable

Competing interests

The authors declare that they have no competing interests.

Author details

[1]Affiliated Hospital of Qinghai University, Affiliated Cancer Hospital of Qinghai University, Xining 810000, China. [2]Shouguang Hospital of Traditional Chinese Medicine, Weifang 262700, China. [3]Peking University Cancer Hospital and Institute, Beijing 100142, China. [4]The Fifth People's Hospital of Qinghai Province, Xining 810000, China.

References

1. Persson C, Sjöblom T, Groen A, Kappert K, Engström U, Hellman U, et al. Preferential oxidation of the second phosphatase domain of receptor-like PTP-α revealed by an antibody against oxidized protein tyrosine phosphatases. Proc Natl Acad Sci U S A. 2004;101:1886–91.
2. Hojjat-Farsangi M. Small-molecule inhibitors of the receptor tyrosine kinases: promising tools for targeted cancer therapies. Int J Mol Sci. 2014;15:13768–801.
3. Hubbard SR, Miller WT. Receptor tyrosine kinases: mechanisms of activation and signaling. Curr Opin Cell Biol. 2007;19:117–23.
4. Arora A, Scholar EM. Role of tyrosine kinase inhibitors in cancer therapy. J Pharmacol Exp Ther. 2005;315:971–9.
5. Ferguson FM, Gray NS. Kinase inhibitors: the road ahead. Nat Rev Drug Discov. 2018;17:353–77.
6. Hasskarl J. Sorafenib. Small molecules in oncology. Springer: Berlin; 2014;2: 61–70.
7. Chow LQM, Eckhardt SG. Sunitinib: from rational design to clinical efficacy. J Clin Oncol. 2007;25:884–96.
8. Escudier B, Eisen T, Stadler WM, Szczylik C, Oudard S, Staehler M, et al. Sorafenib for treatment of renal cell carcinoma: final efficacy and safety results of the phase III treatment approaches in renal cancer global evaluation trial. J Clin Oncol. 2009;27:3312–8.
9. Motzer RJ, Hutson TE, Tomczak P, Michaelson MD, Bukowski RM, Oudard S, et al. Overall survival and updated results for sunitinib compared with interferon alfa in patients with metastatic renal cell carcinoma. J Clin Oncol. 2009;27:3584–90.
10. Li J, Qin S, Xu R, Yau TC, Ma B, Pan H, et al. Regorafenib plus best supportive care versus placebo plus best supportive care in Asian patients with previously treated metastatic colorectal cancer (CONCUR): a randomised, double-blind, placebo-controlled, phase 3 trial. Lancet Oncol. 2015;16:619–29.
11. Grothey A, Van Cutsem E, Sobrero A, Siena S, Falcone A, Ychou M, et al. Regorafenib monotherapy for previously treated metastatic colorectal cancer (CORRECT): an international, multicentre, randomised, placebo-controlled, phase 3 trial. Lancet. 2013;381:303–12.
12. van der Graaf WT, Blay JY, Chawla SP, Kim DW, Bui-Nguyen B, Casali PG, et al. Pazopanib for metastatic soft-tissue sarcoma (PALETTE): a randomised, double-blind, placebo-controlled phase 3 trial. Lancet. 2012;379:1879–86.
13. Margaret von Mehren, R. Lor Randall, Robert S. Benjamin, Sarah Boles, Marilyn M. Bui, Kristen N. Ganjoo, et al. National comprehensive cancer network soft tissue sarcoma guidelines. Version 2. 2018, 2018.
14. Casali PG, Abecassis N, Bauer S, Biagini R, Bielack S, Bonvalot S, et al. Soft tissue and visceral sarcomas: ESMO–EURACAN Clinical Practice Guidelines for diagnosis, treatment and follow-up. Ann Oncol. 2018;00:1–11. https://doi.org/10.1093/annonc/mdy096. [Epub ahead of print].
15. Lewin J, Puri A, Quek R, Ngan R, Alcasabas AP, Wood D, et al. Management of sarcoma in the Asia-Pacific region: resource-stratified guidelines. Lancet Oncol. 2013;14:e562–70.
16. Xie C, Wan X, Quan H, Zheng M, Fu L, Li Y, et al. Preclinical characterization of anlotinib, a highly potent and selective vascular endothelial growth factor receptor-2 inhibitor. Cancer Sci. 2018;109:1207–19.
17. Taurin S, Yang CH, Reyes M, Cho S, Jarboe EA, Werner TL, et al. Abstract 3244: treatment of endometrial cancer cells with a new small tyrosine kinase inhibitor targeting mutated fibroblast growth factor receptor-2. Cancer Res. 2017;77(13 Supplement):3244.
18. Lin B, Song X, Yang D, Bai D, Yao Y, Lu N, et al. Anlotinib inhibits angiogenesis via suppressing the activation of VEGFR2, PDGFRβ and FGFR1. Gene. 2018;654:77–86.
19. Taurin S, Yang CH, Reyes M, Cho S, Coombs DM, Jarboe EA, et al. Endometrial cancers harboring mutated fibroblast growth factor receptor 2 protein are successfully treated with a new small tyrosine kinase inhibitor in an orthotopic mouse model. Int J Gynecol Cancer. 2018;28:152–60.
20. Zhong CC, Chen F, Yang JL, Jia WW, Li L, Cheng C, et al. Pharmacokinetics and disposition of anlotinib, an oral tyrosine kinase inhibitor, in experimental animal species. Acta Pharmacol Sin. 2018;39:1048–63.
21. Sun Y, Niu W, Du F, Du C, Li S, Wang J, et al. Safety, pharmacokinetics, and antitumor properties of anlotinib, an oral multi-target tyrosine kinase

inhibitor, in patients with advanced refractory solid tumors. J Hematol Oncol. 2016;9:105.

22. Werner TL, Kannapel E, Chen J, Chen M, Cohen A L. Safety and PK results from a phase Ib study of AL3818 (anlotinib) hydrochloride in subjects with ovarian, cervical, and endometrial cancers. J Clin Oncol. 2017;35(15_suppl):e17071.

23. Sun W, Wang Z, Chen R, Huang C, Sun R, Hu X, et al. Influences of anlotinib on cytochrome P450 enzymes in rats using a cocktail method. Biomed Res Int. 2017;2017:3619723.

24. van Erp NP, Gelderblom H, Guchelaar HJ. Clinical pharmacokinetics of tyrosine kinase inhibitors. Cancer Treat Rev. 2009;35:692–706.

25. Han B, Li K, Zhao Y, Li B, Cheng Y, Zhou J, et al. Anlotinib as a third-line therapy in patients with refractory advanced non-small-cell lung cancer: a multicentre, randomised phase II trial (ALTER0302). Br J Cancer. 2018;118: 654–61.

26. Han B, Li K, Wang Q, et al. Third-line treatment: a randomized, double-blind, placebo-controlled phase III ALTER-0303 study—efficacy and safety of anlotinib treatment in patients with refractory advanced NSCLC. J Clin Oncol. 2017;35(15_suppl):9053.

27. Han B, Li K, Wang Q, Zhao Y, Zhang L, Shi J, et al. Efficiency of anlotinib as 3rd line treatment in patients with different EGFR gene status, an exploratory subgroup analysis of ALTER0303 trial. J Thorac Oncol. 2017;12:S2275.

28. Li K, Han B, Wang Q, Zhang L, Shi J, Wang Z, et al. OS outcomes to anlotinib in patients (pts) with refractory NSCLC of both wild-type (WT) and mutant EGFR. J Clin Oncol. 2018;36(15_suppl):e21013.

29. Cheng Y, Han B, Li K, Wang Q, Zhang L, Shi J, et al. Subgroup analysis of histology in ALTER0303: anlotinib hydrochloride as 3rd line and further line treatment in refractory advanced NSCLC patients (pts). J Clin Oncol. 2018; 36(15_suppl):9080.

30. Shi J, Han B, Li K, Wang Q, Zhang L, Wang Z, et al. Subgroup analysis of elderly patients (pts) in ALTER0303: Anlotinib hydrochloride as 3rd-line and further line treatment in refractory advanced NSCLC pts from a randomized, double-blind, placebo-controlled phase III ALTER0303 trial. J Clin Oncol. 2018;36(15_suppl):e21181.

31. Wang Q, Han B, Li K, Zhang L, Shi J, Wang Z, et al. Efficiency of anlotinib as 3rd line treatment in patients (pts) from a randomized, double-blind, placebo-controlled phase III trial, an exploratory subgroup analysis of ALTER0303 trial for the previous therapy strategy effect. J Clin Oncol. 2018; 36(15_suppl):e21182.

32. China Food and Drug Administration, Approved drugs, Anlotinib [internet]. http://app1.sfda.gov.cn/datasearch/face3/base.jsp?tableId=25&tableName=TABLE25&title=%E5%9B%BD%E4%BA%A7%E8%8D%AF%E5%93%81&bcId=124356560303886909015737447882. Accessed 8 May 2018.

33. Y. Cheng, Y. Wu, S. Lu, C. Zhou, C. Wang, L. Wang, et al. Chinese Society of Clinical Oncology (CSCO) guidelines for diagnosis and treatment of primary lung cancer. Version 1. 2018, 2018.

34. Sleijfer S, Ray-Coquard I, Papai Z, Le Cesne A, Scurr M, Schöffski P, et al. Pazopanib, a multikinase angiogenesis inhibitor, in patients with relapsed or refractory advanced soft tissue sarcoma: a phase II study from the European organisation for research and treatment of cancer-soft tissue and bone sarcoma group (EORTC study 62043). J Clin Oncol. 2009;27:3126–32.

35. Cassier PA, Gelderblom H, Stacchiotti S, Thomas D, Maki RG, Kroep JR, et al. Efficacy of imatinib mesylate for the treatment of locally advanced and/or metastatic tenosynovial giant cell tumor/pigmented villonodular synovitis. Cancer. 2012;118:1649–55.

36. Stacchiotti S, Negri T, Libertini M, Conca E, Castelli C, Tazzari M, et al. Sunitinib malate in solitary fibrous tumor (SFT). Ann Oncol. 2012;23:3171–9.

37. Valentin T, Fournier C, Penel N, Bompas E, Chaigneau L, et al. Sorafenib in patients with progressive malignant solitary fibrous tumors: a subgroup analysis from a phase II study of the French Sarcoma Group (GSF/GETO). Investig New Drugs. 2013;31:1626–7.

38. Butrynski JE, D'Adamo DR, Hornick JL, Dal Cin P, Antonescu CR, Jhanwar SC, et al. Crizotinib in ALKrearranged inflammatory myofibroblastic tumor. N Engl J Med. 2010;363:1727–33.

39. Shaw AT, Kim DW, Mehra R, Tan DS, Felip E, Chow LQ, Camidge DR, et al. Ceritinib in ALK-rearranged non-small-cell lung cancer. N Engl J Med. 2014; 370:1189–97.

40. Tap WD, Jones RL, Van Tine BA, Chmielowski B, Elias AD, Adkins D, et al. Olaratumab and doxorubicin versus doxorubicin alone for treatment of soft-tissue sarcoma: an open-label phase 1b and randomised phase 2 trial. Lancet. 2016;388:488–97.

41. Agulnik M, Yarber JL, Okuno SH, von Mehren M, Jovanovic BD, Brockstein BE, et al. An open-label, multicenter, phase II study of bevacizumab for the treatment of angiosarcoma and epithelioid hemangioendotheliomas. Ann Oncol. 2013;24:257–63.

42. Chi Y, Sun Y, Cai J, Yao Y, Hong X, Fang Z, et al. Phase II study of anlotinib for treatment of advanced soft tissues sarcomas. J Clin Oncol. 2016;34(15_suppl):11005.

43. Stacchiotti S, Negri T, Zaffaroni N, Palassini E, Morosi C, Brich S, et al. Sunitinib in advanced alveolar soft part sarcoma: evidence of a direct antitumor effect. Ann Oncol. 2011;22:1682–90.

44. Chi Y, Yao Y, Wang S, Huang G, Cai Q, Shang G, et al. Anlotinib for metastasis soft tissue sarcoma: a randomized, double-blind, placebo-controlled and multi-centered clinical trial. J Clin Oncol. 2018;36(15_suppl):11503.

45. Sternberg CN, Davis ID, Mardiak J, Szczylik C, Lee E, Wagstaff J, et al. Pazopanib in locally advanced or metastatic renal cell carcinoma: results of a randomized phase III trial. J Clin Oncol. 2010;28:1061–8.

46. Motzer RJ, Hutson TE, Tomczak P, Ecklund DJ, Klingner EA, Yankey JW, et al. Sunitinib versus interferon alfa in metastatic renal-cell carcinoma. N Engl J Med. 2007;356:115–4.

47. Choueiri TK, Halabi S, Sanford BL, Hahn O, Michaelson MD, Walsh MK, et al. Cabozantinib versus sunitinib as initial targeted therapy for patients with metastatic renal cell carcinoma of poor or intermediate risk: the Alliance A031203 CABOSUN trial. J Clin Oncol. 2017;35:591–7.

48. Hutson TE, Lesovoy V, Al-Shukri S, Stus VP, Lipatov ON, Bair AH, et al. Axitinib versus sorafenib as first-line therapy in patients with metastatic renal-cell carcinoma: a randomised open-label phase 3 trial. Lancet Oncol. 2013;14:1287–94.

49. Motzer RJ, Hutson TE, Ren M, Dutcus C, Larkin J. Independent assessment of lenvatinib plus everolimus in patients with metastatic renal cell carcinoma. Lancet Oncol. 2016;17:e4–5.

50. Zhou AP, Bai Y, Song Y, Li H, Xie X, Ren XB, et al. Anlotinib in metastatic renal cell carcinoma (mRCC) with a previous anti-VEGFR TKI: preliminary results from a multicenter, phase II trial. J Clin Oncol. 2016;34(15_suppl): e16082.

51. Zhou AP, Ma J, Bai Y, Song Y, Li H, Xie X, et al. Anlotinib versus sunitinib as first line treatment for metastatic renal cell carcinoma (mRCC): preliminary results from a randomized phase II clinical trial. J Clin Oncol. 2016;34(15_suppl):4565.

52. Brose MS, Nutting CM, Jarzab B, Libby P, Thuren T, Glynn RJ, et al. Sorafenib in radioactive iodine-refractory, locally advanced or metastatic differentiated thyroid cancer: a randomised, double-blind, phase 3 trial. Lancet. 2014;384: 319–28.

53. Carr LL, Mankoff DA, Goulart BH, Eaton KD, Capell PT, Kell EM, et al. Phase II study of daily sunitinib in FDG-PET-positive, iodine-refractory differentiated thyroid cancer and metastatic medullary carcinoma of the thyroid with functional imaging correlation. Clin Cancer Res. 2010;16:5260–8.

54. Elisei R, Schlumberger MJ, Muller SP, Schöffski P, Brose MS, Shah MH, et al. Cabozantinib in progressive medullary thyroid cancer. J Clin Oncol. 2013;31: 3639–46.

55. Wells SA Jr, Robinson BG, Gagel RF, Dralle H, Fagin JA, Santoro M, et al. Vandetanib in patients with locally advanced or metastatic medullary thyroid cancer: a randomized, double-blind phase III trial. J Clin Oncol. 2012; 30:134–41.

56. Bible KC, Suman VJ, Molina JR, Smallridge RC, Maples WJ, Menefee ME, et al. Efficacy of pazopanib in progressive, radioiodine-refractory, metastatic differentiated thyroid cancers: results of a phase 2 consortium study. Lancet Oncol. 2010;11:962–72.

57. Sun Y, Chi Y, Tang P, Gao M, Ji Q, Li Z, et al. Phase II study of anlotinib for treatment of advanced medullary thyroid carcinoma. J Clin Oncol. 2016; 34(15_suppl):6015.

58. Beck J, Procopio G, Bajetta E, Keilholz U, Negrier S, Szczylik C, et al. Final results of the European Advanced Renal Cell Carcinoma Sorafenib (EU-ARCCS) expanded-access study: a large open-label study in diverse community settings. Ann Oncol. 2011;22:1812–23.

59. Stadler WM, Figlin RA, McDermott DF, Dutcher JP, Knox JJ, Miller WH, et al. Safety and efficacy results of the advanced renal cell carcinoma sorafenib expanded access program in North America. Cancer. 2010;116:1272–80.

60. Gore ME, Szczylik C, Porta C, Bracarda S, Bjarnason GA, Oudard S, et al. Safety and efficacy of sunitinib for metastatic renal-cell carcinoma: an expanded-access trial. Lancet Oncol. 2009;10:757–63.

61. Qi WX, Shen Z, Tang LN, Yao Y. Risk of arterial thromboembolic events with vascular endothelial growth factor receptor tyrosine kinase inhibitors: an up-to-date meta-analysis. Crit Rev Oncol Hematol. 2014;92:71–82.

62. Liu Z, Wang J, Meng Z, Wang X, Zhang C, Chen J, et al. Analysis on ALTER0303 trial: aCECs level may correlate with metastases burden and predict PFS of Anlotinib in advanced NSCLC. J Thorac Oncol. 2017;12: S2234–5.

63. Han B, Zhao Y, Li K, Wang J, Wang Q, Zhang L, et al. P3. Blood samples NGS for baseline molecular signature of anotinib treated advanced NSCLC patients in ALTER0303 trial. J Thorac Oncol. 2017;12:S2279.

64. Wilke H, Muro K, Van Cutsem E, Oh SC, Bodoky G, Shimada Y, et al. Ramucirumab plus paclitaxel versus placebo plus paclitaxel in patients with previously treated advanced gastric or gastro-oesophageal junction adenocarcinoma (RAINBOW): a double-blind, randomised phase 3 trial. Lancet Oncol. 2014;15:1224–35.

65. Garon EB, Ciuleanu TE, Arrieta O, Prabhash K, Syrigos KN, Goksel T, et al. Ramucirumab plus docetaxel versus placebo plus docetaxel for second-line treatment of stage IV non-small-cell lung cancer after disease progression on platinum-based therapy (REVEL): a multicentre, double-blind, randomised phase 3 trial. Lancet. 2014;384:665–73.

66. Vanneman M, Dranoff G. Combining immunotherapy and targeted therapies in cancer treatment. Nat Rev Cancer. 2012;12:237–51.

67. Hughes PE, Caenepeel S, Wu LC. Targeted therapy and checkpoint immunotherapy combinations for the treatment of cancer. Trends Immunol. 2016;37:462–76.

10

Targeting WEE1 to enhance conventional therapies for acute lymphoblastic leukemia

Andrea Ghelli Luserna Di Rorà[1*], Neil Beeharry[3,6], Enrica Imbrogno[1], Anna Ferrari[1], Valentina Robustelli[1], Simona Righi[1], Elena Sabattini[1], Maria Vittoria Verga Falzacappa[2], Chiara Ronchini[2], Nicoletta Testoni[1], Carmen Baldazzi[1], Cristina Papayannidis[1], Maria Chiara Abbenante[1], Giovanni Marconi[1], Stefania Paolini[1], Sarah Parisi[1], Chiara Sartor[1], Maria Chiara Fontana[1], Serena De Matteis[4], Ilaria Iacobucci[1,7], Pier Giuseppe Pelicci[2], Michele Cavo[1], Timothy J. Yen[3] and Giovanni Martinelli[5]

Abstract

Background: Despite the recent progress that has been made in the understanding and treatment of acute lymphoblastic leukemia (ALL), the outcome is still dismal in adult ALL cases. Several studies in solid tumors identified high expression of WEE1 kinase as a poor prognostic factor and reported its role as a cancer-conserving oncogene that protects cancer cells from DNA damage. Therefore, the targeted inhibition of WEE1 kinase has emerged as a rational strategy to sensitize cancer cells to antineoplastic compounds, which we evaluate in this study.

Methods: The effectiveness of the selective WEE1 inhibitor AZD-1775 as a single agent and in combination with different antineoplastic agents in B and T cell precursor ALL (B/T-ALL) was evaluated in vitro and ex vivo studies. The efficacy of the compound in terms of cytotoxicity, induction of apoptosis, and changes in gene and protein expression was assessed using different B/T-ALL cell lines and confirmed in primary ALL blasts.

Results: We showed that *WEE1* was highly expressed in adult primary ALL bone marrow and peripheral blood blasts ($n = 58$) compared to normal mononuclear cells isolated from the peripheral blood of healthy donors ($p = 0.004$). Thus, we hypothesized that WEE1 could be a rational target in ALL, and its inhibition could enhance the cytotoxicity of conventional therapies used for ALL. We evaluated the efficacy of AZD-1775 as a single agent and in combination with several antineoplastic agents, and we elucidated its mechanisms of action. AZD-1775 reduced cell viability in B/T-ALL cell lines by disrupting the G2/M checkpoint and inducing apoptosis. These findings were confirmed in human primary ALL bone marrow and peripheral blood blasts ($n = 15$). In both cell lines and primary leukemic cells, AZD-1775 significantly enhanced the efficacy of several tyrosine kinase inhibitors (TKIs) such as bosutinib, imatinib, and ponatinib, and of chemotherapeutic agents (clofarabine and doxorubicin) in terms of the reduction of cell viability, apoptosis induction, and inhibition of proliferation.

Conclusions: Our data suggest that WEE1 plays a role in ALL blast's survival and is a bona fide target for therapeutic intervention. These data support the evaluation of the therapeutic potential of AZD-1775 as chemo-sensitizer agent for the treatment of B/T-ALL.

Keywords: Acute lymphoblastic leukemia, WEE1 inhibitor, Chemo-sensitizer agent, G2/M checkpoint

* Correspondence: andrea.ghelliluserna@studio.unibo.it
[1]Department of Experimental, Diagnostic and Specialty Medicine, Institute of Hematology "L. e A. Seràgnoli", University of Bologna, Via Massarenti 9, 40138 Bologna, Italy
Full list of author information is available at the end of the article

Background

Although many progresses have been made in understanding the pathogenesis of ALL and in improving outcome, response rates are still unsatisfied in adult patients with a 5-year survival rate of less than 35%. To date, the therapeutic options, with the exclusion of drugs against particular genetic alterations (*BCR-ABL1* fusion or *BCR-ABL1*-like alterations), are still mainly based on conventional chemotherapy especially for the induction phase [1–11]. Therefore, there is a clinical need to identify novel targets for more effective therapies and/or improve the effectiveness of the conventional treatments in order to increase the survival rates of adult patients with ALL. It is well established that eukaryotic cells respond to DNA damage by activating specific pathways, collectively termed DNA damage response (DDR) [12–14]. DDR, therefore, refers to a network of biological processes that are activated by aberrant DNA structures generated upon DNA damage, including cell cycle checkpoints, DNA repair mechanisms, cell death, and senescence [15]. The WEE1 kinase is a key player in the DDR process and acts to inhibit mitotic entry in cells with damaged DNA. This is achieved by WEE1-mediated inhibitory phosphorylation on key residues of CDK1 and 2 kinases [16–20]. Several studies speculated on the importance of WEE1 expression in cancer cells ascribing a dual biological role as a tumor suppressor, whose loss promotes the accumulation of genetic aberrations on pre-neoplastic lesions, or as a cancer-conserving oncogene, whose expression protects cancer cells from DNA damage and aberrant mitosis [21–25]. Moreover, different cancer cells depend on the expression of WEE1 for survival as shown by the effectiveness of a selective WEE1 inhibitor [26]. Due to the above-mentioned crucial biological roles, and the relationship between high expression of *WEE1* and poor prognosis in several kinds of tumors [25, 27], selective WEE1 inhibitors (PD0166285, PD0407824, and AZD-1775) have been developed [26, 28–37]. Several preclinical and clinical studies (clinicaltrials.gov; NCT02341456; NCT03012477; NCT03315091; NCT01748825), mostly focused on solid tumors, demonstrated the efficacy of AZD-1775 not only as a single agent but also in combination with DNA damaging drugs or different targeted inhibitors in several cancer models [37–39]. Several studies demonstrate that AZD-1775 is a powerful approach to override chemoresistance in different tumor models. For instance, it has been shown that AZD1775 increased the sensitivity to cisplatin and gemcitabine (both DNA damaging agents) by overriding the G2/M checkpoint and force cancer cells with defective DNA replication to inappropriately enter mitosis and die via mitotic catastrophe [40, 41]. Combinatorial studies can be used to exploit tumor resistance to AZD-1775. Indeed, AZD1775-resistant small cell lung cancer models were shown to have elevated expression of

AXL, pS6, and MET genes that a WEE1/AXL or WEE1/mTOR inhibitor combination could overcome the resistance in vitro and in vivo [42]. Despite the promising data from studies using solid tumor models, few studies have investigated the mechanisms of the action of AZD-1775 and its efficacy in hematological malignances especially in acute leukemia [35–38]. In the present study, we provide evidence that WEE1 represents a rational therapeutic target in ALL. First, we evaluated the levels of expression of *Wee1* mRNA in a cohort of 58 ALL primary samples, and then the effectiveness of AZD-1775, as monotherapy and in combination with different drugs normally used as a standard of care for adult ALL patients.

Methods
Drugs and cell lines

AZD-1775 was purchased from MedChemexpress. Clofarabine, doxorubicin, imatinib, and ponatinib were obtained from Sigma-Aldrich. Bosutinib (Bos) was purchased from Tocris, and Bosutinib isomer (Bos-I) was purchased from LC Labs. Human B and T cell precursor ALL (B/T-ALL) cell lines (B-ALL: BV-173, SUP-B15, REH, NALM-6, NALM-19; T-ALL: MOLT-4, RPMI-8402, CCRF-CEM) were cultured in RPMI-1640 (Invitrogen) with 1% L-glutamine (Sigma-Aldrich), penicillin (100 U/ml, Gibco), and streptomycin (100 μg/ml, Gibco) supplemented with 10–20% fetal bovine serum (FBS, Gibco). All the cell lines were purchased from Deutsche Sammlung von Mikroorganismen und Zellkulturen GmbH (DSMZ) website (https://www.dsmz.de).

Primary leukemic cells and treatment

To assess the effect of AZD-1775 in primary samples, upon written informed consent, primary leukemic cells with > 70% of blasts were isolated from the peripheral blood and bone marrow of adult ALL cases ($n = 15$, Additional file 1: Table S1) and treated ex vivo with increasing concentration of the test drug. The study was performed in accordance with the principles laid down in the Declaration of Helsinki. Primary cells Lymphoprep-isolated (Nycomed UK, Birmingham) were seeded in 6-well plates at 1×10^6 cells/ml in RPMI-1640 supplemented with 20% FBS and treated with AZD-1775 (2.5, 5, and 10 μM) for 24 h. In order to evaluate the cytotoxicity of the compound on non-leukemic cells, mononuclear cells (MNCs) isolated, upon written informed consent, from the peripheral blood of healthy donors ($n = 5$) were incubated in 6-well plates at 1×10^6 cells/ml in RPMI-1640 with 20% FBS and treated with AZD-1775 at the same concentration reported above for 24 h. For drug combination studies, cells were incubated with increasing concentrations of AZD-1775 and a fixed dose of clofarabine (500 nM) or Bos (1 μM) for 24 h. The number of viable cells was detected by trypan blue exclusion dye (Sigma-Aldrich).

Immunohistochemistry analysis

Bone marrow specimens were fixed in B5 solution for 2 h, soaked in 70% alcohol for at least 30 min, and then decalcified in an EDTA-based solution for 2.5 h. Sections of 3 μm thickness were cut for histological examination (H&E, Giemsa, Gomori silver impregnation) and immunohistochemistry. For diagnostic purpose, the following antibodies were applied in all cases: anti-CD79a (clone JCB, dilution 1:50, DakoCytomation, Glostrup, Denmark), anti-PAX5 (clone DAK-Pax5, dilution 1:60, DakoCytomation), anti-CD20 (clone L26, dilution 1:300, DakoCytomation), anti-CD10 (clone 56C6, dilution 1:50, Leica Biosystem), anti-CD34 (clone QBEnd/10, dilution 1:100, Leica Biosystem), and anti-TdT (clone EP266, dilution 1:40, DakoCytomation). Antigens were retrieved with the PT-link (PT100/PT101, DakoCytomation) and the EnVision Flex Target Retrieval Solution High pH (K8004, DakoCytomation) at 92 °C or 80 °C for 5 min. For the study, the Wee1 antibody was applied in 7/58 bone marrow biopsies available at the Unit of Haemolymphopathology, Bologna. This antibody (clone B-11, 1:30, Santa Cruz Biotechnology, CA, USA) was applied on pre-exposing slides soaked in a Tris-EDTA pH 9 solution at 1 min heating in a pressure cooker. Immunohistochemistry was performed on an Autostainer Plus platform (DakoCytomation), incubating primary antibody at room temperature for 30 min; the reaction was detected by the Dako Real Detection Systems Alkaline Phosphatase/RED Rabbit/Mouse Kit (K 5005, DakoCytomation). Double staining was performed using the Dako Real Detection Systems Alkaline Phosphatase/RED Rabbit/Mouse Kit (K 5005, DakoCytomation) to reveal anti-CD79 and the Dako Real EnVision Detection System, Peroxidase/DAB, Rabbit/Mouse (K5007, DakoCytomation) to highlight anti-Wee1. All slides were counterstained with Gill's hematoxylin.

Cell viability and cell proliferation assay

In order to assess cell viability, cells were seeded into 96-well plates at 0.5×10^6 cells/ml and incubated with AZD-1775 (6 to 5000 nM, dilution 1:3 media) for 24, 48, and 72 h. Cell viability was then determined using MTS Cell Proliferation Assay Kit (Promega). For the drug combination index assay, cells were treated simultaneously with increasing concentration of the two test drugs for 24, 48, and 72 h. The additive, synergistic, and antagonistic effect of the drug combinations was evaluated using Compusyn Software where combination index (CI) < 1 synergism, CI = 1 additivity, and CI > 1 antagonism. To assess the proliferation ability, cell lines were seeded in 6-well plates at a concentration of 0.2×10^6 cells/ml and counted every 24 h for 4 days of continuous drug exposure. All drug treatments were performed in triplicate, and independent experiments were performed at least three times.

Light and fluorescence microscopy analyses

To investigate potential macroscopic modifications of cell morphology, cells (primary and cell lines) were seeded in 6-well plates at 0.5×10^5 cells/ml and incubated with increasing concentration of AZD-1775 for 24 h. Cells were harvested, spun down (10 min at 200 g) onto glass slips using a Cytospin™ centrifuge (Thermofisher), and then stained with the May-Grünwald Giemsa solutions (Sigma-Aldrich). The slides were analyzed using an optical microscope AXIOVERT 40 CFL and the pictures analyzed using AxioVision Rel.4.7 software. For the immunofluorescence analysis, BV-173 cells were seeded to poly-D-lysine-coated coverslips, fixed with 4% paraformaldehyde (PFA) and stained at 37 °C with an anti-phospho-Ser/Thr-Pro MPM-2 antibody FITC conjugated (Millipore Sigma). Coverslips were, then, mounted on glass slides using a mounting media with DAPI (4′,6-diamidino-2-phenylindole) (Prolong Gold with DAPI, Invitrogen). Immunofluorescence analyses were performed using the AXIOVERT 40 CFL microscope and the picture analyzed using AxioVision Rel.4.7 software.

Flow cytometry

All analyses were performed using the flow cytometer Facs CantoII (BD). Apoptosis was performed using Annexin V/propidium iodide (PI) according to the manufacturer's instructions (Roche). Cells were seeded in 12-well plates at 0.5×10^5 cells/ml with AZD-1775 (at IC_{50}, IC_{25}, and $IC_{12.5}$) for 24 h at 37 °C. The percentage of Annexin V/PI-positive cells was determined by assaying a minimum of 10,000 cells. The mean percentage of Annexin V/PI-positive cells and standard error measurements were calculated from at least two independent experiments. Cell cycle analyses were performed using the PI staining mix (BD). Cells were seeded in a 24-well plate at a concentration of 0.5×10^6 cells per well and treated with AZD-1775 (IC_{50}) for 24 h. After 24 h of incubation, the cells were harvested and washed with cold PBS. After washing with PBS, the cells were fixed using ethanol 70% and stored at -20 °C for 24 h. After the fixation period, the ethanol was removed by one wash in PBS, and the cells were incubated for 30 min at 37 °C with the PI staining mix. The quantitative analyses were performed using Flowing and ModfiT software (Verity Software House).

Immunoblotting

Immunoblotting analyses were performed using Mini-Protean TGX stain-free precast gels, blotted to nitrocellulose membranes (Bio-Rad Trans-blot turbo transfer pack) and incubated overnight with the following anti-bodies: Chk1 (#2345S), pChk1 (Ser317) (#2344S), pChk1 (ser296) (#2349), Cdc2 (#9112S), pCdc2 (Tyr15) (#4539S), Cdc25C (#4688), Cdc25B (#9525), CCNB1 (#4138), CDKN1A (#2947), pH2A.X (Ser139) (#2577S), MYT1 (#4282), p-c-ABL (Tyr245) (#2868), and Rad51 (#8875) from Cell Signaling. Antibody to CCNB2 (ab18250) was from Abcam. Antibody to β-actin was from Sigma (St. Louis, MO). Finally, all the antibodies were detected using the enhanced chemiluminescence kit ECL (GE) and the compact darkroom ChemiDoc-It (UVP).

Quantitative PCR and gene expression

To evaluate how AZD-1775 affects the gene expression of different components of the G2/M checkpoint, cell lines (BV-173 and CCRF-CEM) and primary cells were treated for 12 h with increasing concentration of AZD-1775 at approximately their IC_{50}. The treatment was performed for 12 h in order to highlight the effect of the compound on gene expression before inducing overt cytotoxicity. After the period of incubation, the cells were harvested and the total RNA was extracted using Maxwell simply RNA Blood kit (Promega), and 1 μg of each RNA sample (quantified by ND1000 Spectrophotometer) was reverse transcribed using iScript Advanced cDNA Synthesis kit for RT-qPCR (Bio-Rad). For the quantification of G2/M checkpoint genes, the commercial 96-well PrimePCR plates (DNA damage DNA-ATM/ATR regulation of G2/M checkpoint, Bio-Rad) were employed according to the instructions of the manufacturer: SsoAdvanced Universal Sybr Green Supermix (Bio-Rad) and LightCycler 480 System amplification protocol (Roche Diagnostics, Mannheim, Germany). Data analysis was performed with PrimePCR analysis software (Bio-Rad).

Gene expression profile

Gene expression profiling on 58 adult ALL patient samples (Additional file 1: Table S1) and on 7 MNCs samples obtained from the peripheral blood of seven healthy donors was performed using Affymetrix GeneChip Human Transcriptome Array 2.0 (Affymetrix Inc., Santa Clara, CA, USA; currently ThermoFisher Scientific) following the manufacturers' instructions. In particular, we analyzed 33 BCR-ABL1-negative (27 at the time of diagnosis and six unpaired relapses) and 25 BCR-ABL1-positive (17 at the time of diagnosis, eight unpaired relapses) samples. Raw data were normalized with Expression Console Software 1.4 (Affymetrix Inc.; currently ThermoFisher Scientific) by using the gene-level SST RMA algorithm.

Statistical analysis

Data were presented as the mean ± standard deviation (SD) from at least three biological replicates. Two-tailed

t test or one-way ANOVA test were used to analyze the statistical significance between the groups. p value < 0.05 was considered a significant difference. Statistical analysis was performed with Graphpad5 software (GraphPad Inc., San Diego, CA, USA).

Results

Wee1 transcript is highly expressed in ALL primary samples

Gene expression analysis revealed that Wee1 is highly expressed in adult ALL samples ($n = 58$, 44 at diagnosis and 14 at unpaired relapses) compared to normal mononuclear cells (MNCs) ($p = 0.0046$) (Fig. 1a). Among different leukemia subtypes, Wee1 was significantly higher in BCR-ABL1-negative samples (diagnosis $p = 0.0061$; relapse $p = 0.005$) than in BCR-ABL1-positive samples (diagnosis ns; relapse $p = 0.01$) compared with normal MNCs (Fig. 1b) (Additional file 1: Table S1). To correlate the level of Wee1 transcript with its protein levels, immunohistochemistry analyses were performed on eight ALL samples. In the bone marrow biopsies, all cases were confirmed by immunohistochemistry as B cell precursor lymphoblastic leukemias (B-ALL); upon CD20 reactivity, three cases were staged as pro-B-ALL (CD20-negative) and four as pre-B-ALL (CD20-positive). Regarding the WEE1 staining, in the reactive bone marrow sections, the protein revealed moderate to strong nuclear and/or nuclear-cytoplasmic staining in a subset of cells morphologically referable as myeloid immature precursors and, more rarely, in the nuclei of the megakaryocytes (Fig. 1c). In the neoplastic blasts, the WEE1 protein localized in the nuclear and/or nuclear-cytoplasmic compartments. The percentage of positive cells was defined in relation to the comparison of CD79a staining in leukemic blasts. Two bone marrow samples turned out to be negative for WEE1 staining on leukemic blasts (ALL_34 and ALL_52); while in the remaining five samples, the percentage of positive blasts ranged from 20% (ALL_26 and ALL_47) to 50% (ALL_35) and to more than 75% (ALL_48 and ALL_22) (Fig. 1d) of the blastic population. In the two cases with 20% positivity, a double staining WEE1/CD79a was performed to correctly assess the amount of double-stained cells (Fig. 1e). These results suggest that given the association of WEE1 abundance in ALL relative to normal cells, WEE1 can be considered a logical therapeutic target.

AZD-1775 reduces cell viability and induces apoptosis in ALL cell lines

Having established that the abundance of WEE1 is significantly higher in primary ALL blasts than normal MNCs, this raised the possibility that ALL cells may be reliant on WEE1 for survival. We therefore evaluated the efficacy of a selective WEE1 inhibitor (AZD-1775)

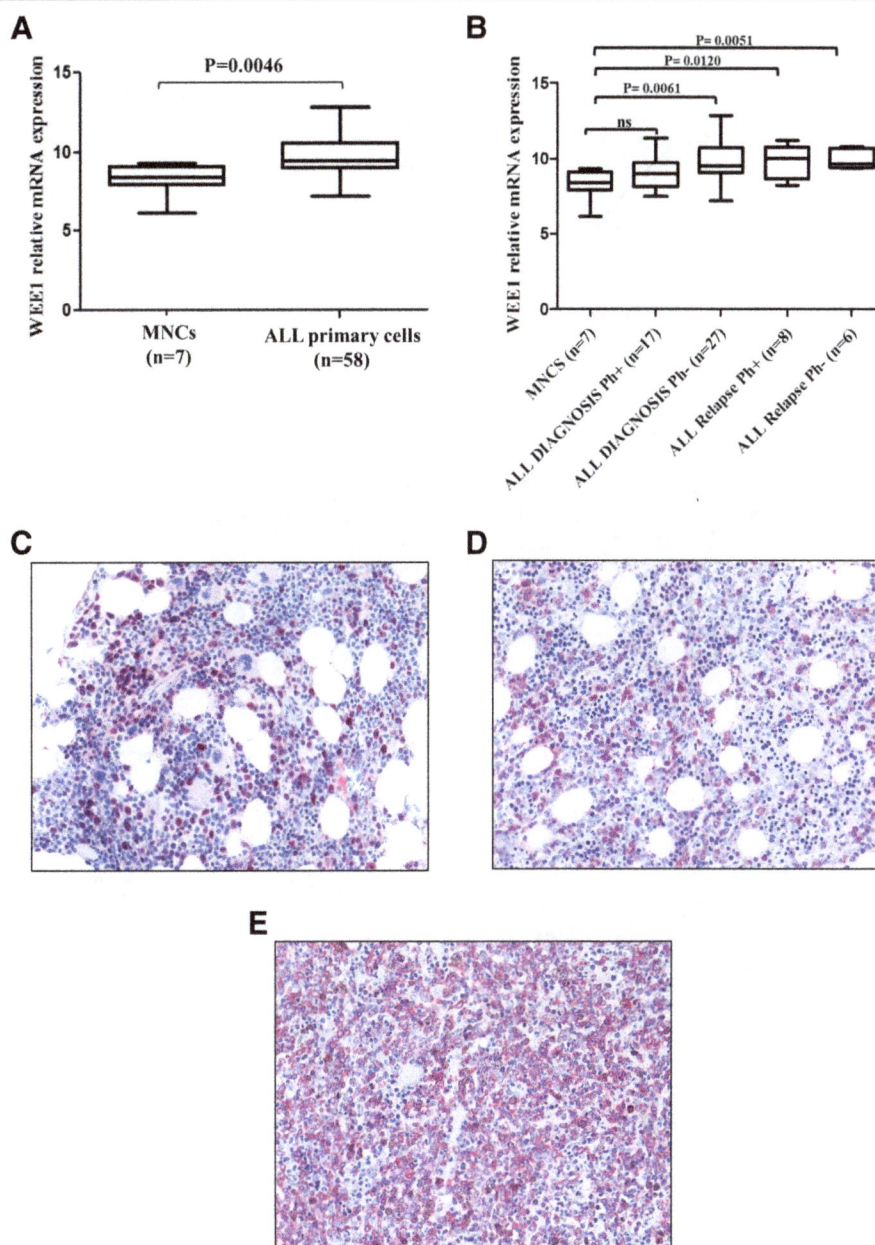

Fig. 1 WEE1 overexpression in ALL samples. **a** WEE1 transcript levels in samples isolated from adult ALL ($n = 58$) and in MNCs ($n = 7$) from peripheral blood of healthy donors. One-way ANOVA test was performed to confirm the statistical significance of the differences. Results are expressed as Log10 2exp[−(ΔΔCt). **b** WEE1 transcript levels in samples isolated from adult *BCR-ABL1*-positive (Ph+) ALL at diagnosis ($n = 17$), adult *BCR-ABL1*-negative (Ph−) ALL at diagnosis ($n = 27$), adult *BCR-ABL1*-positive ALL at relapse (unpaired, $n = 8$), adult *BCR-ABL1*-negative ALL at relapse (unpaired, $n = 6$), and in MNCs ($n = 7$) from the peripheral blood samples of healthy donors. Results are expressed as Log10 2exp[−(ΔΔCt). **c** Immunohistochemistry analysis of a reactive bone marrow sample; WEE1 is positive at moderate to strong intensity in morphologically typical myeloid precursors ($\times 20$). **d** Immunohistochemistry analysis of leukemic blasts scattered in the interstitium and positive for WEE1 ($\times 20$). **e** Leukemic blasts are widely positive for the B cell marker CD79a (red) while those positive for WEE1 (brown) are much fewer, as shown by the few scattered double-stained blasts ($\times 20$)

on ALL cell lines. AZD-1775 as a single agent reduced cell viability in a dose- and time-dependent manner in a panel of eight ALL cell lines (Fig. 2a, Additional file 2: Figure S1A and B). Consistent with our previous results using inhibitors that target Chk1 and Chk2 checkpoint kinases [43, 44], the sensitivity to AZD-1775 did not correlate with leukemia subtypes, karyotype, or with the basal expression of WEE1 (data not shown). We next treated BV-173 (*BCR-ABL1*-positive B-ALL), NALM-6 (*BCR-ABL1*-negative B-ALL), MOLT-4 (T-ALL), and

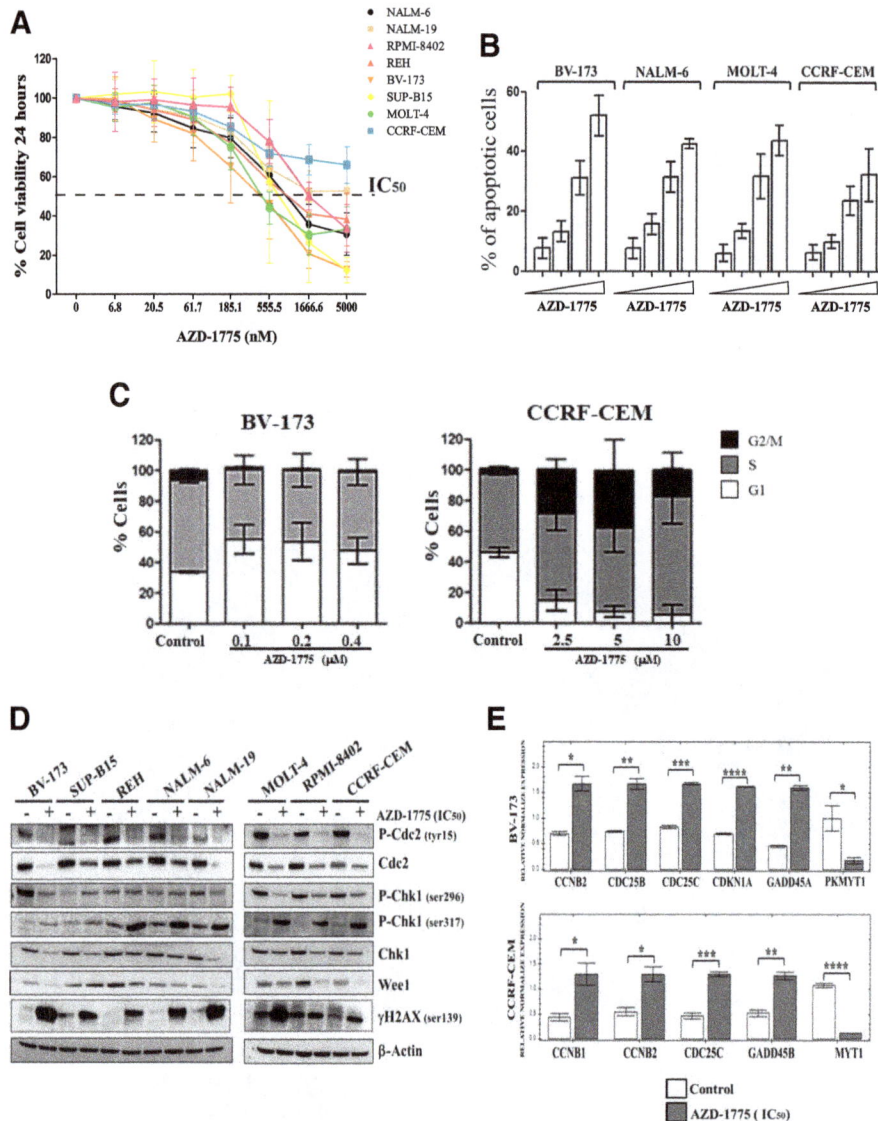

Fig. 2 AZD-1775 overrides the G2/M checkpoint and induces mitosis in B/T-ALL cell lines. **a** Viability analyses in ALL cell lines incubated for 24 h with AZD-1775 (6 to 5000 nM). The percentage of viable cells is depicted as a percentage of untreated controls. **b** Apoptosis analyses in BV-173, NALM-6, MOLT-4, and CCRF-CEM cells after 24 h of incubation with AZD-1775 (for each cell line: IC_{50}, IC_{25}, and $IC12.5$). The percentage of apoptotic cells was detected after Annexin V/propidium iodide staining. **c** Cell cycle analysis of BV-173 and CCRF-CEM cell line incubated for 24 h with increasing concentration of AZD-1775. **d** Representative immunoblots showing the expression of key proteins of the WEE1 pathway after treatment with AZD-1775 (IC_{50} for each cell line) for 24 h of the indicated cells lines. β-actin was used for loading normalization. **e** Quantitative mRNA analysis of six representative genes of 24 G2/M checkpoint genes analyzed. The white columns represent the controls and the gray columns represent the samples treated with AZD-1775 (IC_{50}) for 12 h of the indicated cell lines. Results are expressed as Log10 2exp[−(ΔΔCt)

CCRF-CEM (T-ALL) cells with AZD-1775 for 24 h at the IC_{50}, IC_{25}, and $IC_{12.5}$ for each cell line and determined the percentage of apoptotic cells using flow cytometry. In all cell lines, AZD-1775 induced apoptosis in a dose-dependent manner (Fig. 2b).

AZD-1775 changes the cell cycle profile and activates the DNA damage response pathway in ALL cell lines

Given the known role of WEE1 in cell cycle regulation, we next determined whether AZD-1775 adversely affected

cell cycle progression. Cell cycle analysis showed that the treatment with AZD-1775 (IC_{50}) for 24 h increased the percentage of cells in G1 phase in BV-173 cell line. Conversely, in CCRF-CEM, we observed a progressive increase in the percentage of cells accumulating in S and G2/M (Fig. 2c). A shorter treatment (12 h) highlighted that in BV-173, AZD-1775 increased the percentage of cells in S phase whereas in CCRF-CEM the percentage in S and G2/M (Additional file 2: Figure S1c). Immunoblotting analysis was conducted to investigate the effects of

AZD-1775 on the cell cycle checkpoint and on the DNA damage induction. AZD-1775 treatment reduced phospho-CDC2 Tyr[15], confirming the inhibition of WEE1 activity [45], and also reduced the basal amount of the protein in all treated samples. Since the G2/M checkpoint is mostly regulated by the activity of CHK1, which cooperates with WEE1 in the regulation of the activity of CDC2-Cyclin B1 complex [45], the expression of this kinase was evaluated in all samples. The expression of phospho-CHK1 Ser[317], a marker of CHK1 activation in response to DNA damage, was increased in all treated cells while the expression of the total abundance of CHK1 was heterogeneously modified (Fig. 2d). To better understand how AZD-1775 impairs the G2/M checkpoint, quantitative PCR analysis of 24 genes involved in the G2/M checkpoint was performed on the most sensitive (BV-173) and less sensitive (CCRF-CEM) cell lines incubated for 12 h with AZD-1775 at the previously established IC_{50}. In both cell lines, *CCNB2* ($p = 0.05$) and *CDC25C* ($p = 0.001$) were significantly upregulated while *MYT1* (*PKMYT1*) was significantly downregulated (BV-173 $p = 0.05$; CCRF-CEM $p = 0.0001$). Moreover, while both cell lines showed an increase in genes involved in cell cycle and apoptosis, the specific genes were different: in BV-173 cells, the treatment upregulated the expression of *CDKN1A* (cell cycle) and *GADD45A* (apoptosis), while in CCRF-CEM, the treatment upregulated the expression of *CCNB2* (cell cycle) and *GADD45B* (apoptosis) (Fig. 2e). Immunoblotting analyses of BV-173 cells partially confirmed the changes showed by the gene expression analyses. Indeed, AZD-1775 upregulated the protein expression levels of CDKN1A, CDC25C, CDC25B, and CCNB2, but no reduction of MYT1 was detected (Additional file 2: Figure S1C). Interestingly, in BV-173 cells, the treatment increased the amount of the mitotic isoform of MYT1, but this data was not associated with a concomitant increase of cells in G2/M phase, as observed from the cell cycle analysis. Finally, in contrast to the effect on GADD45A transcript, the abundance of protein was reduced upon drug treatment (Additional file 2: Figure S1C). We correlated the effect on gene transcription with the perturbation on cell cycle profile in BV-173 and CCRF-CEM after 12 h of treatment (IC_{50}). For both cell lines, the treatment induced a slight increase in the S phase cells. Only CCRF-CEM cells exhibited a significant increase in cells in the G2/M phase. The G2/M phase delay of CCRF-CEM cells is consistent with the upregulation of transcripts involved in the cell cycle regulation such as *CCNB1*, *CCNB2*, and *CDC25C*. For BV-173 cells, the increase in the S phase cells was confirmed by the upregulation of *CDC25B* which act on late S phase prior to CDC25C for the induction of the G2 transition [46, 47](Additional file 2: Figure S1D). Finally, in order to confirm the induction of DNA damage and to evaluate the potential mechanism of cell death, different immunofluorescence analyses were performed looking at the marker of DNA damage, phospho-γH2AX, and the marker of mitosis, phospho-MPM2. The MPM2 antibody recognizes a phospho-amino acid-containing epitope (peptides containing LTPLK and FTPLQ domains) present on more than 50 proteins of M phase eukaryotic cells [48]. Cells treated with AZD-1775 showed a significantly greater number of apoptotic bodies positive for MPM2, suggesting that apoptosis occurred during mitosis (Additional file 2: Figure S1E).

AZD-1775 reduces the cell viability of primary leukemic samples

The efficacy of AZD-1775 used at 2.5, 5, and 10 μM for 24 h was then evaluated ex vivo on primary leukemic cells isolated from the bone marrow and peripheral blood of adult ALL patients ($n = 13$, Additional file 1: Table S2) and on normal MNCs isolated from the peripheral blood samples of healthy donors ($n = 5$). AZD-1775 reduced the cell viability in a dose-dependent manner in all primary samples but did not affect the viability of normal MNCs (Fig. 3a, Additional file 2: Figure S1F). Despite the small number of samples tested, the sensitivity to AZD-1775 as a single agent apparently did not correlate with the leukemic subtypes (*BCR-ABL1*-positive versus *BCR-ABL1*-negative ALL patients) nor with the progression of the disease (diagnosis versus relapses). The ex vivo response to AZD-1775 of six primary leukemic samples was correlated with the basal expression of the 24 genes involved in the G2/M checkpoint. The samples were divided into three groups: high responders (IC_{50} within 5 μM), intermediate (IC_{50} within 10 μM), and poor ($IC_{50} > 10$ μM), and the gene expression profile was compared with that from MNCs. Analysis revealed that three genes were significantly overexpressed in the high responders group in comparison with the other three groups: *CHK1* ($p = 0.02$), *GADD45A* ($p = 0.01$), and *MYT1* ($p = 0.004$) (Fig. 3b, Additional file 1: Table S3). We evaluated the expression of phospho-CHK1 Ser[317], phospho-CDC2 Tyr[15], CDC2, and γ-H2AX in two ALL cases (1# and 6#) and the MNCs of one healthy donor (donor 4) after treatment with AZD-1775 at the same concentration reported above. The inhibitor reduced the expression of phospho-CDC2 Tyr[15] while increased the amount of γH2AX in the leukemic samples but not on normal cells (only a mild increase of γH2AX was observed over baseline). Surprisingly, the treatment induced an increase of phospho-CHK1 Ser[317] expression in sample 1# and in donor 4 but not in sample 6# (Fig. 3d). In addition, AZD-1775 significantly altered the morphology of the nuclei only in the primary leukemic samples, increasing the number of micro/macronuclei and of DNA bridges. All the nuclear alterations were restricted to leukemic samples (Fig. 3d). Our findings in the primary samples are

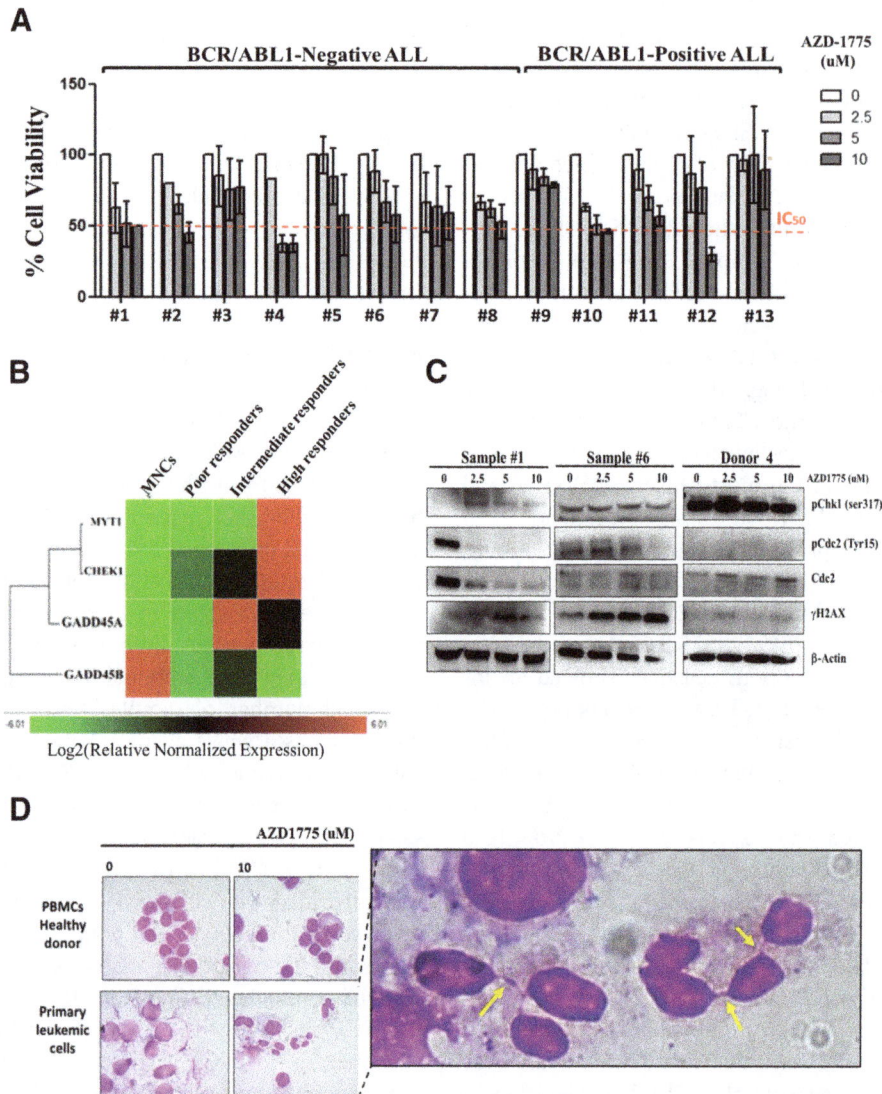

Fig. 3 AZD-1775 reduces the cell viability of primary leukemic samples. **a** Cell viability analysis on primary leukemic cells isolated from 13 adult ALL patients treated with AZD-1775 (2.5, 5, and 10 uM) for 24 h. Viable cells are depicted relative to the untreated controls. **b** Quantitative mRNA analyses of 24 genes of the G2/M checkpoint. The basal gene expression of MNCs samples (n = 3) was compared with the basal gene expression of poor (n = 3), intermediate (n = 2), and high (n = 2) responders to AZD-1775 (ex vivo). Clustergram with a color indicative of the degree of upregulation (red) or downregulation (green). Targets with similar regulation cluster together. **c** Immunoblotting analyses of primary leukemic cells (n = 2, samples #1 and #6) and MNCs (n = 1, donor 4) treated with AZD-1775 (2.5, 5, and 10 uM) for 24 h and then stained for markers of WEE1 functional inhibition (phospho-CDC2) and induction of DNA damages (phospho-CHK1 and phospho-γH2AX). β-actin was used for loading normalization. **d** Light microscopy analysis of normal MNCs and primary leukemic cells treated with AZD-1775 (10uM) for 24 h and then stained with May-Grünwald Giemsa solutions. In the figure, the yellow arrows indicate DNA bridges induced by the treatment. Controls in all panels are cells treated with DMSO 0.1%. Representative images are shown at × 100 magnification

consistent with those observed in the cell lines, suggesting a consistent mechanism of cell death.

AZD-1775 sensitizes leukemia cells to clofarabine and other genotoxic agents

The current therapeutic approaches for both *BCR-ABL1*-positive/negative ALL patients are based on conventional chemotherapy with or without targeted therapeutics (for example, tyrosine kinase inhibitors,

TKIs), especially during the induction phase [3, 49]. The findings demonstrating that AZD-1775 can act to increase the efficacy of DNA damaging drugs, i.e., can act as a chemo-sensitizer agent [36, 37, 50], promoted us to evaluate whether AZD-1775 could also play a role as a chemo-sensitizer with drugs routinely used in clinical practice for ALL patients. Different ALL cell lines were treated for 24, 48, and 72 h with increasing concentration of AZD-1775 (from 6 to 5000 nM) in combination

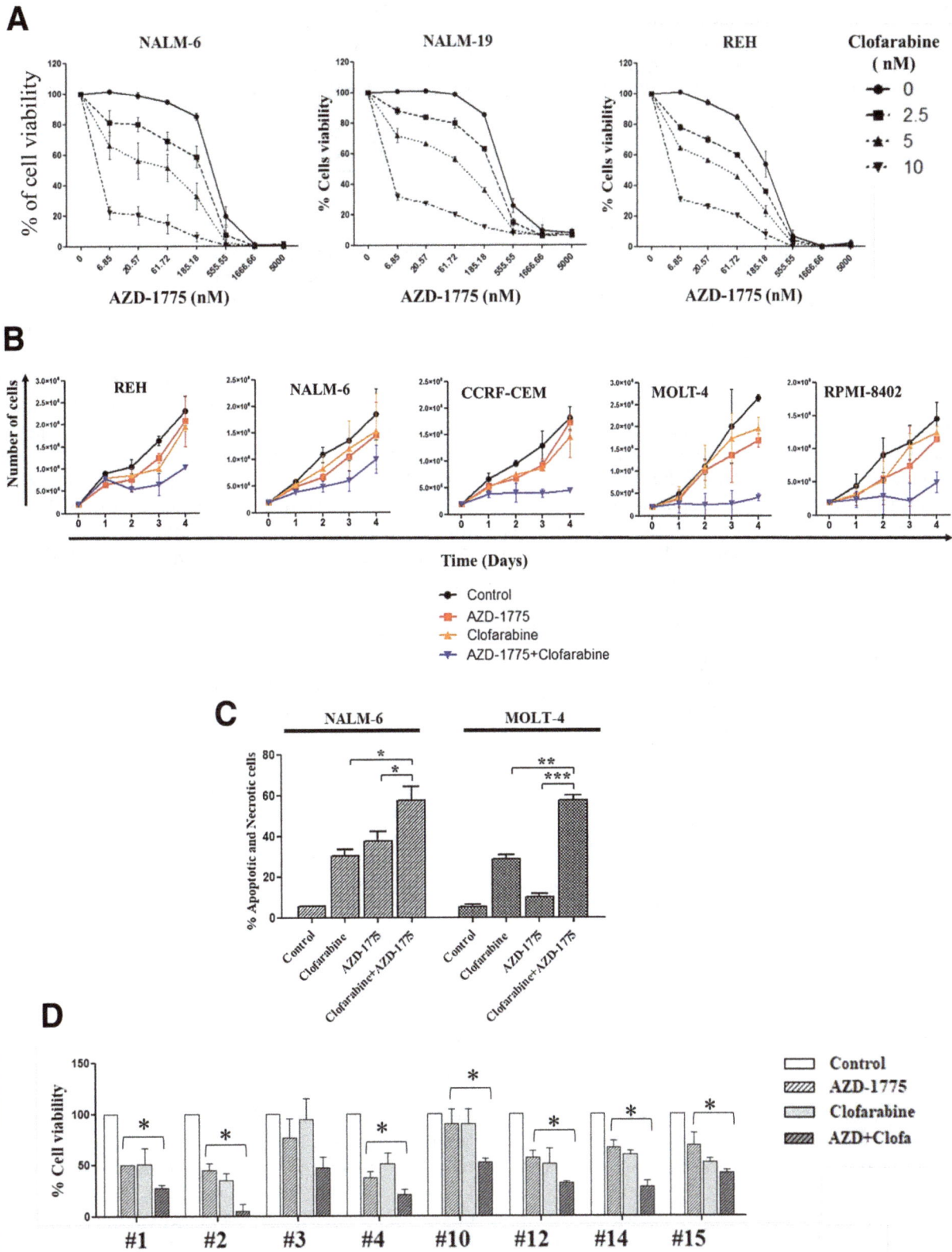

Fig. 4 (See legend on next page.)

(See figure on previous page.)
Fig. 4 AZD-1775 enhances the toxicity of antineoplastic compounds on ALL cell lines and primary cells. **a** Cell viability analyses of NALM-6, NALM-19, and REH cell lines incubated with AZD-1775 (6 to 5000 nM, dilution rate 1:3) and clofarabine (2.5, 5, and 10 nM) for 72 h. Viable cells are depicted relative to the untreated controls. Data were used to determine the CI values. **b** Growth curve of REH, NALM-6, CCRF-CEM, MOLT-4, and RPMI-8402 treated for 4 days with AZD-1775 (185 nM) and clofarabine (REH, NALM-6, and RPMI-8402 10 nM; CCRF-CEM and MOLT-4 20 nM). The number of viable cells was evaluated in the different groups every 24 h. **c** Apoptosis analyses of NALM-6 and MOLT-4 cell lines after 24 h of incubation with AZD-1775 (185 nM) and clofarabine (MOLT-4 20 nM and NALM-6 10 nM). The percentage of apoptotic cells was detected after Annexin V/propidium iodide staining. **d** Cell viability analysis on primary leukemic cells isolated from eight adult ALL patients treated with AZD-1775 (5 uM) and clofarabine (500 nM) for 24 h. Viable cells are depicted as percentage of the untreated controls. $*p \leq 0.05$, $**p \leq 0.01$, $***p \leq 0.001$

with increasing concentration of the antimetabolite clofarabine (NALM-6, NALM-19, REH: 2.5, 5, 10 nM, respectively; CCRF-CEM, MOLT-4, and RPMI-8402: 5, 10, 20 nM, respectively). Combination index (CI) analyses were performed on each cell line to determine any synergism, additivity, or antagonism of the different drug combinations. However, AZD-1775 generally acted with clofarabine in synergism (Fig. 4a; Table 1 for CI summary). Based on the results of the CI analyses, MOLT-4 and NALM-6 cell lines were treated with AZD-1775 (185 nM) in combination with clofarabine (MOLT-4 20 nM and NALM-6 10 nM), and cell proliferation was assessed. The combined treatment for 4 days induced a reduction in proliferation of B/T-ALL cell lines with the most dramatic results observed in MOLT-4, CCRF-CEM, and RPMI-8402 cell lines (Fig. 4b). Similar results on the reduction of proliferation were obtained with AZD-1775 in combination with the topoisomerase 2 inhibitor, doxorubicin, which also results in DNA damage (Additional file 2: Figure S2A). We next evaluated if the reduction of cell viability and proliferation was due to the induction of apoptosis. In both cell lines, the combination significantly increased the percentage of apoptotic cells, in comparison with the effect of clofarabine (MOLT-4, $p = 0.0029$; NALM-6, $p = 0.0171$) or AZD-1775 (MOLT-4, $p = 0.0008$; NALM-6, $p = 0.0377$) as single agents (Fig. 4c). We also confirmed the efficacy of the combined treatment on primary cells isolated from eight adult *BCR-ABL1*-negative ALL patients, with the exception of sample #3, in comparison with the effect of the single agent treatments ($p < 0.05$) (Fig. 4d).

AZD-1775 sensitizes leukemic cells to the tyrosine kinase inhibitors

The chemo-sensitizing activity of AZD-1775 was also assessed in combination with different TKIs, which represent the frontline therapy for the treatment of *BCR-ABL1*-positive ALL and chronic myeloid leukemia (CML) patients [51–54]. Specifically, we explored the effect of AZD-1775 in combination with bosutinib (Bos), which is approved by the FDA for newly diagnosed *BCR-ABL1*-positive CML. In addition, we evaluated a structural isomer of bosutinib (hence named as Bos-I). We decided to combine TKIs with AZD-1775 as we

previously showed that both Bos and Bos-I had off-target inhibitory activity on WEE1 and CHK1 kinases (albeit greater inhibitory activity is observed for Bos-I versus Bos) [28, 55] and also that this compound can sensitize pancreatic tumor cells to the anti-metabolite gemcitabine [28]. The efficacy of the two isomers as a single agent was performed on the panel of ALL cell lines. Both compounds reduced the viability of ALL cell lines, although Bos-I resulted in more potent anti-proliferative activity than Bos on *BCR-ABL1*-negative cell lines (Additional file 2: Figure S2B). The combination of Bos (subtoxic concentration) with AZD-1775 using increasing concentration (from 6 to 5000 nM, 1:3 dilution series) for 24 and 48 h reduced the cell viability not only of *BCR-ABL1*-positive cell lines but also of different *BCR-ABL1*-negative cell lines. Interestingly, this combination had a stronger effect on *BCR-ABL1*-positive cell lines than on the combination between AZD-1775 and Bos-I (Fig. 5a). However, in *BCR-ABL1*-negative cell lines, the combination of AZD-1775 with Bos-I had a greater effect on reducing cell viability in comparison with Bos (Fig. 5b; Tables 2 and 3 for CI summary). To investigate the effect of the drugs on apoptosis induction and proliferation, BV-173 and NALM-6 were treated for 24 h with AZD-1775 (185 nM) and sublethal concentrations of Bos or Bos-I (BV-173 50 nM and NALM-6 2uM). The comparison of the two combinations showed that AZD-1775 combined with Bos significantly increased the percentage of apoptotic cells in *BCR-ABL1*-positive BV-173 cells. In contrast, AZD-1775 combined with Bos-I was more effective in inducing apoptosis of *BCR-ABL1*-negative NALM-6 cells (Fig. 5c). Similar results were observed on the inhibition of cell proliferation (Fig. 5d). To expand upon the data of the synergism between AZD-1775 and TKIs on *BCR-ABL1*-positive cells, we tested other TKIs indicated for CML and ALL. Different combination index analyses using increasing concentration of AZD-1775 (from 6 to 5000 nM; dilution 1:3) in combination with ponatinib (25, 50, and 100 nM) or imatinib (250, 500, and 1000 nM) were performed on BV-173 for 24 and 48 h and showed comparable results in terms of synergy (Additional file 2: Figure S2D; Table 4 for CI summary). To explain the biological reasons for the synergic effect between AZD-1775 and the TKIs,

Table 1 Combination index values of AZD-1775 in combination with clofarabine

			24 h			48 h			72 h		
			Clofarabine (nM)			Clofarabine (nM)			Clofarabine (nM)		
	Cell lines		2.5	5	10	2.5	5	10	2.5	5	10
REH	AZD-1775 (nM)	6.9	0.70	0.80	0.95	0.61	0.88	0.99	0.78	1.07	1.12
		20.6	0.80	0.70	0.94	0.85	0.95	1.06	0.78	1.02	1.15
		61.7	1.32	0.70	0.91	1.61	1.38	1.05	0.90	1.10	1.09
		185.2	1.64	0.70	0.82	2.56	2.02	0.92	1.26	1.09	0.81
		555.6	0.89	0.46	0.65	1.00	0.82	0.55	0.43	0.24	0.29
		1666.7	1.10	0.43	0.76	0.33	0.34	0.34	0.62	0.64	0.68
		5000.0	2.23	1.11	0.77	1.00	0.26	1.01	1.81	1.83	1.88
NALM-6	AZD-1775 (nM)	6.9	0.24	0.45	0.55	0.60	0.46	0.75	0.73	1.06	1.15
		20.6	0.20	0.30	0.49	0.49	0.56	0.96	0.76	1.02	1.17
		61.7	0.26	0.22	0.39	0.66	0.76	0.93	0.84	1.08	1.14
		185.2	0.45	0.34	0.33	1.99	1.31	0.80	1.24	1.16	0.97
		555.6	0.63	0.39	0.27	1.38	0.93	0.66	0.85	0.66	0.57
		1666.7	0.55	0.36	0.33	9.87	0.84	1.04	0.20	0.26	0.37
		5000.0	0.84	0.64	0.71	2.05	1.98	2.19	0.49	0.55	0.66
NALM-19	AZD-1775 (nM)	6.9	0.46	0.54	0.85	0.52	0.59	0.81	1.02	1.20	1.09
		20.6	0.45	0.43	0.60	0.35	0.54	0.68	1.00	1.18	1.08
		61.7	0.56	0.39	0.62	0.38	0.41	0.43	0.91	1.01	0.92
		185.2	0.73	0.32	0.44	0.49	0.35	0.20	0.91	0.79	0.73
		555.6	0.60	0.21	0.32	0.20	0.14	0.18	0.53	0.50	0.74
		1666.7	0.68	0.27	0.41	0.21	0.15	0.27	0.69	0.75	1.10
		5000.0	1.39	0.76	0.69	0.56	0.53	0.70	1.75	1.79	2.43
RPMI-8402	AZD-1775 (nM)	6.9	0.21	0.26	0.50	0.23	0.36	1.39	8.20	1.23	1.46
		20.6	0.14	0.24	0.63	0.34	0.42	11.91	0.69	0.78	1.43
		61.7	0.22	0.21	0.62	0.77	0.53	3.17	0.55	0.83	1.26
		185.2	0.41	0.26	0.81	1.48	1.43	2.37	0.66	0.80	0.73
		555.6	0.57	0.36	0.54	0.95	0.61	0.48	0.43	0.41	0.08
		1666.7	0.60	0.38	0.32	0.55	0.33	0.21	0.28	0.10	0.12
		5000.0	0.37	0.26	0.05	0.09	0.02	0.04	0.22	0.24	0.26
			5	10	20	5	10	20	5	10	20
	Cell lines										
CCRF-CEM	AZD-1775 (nM)	6.9	0.01	0.02	0.23	0.74	1.13	1.15	1.01	1.61	1.06
		20.6	0.01	0.01	0.08	0.92	2.29	1.30	0.43	2.41	1.02
		61.7	0.01	0.01	0.02	0.64	1.07	0.70	4.20	4.81	0.98
		185.2	0.01	0.01	0.02	1.13	0.78	0.29	0.91	0.83	0.76
		555.6	0.01	0.01	0.01	0.20	0.19	0.22	0.39	0.51	0.72
		1666.7	0.05	0.06	0.09	0.44	0.42	0.45	0.80	0.94	1.08
		5000.0	0.42	0.45	0.30	1.40	1.22	0.96	2.02	2.11	1.87
MOLT-4	AZD-1775 (nM)	6.9	0.00	0.09	0.25	1.62	8.99	8.15	1.00	1.03	1.27
		20.6	0.11	0.15	0.32	2.26	0.85	10.07	0.80	1.14	1.02
		61.7	0.32	0.24	0.40	0.69	0.75	0.55	0.95	1.19	0.62
		185.2	0.57	0.27	0.23	1.24	0.94	0.43	0.81	0.53	0.26

Table 1 Combination index values of AZD-1775 in combination with clofarabine *(Continued)*

	24 h			48 h			72 h		
	Clofarabine (nM)			Clofarabine (nM)			Clofarabine (nM)		
555.6	0.31	0.16	0.18	0.88	0.61	0.40	0.00	0.11	0.12
1666.7	0.40	0.28	0.30	1.31	1.42	0.42	0.31	0.31	0.32
5000.0	1.61	1.76	1.66	6.06	5.49	5.24	0.92	2.04	0.93

The table reports the Combination Index (CI) value for each combination of drugs. CI < 1 indicates synergism, CI = 1 indicates additivity and CI > 1 indicates antagonism

immunoblotting analysis was performed on BV-173 cell line. The combination treatment of AZD-1775 (185 nM) and bosutinib (50 nM) enhanced γH2AX, the marker of DNA damage. The combination also perturbed the G2/M checkpoint as evidenced by the combined effect on reducing phospho-CDC2 (Tyr15) in comparison with the single treatments. Different studies showed that the oncogenic BCR/ABL tyrosine kinase facilitates the repair of DNA double-strand breaks (DSBs) through the stimulation of the homologous recombination (HR) repair [56]. It also has been established that AZD-1775 impairs HR repair through forced activation of CDC2 [57]. Based on this knowledge, the synergism of the combination could be related to the impairment of the DNA repair machinery. Consistent with this notion, the combination treatment additively reduced the amount of RAD51 protein master regulator of DSB repair to the HR repair [58]. In addition, the putative effect of AZD-1775 on altering BCR/ABL1 functionality was evaluated by looking at the expression of phospho-BCR/ABL (tyr245) fusion protein. Indeed, no effect of AZD-1775 was seen on BCR/ABL1 levels (Fig. 5e). Finally, we observed that AZD-1775 sensitized also the primary cells isolated from two BCR-ABL1-positive ALL patients to the TKIs (Fig. 5f), in concordance with our data in cell lines, suggesting a consistent mechanism of action.

Discussion

The inhibition of the DDR is a promising therapeutic strategy to sensitize tumor cells to an additional therapeutic compound, with the goal to improve response rates for the treatment of various cancers. Indeed, this rational approach is being thoroughly investigated in clinical studies with over 15 trials currently evaluating the efficacy of a DDR-inhibitor in combination with DNA damaging agents. For example, AZD-1775 is being evaluated in combination with cisplatin for breast cancer (NCT03012477) or with carboplatin and paclitaxel for squamous cell lung cancer (NCT02513563). Nonetheless, no trial has been yet registered to assess this approach to treat ALL. Our group has previously reported the efficacy of different CHK1/CHK2 inhibitors as a single agent and in combinations in primary ALL samples [43], suggesting that this approach might be amenable for the treatment of ALL in a clinical setting. Following

this line of thought, we asked whether other DDR targets in ALL may also be efficaciously inhibited. Here, we focused on WEE1, since we observed that *WEE1* is highly expressed in primary leukemic samples from adult ALL patients and, in particular, in the relapsed samples, confirming previous data in solid tumors from multiple studies [24, 27, 59–62]. Moreover, the significance of *Wee1* expression in ALL is further exemplified by the data from the CCLE database [63] showing that out of twenty profiled indications, B-ALL and T-ALL have the fourth and fifth highest expression of *Wee1* mRNA, respectively (Additional file 2: Figure S3A). Regarding the correlation between Wee1 mRNA and protein expression, in 5/7 cases, our results provide concordant data and suggest that a 50% cutoff of WEE1-positive blasts may reliably indicate upregulated Wee1 mRNA; in addition, the WEE1 immunohistochemical negativity always corresponds to Wee1 mRNA downregulation. It is tempting to speculate that these data, together with our previous findings [43, 44], suggest that in primary leukemic cells, the expression of several DDR genes may be fundamental to sustain the genetic instability, to overcome the inhibitory signal of DNA damage checkpoint activation, and to promote proliferation [26]. Indeed, the bypass of the DNA damage checkpoint activation by pharmacological inhibition of WEE1 led to the increased DNA damage (as measured by γ-H2AX), drastically reduced cell viability, inhibited the proliferation rate, and induced apoptosis both in ALL cell lines and primary leukemic blasts. Considering the effect of AZD-1775 on perturbation of the cell cycle (increase of cells in S and G2/M phases) and on cell death, we hypothesize that the induction of cell death must occur during late S phase or mitosis. Indeed, in the primary leukemic samples, we observed the appearance of DNA bridges, which are markers of aberrant mitosis, and we found that the apoptotic bodies were strongly positive for the phospho-MPM2 marker.

It has been established that, in order to prevent premature entry in mitosis, CDK1 is maintained in an inactive state by WEE1 through phosphorylation on tyrosine 15 and, subsequently, by MYT1 (PKMYT1) through phosphorylation on threonine 14 [64]. The importance of MYT1 has not yet been fully understood, especially in

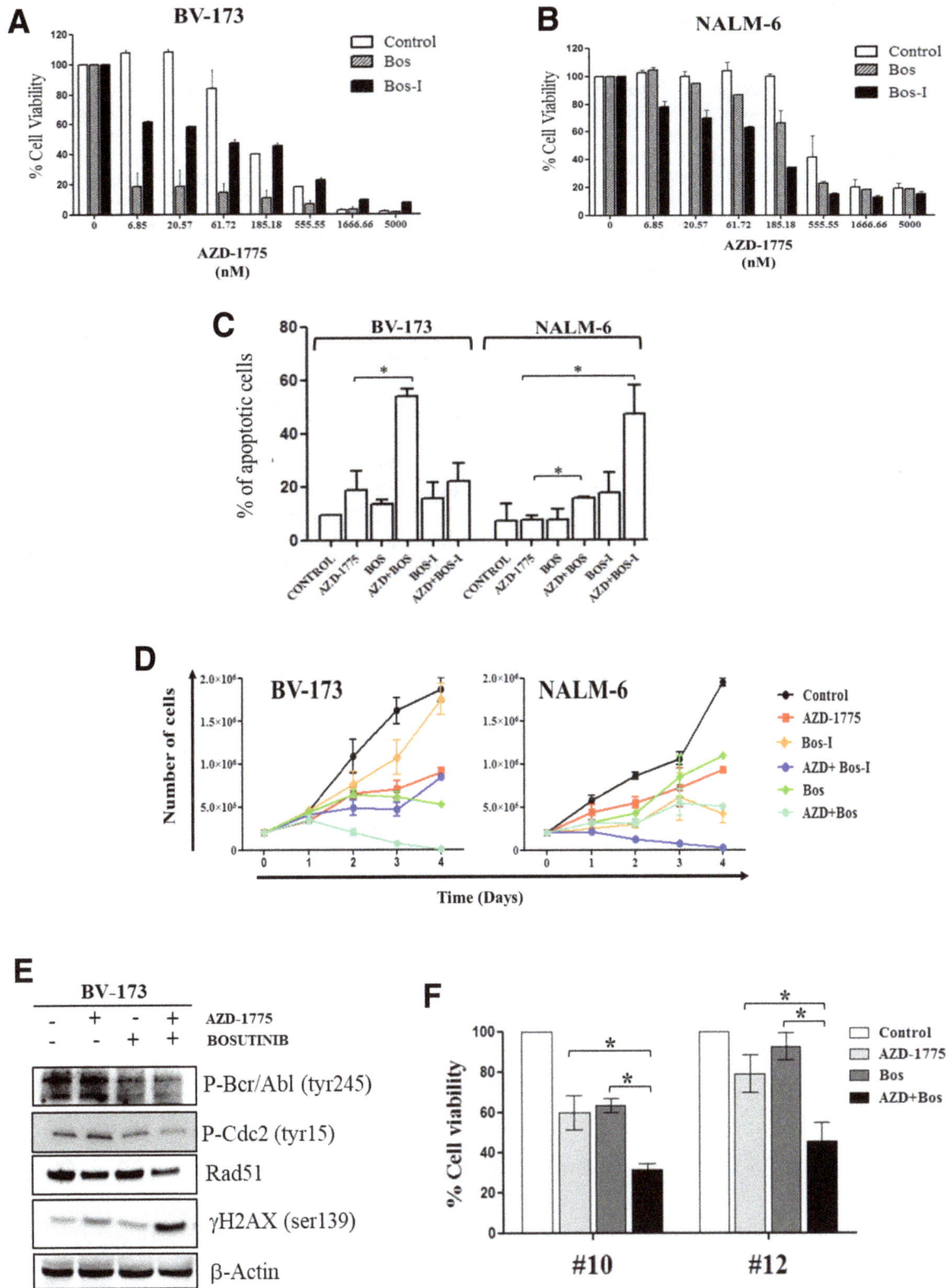

Fig. 5 (See legend on next page.)

(See figure on previous page.)
Fig. 5 AZD-1775 enhances the toxicity of tyrosine kinase inhibitors in ALL cell lines and leukemia primary samples. **a** Cell viability analyses of BV-173 cell line incubated simultaneously with AZD-1775 (6 to 5000 nM, dilution rate 1:3) and with bosutinib authentic (50 nM) or bosutinib isomer (50 nM) for 48 h. In the graph: AZD-1775 (control, white columns), bosutinib (Bos, gray columns), and bosutinib isomer (Bos-I, black columns). The percentage of viable cells is depicted relative to the untreated controls. Data were used to determine CI values. **b** Cell viability analyses of NALM-6 cell line incubated with AZD-1775 (6 to 5000 nM, dilution rate 1:3) and with bosutinib authentic (2 uM) or bosutinib isomer (2 uM) for 72 h. In the graph: AZD-1775(control, white columns), bosutinib (Bos, gray columns), and bosutinib isomer (Bos-I, black columns). The number of viable cells is depicted as a percentage of the untreated controls. Data were used to determine CI values. **c** Apoptosis analyses of BV-173 and NALM-6 cells after 24 h of incubation with AZD-1775 (185 nM) and bosutinib authentic/isomer (BV-173 50 nM; NALM-6 2 uM). The percentage of apoptotic cells was detected after Annexin V/propidium iodide staining. **d** Growth curve of BV-173 and NALM-6 treated for 4 days with AZD-1775 (185 nM) and bosutinib authentic/bosutinib isomer (BV-173 50 nM; NALM-6 2 uM). **e** Immunoblotting analysis of BV-173 treated with AZD-1775 (185 nM) and bosutinib (50 nM) for 24 h. β-actin was used for loading normalization. **f** Cell viability analysis in primary leukemic cells isolated from two adult *BCR-ABL1*-positive ALL patients treated with AZD-1775 (5 uM) and bosutinib authentic (2 uM) for 24 h. The percentage of viable cells is depicted relative to the untreated controls. Controls in all panels are cells treated with DMSO 0.1%. *$p \leq 0.05$

cancer cells. Here, we report that in our ALL cohort, *MYT1* gene is highly expressed in relapsed *BCR-ABL1*-positive/negative ALL samples in comparison with normal MNCs (Additional file 2: Figure S1F). Moreover, in the ex vivo drug treatment, the samples highly sensitive to AZD-1775 showed a higher level of expression of *MYT1* ($p = 0.004$) in comparison with the intermediate, poor, and MNCs groups. While the significance of this finding is beyond the scope of this study, it does hint at MYT1 playing a role in ALL. In agreement with the results by Tibes and colleagues [61], our data demonstrated that WEE1 inhibition leads to chemo-sensitization in ALL cell lines and in primary leukemic samples, albeit using a different approach. In that study, an unbiased RNAi screen looking

for sensitizers to cytarabine identified WEE1 as the top hit, and the authors further validated these results using AZD-1775. Additionally, they found that sensitization occurred in AML and CML cell lines, suggesting the use of these rational drug combinations with WEE1 inhibitor in other hematological indications.

In *BCR-ABL1*-positive ALL samples, the concomitant inhibition of WEE1 and *BCR-ABL1* resulted in a significant inhibition of cell viability and proliferation as well as induction of apoptosis. Consistently, taking advantage of the different kinase inhibitory profiles of Bos and Bos-I toward WEE1 [28], Bos-I results in approximately tenfold more potent synergistic activity. It is interesting to note that Bos-I displayed greater synergistic activity in

Table 2 Combination index values of AZD-1775 in combination with bosutinib (Bos) on *BCR-ABL1*-positive cell lines

			24 h BOS (nM)			48 h BOS (nM)		
	Cell line		10	25	50	10	25	50
BV-173	AZD-1775 (nM)	6.9	0.95	1.11	0.99	1.45	1.03	1.27
		20.6	1.03	1.21	1.01	1.59	0.98	1.29
		61.7	0.73	0.86	0.62	0.88	0.72	1.08
		185.2	0.71	0.77	0.71	0.59	0.65	1.01
		555.6	1.26	0.75	0.61	0.85	0.78	1.03
		1666.7	1.14	0.92	0.81	1.08	1.08	1.24
		5000.0	1.82	1.71	1.58	2.44	1.86	2.02
	Cell line		500	1000	2000	500	1000	2000
SUP-B15	AZD-1775 (nM)	6.9	0.52	0.96	1.23	0.59	0.84	1.23
		20.6	0.64	0.72	1.11	0.61	0.99	0.98
		61.7	0.7	1.36	0.91	0.73	0.83	0.89
		185.2	1.05	1.51	0.79	0.79	0.88	0.79
		555.6	1.07	1.3	1.14	1.18	1.22	1
		1666.7	0.44	0.54	0.46	0.5	0.55	0.54
		5000.0	0.51	0.49	0.4	0.41	0.41	0.31

The table reports the Combination Index (CI) value for each combination of drugs. CI < 1 indicates synergism, CI = 1 indicates additivity and CI > 1 indicates antagonism

Table 3 Combination index values of AZD-1775 in combination with bosutinib isomer (Bos-I) on *BCR-ABL1*-negative cell lines

			24 h			48 h			72 h		
			Bosutinib isomer (nM)			Bosutinib isomer (nM)			Bosutinib isomer (nM)		
	Cell line		500	1000	2000	500	1000	2000	500	1000	2000
NALM-6	AZD-1775 (nM)	6.9	0.57	0.69	0.79	0.62	1.00	1.21	0.59	0.79	1.14
		20.6	0.33	0.48	0.64	0.65	0.81	1.07	0.47	0.68	0.99
		61.7	0.35	0.39	0.65	0.67	0.65	0.97	0.68	0.73	0.93
		185.2	0.48	0.41	0.41	0.91	0.65	0.68	0.89	0.73	0.63
		555.6	0.63	0.43	0.36	0.54	0.45	0.47	0.41	0.40	0.48
		1666.7	0.67	0.51	0.41	0.65	0.66	0.68	0.53	0.59	0.66
		5000.0	1.65	1.43	1.21	1.58	1.61	1.62	1.42	1.43	1.52
	Cell lines		250	500	1000	250	500	1000	250	500	1000
NALM-19	AZD-1775 (nM)	6.9	0.43	0.75	1.01	1.99	2.94	0.20	0.19	0.28	0.35
		20.6	0.38	0.47	0.63	1.53	1.15	0.12	0.24	0.29	0.28
		61.7	0.19	0.27	0.23	0.20	0.12	0.09	0.44	0.48	0.31
		185.2	0.27	0.24	0.24	0.42	0.23	0.15	0.67	0.48	0.26
		555.6	0.38	0.31	0.28	0.41	0.31	0.25	0.29	0.28	0.21
		1666.7	0.76	0.68	0.69	0.82	0.72	0.69	0.47	0.44	0.38
		5000.0	1.78	1.95	1.77	2.04	2.09	1.93	1.19	1.30	1.13
MOLT-4	AZD-1775 (nM)	6.9	1.23	0.93	1.11	0.99	1.03	1.28	0.67	1.22	1.26
		20.6	0.78	0.61	0.78	0.85	0.89	1.07	0.74	0.89	1.07
		61.7	0.77	0.53	0.43	0.62	0.63	0.71	0.91	0.85	0.77
		185.2	0.53	0.40	0.23	0.39	0.35	0.34	0.35	0.37	0.53
		555.6	0.22	0.25	0.21	0.34	0.40	0.50	0.35	0.43	0.67
		1666.7	0.40	0.60	0.65	0.95	1.12	1.14	0.92	0.96	1.17
		5000.0	2.46	2.25	3.02	3.06	3.26	3.49	3.54	3.30	3.52
	Cell line		2000	5000	10000	2000	5000	10000	2000	5000	10000
CCRF-CEM	AZD-1775 (nM)	6.9	0.75	0.78	0.84	0.75	0.78	0.84	1.06	0.65	0.39
		20.6	0.38	0.62	0.79	0.38	0.62	0.79	1.21	0.57	0.52
		61.7	0.27	0.54	0.74	0.27	0.54	0.74	0.53	0.49	0.52
		185.2	0.26	0.46	0.58	0.26	0.46	0.58	0.28	0.43	0.49
		555.6	0.25	0.65	0.53	0.25	0.65	0.53	0.35	0.49	0.37
		1666.7	0.84	0.93	0.81	0.84	0.93	0.81	0.66	0.79	0.46
		5000.0	3.13	2.76	0.99	3.13	2.76	0.99	2.08	1.97	0.88

The table reports the Combination Index (CI) value for each combination of drugs. CI < 1 indicates synergism, CI = 1 indicates additivity and CI > 1 indicates antagonism

BCR-ABL1-negative (not Ph-like) cell lines than Bos. We hypothesize that the observed synergy derived from the combined treatment of AZD-1775 with the two TKI compounds is not mediated through their on-target activity toward Src and Abl as this is similar between the two compounds [28]. Indeed, this notion is consistent with the finding that AZD-1775 synergizes with imatinib and ponatinib. One possible explanation of the synergism between AZD-1775 and TKIs comes from the effect of BCR-ABL fusion protein on G2/M checkpoint and DNA repair in leukemic cells [56, 65–67]. In this scenario, the synergism of the combination may be due to the effect of the two classes of inhibitors on the G2/M checkpoint stability and on the functionality of the DNA repair pathway.

Conclusions

Our findings suggest that WEE1 may play a role in the leukemogenesis and in the proliferation of ALL blasts. The inhibition of WEE1, in monotherapy or in

Table 4 Combination index values of AZD-1775 in combination with ponatinib and imatinib on BV-173 cell lines

			24 h			48 h		
			Ponatinb (nM)			Ponatinb (nM)		
Cell line			25	50	100	25	50	100
BV-173	AZD-1775 (nM)	6.9	0.39	0.57	1.16	0.29	0.31	0.67
		20.6	0.34	0.59	1.04	0.33	0.34	0.50
		61.7	0.33	0.55	0.99	0.16	0.17	0.56
		185.2	0.31	0.49	0.90	0.06	0.11	0.48
		555.6	0.47	0.53	0.83	0.02	0.07	0.20
		1666.7	0.53	0.58	0.86	0.01	0.01	0.12
		5000.0	1.23	1.33	1.38	0.06	0.07	0.15
			Imatinib (nM)			Imatinib (nM)		
Cell line			250	500	1000	250	500	1000
BV-173	AZD-1775 (nM)	6.9	0.39	0.41	0.62	0.41	0.03	0.02
		20.6	0.58	0.43	0.69	0.43	0.04	0.03
		61.7	0.32	0.33	0.39	0.18	0.06	0.05
		185.2	0.23	0.31	0.47	0.15	0.07	0.05
		555.6	0.50	0.44	0.48	0.11	0.08	0.07
		1666.7	0.57	0.50	0.53	0.07	0.20	0.17
		5000.0	1.05	1.18	1.21	0.61	1.19	1.56

The table reports the Combination Index (CI) value for each combination of drugs. CI < 1 indicates synergism, CI = 1 indicates additivity and CI > 1 indicates antagonism

combination with different antineoplastic agents, results in a significant reduction of cell viability and apoptosis induction. Although additional in vivo studies should be performed to enforce our results, it has been shown that in ALL models, there is a good correlation of drug studies using ex vivo ALL primary cells and then testing them in vivo model (PDX) [68]. These data lay the basis for evaluation of AZD-1775 as a chemo-sensitizer in the clinic for the treatment of ALL.

Additional files

Additional file 1: Table S1. Patient's characteristic of gene expression cohort. Table S2. Patient's characteristic ex vivo AZD-1775 treatment in single agent or in combination. Table S3. Quantitative analyses of G2/M checkpoint-related genes. Differential gene expression of 24 genes involved in the regulation of the G2/M checkpoint of primary leukemic cells in comparison to normal mononuclear cells (MNCs). In the table, the primary leukemic samples have been divided into three groups based on the ex vivo sensitivity to AZD-1775. Very good $IC_{50} < 5uM$; good $IC_{50} < 10uM$; poor $IC_{50} > 10$ uM. (PDF 253 kb)

Additional file 2: Figure S1. Efficacy of AZD-1775 used as single agent. A) The graph shows the IC_{50} values of B/T-ALL cell lines treated with AZD-1775 for 24, 48, and 72 h. B) Cell viability analysis on CCRF-CEM cell lines showing the effect of high doses of AZD-1775. The percentage of viable cells is depicted relative to untreated controls. C) Immunoblot analysis on BV-173 treated with AZD-1775 (IC_{50}) for 12 h. D) Cell cycle analysis in BV-173 and CCRF-CEM cell lines treated with AZD-1775 (IC_{50}) for 12 h. E) Immunofluorescence analysis of BV-173 cells treated with

AZD-1775 (IC_{50}) for 12 h and, then, stained with DAPI and phospho-MPM2. In the picture, a cell dying in mitosis is reported with apoptotic bodies strongly positive for phospho-MPM2 antibody. Representative images are shown at × 100 magnification. F) Viability of mononuclear cells isolated from the peripheral blood of 5 healthy donors incubated with increasing concentration of AZD-1775 (2.5, 5, and 10 uM) for 24 h. G) MYT1 transcript levels in samples isolated from adult BCR-ABL1-positive ALL at diagnosis ($n = 17$), adult BCR-ABL1-negative ALL at diagnosis ($n = 27$), adult BCR-ABL1-positive ALL at relapse (unpaired, $n = 8$), adult BCR-ABL1-negative ALL at relapse (unpaired, $n = 6$), and in MNCs ($n = 7$) from the peripheral blood of healthy donors. One-way ANOVA test was performed to assess statistical significance. Results are expressed as Log10 2 exp.[−(ΔΔCt). **Figure S2.** AZD-1775 in combination with chemotherapy agents and tyrosine kinase inhibitors. A) Growth curve of BV-173 and REH cell lines treated for 4 days with AZD-1775 (185 nM) and doxorubicin (25 nM). B) Viability analyses in ALL cell lines incubated for 24 h with Bos or Bos-I (6 to 5000 nM). The percentage of viable cells is depicted relative to untreated controls. C) Cell viability analysis of BV-173 cell line treated with AZD-1775 (6 to 5000 nM, dilution rate 1:3) and with ponatinib (25, 50, 100 nM) or imatinib (250, 500, and 1000 nM) for 24 h. The percentage of viable cells is depicted relative to untreated controls, 0.1%. **Figure S3**. Wee1 mRNA expression across different cancer types from the Cancer Cell Line Encyclopedia (CCLE) database. A) Box plots showing the level of expression of Wee1 mRNA in different tumor samples, extracted from CCLE [63]. The red arrows point to B/T-ALL samples. Boxes define the 25th and the 75th percentiles, horizontal line within the boxes indicates the median, and whiskers define the 10th and the 90th percentiles. (PDF 1918 kb)

Abbreviations

ALL: Acute lymphoblastic leukemia; BOS: Bosutinib; BOS-I: Bosutinib isomer; CCNB1/B2: Cyclin B1/B2; CDC2: Cell division cycle protein 2 homolog; CDC25: Cell division cycle 25; CHK1: Checkpoint kinase 1; CHK2: Checkpoint kinase 2; DDR: DNA damage response; MNC: Mononuclear cell; MPF: Mitotic promoting factor; MYT1 (PK MYT1): Membrane-associated tyrosine/threonine 1; TKI: Tyrosine kinase inhibitor

Acknowledgements

TJY acknowledges the core-supported facilities for flow cytometry, cell culture, and biological imaging.

Funding

The research leading to these results has received funding from the European Union Seventh Framework Programme [FP7/2007-2013] under Grant Agreement no. 306242-NGS-PTL. Supported by: EuropeanLeukemiaNet, Associazione italiana leucemie (AIL), AIRC, Fondazione del Monte di Bologna e Ravenna, and University of Bologna (Phd school Scienze Biomediche). TJY is supported by NIH grants CA191956, CA006927, and DoD W81XWH-17-1-0136 and appropriations from the Commonwealth of Pennsylvania and the Greenberg Foundation.

Authors' contributions

AGLDR designed the experiments, analyzed the data, and wrote the manuscript. AGLDR, NB, II, TJY, and GM coordinated the research. AGLDR, EI, AF, VR, SR, ES, MVFF, CS, CR, NT, CB, and SDM performed the laboratory work for this study. CP, MCA, StP, SP, MCF, and GiM contributed to the sample collection. AGLDR, II, TJY, and GM contributed to the data interpretation. MC coordinated the clinical activities. All authors read and approved the final manuscript.

Consent for publication

Not applicable

Competing interests

GM has competing interests with Novartis, BMS, Roche, Pfizer, ARIAD, MSD.

Author details

[1]Department of Experimental, Diagnostic and Specialty Medicine, Institute of Hematology "L. e A. Seràgnoli", University of Bologna, Via Massarenti 9, 40138 Bologna, Italy. [2]Laboratory of Clinical Genomics, European Institute of Oncology, Milan, Italy. [3]Cancer Biology Program, Fox Chase Cancer Center, Philadelphia, PA, USA. [4]Biosciences Laboratory, Istituto Scientifico Romagnolo per lo Studio e la Cura dei Tumori (IRST) IRCCS, Meldola, Italy. [5]Istituto Scientifico Romagnolo per lo Studio e la Cura dei Tumori (IRST) IRCCS, Meldola, Italy. [6]LAM Therapeutics, Guilford, CT, USA. [7]Department of Pathology, St. Jude Children's Research Hospital, Memphis, TN, USA.

References

1. Onciu M. Acute lymphoblastic leukemia. Hematol Oncol Clin North Am. 2009;23(4):655–74.
2. Fielding AK. Current therapeutic strategies in adult acute lymphoblastic leukemia. Hematol Oncol Clin North Am. 2011;25(6):1255–79.
3. Narayanan S, Shami PJ. Treatment of acute lymphoblastic leukemia in adults. Crit Rev Oncol Hematol. 2012;81:94–102.
4. Lech-Maranda E, Korycka A, Robak T. Clofarabine as a novel nucleoside analogue approved to treat patients with haematological malignancies: mechanism of action and clinical activity. Mini Rev Med Chem. 2009;9:805–12.
5. Hunger SP, Mullighan CG. Redefining ALL classification: toward detecting high-risk ALL and implementing precision medicine. Blood. 2015;125:3977–88.
6. Hoelzer D. Personalized medicine in adult acute lymphoblastic leukemia. Haematologica. 2015;100:855–8.
7. Larson S, Stock W. Progress in the treatment of adults with acute lymphoblastic leukemia. Curr Opin Hematol. 2008;15:400–7.
8. Fedorov VD, Upadhyay VA, Fathi AT. The approach to acute lymphoblastic leukemia in older patients: conventional treatments and emerging therapies. Curr Hematol Malig Rep. 2016;11:165–74.
9. Kantarjian H, Thomas D, Jorgensen J, Jabbour E, Kebriaei P, Rytting M, York S, Ravandi F, Kwari M, Faderl S, Rios MB, Cortes J, Fayad L, Tarnai R, Wang SA, Champlin R, Advani A, O'Brien S. Inotuzumab ozogamicin, an anti-CD22-calecheamicin conjugate, for refractory and relapsed acute lymphocytic leukaemia: a phase 2 study. Lancet Oncol. 2012;13:403–11.
10. Portell CA, Wenzell CM, Advani AS. Clinical and pharmacologic aspects of blinatumomab in the treatment of B-cell acute lymphoblastic leukemia. Clinical Pharmacology: Advances and Applications. 2013;(SUPPL 1):5–11.
11. Davila ML, Riviere I, Wang X, Bartido S, Park J, Curran K, Chung SS, Stefanski J, Borquez-Ojeda O, Olszewska M, Qu J, Wasielewska T, He Q, Fink M, Shinglot H, Youssif M, Satter M, Wang Y, Hosey J, Quintanilla H, Halton E, Bernal Y, Bouhassira DCG, Arcila ME, Gonen M, Roboz GJ, Maslak P, Douer D, Frattini MG, Giralt S, et al. Efficacy and toxicity management of 19-28z {CAR} {T} cell therapy in {B} cell acute lymphoblastic leukemia. Sci Transl Med. 2014;6:224ra25.
12. Jackson SP, Bartek J. The DNA-damage response in human biology and disease. Nature. 2009;461:1071–8.
13. Harper JW, Elledge SJ. The DNA damage response: ten years after. Mol Cell. 2007;28:739–45.
14. Giglia-Mari G, Zotter A, Vermeulen W. DNA damage response. Cold Spring Harb Perspect Biol. 2011;3:1–19.
15. Manic G, Obrist F, Sistigu A, Vitale I. Trial watch: targeting ATM–CHK2 and ATR–CHK1 pathways for anticancer therapy. Mol Cell Oncol. 2015;2: e1012976.
16. Finn K, Lowndes NF, Grenon M. Eukaryotic DNA damage checkpoint activation in response to double-strand breaks. Cell Mol Life Sci. 2012;69:1447–73.
17. Sørensen CS, Syljuåsen RG. Safeguarding genome integrity: the checkpoint kinases ATR, CHK1 and WEE1 restrain CDK activity during normal DNA replication. Nucleic Acids Res. 2012;40:477–86.
18. Smith J, Mun Tho L, Xu N, Gillespie DA: The ATM-Chk2 and ATR-Chk1 pathways in DNA damage signaling and cancer. Volume 108; 2010(C).

19. Cuadrado M, Martinez-Pastor B, Murga M, Toledo LI, Gutierrez-Martinez P, Lopez E, Fernandez-Capetillo O. ATM regulates ATR chromatin loading in response to DNA double-strand breaks. J Exp Med. 2006;203: 297–303.
20. Hochegger H, Takeda S, Hunt T. Cyclin-dependent kinases and cell-cycle transitions: does one fit all? Nat Rev Mol Cell Biol. 2008;9:910–6.
21. Masaki T, Shiratori Y, Rengifo W, Igarashi K, Yamagata M, Kurokohchi K, Uchida N, Miyauchi Y, Yoshiji H, Watanabe S, Omata M, Kuriyama S. Cyclins and cyclin-dependent kinases: comparative study of hepatocellular carcinoma versus cirrhosis. Hepatology. 2003;37:534–43.
22. Blenk S, Engelmann JC, Pinkert S, Weniger M, Schultz J, Rosenwald A, Müller-Hermelink HK, Müller T, Dandekar T. Explorative data analysis of MCL reveals gene expression networks implicated in survival and prognosis supported by explorative CGH analysis. BMC Cancer. 2008;8:106.
23. Kiviharju-af Hällström TM, Jäämaa S, Mönkkönen M, Peltonen K, Andersson LC, Medema RH, Peehl DM, Laiho M. Human prostate epithelium lacks Wee1A-mediated DNA damage-induced checkpoint enforcement. Proc Natl Acad Sci U S A. 2007;104:7211–6.
24. De Witt Hamer PC, Mir SE, Noske D, Van Noorden CJF, Würdinger T. WEE1 kinase targeting combined with DNA-damaging cancer therapy catalyzes mitotic catastrophe. Clin Cancer Res. 2011;17:4200–7.
25. Magnussen GI, Holm R, Emilsen E, Rosnes AKR, Slipicevic A, Flørenes VA. High expression of Wee1 is associated with poor disease-free survival in malignant melanoma: potential for targeted therapy. PLoS One. 2012;7:e38254.
26. Vriend LEM, De Witt Hamer PC, Van Noorden CJF, Würdinger T. WEE1 inhibition and genomic instability in cancer. Biochimica et Biophysica Acta - Reviews on Cancer. 2013;1836:227–35.
27. Magnussen GI, Hellesylt E, Nesland JM, Trope CG, Flørenes VA, Holm R. High expression of wee1 is associated with malignancy in vulvar squamous cell carcinoma patients. BMC Cancer. 2013;13:288.
28. Beeharry N, Banina E, Hittle J, Skobeleva N, Khazak V, Deacon S, Andrake M, Egleston BL, Peterson JR, Astsaturov I, Yen TJ. Re-purposing clinical kinase inhibitors to enhance chemosensitivity by overriding checkpoints. Cell Cycle. 2014;13:2172–91.
29. Panek RL, Lu GH, Klutchko SR, Batley BL, Dahring TK, Hamby JM, Hallak H, Doherty AM, Keiser JA. In vitro pharmacological characterization of PD 166285, a new nanomolar potent and broadly active protein tyrosine kinase inhibitor. J Pharmacol Exp Ther. 1997;283:1433–44.
30. Wang Y, Li J, Booher RN, Kraker A, Lawrence T, Leopold WR, Sun Y. Radiosensitization of p53 mutant cells by PD0166285, a novel G2 checkpoint abrogator. Cancer Res. 2001;61:8211–7.
31. Hirai H, Iwasawa Y, Okada M, Arai T, Nishibata T, Kobayashi M, Kimura T, Kaneko N, Ohtani J, Yamanaka K, Itadani H, Takahashi-Suzuki I, Fukasawa K, Oki H, Nambu T, Jiang J, Sakai T, Arakawa H, Sakamoto T, Sagara T, Yoshizumi T, Mizuarai S, Kotani H. Small-molecule inhibition of Wee1 kinase by MK-1775 selectively sensitizes p53-deficient tumor cells to DNA-damaging agents. Mol Cancer Ther. 2009;8:2992–3000.
32. Hirai H, Arai T, Okada M, Nishibata T, Kobayashi M, Sakai N, Imagaki K, Ohtani J, Sakai T, Yoshizumi T, Mizuarai S, Iwasawa Y, Kotani H. MK-1775, a small molecule Wee1 inhibitor, enhances antitumor efficacy of various DNA-damaging agents, including 5-fluorouracil. Cancer Biol Ther. 2010;9:514–22.
33. Bridges KA, Hirai H, Buser CA, Brooks C, Liu H, Buchholz TA, Molkentine JM, Mason KA, Meyn RE. MK-1775, a novel wee1 kinase inhibitor, radiosensitizes p53-defective human tumor cells. Clin Cancer Res. 2011;17:5638–48.
34. Kreahling JM, Gemmer JY, Reed D, Letson D, Bui M, Altiok S. MK1775, a selective Wee1 inhibitor, shows single-agent antitumor activity against sarcoma cells. Mol Cancer Ther. 2012;11:174–82.
35. Qi W, Xie C, Li C, Caldwell J, Edwards H, Taub JW, Wang Y, Lin H, Ge Y. CHK1 plays a critical role in the anti-leukemic activity of the wee1 inhibitor MK-1775 in acute myeloid leukemia cells. J Hematol Oncol. 2014;7:53.
36. Qi W, Zhang W, Edwards H, Chu R, Madlambayan GJ, Taub JW, Wang Z, Wang Y, Li C, Lin H, Ge Y. Synergistic anti-leukemic interactions between panobinostat and MK-1775 in acute myeloid leukemia ex vivo. Cancer Biol Ther. 2015;16(12):1784–93.
37. Ford JB, Baturin D, Burleson TM, Van Linden AA, Kim Y, Porter CC. AZD1775 sensitizes T cell acute lymphoblastic leukemia cells to cytarabine by promoting apoptosis over DNA repair. Oncotarget. 2015;6(29):28001–10.
38. Zhou L, Zhang Y, Chen S, Kmieciak M, Leng Y, Lin H, Rizzo KA, Dumur CI, Ferreira-Gonzalez A, Dai Y, Grant S. A regimen combining the Wee1 inhibitor AZD1775 with HDAC inhibitors targets human acute myeloid leukemia cells harboring various genetic mutations. Leukemia. 2015;29(4):807–18.

39. Van Linden AA, Baturin D, Ford JB, Fosmire SP, Gardner L, Korch C, Reigan P, Porter CC. Inhibition of Wee1 sensitizes cancer cells to antimetabolite chemotherapeutics in vitro and in vivo, independent of p53 functionality. Mol Cancer Ther. 2013;12:2675–84.

40. Geenen JJJ, Schellens JHM. Molecular pathways: targeting the protein kinase Wee1 in cancer. Clin Cancer Res. 2017;23:4540–4.

41. Rajeshkumar NV, De Oliveira E, Ottenhof N, Watters J, Brooks D, Demuth T, Shumway SD, Mizuarai S, Hirai H, Maitra A, Hidalgo M. MK-1775, a potent Wee1 inhibitor, synergizes with gemcitabine to achieve tumor regressions, selectively in p53-deficient pancreatic cancer xenografts. Clin Cancer Res. 2011;17:2799–806.

42. Sen T, Tong P, Diao L, Li L, Fan Y, Hoff J, Heymach JV, Wang J, Byers LA. Targeting AXL and mTOR pathway overcomes primary and acquired resistance to WEE1 inhibition in small-cell lung cancer. Clin Cancer Res. 2017;23:6239–54.

43. Di Rorà AGL, Iacobucci I, Imbrogno E, Papayannidis C, Derenzini E, Ferrari A, Guadagnuolo V, Robustelli V, Parisi S, Sartor C, Abbenante MC, Paolini S, Martinelli G. Prexasertib, a Chk1/Chk2 inhibitor, increases the effectiveness of conventional therapy in B-/T- cell progenitor acute lymphoblastic leukemia. Oncotarget. 2016;7

44. Iacobucci I, Di RAG, Falzacappa MV, Agostinelli C, Derenzini E, Ferrari A, Papayannidis C, Lonetti A, Righi S, Imbrogno E, Pomella S, Venturi C, Guadagnuolo V, Cattina F, Ottaviani E, Abbenante MC, Vitale A, Elia L, Russo D, Zinzani PL, Pileri S, Pelicci PG, Martinelli G. In vitro and in vivo single-agent efficacy of checkpoint kinase inhibition in acute lymphoblastic leukemia. J Hematol Oncol. 2015;8:125.

45. Perry JA, Kornbluth S. Cdc25 and Wee1: analogous opposites? Cell Div. 2007;2:12.

46. Cazales M, Schmitt E, Montembault E, Dozier C, Prigent C, Ducommun B. CDC25B phosphorylation by Aurora-A occurs at the G2/M transition and is inhibited by DNA damage. Cell Cycle. 2005;4:1233–8.

47. Donzelli M, Draetta GF. Regulating mammalian checkpoints through Cdc25 inactivation. EMBO Rep. 2003;4:671–7.

48. Tapia C, Kutzner H, Mentzel T, Savic S, Baumhoer D, Glatz K. Two mitosis-specific antibodies, MPM-2 and phospho-histone H3 (Ser28), allow rapid and precise determination of mitotic activity. Am J Surg Pathol. 2006;30:83–9.

49. Faderl S, O'Brien S, Pui C-H, Stock W, Wetzler M, Hoelzer D, Kantarjian HM. Adult acute lymphoblastic leukemia: concepts and strategies. Cancer. 2010; 116:1165–76.

50. Zhou L, Zhang Y, Chen S, Kmieciak M, Leng Y, Lin H, Rizzo KA, Dumur CI, Ferreira-Gonzalez A, Dai Y, Grant S. A regimen combining the Wee1 inhibitor AZD1775 with HDAC inhibitors targets human acute myeloid leukemia cells harboring various genetic mutations. Leukemia. 2015;29:807–18.

51. Puttini M, Coluccia AML, Boschelli F, Cleris L, Marchesi E, Donella-Deana A, Ahmed S, Redaelli S, Piazza R, Magistroni V, Andreoni F, Scapozza L, Formelli F, Gambacorti-Passerini C. In vitro and in vivo activity of SKI-606, a novel Src-Abl inhibitor, against imatinib-resistant Bcr-Abl+ neoplastic cells. Cancer Res. 2006;66:11314–22.

52. Kantarjian HM, Cortes JE, Kim DW, Khoury HJ, Brümmendorf TH, Porkka K, Martinelli G, Durrant S, Leip E, Kelly V, Turnbull K, Besson N, Gambacorti-Passerini C. Bosutinib safety and management of toxicity in leukemia patients with resistance or intolerance to imatinib and other tyrosine kinase inhibitors. Blood. 2014;123:1309–18.

53. Chiaretti S, Foà R. Management of adult Ph-positive acute lymphoblastic leukemia. Hematology Am Soc Hematol Educ Program. 2015;2015:406–13.

54. Liu-Dumlao T, Kantarjian H, Thomas DA, O'Brien S, Ravandi F. Philadelphia-positive acute lymphoblastic leukemia: current treatment options. Curr Oncol Rep. 2012;14:387–94.

55. Levinson NM, Boxer SG. Structural and spectroscopic analysis of the kinase inhibitor bosutinib and an isomer of bosutinib binding to the Abl tyrosine kinase domain. PLoS One. 2012;7

56. Slupianek A, Hoser G, Majsterek I, Bronisz A, Malecki M, Blasiak J, Fishel R, Skorski T. Fusion tyrosine kinases induce drug resistance by stimulation of homology-dependent recombination repair, prolongation of G(2)/M phase, and protection from apoptosis. Mol Cell Biol. 2002;22:4189–201.

57. Krajewska M, Heijink AM, Bisselink YJWM, Seinstra RI, Silljé HHW, De Vries EGE, Van Vugt MATM. Forced activation of Cdk1 via wee1 inhibition impairs homologous recombination. Oncogene. 2013;32:3001–8.

58. Baumann P, West SC. Role of the human RAD51 protein in homologous recombination and double-stranded-break repair. Trends Biochem Sci. 1998; 23:247–51.

59. Mir SE, De Witt Hamer PC, Krawczyk PM, Balaj L, Claes A, Niers JM, Van Tilborg AAG, Zwinderman AH, Geerts D, Kaspers GJL, Peter Vandertop W, Cloos J, Tannous BA, Wesseling P, Aten JA, Noske DP, Van Noorden CJF, Würdinger T. In silico analysis of kinase expression identifies WEE1 as a gatekeeper against mitotic catastrophe in glioblastoma. Cancer Cell. 2010;18:244–57.

60. PosthumaDeBoer J, Würdinger T, Graat HCA, van Beusechem VW, Helder MN, van Royen BJ, Kaspers GJL. WEE1 inhibition sensitizes osteosarcoma to radiotherapy. BMC Cancer. 2011;11:156.

61. Tibes R, Bogenberger JM, Chaudhuri L, Hagelstrom RT, Chow D, Buechel ME, Gonzales IM, Demuth T, Slack J, Mesa RA, Braggio E, Yin HH, Arora S, Azorsa DO. RNAi screening of the kinome with cytarabine in leukemias. Blood. 2012;119:2863–72.

62. Music D, Dahlrot RH, Hermansen SK, Hjelmborg J, de Stricker K, Hansen S, Kristensen BW. Expression and prognostic value of the WEE1 kinase in gliomas. J Neuro-Oncol. 2016;127:381–9.

63. Barretina J, Caponigro G, Stransky N, Venkatesan K, Margolin AA, Kim S, Wilson CJ, Lehár J, Kryukov GV, Sonkin D, Reddy A, Liu M, Murray L, Berger MF, Monahan JE, Morais P, Meltzer J, Korejwa A, Jané-Valbuena J, Mapa FA, Thibault J, Bric-Furlong E, Raman P, Shipway A, Engels IH, Cheng J, Yu GK, Yu J, Aspesi P, De Silva M, et al. The Cancer Cell Line Encyclopedia enables predictive modelling of anticancer drug sensitivity. Nature. 2012;483:603–7.

64. Schmidt M, Rohe A, Platzer C, Najjar A, Erdmann F, Sippl W. Regulation of G2/M transition by inhibition of WEE1 and PKMYT1 kinases. Molecules. 2017;22:2045.

65. Skorski T. BCR/ABL regulates response to DNA damage: the role in resistance to genotoxic treatment and in genomic instability. Oncogene. 2002;21(56 REV. ISS. 7):8591–604.

66. Bedi A, Barber JP, Bedi GC, el Deiry WS, Sidransky D, Vala MS, Akhtar AJ, Hilton J, Jones RJ. BCR-ABL-mediated inhibition of apoptosis with delay of G2/M transition after DNA damage: a mechanism of resistance to multiple anticancer agents. Blood. 1995;86:1148–58.

67. Slupianek A, Schmutte C, Tombline G, Nieborowska-Skorska M, Hoser G, Nowicki MO, Pierce AJ, Fishel R, Skorski T. BCR/ABL regulates mammalian RecA homologs, resulting in drug resistance. Mol Cell. 2001;8:795–806.

68. Zhang Q, Shi C, Han L, Jain N, Roberts KG, Ma H, Cai T, Cavazos A, Tabe Y, Jacamo RO, Mu H, Zhao Y, Wang J, Wu S-C, Cao F, Zeng Z, Zhou J, Mi Y, Jabbour EJ, Levine R, Tasian SK, Mullighan CG, Weinstock DM, Fruman DA, Konopleva M. Inhibition of mTORC1/C2 signaling improves anti-leukemia efficacy of JAK/STAT blockade in CRLF2 rearranged and/or JAK driven Philadelphia chromosome-like acute B-cell lymphoblastic leukemia. Oncotarget. 2018;9:8027–41.

11

A cytoplasmic long noncoding RNA LINC00470 as a new AKT activator to mediate glioblastoma cell autophagy

Changhong Liu[1,2,3,4], Yan Zhang[1,2,3,4], Xiaoling She[5], Li Fan[6], Peiyao Li[1,2,3,4], Jianbo Feng[1,2,3,4], Haijuan Fu[1,2,3,4], Qing Liu[7], Qiang Liu[8], Chunhua Zhao[1,2,3,4], Yingnan Sun[1,2,3,4] and Minghua Wu[2,3,4*]

Abstract

Background: Despite the overwhelming number of investigations on AKT, little is known about lncRNA on AKT regulation, especially in GBM cells.

Methods: RNA-binding protein immunoprecipitation assay (RIP) and RNA pulldown were used to confirm the binding of LINC00470 and fused in sarcoma (FUS). Confocal imaging, co-immunoprecipitation (Co-IP) and GST pulldown assays were used to detect the interaction between FUS and AKT. EdU assay, CCK-8 assay, and intracranial xenograft assays were performed to demonstrate the effect of LINC00470 on the malignant phenotype of GBM cells. RT-qPCR and Western blotting were performed to test the effect of LINC00470 on AKT and pAKT.

Results: In this study, we demonstrated that LINC00470 was a positive regulator for AKT activation in GBM. LINC00470 bound to FUS and AKT to form a ternary complex, anchoring FUS in the cytoplasm to increase AKT activity. Higher pAKT activated by LINC00470 inhibited ubiquitination of HK1, which affected glycolysis, and inhibited cell autophagy. Furthermore, higher LINC00470 expression was associated with GBM tumorigenesis and poor patient prognosis.

Conclusions: Our findings revealed a noncanonical AKT activation signaling pathway, i.e., LINC00470 directly interacts with FUS, serving as an AKT activator to promote GBM progression. LINC00470 has an important referential significance to evaluate the prognosis of patients.

Keywords: LncRNA, AKT activation, Oncogene, GBM

Background

AKT is a serine/threonine kinase, also known as protein kinase B, which plays critical roles in diverse cellular processes such as proliferation, autophagy, metabolism, and survival [1–4]. Aberrant AKT activation causes a wide variety of disorders including diabetes, neurodegenerative syndromes, and various types of cancers. AKT is well established as the predominant PI3K effector in many cell types [5]. Many cancer genetic alterations deregulate cell signaling pathways and exert their oncogenic effects in part through the PI3K/AKT pathway [6, 7]. Hence, there is a particularly intimate relationship between the activation of the AKT signaling pathway and tumorigenesis. Activation of PI3K results in the phosphorylation of two key residues on AKT, i.e., Thr308 in the activation motif and Ser473 in a C-terminal hydrophobic motif [7, 8]. AKT can translocate from the plasma membrane to intracellular compartments, including the cytoplasm and nucleus where it phosphorylates substrates [9, 10]. Growth factors stimulate phosphorylated AKT to translocate from the cytoplasm to the nucleus [11] where AKT can be phosphorylated and activated [12]. For example, nuclear AKT phosphorylates members of the Foxo subfamily of forkhead transcription factors, promoting nuclear exclusion and thereby inhibiting the transcription of death genes [13, 14]. Evidence indicates that a number of positive regulators, including regulatory proteins (such

* Correspondence: wuminghua554@aliyun.com
[2]Cancer Research Institute, School of Basic Medical Science, Central South University, Changsha 410078, Hunan, China
[3]Key Laboratory of Carcinogenesis and Cancer Invasion, Ministry of Education, Changsha 410078, Hunan, China
Full list of author information is available at the end of the article

as PI3K, PTEN, PDK1) [15–17], miRNAs (such as miRNA-7, miRNA-379, and miRNA-126) [18–21], and long noncoding RNAs (lncRNAs, such as LINK-A, lncRNA OIP5-AS1, and MALAT1), promote the over-activation of AKT signaling [22–24]. Until now, the underlying mechanism of AKT in the GBM was not fully understood despite many years of investigation.

Recent studies have revealed the regulatory potential of many lncRNAs involved in numerous physiological and pathological processes [25]. LncRNAs have regulatory roles in gene expression at both transcriptional and post-transcriptional levels in diverse cellular contexts and biological processes [26]. LncRNAs are responsible for nuclear structure integrity and can regulate the expression of either nearby genes (acting in *cis* in the nucleus) or genes elsewhere in cells (acting in *trans* in the nucleus or cytoplasm) by interacting with proteins, RNA, and DNA [27–29]. LncRNAs operate through distinct modes, such as signals, scaffolds for protein-protein interactions, molecular decoys, or guides, to target elements in the genome [30, 31]. In addition, new types of lncRNAs are likely to be discovered through integrated approaches. For example, sno-lncRNA can form a nuclear accumulation that is enriched in RNA-binding proteins [32].

LINC00470 (also known as C18orf2) is a long non-coding RNA located in chromosome band 18p11.32 between RP11-16P11 and RP11-732L14 [33, 34]. Its alternative splicing of seven exons generates four transcripts. Our previous data demonstrated that LINC00470 expression levels in astrocytoma were significantly higher than those in normal brain tissues [35]. However, the role of LINC00470 remains to be elucidated; in particular, it is not known whether lncRNAs are involved in the regulation of AKT activity in GBM.

In this study, we found that (1) LINC00470 is a positive regulator of AKT activation and it inhibited the nuclear translocation of phosphorylated AKT; (2) LINC00470 directly bound FUS and anchored FUS in the cytoplasm, resulting in FUS activation; (3) LINC00470 interacted with FUS and AKT to form a stable complex; and (4) LINC00470 decreased the ubiquitination of HK1, which affected glycolysis by positively regulating AKT activation in GBM tumorigenesis.

Methods

Primary tumor cell culture and cell lines

A primary tumor cell culture was performed as previously described [36]. Astrocytoma cell lines U251 and U87 were bought from cell banks of the Chinese Academy of Sciences (Shanghai, China). All astrocytoma cell lines were subjected to a short tandem repeat (STR) test. U251 and primary tumor cells were cultured in DMEM high-glucose medium with 10% FBS and a 1% antibiotic-antimycotic

solution (Gibco, Grand Island, NY, USA), while U87 cells were cultured in MEM medium with 10% FBS and 1% antibiotic-antimycotic solution at 37 °C and 5% CO_2.

Antibodies and reagents

The following primary antibodies were used: AKT (rabbit, Proteintech, 10176-2-AP, WB1:1500, IP:1:250, RIP:1:100); FUS (rabbit, Abcam, ab23439, WB1:2000, IP1: 200, RIP1:100); phospho-Akt (Ser473) (rabbit, Cell Signaling, #4060, WB1:1500); phospho-Akt (Thr308) (rabbit, Cell Signaling, #13038, WB1:1500); hexokinase I (rabbit, Cell Signaling, #2024, WB1:1000); hexokinase II (rabbit, Cell Signaling, #2867, WB1:1000); Flag (mouse, Sigma-Aldrich, F1804, IP 1:200); GAPDH (mouse, Sangon, D190090, WB 1:5000); H3 (rabbit, Beyotime, AH433, WB 1:500); and p53 (mouse, Active Motif, 39739, WB 1:1000, RIP 1:150). MK-2206 2HCl (S1078) was purchased from Selleck.

LncRNA, siRNAs, and transfection

Cell transfection was performed using Lipofectamine 3000 (Invitrogen-Life Technologies, Carlsbad, CA, USA) per the manufacturer's instructions.

RNA isolation and RT-qPCR

This procedure was carried out as previously described. The following primers were used: LINC00470: F: 5′-CGTA AGGTGACGAGGAGCTG-3′, R: 5′-GGGGAATGGCTT TTGGGTCA-3′; AKT: F: 5′-GAAGGACGGGAGCAGG C-3′, R: 5′-AAGGTGCGTTCGATGACAGT-3′; and GAP DH: F: 5′-AATGGGCAGCCGTTAGGAAA-3′, R: 5′-GC GCCCAATACGACCAAATC-3′.

Western blotting

Details of Western blotting were previously described [37]. Cell lysates were prepared with GLB buffer (10 mM Tris-HCl, pH = 7.5; 10 mM NaCl; 0.5% Triton X-100; 10 mM EDTA) supplemented with protease inhibitor cocktail (Bimake, Houston, TX, USA, B14001) and phosphatase inhibitor (Bimake, B15001). Cytoplasmic and nuclear proteins were prepared with a Nuclear and Cytoplasmic Protein Extraction Kit (Beyotime, p0028). Thirty-microgram proteins were subjected to electrophoresis in different percentages of gels according to the molecular weight of the detected proteins.

Co-immunoprecipitation assay

For the interaction of FUS and AKT, HEK293 cells were transfected with the indicated plasmids and extracted by the addition of lysis buffer. For the immunoprecipitation of endogenous FUS and AKT proteins extracted by the addition of lysis buffer, the soluble supernatants were incubated with the indicated antibodies for 1 h at 4 °C. The immunocomplexes were then precipitated with protein

A-Sepharose CL-4B. The immunocomplexes were washed three times with lysis buffer, eluted by boiling in sample buffer for SDS-PAGE, and then subjected to immunoblot analysis.

Pulldown assay

GST fusion proteins containing various deletions of FUS cytoplasmic domain or deletions of AKT were expressed in U251 cells with the pGEX-4T-2 vector and were purified. The lysate was incubated for 1 h with GST-tagged proteins and glutathione-Sepharose 4B beads. The beads were subsequently washed three times in the lysis buffer containing 1 mM EDTA and 0.5 mM DTT. Precipitates were separated by SDS-PAGE and detected by Western blotting analysis.

Cell viability and EdU assays

This procedure was carried out as previously described [35].

RNA-binding protein immunoprecipitation assay

Approximately 2 μg of the cell extract was mixed with agarose beads, which had already precipitated with the protein antibodies. Beads were washed briefly three times with GLB$^+$ lysis, and the retrieved protein was detected by Western blotting. The co-precipitated RNAs were detected by RT-qPCR.

Intracranial implantation mouse model

All animal experiments were approved by the Animal Care and Use Committee of Central South University. Mouse orthotopic xenograft model was performed as previously described [36]. Six-week SD mice were chosen. Injection of cyclophosphamide once every 2 days. One-centimeter incision was made on the midline, and a 1-mm burr hole was drilled at AP = + 1 mm and MR = − 3 mm from the bregma at the right hemisphere. Ten microliters of 10^7 cell was infused into the brain at a depth of − 5 mm from the dura, at a speed of 1 μl/min.

Statistical analysis

All experiments were analyzed with GraphPad Prism 5 (La Jolla, CA, USA). Differences between the different groups were tested using Student's t test or one-way ANOVA. The relationships between the LINC00470 expression and clinic-pathological parameters were examined using the χ^2 test. The expression of LINC00470 and patients' survival time was analyzed by single factor and multiplicity factor analysis, and OS curves were calculated using the Kaplan-Meier method with the SPSS 15.0 program (SPSS Inc., Chicago, IL, USA). Data are expressed as the mean ± S.E.M. from at least three independent experiments. A probability value $P < 0.05$ was considered statistically significant.

Results

LINC00470 was a positive regulator of AKT activities

A vector construct containing the full-length LINC00470 with EGFP tag was developed and assessed for LINC00470 expression. LINC00470 did not have any detectable protein-coding ability (Additional file 1: Figure S1A and B). To investigate biological processes associated with LINC00470 expression in GBM, Pearson correlation analysis between LINC00470 expression and whole genome profiling were performed in GBM samples by TCGA databases. A total of 1802 gene expressions that correlated with LINC00470 expression are shown in Fig. 1a. To investigate which canonical pathways were significantly dysregulated in GBM groups with LINC00470 expression, Fisher's exact test was used to identify 20 canonical pathways in GBM that included PI3K-AKT signaling (Fig. 1a). These analyses indicated that LINC00470 may be associated with PI3K-AKT signaling. Then, we measured the expression levels of LINC00470, AKT, and p-AKT in GBM cell lines and primary cultured GBM cells by RT-qPCR (Additional file 2: Figure S2A) and Western blotting (Additional file 2: Figure S2B). We found a positive correlation between the expression of LINC00470 and p-AKT. In GBM, LINC00470 and AKT had no correlation (Additional file 2: Figure S2B). Overexpression of LINC00470 upregulated the expression of p-AKT^{T308} and p-AKT^{S473} (Fig. 1b). We designed three kinds of siRNA and selected the best interfering effects for follow-up study (Additional file 3: Figure S3), while knockdown LINC00470 reduced p-AKT^{T308} and p-AKT^{S473} levels (Fig. 1c). We also re-expressed LINC00470 in the LINC00470-KD cells. Expression of LINC00470 was elevated after LINC00470 was re-expressed in the LINC00470-KD cells (Fig. 1d upper) and enhanced the p-AKT^{T308} and p-AKT^{S473} level (Fig. 1d lower panel). However, neither overexpression nor knockdown of LINC00470 affected total AKT and PI3K expression (Fig. 1b, c and Additional file 4: Figure S4). Therefore, we proposed that LINC00470 modulates AKT activities possibly through a previously unidentified mechanism.

FUS interacted with both LINC00470 and AKT to form a ternary complex in the cytoplasm

Bioinformatics (http://starbase.sysu.edu.cn/browseRbpLncRNA.php) predicted FUS, an RNA-binding protein associated with LINC00470, may also bind to AKT. An RIP assay verified the interaction between LINC00470 and FUS (Fig. 2a). A biotin-RNA pulldown assay further confirmed the binding between LINC00470 and FUS (Fig. 2b). Interestingly, RNA-binding protein immunoprecipitation of FUS, but not AKT, specifically retrieved LINC00470 (Fig. 2c). We also performed RIP assay in U87 cells; the result of RIP assay was consistent with that in U251cells (Additional file 5: Figure S5). These results indicated that

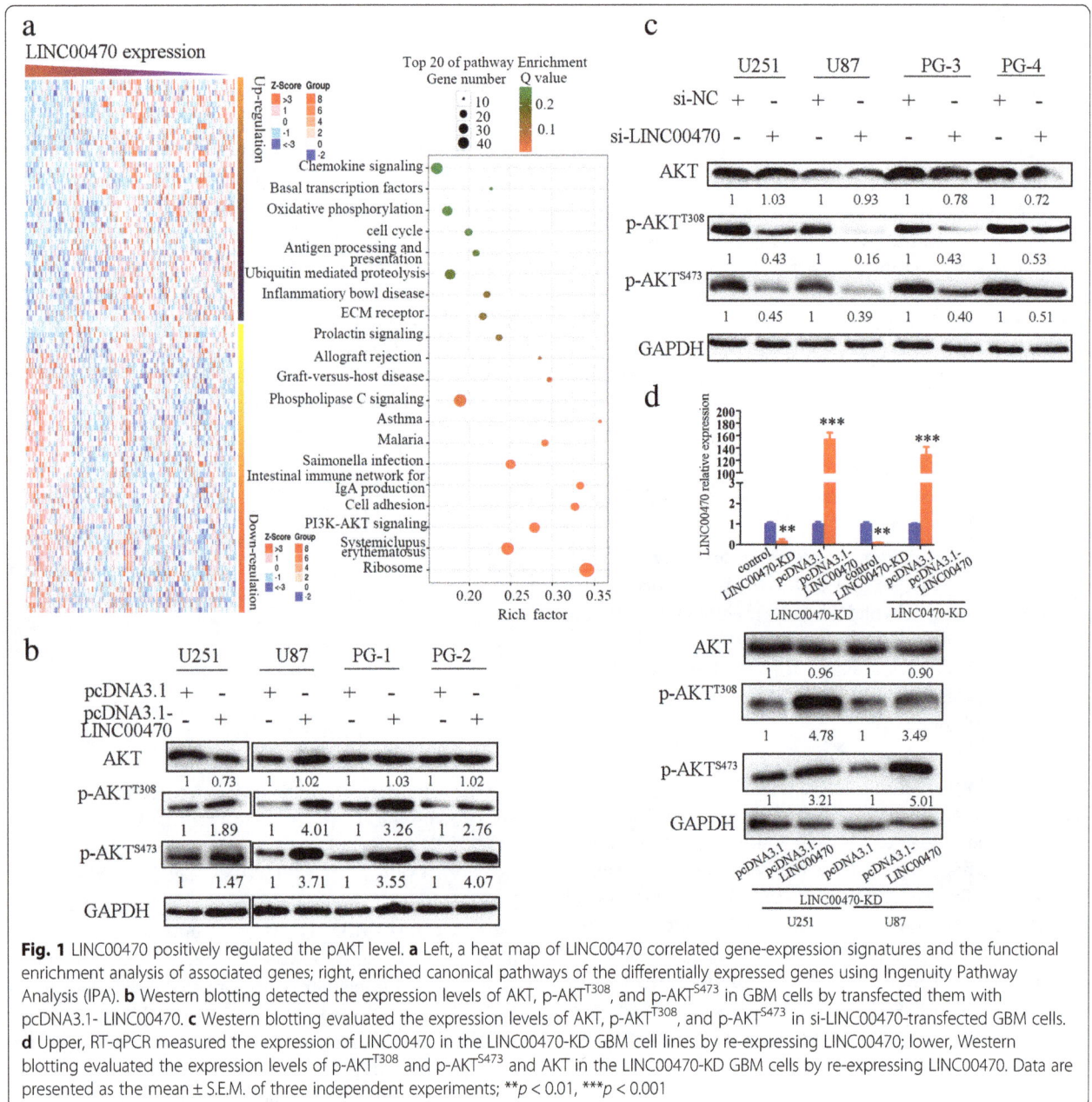

Fig. 1 LINC00470 positively regulated the pAKT level. **a** Left, a heat map of LINC00470 correlated gene-expression signatures and the functional enrichment analysis of associated genes; right, enriched canonical pathways of the differentially expressed genes using Ingenuity Pathway Analysis (IPA). **b** Western blotting detected the expression levels of AKT, p-AKT^{T308}, and p-AKT^{S473} in GBM cells by transfected them with pcDNA3.1- LINC00470. **c** Western blotting evaluated the expression levels of AKT, p-AKT^{T308}, and p-AKT^{S473} in si-LINC00470-transfected GBM cells. **d** Upper, RT-qPCR measured the expression of LINC00470 in the LINC00470-KD GBM cell lines by re-expressing LINC00470; lower, Western blotting evaluated the expression levels of p-AKT^{T308} and p-AKT^{S473} and AKT in the LINC00470-KD GBM cells by re-expressing LINC00470. Data are presented as the mean ± S.E.M. of three independent experiments; **$p < 0.01$, ***$p < 0.001$

FUS interacted with LINC00470, but there was no direct interaction between LINC00470 and AKT.

To examine the simultaneous existence of LINC00470, FUS, and AKT within the same complex, a two-step Co-IP assay was performed using HEK293 cell lysate from cells in which HA-AKT, Flag-FUS, and pcDNA3.1-LINC00470 were co-transfected. LINC00470 was found in the final immunoprecipitation, suggesting that LINC00470, FUS, and AKT form a ternary complex (Fig. 2d). At the same time, we also found LINC00470, FUS, and AKT can form a ternary complex in U251 cells (Additional file 6: Figure S6). In the absence of LINC00470, FUS and AKT were co-localized in the nucleus of HEK293 cells

(Additional file 7: Figure S7 and Fig. 2e). However, overexpression of LINC00470 anchored FUS and AKT in the cytoplasm (Fig. 2e), while with knockdown of LINC00470 in U251 cells, FUS and AKT translocated from the cytoplasm to the nucleus (Fig. 2f). The interactions between FUS and AKT in the cytoplasm of U251 cells were also verified by Western blotting analysis (Fig. 2g left). An RNA pulldown assay showed that the interaction of LINC00470 and AKT disappeared after FUS knockdown in U251 cells (Fig. 2g right). We also found LINC00470 could not affect AKT activation after pcDNA3.1-LINC00470 was transfected into FUS-KD cells (Fig. 2h). The phosphorylated AKT

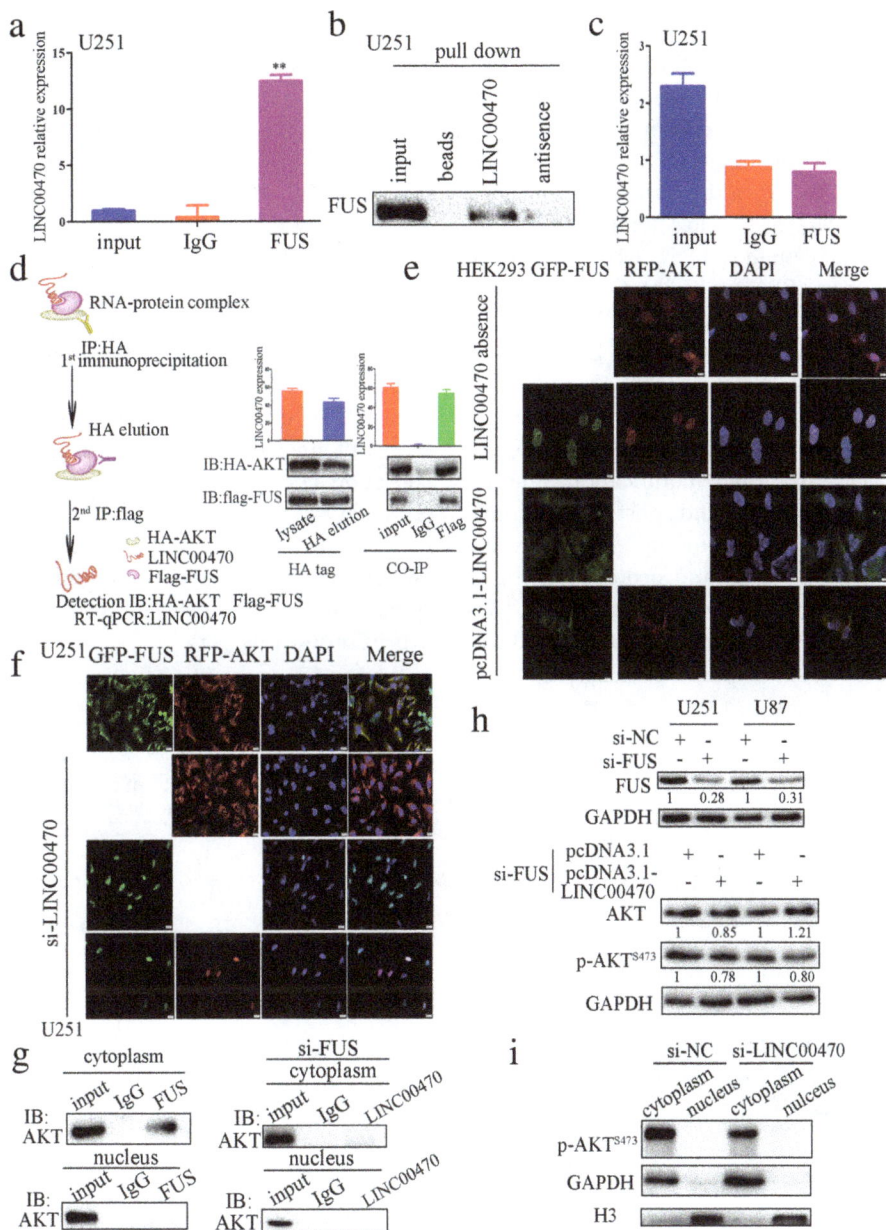

Fig. 2 FUS interacted with LINC00470 and AKT to form a ternary complex in the cytoplasm. **a** The interaction of LINC00470 and FUS was detected through RIP assays in U251 cells. Data are presented as the mean ± S.E.M. of three independent experiments. **$p < 0.01$. **b** RNA pulldown showed binding between LINC00470 and FUS. **c** RIP assays showed that there was no interaction between LINC00470 and AKT in U251 cells. Data are presented as the mean ± S.E.M. of three independent experiments. **d** HEK293 cells were transfected with HA-AKT, Flag-FUS, and pcDNA3.1-LINC00470. Two-step co-immunoprecipitation verified their interaction. The expression levels of LINC00470, AKT, and FUS were measured with RT-qPCR and Western blotting, respectively. **e** The localization of AKT and FUS was detected by immunofluorescence staining in HEK293 cells. **f** The co-localization of AKT and FUS was detected by immunofluorescence staining in U251 cells. **g** Left, the interactions between endogenous FUS and AKT in the cytoplasm and nucleus were measured by co-immunoprecipitation; right, an RNA pulldown assay showed binding between endogenous LINC00470 and AKT in the cytoplasm and nucleus of U251 cells transfected by si-FUS. **h** Western blotting detected the expression of FUS in GBM cells transfected by si-FUS. Expression levels of AKT and p-AKT^{S473} were measured by Western blotting in GBM cells that re-expressed LINC00470 in FUS-KD GBM cells. **i** Western blotting detected the expression levels of p-AKT^{S473} in the cytoplasm and nucleus of U251 cells transfected by si-LINC00470

was reduced in the cytoplasm in LINC00470-knockdown GBM cells (Fig. 2i). The data indicated that LINC00470 promoted the activation of AKT in the cytoplasm by interacting with FUS.

LINC00470 anchored FUS in the cytoplasm and phosphorylated FUS

Next, a series of LINC00470 deletion mutants were constructed to determine the nucleotides in LINC00470 that bind to FUS. An RNA pulldown assay showed that there was an interaction between FUS and LINC00470 mutants (1–300 nt, 1–710 nt, 1–1500 nt, 1–2231 nt, and 100–2231 nt), but no interaction between FUS and other LINC00470 deletion mutants (1–100 nt, 300–2231 nt, 710–2231 nt, 1500–2231 nt, 300–710 nt, 300–1500 nt, and 710–1500 nt) (Fig. 3a), suggesting that the 100–300 nt region of LINC00470 was responsible for its binding to FUS. We also found FUS bound to LINC00470 through its RNA recognition domain (RRM) (Fig. 3b). Confocal fluorescence microscopy indicated that LINC00470 and FUS were mainly co-localized in the cytoplasm in HEK 293 cells after overexpression of LINC00470 (Fig. 3c).

FUS was reported to be continuously shuttling between the nucleus and the cytoplasm [38]. FUS contains multiple post-translational modification sites in the RRM and GGR domain, and post-translational modifications of FUS have profound effects on its binding capacity of DNA, RNA and proteins, changes in protein stability, or subcellular localization [39, 40]. We speculated that LINC00470 may impact FUS subcellular

localization. The nuclear localization of FUS was explored by transient expression of the GFP-FUS fusion plasmid in HEK293 cells (Fig. 3d). When HEK293 cells were co-transfected by pcDNA3.1-LINC00470 and the GFP-FUS fusion plasmid, LINC00470 led to the translocation of FUS from the nucleus to the cytoplasm (Fig. 3d). In GBM cells, the expression of FUS was increased by LINC00470 overexpression and the FUS level was significantly increased in cytoplasm; however, its expression was decreased in the nucleus (Fig. 3e). These data suggested that LINC00470 anchored FUS in the cytoplasm and promoted its expression in the cytoplasm. FUS immunoprecipitation from U251 cells after overexpression of LINC00470 was immunoblotted with anti-phospho-T (threonine phosphorylation) antibodies to assess the level of FUS phosphorylation; LINC00470 promoted phosphorylation of FUS at threonine residues (Fig. 3f). In addition, we also found that LINC00470 was mainly located in the cytoplasm in GBM cells by RNA fluorescence in situ hybridization (Fig. 3g).

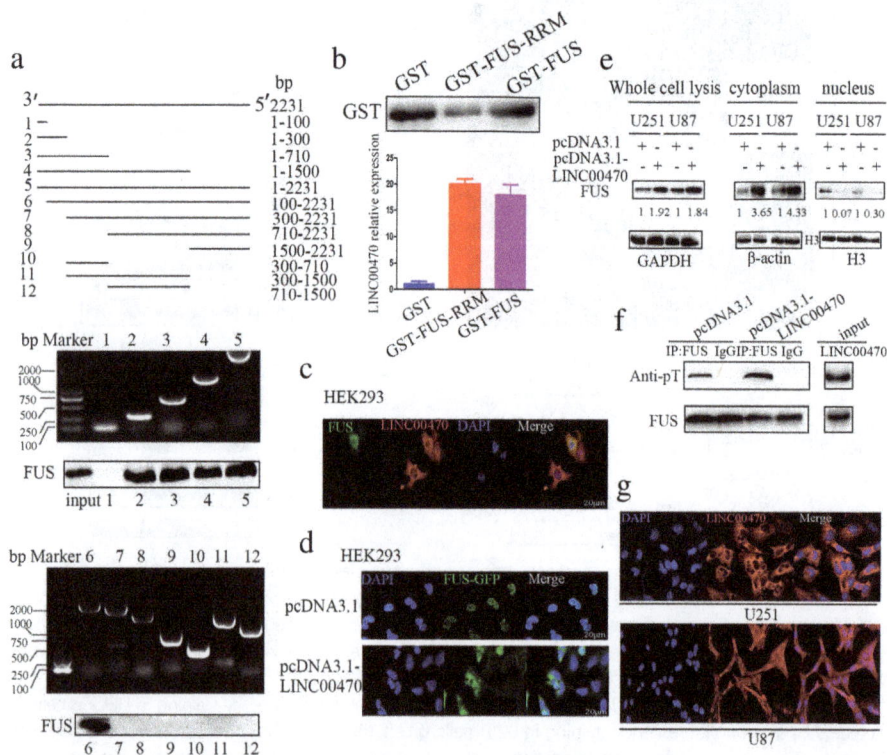

Fig. 3 LINC00470 anchored FUS in the cytoplasm and phosphorylated FUS. a Upper, schematic illustration of substitution mutant constructs of LINC00470; middle and lower, an RNA pulldown assay examined the interaction between FUS and the different mutants of LINC00470. b GST pulldown assays showed that the RRM domain of FUS pulled down LINC00470. c Representative immunofluorescence staining displayed the co-localization of LINC00470 and FUS in the cytoplasm of HEK293 cells after LINC00470 overexpression. Scale bar, 20 μm. d Representative imaging of LINC00470 anchoring FUS in the cytoplasm in HEK293 cells. Scale bar, 20 μm. e Western blotting measured the expression of FUS in whole cell lysis and the cytoplasm and nucleus in U251 cells transfected by pcDNA3.1-LINC00470. f Representative immunoprecipitation analysis detected FUS phosphorylation in U251 cells transfected by pcDNA3.1-LINC00470. FUS immunoprecipitated from U251 cells was immunoblotted with pan-phospho-S/TQ antibodies to assess the phosphorylation level of FUS. g RNA fluorescence in situ hybridization showed the localization of LINC00470 in GBM cells. The nucleus was counterstained with DAPI. Scale bar, 29 μm

FUS bound to AKT and promoted AKT nuclear translocation and activation

The "Scansite 2.0" software was utilized to identify a docking domain (GGR domain) in FUS, which is an AKT kinase-binding site. GFP-FUS and RFP-AKT expression plasmids were co-transfected into HEK293 cells, CO-IP and immunofluorescence suggested there were interactions between FUS and AKT, and both were co-localized in the nucleus of HEK293 cells (Fig. 4a, b). In addition, we confirmed that endogenous AKT interacted with FUS in the cytoplasm of U251 cells (Fig. 4c, d). Next, a fusion protein of the GGR domain mutation in FUS (GST-FUS-GGR domain) was constructed. A GST pulldown assay indicated that AKT was precipitated with the GST-FUS-GGR peptide (Fig. 4e left) and FUS mainly bound with the N domain of AKT (Fig. 4e right). Then, we analyzed the changes in AKT protein levels after silencing FUS. Knockdown of FUS did not affect AKT expression. Similarly, FUS expression was not affected by silencing AKT (Fig. 4f). However, we observed that FUS influenced the subcellular localization of AKT by promoting AKT nuclear translocation and increased AKT activation in the nucleus (Fig. 4g).

LINC00470 decreased ubiquitination of HK1 to affect glycolysis by positively regulating AKT activation

AKT, which is frequently dysregulated in cancer, is a well-established regulator of glucose metabolism [41].

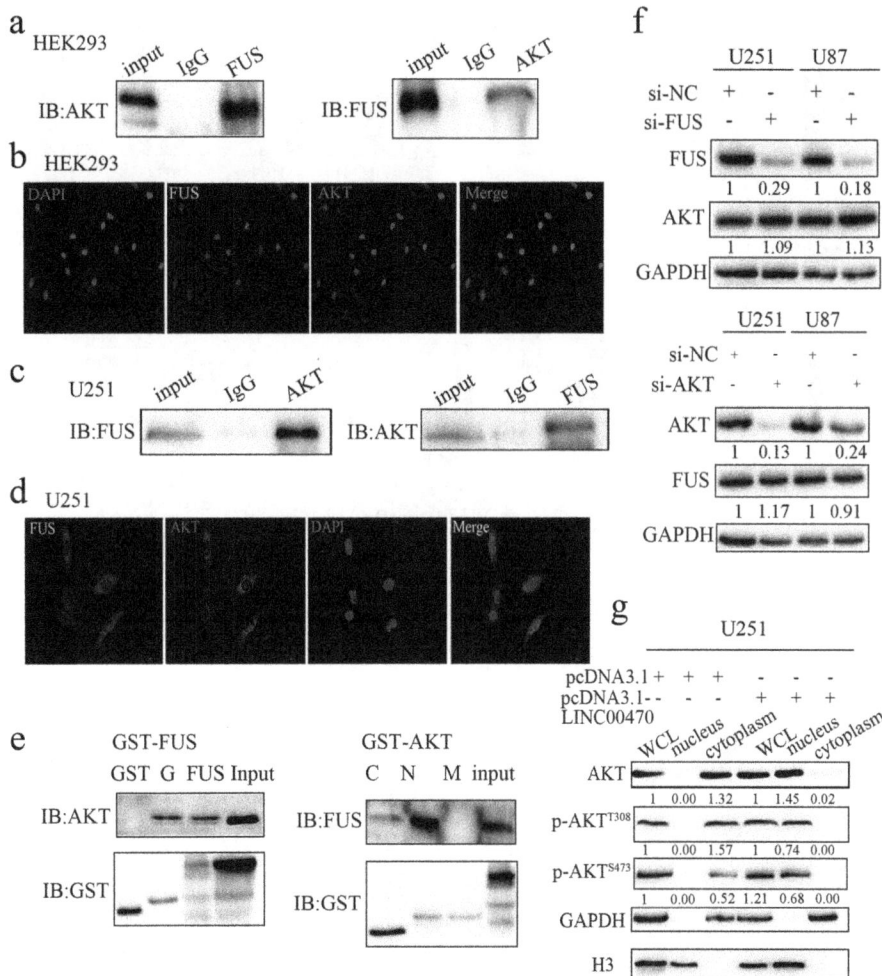

Fig. 4 FUS bound to AKT and promoted AKT activation. **a** Co-IP analysis measured the exogenous interaction between FUS and AKT in HEK293 cells. **b** Representative immunofluorescence staining displayed the co-localization of FUS and AKT in the nucleus of HEK293 cells. **c** Co-IP analysis measured the endogenous interaction between FUS and AKT in U251 cells. **d** Representative immunofluorescence staining displayed the endogenous co-localization of FUS and AKT in the cytoplasm of U251 cells. **e** Left, GST pulldown assays showed that the GGR domain of FUS pulled down AKT; right, GST pulldown assays showed that the N-terminal region of AKT mainly pulled down FUS. **f** Upper, Western blotting measured the expression levels of FUS and AKT in GBM cells transfected by si-FUS; lower, Western blotting measured the expression levels of AKT and FUS in GBM cells transfected with si-AKT. **g** Western blotting measured the expression levels of AKT and pAKT in the whole lysis, cytoplasm, and nucleus of U251 cells transfected by pcDNA3.1-FUS

Its regulation on metabolic processes is required for tumor proliferation, apoptosis, and autophagy [42–44]. Enforcing or silencing LINC00470 expression in GBM cells increased or reduced glycolysis uptake and lactate production, respectively (Fig. 5a, b). Hexokinases catalyze the first and irreversible step of glucose metabolism, i.e., the ATP-dependent phosphorylation of glucose to yield glucose-6-phosphate [45]. Overexpression of LINC00470 increased the total hexokinase activity in U251 cells compared to controls, and HK activity was inhibited after knockdown of LINC00470 in U251 cells (Fig. 5c). HK1 is a major isoform of HK

and is the first key enzyme in the glycolysis pathway [45]. Importantly, the protein expression level of HK1 was markedly increased in response to LINC00470 overexpression (Fig. 5d). In contrast, we found that HK2, another major isoform of HK, was not changed statistically significantly in LINC00470-overexpressed cells (Fig. 5d).

Next, we explored the molecular mechanisms underlying the LINC00470 that affects the activity of HK1. Inhibiting the activity of AKT with MK-2206 resulted in downregulated of HK1 (Fig. 5e). Additionally, we transfected both pcDNA3.1 and pcDNA3.1-LINC00470 vectors into U251

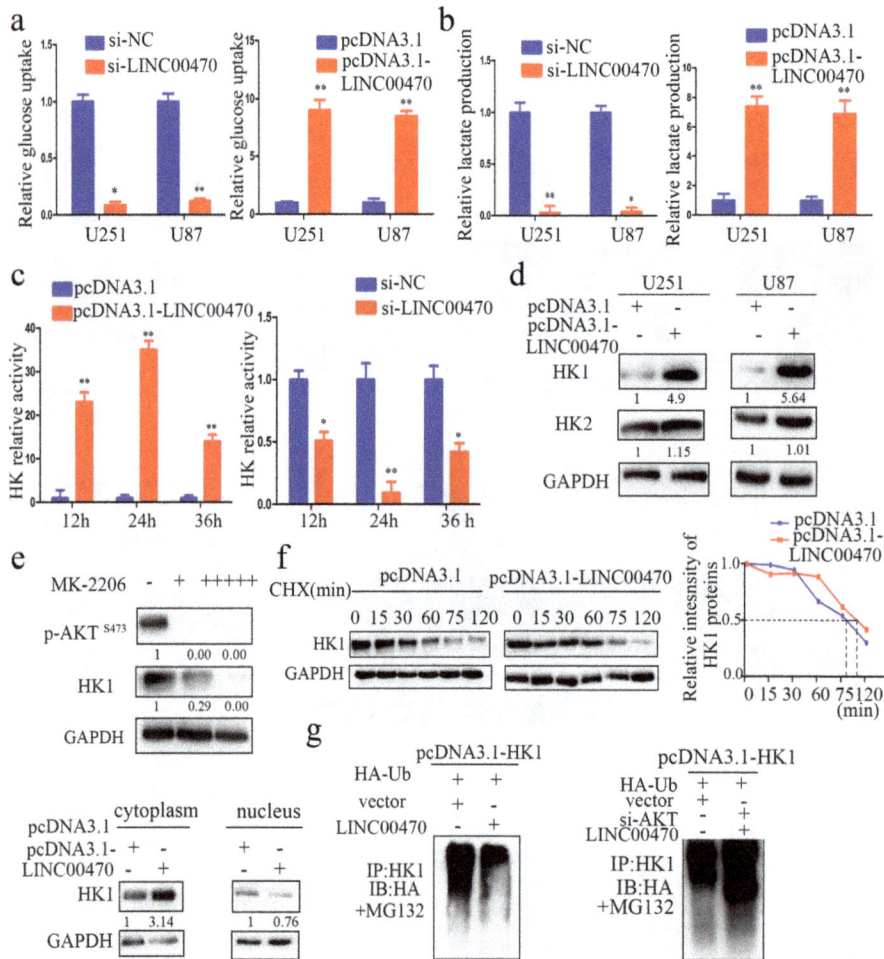

Fig. 5 LINC00470 inhibited HK1 ubiquitination to affect glycolysis by positively regulating AKT activation. **a** RT-qPCR measured the expression of LINC00470 in the GBM cell lines; GBM cells were transfected with si-LINC00470 or pcDNA3.1-LINC00470. Data are presented as the mean ± S.E.M. of three independent experiments; *$p < 0.05$, **$p < 0.01$. **b** Relative levels of glucose uptake and lactate production were detected in GBM cells. GBM cells were transfected with si-LINC00470 or pcDNA3.1-LINC00470. Data are presented as the mean ± S.E.M. of three independent experiments; *$p < 0.05$, **$p < 0.01$. **c** HK activity was measured at different time points after GBM cells were transfected with pcDNA3.1-LINC00470 or si-LINC00470. Data are presented as the mean ± S.E.M. of three independent experiments; **$p < 0.01$, ***$p < 0.001$. **d** Western blotting detected the expression levels of HK1 and HK2 in GBM cells transfected by LINC00470. **e** Upper, Western blotting detected the expression levels of p-AKT^{S473} and HK1 in U251 cells. The cells were treated with different concentrations of AKT inhibitor (MK-2206; +, 1 μM; +++++, 5 μM); lower, Western blotting detected the expression levels of HK1 in the cytoplasm and nucleus in U251 cells transfected by pcDNA3.1-LINC00470. **f** The half-life of HK1 was assessed in U251 cells. Cells were transfected with pcDNA3.1-LINC00470. **g** The relative amount of ubiquitination HK1 was determined by a ubiquitination assay in U251 cells transfected by LINC00470 or si-AKT and LINC00470

cells, then analyzed the protein levels of HK1 in the cytoplasm and nucleus. HK1 expression increased in the cytoplasm under different experimental conditions; concomitantly, HK1 expression in the nucleus did not change significantly (Fig. 5e). To determine how HK1 protein changed, we treated U251 cells with cycloheximide (CHX) and analyzed the stability of HK1 in response to LINC00470 overexpression. The half-life of

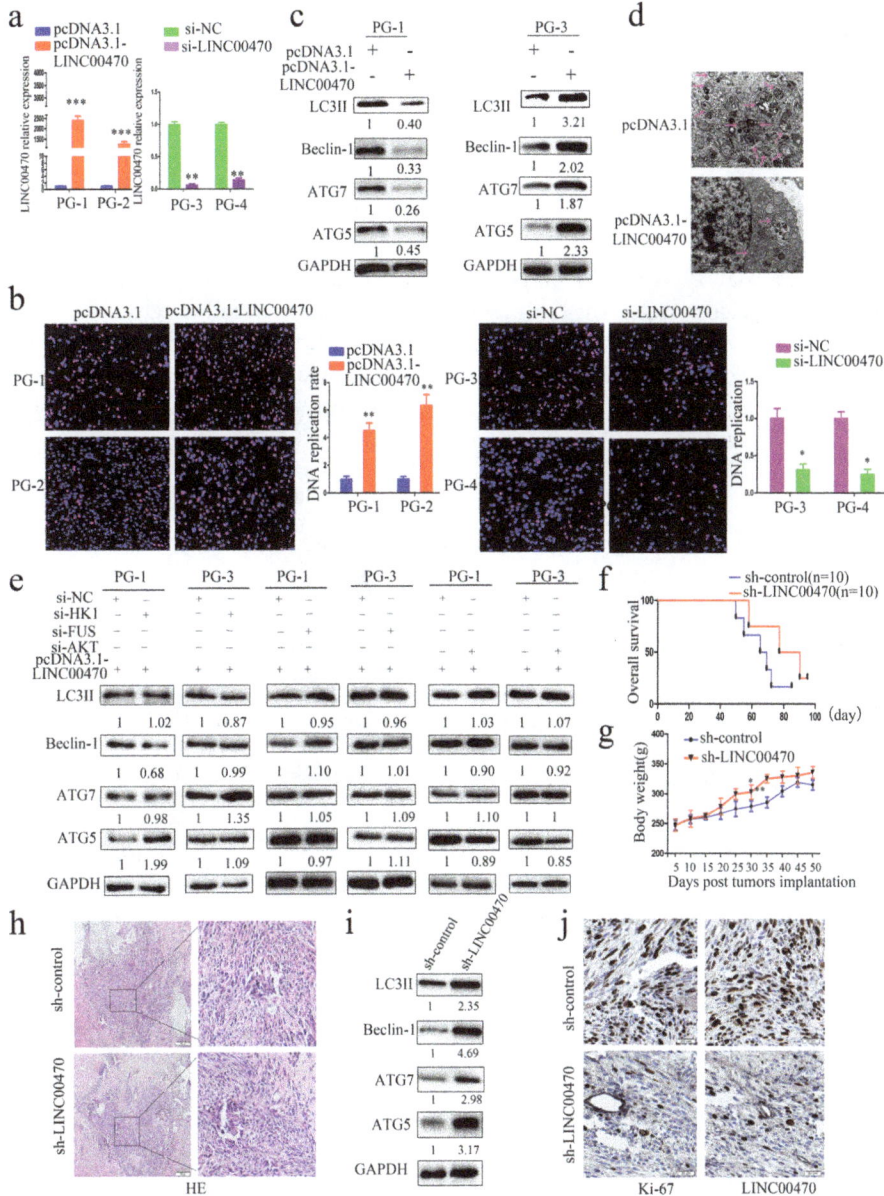

Fig. 6 LINC00470 promoted the tumorigenesis of GBM cells. **a** Expression levels of LINC00470 were measured by RT-qPCR in primary cultured GBM cells (LINC00470 had relatively low expression in PG-1 and PG-2; LINC00470 had relatively high expression in PG-3 and PG-4). Primary cultured GBM cells were transfected with si-LINC00470 or pcDNA3.1-LINC00470. Data are presented as the mean ± S.E.M. of three independent experiments; $**p < 0.01$, $***p < 0.001$. **b** An EDU assay was applied to assess cell proliferation of primary cultured GBM cells. Primary cultured GBM cells were transfected with pcDNA3.1-LINC00470 or si-LINC00470. **c** Western blotting measured the expression levels of autophagy marker LC3, beclin-1, ATG7, and ATG5 in PG-1 and PG-3 cells. The cells were transfected with pcDNA3.1-LINC00470 or si-LINC00470. **d** Electron microscopy detected the autophagy of U251 cells transfected with pcDNA3.1-LINC00470. **e** Western blotting measured the expression levels of autophagy marker LC3, beclin-1, ATG7, and ATG5 in PG-1 and PG-3 cells. The cells were transfected with si-HK1, si-FUS or si-AKT. **f** Survival analysis showed that Sprague Dawley rats transplanted with U251-sh-LINC00470 cells have longer overall survival. **g** Tumor growth for U251-sh-control and U251-sh-LINC00470 in Sprague Dawley rats.$*p < 0.05$, $**p < 0.01$. **h** H&E staining showed the volume and morphology of tumors in mice transplanted with U251-sh-LINC00470 cells. The white circle represents the size of the tumor. **i** Western blotting measured the expression levels of the autophagy marker LC3, beclin-1, ATG7, and ATG5 in intracranial transplanted tumors. **j** Expression of Ki-67 and LINC00470 in intracranial transplanted tumors was detected by immunohistochemical staining or in situ hybridization, respectively

HK1 was much longer in LINC00470-overexpressed cells than that in controls (Fig. 5f). We further explored the mechanism of AKT-mediated HK1 regulation and found lower HK1 ubiquitination levels in LINC00470-transfected cells treated with MG132, and a restoration experiment was performed by knocking down AKT. We found that the ubiquitination level of HK1 was rescued (Fig. 5g). Together, these observations suggested that LINC00470 affected the ubiquitination and expression of HK1 through activating AKT.

LINC00470 is an onco-RNA, and it induced the malignant characteristics of GBM cells

The above data suggested that LINC00470 plays an important role in GBMs. Accordingly, the primary cultured cells were used to evaluate the functions of LINC00470. As shown in Additional file 7: Figure S7, there was relatively low expression of LINC00470

in PG-1 and PG-2 cells and relatively high expression of LINC00470 in PG-3 and PG-4 cells. Therefore, we expected overexpression of LINC00470 in PG-1 and PG-2 cells and knockdown of LINC00470 in PG-3 and PG-4 cells (Fig. 6a). We found overexpression of LINC00470 contributed to the proliferation of PG1 and PG2 cells by CCK-8 assay (Fig. 6b and Additional file 8: Figure S8). Knockdown of LINC00470 in PG-3 and PG-4 cells decreased cell proliferation (Fig. 6b and Additional file 8: Figure S8). Autophagy primarily promoted the progression of cancers [46, 47]. We also found that, in PG-1 cells, overexpression of LINC00470 inhibited the levels of autophagy (Fig. 6c, d), and in PG-3 cells, knockdown of LINC00470 promoted the levels of autophagy (Fig. 6c).

To evaluate whether glycolysis activation serves as an upstream mechanism for LINC00470-mediated autophagy, we monitored the markers of autophagy by knockdown of HK1, FUS, and AKT, respectively. The

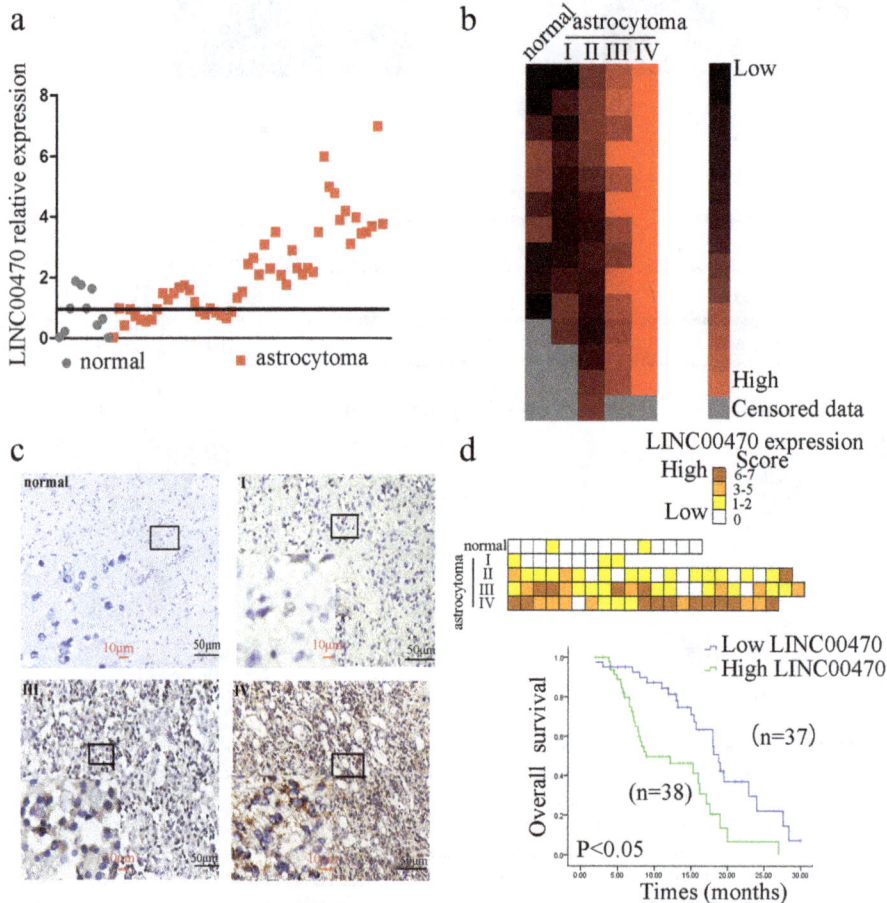

Fig. 7 LINC00470 was an independent prognostic factor in astrocytoma patients. **a** RT-qPCR detected the expression levels of LINC00470 in normal brain tissues and astrocytoma. **b** RT-qPCR measured the expression levels of LINC00470 in astrocytoma with different WHO grades of astrocytoma. **c** The expression levels of LINC00470 were detected in astrocytoma tissues via in situ hybridization. Black scale bars, 50 μm; red scale bars, 10 μm. **d** Upper, the score of in situ hybridization in astrocytoma tissues; lower: Kaplan-Meier analysis for overall survival in 75 astrocytomas in high- and low-risk groups based on LINC00470 expression levels

results showed that when HK1, FUS, or LINC00470 was knocked down, the autophagy level of GBM did not decrease. These results suggested that LINC00470 affected autophagy that was required for HK1, FUS, and AKT (Fig. 6e). At the same time, we applied an intracranial orthotopic transplanted model to evaluate whether LINC00470 mediated GBM tumorigenesis. Compared to mice transplanted with U251-sh-control cells, mice transplanted with U251-sh-LINC00470 cells exhibited longer survival (Fig. 6f), gained more weight (Fig. 6g), and had smaller tumors (Fig. 6h). Knockdown of LINC00470 significantly increased the autophagy levels and decreased the expression of Ki-67 and LINC00470 in an intracranial orthotopic transplanted model (Fig. 6i, j).

LINC00470 was an independent prognostic factor in astrocytoma patients

To further evaluate the clinical significance of LINC00470 in astrocytomas, including GBMs, we found that the levels of LINC00470 were significantly increased in astrocytoma tissues ($n = 60$) compared with normal brain tissues ($n = 12$) by RT-qPCR (Fig. 7a), especially in high-grade astrocytomas (Fig. 7b). We next measured LINC00470 levels in a panel of 75 astrocytoma tissues and 15 normal brain tissues by in situ hybridization (Fig. 7c). The results were consistent with those of RT-qPCR (Fig. 7a).

Subsequently, we conducted a univariate cox regression analysis using clinical variables for astrocytoma patients and found that expression of LINC00470, astrocytoma grade, patients' age, and the astrocytoma location were statistically associated with overall survival (Table 1). The multivariate cox proportional hazards model indicated that LINC00470 expression and astrocytoma grades were independently associated with overall survival (hazard ratio [HR] = 2.876, $P = 0.02$; HR = 1.892, $P = 0.044$; respectively) (Table 2). The results showed that LINC00470 was an independent prognostic factor in astrocytoma patients.

The patients were divided into high or low LINC00470 expression groups according to the ISH scores. Kaplan-Meier analysis of the 75 patients with astrocytoma revealed that high LINC00470 expression levels significantly correlated with shorter survival times (Fig. 7d). High LINC00470 expression was significantly associated with a poor prognosis of astrocytoma patients.

Discussion

Previous studies have shown multiple signaling pathways that are misregulated in human glioblastomas, such as RTK/PI3K/AKT/Foxos signaling pathway, p53, and Rb1 tumor suppressor pathways [48]. Given the

Table 1 Correlation between the clinicopathological factors and expression of LINC00470 in astrocytoma

Characteristic	Total(N=75)	LINC00470 high expression	LINC00470 low expression
Histologic grade*-no.(%)			
Astrocytoma			
I	9(12)	3(33)	6(67)
II	27(36)	14(52)	13(48)
III	18(24)	13(72)	15(28)
IV	21(28)	17(81)	4(19)
Sex-no.(%)			
Male	39(52)	17(44)	22(56)
Female	36(48)	21(58)	15(42)
Age*-no.(%)			
≤42	31(41)	10(33)	21(67)
>42	44(54)	35(80)	9(20)
Tumor location*-no./total no.(%)			
Frontal lobe	23/72(32)	9/23(39)	14/23(61)
Parietal lobe	19/72(26)	6/19(32)	13/19(68)
Temporal lobe	13/72(19)	10/13(77)	3/13(23)
Brainstem	3/72(4)	2/3(66)	1/3(34)
others	14/72(19)	7/17(50)	7/17(50)
Laterality-no./total no.(%)			
Left	32/72(44)	15/33(47)	17/33(53)
Right	25/72(35)	10/26(38)	16/26(62)
others	15/72(21)	7/16(43)	9/16(57)
Presenting symptom-no./total no.(%)			
Seizure	38/70(54)	21/38(55)	17/38(45)
Headache	12/70(17)	6/12(50)	6/12(50)
Sensory or visual change	9/70(13)	5/9 (56)	4/9(44)
Mental statue change	11/70(16)	6/11(55)	5/11(45)

Categorical distributions were compared with the use of Fisher's exact test.
*P<0.01 for the difference among the molecular subtypes.

complexity and redundancy of the signaling networks associated with glioma, targeting of critical oncogenic pathways might constitute a promising treatment approach [49]. For example, S109 treatment disturbed three pathways in glioma including the RTK/AKT/Foxos signaling pathway and the p53 and Rb1 tumor-suppressor pathways [48]. Although a multitude of studies have demonstrated the importance of PI3K in the activation of AKT, there have been reports suggesting that AKT activation can proceed in a manner that is independent of PI3K [2]. In the present study, we provided the evidence that LINC00470 was required for AKT cytoplasm activation and the interaction of LINC00470 and FUS was

Table 2 Summary of multivariate analysis of Cox proportional hazards model for survival of patients with astrocytoma

Variable	Univarible Regression		Multivariable Regression	
	HR	P	HR	P
Gender(Female vs. Male)	1.23	0.244	1.150	0.593
Age	1.46	0.332	1.398	0.475
Grade				
I+II vs. III + IV	1.741	0.051	1.892	0.044
Tumor location	1.021	0.871	1.566	0.111
Laterality	1.381	0.211	1.522	0.169
Presenting symptom	0.721	0.879	0.901	0.351
HighLINC00470 expression	2.113	0.030	2.876	0.021

critical for AKT activation. Our results provided a new mechanism for AKT activity regulation, and we uncovered noncanonical AKT activation signaling by long non-coding RNA.

Recently, the study of lncRNAs has become important, with emerging evidence indicating that lncRNAs function as oncogenes and tumor suppressors, thus having an impact on one or more of the cancer hallmarks [50, 51]. The roles of a small number of lncRNAs such as HOTAIR, H19, and MALAT1 have been depicted in cancers, but little is known about LINC00470. Our study suggested an oncogenic role for LINC00470 in GBM. This was based on the following lines of evidence: (1) LINC00470 was upregulated in GBM and its expression was positively correlated with p-AKT; (2) ectopic expression of LINC00470 or knockdown of LINC00470 increased or suppressed AKT activity and tumor cell proliferation, respectively; and (3) re-expression

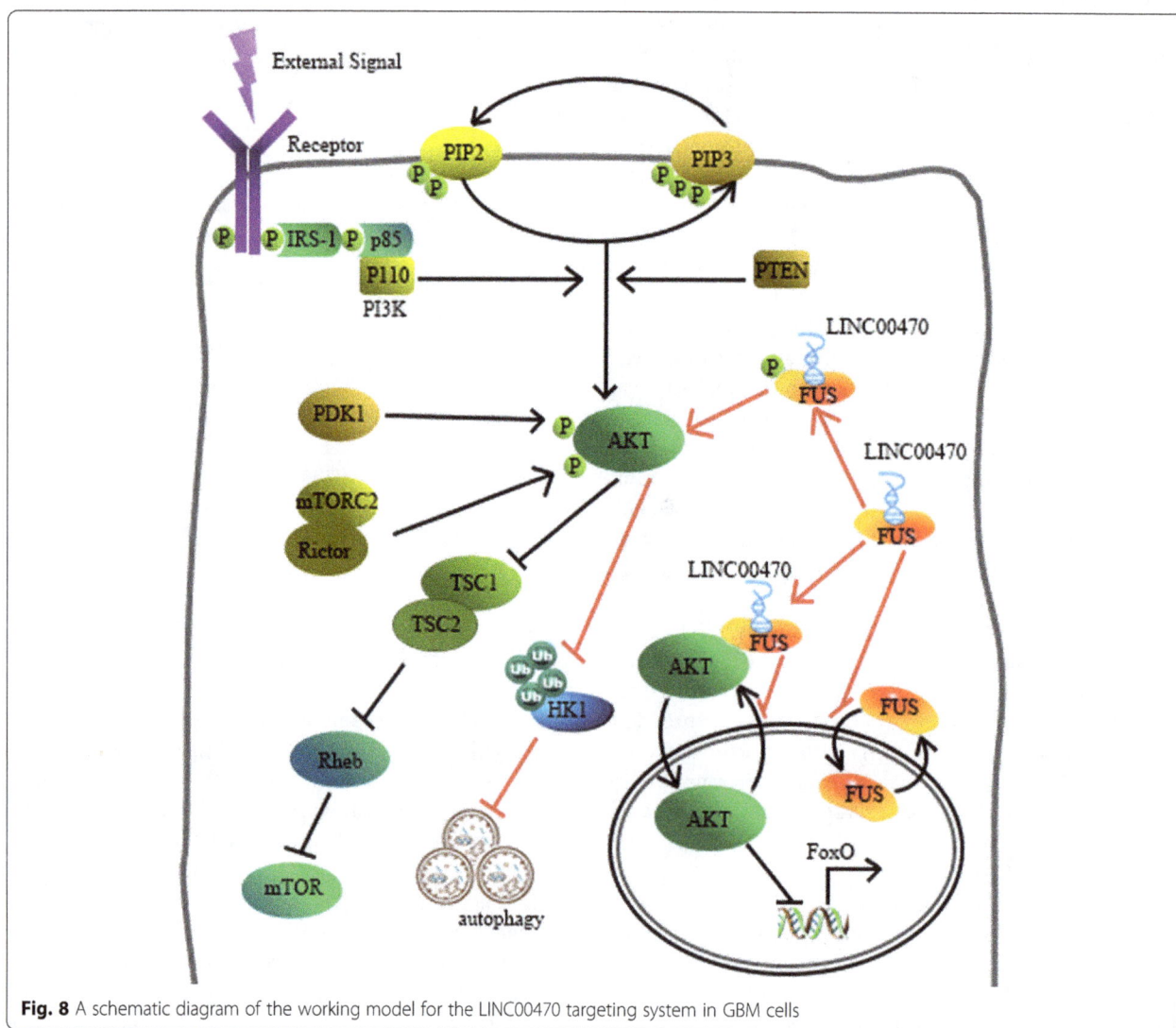

Fig. 8 A schematic diagram of the working model for the LINC00470 targeting system in GBM cells

of LINC00470 in LINC00470-KO cells was able to restore AKT activation.

FUS is a member of the Ewing's sarcoma family of proteins that appears to translocate from the cytoplasm to the nucleus [52], and it is phosphorylated in response to radiotherapy [53]. However, to date, there is no evidence that lncRNAs can regulate FUS localization and activation. Our study demonstrated that FUS was a new binding partner of LINC00470. LINC00470 bound FUS, anchored it in the cytoplasm, and increased FUS expression in the cytoplasm to activate it. Our results not only revealed that FUS could be used as molecular scaffolding that bound LINC00470 and AKT but also upregulated phosphorylated AKT. In HEK293 cells with the absence of LINC00470, FUS was mainly located in the nucleus, and it transported AKT to the nucleus. However, in GBM cells, LINC00470 prevented FUS from transporting to the nucleus, so AKT was also activated and anchored in the cytoplasm. High levels of p-AKT decreased ubiquitination of HK1, so that the HK1 protein degradation rate was inhibited, and a higher level of HK1 affected glycolysis and inhibited cell autophagy. Our results further suggested that LINC00470 mediated AKT activation, at least in part, through interaction with FUS.

Finally, we confirmed the prognostic value of LINC00470 and that the high level expression of LINC00470 was an unfavorable prognosis marker for astrocytoma patients. Patients with high expression of LINC00470 had shorter survival times than those with low expression of LINC00470.

Conclusions

To summarize, we first demonstrated the function of LINC00470 in GBM and manifested a new regulatory mechanism for AKT activation. These results will provide a theoretical and experimental basis for verifying the mechanism of GBM carcinogenesis and identifying biomarkers for the early diagnosis and prognosis in GBM (Fig. 8).

Additional files

Additional file 1: Bioinformatics analyses of evolutional conservation and protein-coding potential of LINC00470. A: the analysis of protein coding potential of LINC00470 using tools provided by the Peking University Center for Bioinformatics (cpc.cbi.pku.edu.cn/programs/run_cpc.jsp) shows LINC00470 lack of protein-coding capability. B: plasmids as schematically shown at left were transfected to HEK293 cells (right). Immunoblotting using antibody specific to ERK and fluorescent imaging showed that LINC0040-EGFP plasmid did not express GFP. (DOCX 755 kb)

Additional file 2: The relationship between LINC00470, AKT, and p-AKT. A: RT-qPCR and Western blotting measured the expression of LINC00470 and AKT in GBM cell lines and primary GBM cells. Data presented as mean ± S.E.M. of three independent experiments. B: Western blotting measured the expression of AKT and p-AKT in GBM cell lines and primary

GBM cells. Data showed positive correlation between the expression of LINC00470 and p-AKT in GBM. (DOCX 302 kb)

Additional file 3: Effect of LINC00470 knockdown in GBM cells. RT-qPCR measured the expression of LINC00470 in GBM cell lines and primary GBM cells. Data presented as mean ± S.E.M. of three independent experiments. (DOCX 168 kb)

Additional file 4: The expression of PI3K in GBM cells. The expression of PI3K was measured by Western blotting in GBM cells. (DOCX 204 kb)

Additional file 5: The associate between LINC00470, FUS, and AKT in U87 cells. A: the interaction of LINC00470 and FUS was detected through RIP assays in U87 cells. Data are presented as the mean ± S.E.M. of three independent experiments. **$p < 0.01$. B: RNA pulldown showed binding between LINC00470 and FUS. Data are presented as the mean ± S.E.M. of three independent experiments. C: RIP assays showed that there was no interaction between LINC00470 and AKT in U87 cells. Data are presented as the mean ± S.E.M. of three independent experiments. (DOCX 264 kb)

Additional file 6: LINC00470, FUS, and AKT can form a ternary complex in U251 cells. The expression levels of LINC00470, AKT, and FUS were measured by RT-qPCR and Western blotting, respectively. Data presented as mean ± S.E.M. of three independent experiments. (DOCX 1262 kb)

Additional file 7: The expression levels of LINC00470 in GBM cells. The expression levels of LINC00470 were measured by RT-qPCR. Data presented as mean ± S.E.M. of three independent experiments. (DOCX 129 kb)

Additional file 8: LINC00470 promoted GBM cell proliferation. CCK8 assay was performed to determine the viability of primary GBM cells. Primary GBM cells were transfected with si-NC and si-LINC00470, pcDNA3.1, and pcDNA3.1-LINC00470, respectively.*$p < 0.05$, **$p < 0.01$. (DOCX 935 kb)

Abbreviations
ANOVA: Analysis of variance; CCK-8: Cell counting kit-8; cDNA: Complementary deoxyribonucleic acid; Co-IP: Co-immunoprecipitation; GBM: Glioblastoma; GFP: Green fluorescent protein; LINC00470: Long intergenic non-protein coding RNA 470; RFP: Red fluorescent protein; RT-qPCR: Quantitative real-time polymerase chain reaction; siRNA: Small interference RNA

Acknowledgements
The authors thank Ph.D. WeiGuo Ren for his kind help in plasmid construction and Ph.D. Gang Xu and ZeYou Wang for their excellent technical assistance.

Funding
This work was supported by the National Science Foundation of China under grant number 81272297, National Key Technology Research and Development program of the Ministry of Science and Technology of China under grant number 2014BAI04B02, 111 Project under grant number 111-2, and Graduate Research and Innovation Projects of Central South University under grant number 2017zzts012.

Authors' contributions
MW and CL designed the study. CL, YZ, XS, PL, JF, HF, and CZ conducted the experiments. QL and QL acquired and managed patients and provided facilities. MW and CL wrote the article. FL revised of the manuscript. All authors read and approved the final manuscript.

Competing interests
The authors declare that they have no competing interests.

Author details
[1]Hunan Provincial Tumor Hospital and the Affiliated Tumor Hospital of Xiangya Medical School, Central South University, Changsha 410006, Hunan, China. [2]Cancer Research Institute, School of Basic Medical Science, Central South University, Changsha 410078, Hunan, China. [3]Key Laboratory of Carcinogenesis and Cancer Invasion, Ministry of Education, Changsha 410078, Hunan, China. [4]Key Laboratory of Carcinogenesis, Ministry of Health, Changsha 410078, Hunan, China. [5]Second Xiangya Hospital, Central South University, Changsha 410011, Hunan, China. [6]Department of Biochemistry, University of California, Riverside, CA 92521, USA. [7]Xiangya Hospital, Central South University, Changsha 410008, Hunan, China. [8]Third Xiangya Hospital, Central South University, Changsha 410013, Hunan, China.

References

1. Wang RC, Wei Y, An Z, Zou Z, Xiao G, Bhagat G, et al. Akt-mediated regulation of autophagy and tumorigenesis through Beclin 1 phosphorylation. Science. 2012;338:956–9.

2. Manning BD, Toker AAKT. PKB Signaling: Navigating the Network. Cell. 2017;169:381–405.

3. Vasudevan KM, Garraway LA. AKT signaling in physiology and disease. Curr Top Microbiol Immunol. 2010;347:105–33.

4. Massihnia D, Avan A, Funel N, Maftouh M, van Krieken A, Granchi C, et al. Phospho-Akt overexpression is prognostic and can be used to tailor the synergistic interaction of Akt inhibitors with gemcitabine in pancreatic cancer. J Hematol Oncol. 2017;10:9.

5. Zhang Y, Kwok-Shing NP, Kucherlapati M, Chen F, Liu Y, Tsang YH, et al. A Pan-Cancer Proteogenomic Atlas of PI3K/AKT/mTOR Pathway Alterations. Cancer Cell. 2017;31:820–32.

6. Fan CD, Lum MA, Xu C, Black JD, Wang X. Ubiquitin-dependent regulation of phospho-AKT dynamics by the ubiquitin E3 ligase, NEDD4-1, in the insulin-like growth factor-1 response. J Biol Chem. 2013;288:1674–84.

7. Delaloge S, DeForceville L. Targeting PI3K/AKT pathway in triple-negative breast cancer. Lancet Oncol. 2017;18:1293–4.

8. Castel P, Ellis H, Bago R, Toska E, Razavi P, Carmona FJ, et al. PDK1-SGK1 Signaling Sustains AKT-Independent mTORC1 Activation and Confers Resistance to PI3Kalpha Inhibition. Cancer Cell. 2016;30:229–42.

9. Miura H, Matsuda M, Aoki K. Development of a FRET biosensor with high specificity for Akt. Cell Struct Funct. 2014;39:9–20.

10. Gao X, Lowry PR, Zhou X, Depry C, Wei Z, Wong GW, et al. PI3K/Akt signaling requires spatial compartmentalization in plasma membrane microdomains. Proc Natl Acad Sci U S A. 2011;108:14509–14.

11. Li T, Wang G. Computer-aided targeting of the PI3K/Akt/mTOR pathway: toxicity reduction and therapeutic opportunities. Int J Mol Sci. 2014;15:18856–91.

12. Wang R, Brattain MG. AKT can be activated in the nucleus. Cell Signal. 2006;18:1722–31.

13. Zhan L, Wang T, Li W, Xu ZC, Sun W, Xu E. Activation of Akt/FoxO signaling pathway contributes to induction of neuroprotection against transient global cerebral ischemia by hypoxic pre-conditioning in adult rats. J Neurochem. 2010;114:897–908.

14. Farhan M, Wang H, Gaur U, Little PJ, Xu J, Zheng WFOXO. Signaling Pathways as Therapeutic Targets in Cancer. Int J Biol Sci. 2017;13:815–27.

15. Gutierrez A, Look AT. NOTCH and PI3K-AKT pathways intertwined. Cancer Cell. 2007;12:411–3.

16. Itoh Y, Higuchi M, Oishi K, Kishi Y, Okazaki T, Sakai H, et al. PDK1-Akt pathway regulates radial neuronal migration and microtubules in the developing mouse neocortex. Proc Natl Acad Sci U S A. 2016;113:E2955–64.

17. Zhao L, Shan Y, Liu B, Li Y, Jia L. Functional screen analysis reveals miR-3142 as central regulator in chemoresistance and proliferation through activation of the PTEN-AKT pathway in CML. Cell Death Dis. 2017;8:e2830.

18. Fang Y, Xue JL, Shen Q, Chen J, Tian L. MicroRNA-7 inhibits tumor growth and metastasis by targeting the phosphoinositide 3-kinase/Akt pathway in hepatocellular carcinoma. Hepatology. 2012;55:1852–62.

19. Sun X, Li J, Sun Y, Zhang Y, Dong L, Shen C, et al. miR-7 reverses the resistance to BRAFi in melanoma by targeting EGFR/IGF-1R/CRAF and inhibiting the MAPK and PI3K/AKT signaling pathways. Oncotarget. 2016;7:53558–70.

20. Zhou F, Nie L, Feng D, Guo S, Luo R. MicroRNA-379 acts as a tumor suppressor in non-small cell lung cancer by targeting the IGF1R-mediated AKT and ERK pathways. Oncol Rep. 2017;38:1857–66.

21. Yang HH, Chen Y, Gao CY, Cui ZT, Yao JM. Protective Effects of MicroRNA-126 on Human Cardiac Microvascular Endothelial Cells Against Hypoxia/Reoxygenation-Induced Injury and Inflammatory Response by Activating PI3K/Akt/eNOS Signaling Pathway. Cell Physiol Biochem. 2017;42:506–18.

22. Lin A, Hu Q, Li C, Xing Z, Ma G, Wang C, et al. The LINK-A lncRNA interacts with PtdIns(3,4,5)P3 to hyperactivate AKT and confer resistance to AKT inhibitors. Nat Cell Biol. 2017;19:238–51.

23. Yang N, Chen J, Zhang H, Wang X, Yao H, Peng Y, et al. LncRNA OIP5-AS1 loss-induced microRNA-410 accumulation regulates cell proliferation and apoptosis by targeting KLF10 via activating PTEN/PI3K/AKT pathway in multiple myeloma. Cell Death Dis. 2017;8:e2975.

24. Jin Y, Feng SJ, Qiu S, Shao N, Zheng JH. LncRNA MALAT1 promotes proliferation and metastasis in epithelial ovarian cancer via the PI3K-AKT pathway. Eur Rev Med Pharmacol Sci. 2017;21:3176–84.

25. Xing Z, Lin A, Li C, Liang K, Wang S, Liu Y, et al. lncRNA directs cooperative epigenetic regulation downstream of chemokine signals. Cell. 2014;159:1110–25.

26. Chen LL. Linking Long Noncoding RNA Localization and Function. Trends Biochem Sci. 2016;41:761–72.

27. Quinn JJ, Chang HY. Unique features of long non-coding RNA biogenesis and function. Nat Rev Genet. 2016;17:47–62.

28. Rinn JL, Chang HY. Genome regulation by long noncoding RNAs. Annu Rev Biochem. 2012;81:145–66.

29. Goff LA, Rinn JL. Linking RNA biology to lncRNAs. Genome Res. 2015;25:1456–65.

30. Wang KC, Yang YW, Liu B, Sanyal A, Corces-Zimmerman R, Chen Y, et al. A long noncoding RNA maintains active chromatin to coordinate homeotic gene expression. Nature. 2011;472:120–4.

31. Flynn RA, Chang HY. Long noncoding RNAs in cell-fate programming and reprogramming. Cell Stem Cell. 2014;14:752–61.

32. Wu H, Yin QF, Luo Z, Yao RW, Zheng CC, Zhang J, et al. Unusual Processing Generates SPA LncRNAs that Sequester Multiple RNA Binding Proteins. Mol Cell. 2016;64:534–48.

33. Stohr H, Mah N, Schulz HL, Gehrig A, Frohlich S, Weber BH. EST mining of the UniGene dataset to identify retina-specific genes. Cytogenet Cell Genet. 2000;91:267–77.

34. Ota T, Suzuki Y, Nishikawa T, Otsuki T, Sugiyama T, Irie R, et al. Complete sequencing and characterization of 21,243 full-length human cDNAs. Nat Genet. 2004;36:40–5.

35. Liu C, Sun Y, She X, Tu C, Cheng X, Wang L, et al. CASC2c as an unfavorable prognosis factor interacts with miR-101 to mediate astrocytoma tumorigenesis. Cell Death Dis. 2017;8:e2639.

36. Yu Z, Sun Y, She X, Wang Z, Chen S, Deng Z, et al. SIX3, a tumor suppressor, inhibits astrocytoma tumorigenesis by transcriptional repression of AURKA/B. J Hematol Oncol. 2017;10:115.

37. Xiaoping L, Zhibin Y, Wenjuan L, Zeyou W, Gang X, Zhaohui L, et al. CPEB1, a histone-modified hypomethylated gene, is regulated by miR-101 and involved in cell senescence in glioma. Cell Death Dis. 2013;4:e675.

38. Nakaya T, Alexiou P, Maragkakis M, Chang A, Mourelatos Z. FUS regulates genes coding for RNA-binding proteins in neurons by binding to their highly conserved introns. Rna. 2013;19:498–509.

39. Kovar H. Dr. Jekyll and Mr. Hyde: The Two Faces of the FUS/EWS/TAF15 Protein Family. Sarcoma. 2011;2011:837474.

40. Lagier-Tourenne C, Polymenidou M, Hutt KR, Vu AQ, Baughn M, Huelga SC, et al. Divergent roles of ALS-linked proteins FUS/TLS and TDP-43 intersect in processing long pre-mRNAs. Nat Neurosci. 2012;15:1488–97.

41. Le Grand M, Berges R, Pasquier E, Montero MP, Borge L, Carrier A, et al. Akt targeting as a strategy to boost chemotherapy efficacy in non-small cell lung cancer through metabolism suppression. Sci Rep. 2017;7:45136.

42. Han F, Xiao QQ, Peng S, Che XY, Jiang LS, Shao Q, et al. Atorvastatin ameliorates LPS-induced inflammatory response by autophagy via AKT/mTOR signaling pathway. J Cell Biochem. 2018;119:1604–15.

43. Mo Q, Hu L, Weng J, Zhang Y, Zhou Y, Xu R, et al. Euptox A Induces G1 Arrest and Autophagy via p38 MAPK- and PI3K/Akt/mTOR-Mediated Pathways in Mouse Splenocytes. J Histochem Cytochem. 2017;65:543–58.

44. Liu C, Liu Z, Li X, Tang X, He J, Lu S. MicroRNA-1297 contributes to tumor growth of human breast cancer by targeting PTEN/PI3K/AKT signaling. Oncol Rep. 2017;38:2435–43.

45. Smith TA. Mammalian hexokinases and their abnormal expression in cancer. Br J Biomed Sci. 2000;57:170–8.

46. Yoshida GJ. Therapeutic strategies of drug repositioning targeting autophagy to induce cancer cell death: from pathophysiology to treatment. J Hematol Oncol. 2017;10:67.
47. Fulda S. Targeting autophagy for the treatment of cancer. Biol Chem. 2018; [Epub ahead of print]
48. Liu X, Chong Y, Tu Y, Liu N, Yue C, Qi Z, et al. CRM1/XPO1 is associated with clinical outcome in glioma and represents a therapeutic target by perturbing multiple core pathways. J Hematol Oncol. 2016;9:108.
49. Akinleye A, Avvaru P, Furqan M, Song Y, Liu D. Phosphatidylinositol 3-kinase (PI3K) inhibitors as cancer therapeutics. J Hematol Oncol. 2013;6:88.
50. Liu D, Zhu Y, Pang J, Weng X, Feng X, Guo Y. Knockdown of long non-coding RNA MALAT1 inhibits growth and motility of human hepatoma cells via modulation of miR-195. J Cell Biochem. 2018;119:1368–80.
51. Chen SW, Zhu J, Ma J, Zhang JL, Zuo S, Chen GW, et al. Overexpression of long non-coding RNA H19 is associated with unfavorable prognosis in patients with colorectal cancer and increased proliferation and migration in colon cancer cells. Oncol Lett. 2017;14:2446–52.
52. Zinszner H, Sok J, Immanuel D, Yin Y, Ron D. TLS (FUS) binds RNA in vivo and engages in nucleo-cytoplasmic shuttling. J Cell Sci. 1997;110(Pt 15): 1741–50.
53. Tan AY, Manley JL. TLS/FUS: a protein in cancer and ALS. Cell Cycle. 2012;11: 3349–50.

12

Ex vivo and in vivo T cell-depleted allogeneic stem cell transplantation in patients with acute myeloid leukemia in first complete remission resulted in similar overall survival: on behalf of the ALWP of the EBMT and the MSKCC

Florent Malard[1,2]* (iD), Myriam Labopin[1], Christina Cho[3,4], Didier Blaise[5], Esperanza B. Papadopoulos[3,4], Jakob Passweg[6], Richard O'Reilly[7,8], Edouard Forcade[9], Molly Maloy[3], Liisa Volin[10], Hugo Castro-Malaspina[3,4], Yosr Hicheri[11], Ann A. Jakubowski[3,4], Corentin Orvain[12], Sergio Giralt[3,4], Mohamad Mohty[1,2], Arnon Nagler[13,14] and Miguel-Angel Perales[3,4,15]*

Abstract

Background: Graft-versus-host disease (GVHD) is one of the leading causes of non-relapse mortality and morbidity after allogeneic hematopoietic stem cell transplantation (allo-HCT).

Methods: We evaluated the outcomes of two well-established strategies used for GVHD prevention: in vivo T cell depletion using antithymocyte globulin (ATG) and ex vivo T cell depletion using a CD34-selected (CD34+) graft. A total of 525 adult patients (363 ATG, 162 CD34+) with intermediate or high-risk cytogenetics acute myeloid leukemia (AML) in first complete remission (CR1) were included. Patients underwent myeloablative allo-HCT using matched related or unrelated donors.

Results: Two-year overall survival estimate was 69.9% (95% CI, 58.5–69.4) in the ATG group and 67.6% (95% CI, 60.3–74.9) in the CD34+ group ($p = 0.31$). The cumulative incidence of grade II–IV acute GVHD and chronic GVHD was higher in the ATG cohort [HR 2.0 (95% CI 1.1–3.7), $p = 0.02$; HR 15.1 (95% CI 5.3–42.2), $p < 0.0001$]. Parameters associated with a lower GVHD-free relapse-free survival (GRFS) were ATG [HR 1.6 (95% CI 1.1–2.2), $p = 0.006$], adverse cytogenetic [HR 1.7 (95% CI 1.3–2.2), $p = 0.0004$], and the use of an unrelated donor [HR 1.4 (95% CI 1.0–1.9), $p = 0.02$]. There were no statistical differences between ATG and CD34+ in terms of relapse [HR 1.52 (95% CI 0.96–2.42), $p = 0.07$], non-relapse mortality [HR 0.96 (95% CI 0.54–1.74), $p = 0.90$], overall survival [HR 1.43 (95% CI 0.97–2.11), $p = 0.07$], and leukemia-free survival [HR 1.25 (95% CI 0.88–1.78), $p = 0.21$]. Significantly, more deaths related to infection occurred in the CD34+ group (16/52 vs. 19/112, $p = 0.04$).

Conclusions: These data suggest that both ex vivo CD34-selected and in vivo ATG T cell depletion are associated with a rather high OS and should be compared in a prospective randomized trial.

Keywords: Acute myeloid leukemia, T cell depletion, CD34-selected graft, Antithymocyte globulin, Allogeneic hematopoietic cell transplantation

* Correspondence: malardf@yahoo.fr; peralesm@mskcc.org
[1]Service d'Hématologie Clinique et Thérapie Cellulaire, AP-HP, Hôpital Saint-Antoine, Paris F-75012, France
[3]Adult Bone Marrow Transplantation Service, Memorial Sloan Kettering Cancer Center, New York, NY, USA
Full list of author information is available at the end of the article

Background

Allogeneic hematopoietic stem cell transplantation (allo-HCT) is the only potentially curative post-remission consolidation treatment for high-risk acute myeloid leukemia (AML) patients [1, 2]. However, preparative regimen-related toxicities and graft-versus-host disease (GVHD) have limited its widespread use. In particular, chronic GVHD (cGVHD) remains the leading cause of late non-relapse mortality (NRM) and morbidity after allo-HCT. Furthermore, the increasing use of G-CSF mobilized peripheral blood stem cells (PBSC) [3], a well-identified risk factor for chronic GVHD [4, 5], is associated with an increased incidence of cGVHD [3, 6]. Therefore, identification of the most effective prevention of GVHD is required to improve patients' outcome after allo-HCT, particularly in the setting of PBSC transplantation.

In vivo graft manipulation with antithymocyte globulin (ATG) [7–13] or alemtuzumab [14] and ex vivo graft manipulation with CD34 selection and T cell depletion [15–19] are strategies that are associated with lower rates of chronic GVHD. Since 2000, five phase III randomized trials have investigated the efficacy of rabbit ATG for GVHD prophylaxis in patients who received myeloablative (MAC) allo-HCT from unrelated or HLA-identical matched donors [7–13]. In all these studies, the use of ATG was associated with a protective effect against cGVHD and in all but one study [12], overall survival (OS) and progression-free survival were not significantly affected [13]. Therefore, in vivo T cell depletion using ATG is now considered a standard for GVHD prevention after PBSC transplantation using related HLA-identical or unrelated donors in many centers. On the other hand, several studies have shown that the use of ex vivo T cell-depleted (TCD) grafts combined with ATG significantly reduces the risk of GVHD without the need for post-transplant immunosuppression [16, 20, 21]. Although several different approaches for T cell depletion of the allograft have been used over the years, more recently, removal of T cells from the graft has routinely been performed through positive selection of CD34+ cells using immunomagnetic beads [22]. To date, no study has compared outcomes in AML patients after myeloablative allo-HCT with ex vivo TCD using CD34 selection or in vivo TCD using ATG. To compare the efficacy of both approaches, we retrospectively evaluated the outcomes of patients with intermediate or high-risk AML in first complete remission (CR1) who underwent myeloablative allo-HCT with either in vivo TCD with ATG within the European group for Blood and Marrow Transplantation (EBMT) centers or ex vivo TCD CD34 selected (CD34+) graft at the Memorial Sloan Kettering Cancer Center (MSKCC).

Methods

Study design and data collection

This retrospective multicenter analysis was performed and approved by the Acute Leukemia Working Party (ALWP) of the EBMT group registry and the institutional review board of the MSKCC. A list of the EBMT participating centers is available online (Additional file 1). The study included all adult patients (age > 18 years) with AML, with intermediate or high-risk cytogenetic, in first morphological CR, who received an in vivo or ex vivo T cell-depleted myeloablative allo-HCT from an HLA matched related (MRD) or unrelated (UD) donor using a peripheral blood stem cell graft between 2005 and 2015. Cytogenetics were classified according to the European Leukemia Net [23]. All allografts were obtained from HLA-A-, HLA-B-, HLA-C-, and HLA-DRB1-matched donors. All patients underwent myeloablative conditioning. Patients at MSKCC received ex vivo TCD graft (CD34+ group, n = 162) after conditioning with one of the following preparative regimens as previously reported: (1) i.v. busulfan (Bu) 0.8 mg/kg/dose for 10 or 12 doses over a 4-day period, melphalan 70 mg/m^2/day for 2 days, and i.v. fludarabine (Flu) 25 mg/m^2/day for 5 days (n = 107); (2) hyperfractionated total body irradiation (TBI) 13.75 Gy over 4 days followed by i.v. thiotepa 5 mg/kg/day for 2 days and i.v. cyclophosphamide (Cy) 60 mg/kg/day for 2 days (n = 45) or i.v. Flu 25 mg/m^2/day for 5 days (n = 10). Peripheral blood grafts underwent CD34 cell selection using the ISOLEX 300i magnetic cell selection system (Baxter, Deerfield, IL), followed by sheep red blood cell-rosette depletion (Isolex-E, n = 53); or CD34+ selection using the CliniMACS CD34 Reagent System (Miltenyi Biotech, Gladbach, Germany) (n = 109). The two approaches provide a similar level of T cell depletion (log10 5.3 with Isolex-E vs. 5.1 with CliniMACS, Jakubowski et al., in preparation). All patients received equine ATG (30 mg/kg total dose, n = 12) or rabbit ATG (thymoglobulin 5 mg/kg total dose, n = 143) to prevent graft rejection, except for those patients receiving a transplant from an HLA-matched related donor and conditioned with hyperfractionated TBI, thiotepa, and Flu (n = 7). No GVHD prophylaxis was administered post-transplantation.

Within the EBMT centers, patients received unmodified grafts and in vivo T cell depletion using rabbit ATG (group ATG, n = 363) after one of the following preparative regimens: (1) Bu 9.6–12.8 mg/kg total dose and i.v. fludarabine (n = 173), (2) Bu 9.6–12.8 mg/kg total dose and i.v. Cy 100–120 mg/kg total dose (n = 129), or (3) high-dose TBI and i.v. Cy 100–120 mg/kg total dose (n = 61). Patients received either thymoglobulin (n = 233) or grafalon (formerly ATG-fresenius, n = 130) for prevention of graft rejection and of GVHD. These patients received post-HCT GVHD prophylaxis consisting of cyclosporine alone (n = 62) or in combination with methotrexate (n = 213) or mycophenolate mofetil (n =

60), tacrolimus in combination with methotrexate ($n = 2$) or sirolimus ($n = 10$) or other combinations ($n = 16$).

Supportive care and antimicrobial prophylaxis were administered according to standard guidelines and include infection prophylaxis for *Pneumocystis jirovecii* and herpes virus. All patients were assessed at least once per week for cytomegalovirus (CMV) and Epstein-Barr virus (EBV) reactivation in the peripheral blood by polymerase chain reaction, to initiate preemptive therapy [24].

Statistical analysis

Endpoints included OS, leukemia-free survival (LFS), cumulative incidence of relapse, NRM, acute and chronic GVHD, and refined GVHD-free relapse-free survival (GRFS) [25]. All outcomes were measured from the time of allo-HCT. OS was based on death, regardless of the cause. LFS was defined as survival with no evidence of relapse. OS and LFS rates were calculated by the Kaplan-Meier estimator. Cumulative incidence functions were used to estimate the probabilities of acute and chronic GVHD, NRM, relapse, and GRFS to accommodate competing risks. NRM and relapse were the competing risks for each other. Patients alive without relapse were censored at the time of last contact. For acute and chronic GVHD, the competing risk was death without the event. For refined GRFS, the events were relapse, grade III–IV acute GVHD, or extensive cGVHD and the competing risk was death without the events [25]. Acute GVHD was defined according to the standard criteria [26]. Due to the retrospective nature of this analysis, NIH cGVHD classification [27] was not available for EBMT centers; therefore, Shulman et al. classification (limited versus extensive) [28] was used for all patients.

Patients' characteristics were compared between the CD34+ and the ATG groups using the chi-square test or the Fisher exact test for categorical variables and the Mann-Whitney test for continuous data. Univariate analyses were performed using the log-rank test for OS and LFS and Gray's test for cumulative incidences. Chronic GVHD was analyzed as a time-dependent variable. For multivariate regression, a Cox proportional hazards model was built. Impact of age was analyzed per decade. Results were expressed as hazard ratio (HR) with 95% confidence interval (CI). All tests were two-sided and the type-1 error rate was fixed at 0.05. Statistical analyses were performed with SPSS 19 (SPSS Inc. /IBM, Armonk, NY) and R 3.0.1 (R Development Core Team, Vienna, Austria) software packages.

Results

Patient and donor characteristics

Patients and transplant characteristics are summarized in Table 1. Patients, in the CD34+ group who were significantly older, were more likely to have a matched related

donor and a Karnofsky performance status < 90% compared to the ATG group. There were no statistically significant differences between groups regarding donor and patient gender, CMV serological status, and cytogenetic risk factor. The median follow-up among surviving patients was 35.4 (range, 2–139) months and was significantly longer in the CD34+ group, 58 (range, 6–139) months, compared to that in the ATG group, 24.5 (range, 2–131) months ($p < 0.001$). As a result, all patients were censored at 2 years for the comparison between groups.

Engraftment

Engraftment was achieved in 362/363 patients (99.7%) in the ATG and 159/162 (98.1%) in the CD34+ group ($p = 0.06$). The median time to neutrophil recovery was significantly longer in the ATG group: 16 (range, 6–34) days compared with 10 (range, 8–20) days in the CD34+ group ($p < 0.0001$).

Overall survival and leukemia-free survival

Univariate and multivariate analyses of transplantation-related events are summarized in Tables 2 and 3, respectively. The Kaplan-Meier estimate of OS at 2 years was 63.9% (95% CI, 58.5–69.4) in the ATG group and 67.6% (95% CI, 60.3–74.9) in the CD34+ group ($p = 0.31$, Fig. 1a). In multivariate analysis, there was no significant difference in OS between the TBI group and the Bu group (HR, 1.43; 95% CI, 0.97–2.11; $p = 0.07$). The only parameters with a significant impact on OS in multivariate analysis were patients' age and cytogenetic status. OS was significantly lower in patients with poor as compared to intermediate-risk cytogenetics (HR, 1.16; 95% CI, 1.11–2.19; $p = 0.009$) and in older patients (HR, 1.15; 95% CI, 1.00–1.34; $p = 0.049$). The Kaplan-Meier estimate of LFS at 2 years was 57.9% (95% CI, 52.4–63.4) in the ATG group and 61.0% (95% CI, 53.4–68.5) in the CD34+ group ($p = 0.29$, Fig. 1b). In multivariate analysis, there was no significant difference in LFS between the ATG and the CD34+ groups (HR, 1.25; 95% CI, 0.88–1.78; $p = 0.21$). The only parameter with a significant impact on LFS in multivariate analysis was cytogenetic status. LFS was significantly lower in patients with poor compared to those with intermediate risk cytogenetics (HR, 1.70; 95% CI, 1.26–2.31).

Relapse

At 2 years, the cumulative incidence of relapse was 30.0% (95% CI, 24.9–35.2) in the ATG group and 21.6% (95% CI, 15.6–28.3) in the CD34+ group ($p = 0.03$, Fig. 1c). In multivariate analysis, there was a trend toward a higher cumulative incidence of relapse in the ATG group (HR, 1.52; 95% CI, 0.96–2.42; $p = 0.07$). The only parameter with a significant impact on relapse incidence in multivariate analysis was cytogenetic risk status: relapse was significantly increased

Table 1 Study population characteristics

Characteristic (%)	ATG (N = 363)	CD34 (N = 162)	p
Patient age, median (range)	46 (19–77)	58 (20–73)	< 0.001
Year of transplant	2012 (2005–2015)	2011 (2005–2015)	
Patient gender			
Male	200 (55%)	90 (56%)	0.92
Female	163 (45%)	72 (44%)	
Female donor to male patient	65 (18%)	37 (23%)	0.19
Karnofsky performance scale			
≥ 90%	258 (76%)	100 (63%)	0.003
< 90%	83 (24%)	59 (37%)	
unknown	22	3	
CMV serologic status			
Seronegative donor-recipient pair	114 (32%)	49 (33%)	0.4
Time from diagnosis to transplant, months (range)	4.9 (1.9–14.3)	4.3 (1.7–11.4)	0.001
Cytogenetic			
Intermediate	259 (71%)	112 (69%)	0.61
Poor	104 (29%)	50 (31%)	
Donor			
Matched related donor	118 (33%)	73 (45%)	0.006
Unrelated donor	245 (67%)	89 (55%)	
Conditioning regimen			
Busulfan + fludarabine	173 (48%)	0	< 0.0001
Busulfan + cycloclophosphamide	129 (36%)	0	
TBI + cyclophosphamide	61 (17%)	0	
Busulafan + fludarabine + melphalan	0	107 (66%)	
TBI + cycloclophosphamide + thiotepa	0	45 (28%)	
TBI + fludarabine + thiotepa	0	10 (6%)	
GVHD prophylaxis			
CsA	62 (17%)	–	–
CsA + MMF	210 (58%)	–	
CsA + MTX	65* (18%)	–	
Tacrolimus + sirolimus	10 (3%)	–	
PT Cy	5 (1%)	–	
Others	11 (3%)	–	
Antithymocyte globuline			
Thymoglobulin (median dose, mg/kg; range)	233 (5; 5–7.5)	143 (5; 2–5)	
Grafalon, (median dose, mg/kg; range)	130 (35; 8–60)	0	
Equine ATG, (median dose, mg/kg; range)	0	12 (30; 15–30)	–
Cells doses			
CD34+ cells, × 10^6/kg (range)	6.13 (1.64–21.2)	8.18 (1.1–31.2)	< 0.0001
CD 3+ cells, × 10^6/kg (range)	213 (1.13–643)	0.002 (0–0.063)	< 0.0001

Abbreviations: TBI total body irradiation, *GVHD* graft versus host disease, *CsA* ciclosporine A, *MMF* mycophenolate mofetil, *PT Cy* post-transplant cyclophosphamide, *NA* not available

*In two patients, CsA have been substituted by tacrolimus

Table 2 Transplant-related events univariate analysis

Characteristic (%)	ATG (N = 363)	CD34 (N = 162)	p
OS at 2 years, months (95% CI)	69.9 (58.5–69.4)	67.6 (60.3–74.8)	0.31
LFS at 2 years, months (95% CI)	57.9 (52.4–63.4)	61.0 (53.4–68.5)	0.29
Cumulative incidence of NRM at 2 years (95% CI)	12.1 (8.9–15.9)	17.4 (12.0–23.6)	0.16
Cumulative incidence of relapse at 2 years (95% CI)	30.0 (24.9–35,2)	21.6 (15.6–28.3)	0.03
Cumulative incidence of grade II–IV aGVHD at 100 days (95% CI)	21.2 (17.1–25.6)	11.3 (7.0–16.8)	0.006
Cumulative incidence of grade III–IV aGVHD at 100 days (95% CI)	6.2 (4–9.1)	1.3 (0.2–4.1)	0.01
Cumulative incidence of cGVHD at 1 year (95% CI)	27.6 (22.8–32.6)	2.5 (0.8–5.8)	< 0.0001
Cumulative incidence of extensive cGVHD at 1 year (95% CI)	11.3 (8.0–15.1)	2.5 (0.8–5.8)	0.001
Cumulative incidence of GRFS at 2 years (95% CI)	47.0 (41.4–52.5)	59.1 (51.5–66.7)	0.003
Cause of death			
GVHD	14 (12%)	5 (10%)	0.36
Infections	19 (17%)	16 (30%)	
Other	20 (18%)	7 (14%)	
Relapse/progression	59 (53%)	24 (46%)	

Abbreviations: *OS* overall survival, *CI* confidence interval. *LFS* leukemia-free survival, *NRM* non-relapse mortality, *aGVHD* acute graft-versus-host disease, *cGVHD* chronic graft versus host disease

in patients with poor compared to intermediate risk cytogenetics (HR, 2.10; 95% CI, 1.46–3.03; $p < 0.0001$). Therefore, a subgroup analysis was performed to separately analyze patients with intermediate and high-risk cytogenetic. In patients with intermediate risk cytogenetic, the 2-year cumulative incidence of relapse was significantly higher in the ATG group compare to the CD34+ group [25.0% (95% CI, 19.5–30.6) versus 11.6% (95% CI, 6.5–18.4)]. In multivariate analysis, TCD approach was the only parameter with an impact on relapse with a significantly higher cumulative incidence of relapse in the ATG group (HR, 2.42; 95% CI, 1.22–4.78; $p = 0.01$). In contrast, in the subgroup of patients with high-risk cytogenetic, TCD approach has no impact on the cumulative incidence of relapse [42.7% (95% CI, 32.1–53.0) in the ATG group versus 44.0% (95% CI, 29.9–57.3)].

Graft-versus-host disease

The day-100 cumulative incidence of grade II–IV and grade III–IV aGVHD were significantly higher in the ATG group, being 21.2% (95% CI, 17.1–25.6) and 6.2% (95% CI, 4–9.1), versus 11.3% (95% CI, 7.0–16.8) and 1.3% (95% CI, 0.2–4.1), respectively, in the CD34+ group ($p = 0.006$ and $p = 0.01$). In multivariate analysis, TCD approach was the only parameter with an impact on aGVHD. The cumulative incidence of grade II–IV aGVHD was significantly higher in the ATG group compared with the CD34+ group (HR, 2.05; 95% CI, 1.12–3.73; $p = 0.02$). At 1 year, the cumulative incidence of cGVHD and extensive cGVHD were significantly higher in the ATG group, being 27.6% and 11.3%, versus 2.5% and 2.5%, respectively, in the CD34+ group ($p < 0.0001$

and $p = 0.001$). In multivariate analysis, TCD approach was the only parameter with an impact on cGVHD. The cumulative incidence of cGVHD was significantly higher in the ATG group compared with the CD34+ group (HR, 15.07; 95% CI, 5.38–42.26; $p < 0.0001$).

Graft-versus-host disease-free relapse-free survival

At 2 years, the cumulative incidence of GRFS was significantly lower in the ATG group, being 47.0% (95% CI, 41.4–52.5) versus 59.1% (95% CI, 53.5–68.5) in the CD34+ groups ($p = 0.003$, Fig. 1d). In multivariate analysis, GRFS was significantly higher in the CD34+ group compared to the ATG group (HR, 1.60; 95% CI, 1.14–2.23; $p = 0.006$). In addition, cytogenetic status and type of donor were also associated with lower GRFS in multivariate analysis.

Non-relapse mortality

At 2 years, the cumulative incidence of NRM was 12.1% (95% CI, 8.9–15.9) in the ATG group and 17.4% (95% CI, 12.0–23.6) in the CD34+ group ($p = 0.16$, Fig. 1e). In multivariate analysis, there was no significant difference in NRM between the ATG and CD34+ groups (HR, 0.96; 95% CI, 0.54–1.74; $p = 0.90$). The only parameter with a significant impact on NRM incidence in multivariate analysis was patient age: NRM significantly increased in older patients (HR, 1.32; 95% CI, 1.03–1.68; $p = 0.02$). NRM was related mainly to infection ($n = 35$) and GVHD ($n = 19$), others causes being hemorrhage ($n = 2$), sinusoidal obstruction syndrome (SOS, $n = 4$), cardiac toxicity ($n = 1$), graft failure ($n = 2$), secondary malignancy ($n = 2$), others ($n = 13$), unknown ($n = 3$). Deaths related to infectious complication were significantly more frequent in the CD34+ group (16/28 versus 19/53 in ATG group, $p =$

Table 3 Transplant-related events multivariate analysis

Outcome	Hazard ratio (95% confidence interval)	p value
Overall survival		
ATG versus CD34	1.43 (0.97–2.11)	0.07
Age per 10 years	1.15 (1.00–1.34)	0.047
Poor versus intermediate cytogenetic	1.16 (1.11–2.19)	0.009
Unrelated versus related donor	1.23 (0.86–1.76)	0.27
Leukemia-free survival		
ATG versus CD34	1.25 (0.88–1.78)	0.21
Age per 10 years	1.03 (0.91–1.17)	0.60
Poor versus intermediate cytogenetic	1.70 (1.26–2.31)	0.0006
Unrelated versus related donor	1.22 (0.88–1.70)	0.23
Non-relapse mortality		
ATG versus CD34	0.96 (0.54–1.74)	0.90
Age per 10 years	1.32 (1.03–1.68)	0.02
Poor versus intermediate cytogenetic	1.08 (0.62–1.90)	0.77
Unrelated versus related donor	1.39 (0.8–2.42)	0.24
Relapse		
ATG versus CD34	1.52 (0.96–2.42)	0.07
Age per 10 years	0.93 (0.80–1.08)	0.31
Poor versus intermediate cytogenetic	2.10 (1.46–3.03)	< 0.0001
Unrelated versus related donor	1.10 (0.73–1.67)	0.63
Grade II-IV acute GVHD		
ATG versus CD34	2.05 (1.12–3.73)	0.02
Age per 10 years	0.99 (0.82–1.18)	0.87
Poor versus intermediate cytogenetic	0.90 (0.56–1.48)	0.66
Unrelated versus related donor	1.87 (1.12–3.09)	0.02
Chronic GVHD		
ATG versus CD34	15.07 (5.38–42.26)	< 0.0001
Age per 10 years	1.13 (0.94–1.36)	0.21
Poor versus intermediate cytogenetic	1.07 (0.66–1.74)	0.79
Unrelated versus related donor	1.58 (0.97–2.56)	0.07
GVHD-free relapse-free survival		
ATG versus CD34	1.60 (1.14–2.34)	0.006
Age per 10 years	1.01 (0.90–1.13)	0.88
Poor versus intermediate cytogenetic	1.65 (1.25–2.18)	0.0004
Unrelated versus related donor	1.42 (1.05–1.93)	0.02

Abbreviations: ATG antithymocyte globulin, *GVHD* graft-versus-host disease

0.045), while there was no difference between groups regarding death related to GVHD (5/28 in CD34+ versus 14/53 in ATG group, $p = 0.41$).

Donor lymphocyte infusion
Similar proportions of patients received DLI post-transplant in both cohorts. In the ATG T cell depletion cohort, 38 (10.5%) patients received DLI for the following indications: mixed chimerism in 8 patients,

relapse in 19 patients, and prophylaxis in 11 patients. In the CD34+ cohort, 19 (11.7%) patients received DLI. The indications were mixed chimerism in 9 patients, relapse in 7 patients, and infection in 3 patients (2 EBV and 1 HHV-6).

Discussion
The optimal goal of allo-HCT is to mediate graft-versus-tumor effect to achieve cure, while sparing

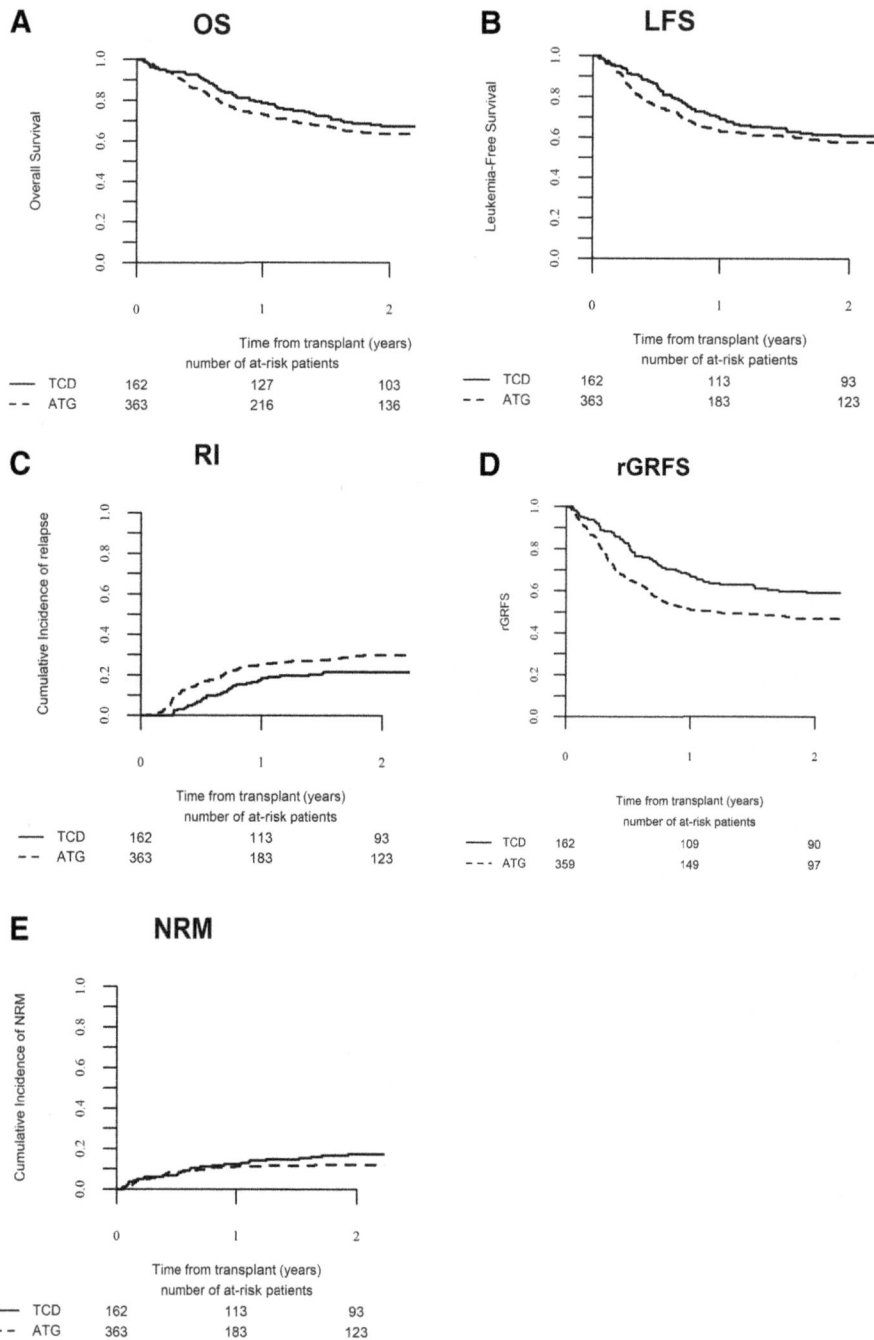

Fig. 1 Outcome after allo-HCT. Overall survival (**a**), leukemia-free survival (**b**), cumulative incidence of relapse (**c**), cumulative incidence of GVHD-free and relapse-free survival (**d**), and cumulative incidence of non-relapse mortality (**e**). OS, overall survival; LFS, leukemia-free survival; RI, relapse incidence, rGRFS, refined GVHD-free relapse-free survival; NRM, non-relapse mortality

patients from severe comorbidity. Over the last decade, patients' outcomes have improved significantly with an improved OS and decreased NRM [3]. However, despite this progress, there has been an increase in the incidence of cGVHD, the leading cause of late NRM and morbidity after allo-HCT [3, 6], associated with the use of unrelated donors and of PBSC grafts [4, 5]. Identification of the best strategy

for cGVHD prevention is of the utmost importance, and while TCD may be a potential strategy, there remains a concern that it may be at the expense of an increased incidence of relapse. The primary objective of this retrospective study was to assess the relative efficacy of two TCD approaches, in vitro TCD using ATG, and ex vivo TCD with CD34 selection, and showed high OS and LFS with both approaches in patients with AML in CR1 transplanted with matched donors after a MAC regimen.

Furthermore, our study confirms that TCD is associated with a low incidence of severe acute and chronic GVHD, with a day 100 cumulative incidence of grade III–IV aGVHD of 6.2% and 1.3% and a 1-year cumulative incidence of extensive cGVHD of 11.3% and 2.5% in the ATG and the CD34+ groups, respectively. The results in the ATG groups are in accordance with previously published prospective randomized trials, with an incidence of grade III–IV aGVHD ranging from 2.4 to 11.7% and an incidence of extensive or moderate to severe cGVHD between 5 and 13% [8–10, 12]. Similarly, in the CD34+ group, the cumulative incidence of severe grade III–IV aGVHD and extensive cGVHD compares favorably to data available from clinical trials. In a prospective randomized trial of ex vivo TCD, Wagner et al. reported a cumulative incidence of grade III–IV aGVHD and overall cGVHD of 19% and 29% [29]; however, TCD in that study was limited to 1 to 2 logs depletion. More recently, with the TCD techniques utilized by the MSKCC group that allow 3 to 4 logs of T cell depletion, Devine et al. reported a cumulative incidence of grade III–IV aGVHD and extensive cGVHD of 4.5% and 6.8%, respectively, in a multicenter prospective phase 2 trial [15]. Overall progress in ex vivo TCD techniques have achieved a very low incidence of GVHD, leading to a significantly lower cumulative incidence of both acute and chronic GVHD in the CD34+ group, translating in a higher GRFS in those patients. It should be noted that the use of CD34 selection incorporates ATG, which is primarily used to promote engraftment by abrogating host T cells, but likely has an effect on residual donor T cells in the CD34-selected graft. This potentially contributes to the low risk of GVHD as well as delayed immune recovery [30]. Finally, use of a matched unrelated donor remains associated with an increase incidence of grade II–IV aGVHD, while there was a trend toward a higher incidence of cGVHD in multivariate analysis, highlighting that TCD, either ex vivo or in vivo, does not completely overcome HLA barrier.

The increased incidence of GVHD seen in the ATG group does not translate in a higher cumulative incidence in NRM in those patients. In fact, there was no difference in the incidence of death related to GVHD between groups (12% in the ATG versus 10% in the CD34 groups), while there was more death related to infections in the CD34 group: 30% versus 17% in the ATG group. Delayed immune recovery after CD34-selected TCD allo-HCT contributes to an increase incidence of infectious complications, which may result in a lack of improvement in OS despite the low incidence of GVHD, compared to unmodified grafts [18, 30–36]. However, the median age in the CD34+ group was over a decade older than the ATG group. Age is a known risk factor for GVHD, NRM and delayed immune reconstitution, and the results of the study need to be considered in the context of this significant age difference between the cohorts.

While use of TCD was thought to be associated with an increase incidence of relapse, relapse incidence remains limited in our study, and no difference between groups was observed in multivariate analysis. This observation is probably related to the intensity of the conditioning regimen administered. Indeed, while in four out of six studies that include exclusively RIC regimen, ATG was associated with an increased risk of relapse, in studies that include MAC or MAC and RIC regimens together, no increase in relapse risk was reported [37]. Similarly, the MSKCC group recently reported a lower incidence of relapse using CD34-selected TCD allo-HCT with MAC compared to RIC [38]. In our study, while there were some differences in conditioning regimen between the two groups, all patients received a MAC regimen. Therefore, the incidences of relapse observed in our study are in accordance with previously published studies, despite the inclusion of one third of patients with poor risk cytogenetic status. Unfortunately, due to its retrospective nature being registry-based study, molecular characteristics were not available for all patients and we were not able to refine our analysis based on these parameters. In addition, the inhomogeneity of ATG doses used in our study may have interfered with patients' outcome. Indeed, while lower ATG exposure is thought to be associated with a higher risk of GVHD, high exposure may produce excessive T cell depletion, leading to delayed immune reconstitution with increased risk of relapse, but also higher NRM, mostly as a result of infections [13]. Therefore, Ayuk et al. reported that use of lower doses of grafalon (30 versus 60 mg/kg) was associated with a lower NRM but had no impact on chronic GVHD and relapse rate after MAC allo-HCT [39]. Furthermore, Locatelli et al. evaluated even lower doses of grafalon (15 versus 30 mg/kg) in a phase III trial and found that they were associated with an improved OS and progression-free survival without significantly increasing the incidence of GVHD [40]. Finally, ATG pharmacokinetics and pharmacodynamics may also have a significant impact on HCT outcomes. For example, while ATG dose is based on patients' weight, Admiraal et al. recently developed a pharmacokinetic model where absolute lymphocyte count at time of ATG administration was the only relevant predictor for ATG pharmacokinetics in adults [41]. Development of such approaches may help to further improve ATG safety and tolerability.

Our study does have some limitations, due in part to its retrospective nature and potential differences in supportive care. One limitation of our study is that all patients from the CD34+ group were treated in a single center highly experienced in this approach, while the ATG group was constituted from a multicenter-based registry. However, inclusion criteria were defined in order to constitute a cohort of patient as homogeneous as possible, CR1

AML patients with a matched donor that received rabbit ATG and a Bu-Cy, Bu-Flu, or Cy-TBI MAC regimen, in order to overcome this limitation and to reduce bias due to disease status and donor type on disease outcome.

Another potential limitation is the broader applicability of CD34 selection given the fact that all patients in the CD34 group were from a single center highly experienced in this approach. However, this approach has previously shown similar results in a multicenter phase 2 trial [15]. Furthermore, a randomized multicenter phase 3 trial is currently comparing this approach to post-transplant cyclophosphamide or tacrolimus and methotrexate in patients with acute leukemia and MDS receiving a MAC transplant from an 8/8 HLA-matched related or unrelated donor (NCT02345850).

Conclusions

Overall, our study shows that NRM, OS, and LFS are similar after ex vivo CD34-selected and in vivo ATG TCD MAC allo-HCT from related/unrelated donors in patients with AML in CR1 and intermediate/high-risk cytogenetic. Notably, the cumulative incidence of acute (total and severe) and chronic GVHD was higher after allo-HCT with ATG, leading to a lower GRFS in those patients. In contrast, stronger immunosuppression in the CD34+ group leads to a higher incidence of infectious related death. Given the high OS seen in patients with AML in CR1 with both approaches, they should be compared in a prospective randomized trial.

Additional file

> **Additional file 1:** List of EBMT contributing centers by decreasing number of patients enrolled in the study. (PDF 38 kb)

Abbreviations
allo-HCT: Allogeneic hematopoietic stem cell transplantation; ALWP: Acute Leukemia Working Party; AML: Acute myeloid leukemia; ATG: Antithymocyte globulin; Bu: Busulfan; cGVHD: Chronic graft-versus-host disease; Cy: Cyclophosphamide; EBMT: European group for Blood and Marrow Transplantation; Flu: Fludarabine; GRFS: GVHD-free relapse-free survival; GVHD: Graft-versus-host disease; HLA: Human leukocyte antigen; HR: Hazard ratio; LFS: Leukemia-free survival; MAC: Myeloablative; MRD: Matched related donor; MSKCC: Memorial Sloan Kettering Cancer Center; NRM: Non-relapse mortality; OS: Overall survival; PBSC: Peripheral blood stem cells; TBI: Total body irradiation; TCD: T cell-depleted; UD: Unrelated donor

Funding
This research was supported in part by National Institutes of Health award number P01 CA23766 and NIH/NCI Cancer Center Support Grant P30 CA008748. The content is solely the responsibility of the authors and does not necessarily represent the official views of the National Institutes of Health.

Authors' contributions
FM, ML, MM, AN, and MAP designed the research and/or analyzed the data. CC, DB, EBP, JP, RO, NM, MM, LV, HCM, YH, AAJ, SF, and SG provided important clinical data. FM wrote the first draft of the manuscript. All authors approved the final version of the manuscript.

Consent for publication
Not applicable.

Competing interests
The authors declare that they have no competing interests.

Author details
[1]Service d'Hématologie Clinique et Thérapie Cellulaire, AP-HP, Hôpital Saint-Antoine, Paris F-75012, France. [2]INSERM, Centre de Recherche Saint-Antoine (CRSA), Sorbonne Université, F-75012 Paris, France. [3]Adult Bone Marrow Transplantation Service, Memorial Sloan Kettering Cancer Center, New York, NY, USA. [4]Department of Medicine, Weill Cornell Medical College, New York, NY, USA. [5]Programme de Transplantation & Therapie Cellulaire, Centre de Recherche en Cancérologie de Marseille, Institut Paoli Calmettes, Marseille, France. [6]University Hospital, Hematology, Basel, Switzerland. [7]Bone Marrow Transplant Service, Department of Pediatrics, Memorial Sloan Kettering Cancer Center, New York, NY, USA. [8]Department of Pediatrics, Weill Cornell Medical College, New York, NY, USA. [9]CHU Bordeaux, Hôpital Haut-leveque, Pessac, France. [10]Stem Cell Transplantation Unit, HUCH Comprehensive Cancer Center, Helsinki, Finland. [11]Département d'Hématologie Clinique, CHU Lapeyronie, Montpellier, France. [12]Service des Maladies du Sang, CHRU, Angers, France. [13]EBMT Paris Study Office/ CEREST-TC, Paris, France. [14]Hematology Division, Chaim Sheba Medical Center, Tel-Hashomer, Israel. [15]Adult Bone Marrow Transplantation Service, Department of Medicine, Memorial Sloan Kettering Cancer Center, 1275 York Avenue, Box 298, New York, NY 10065, USA.

References
1. Dohner H, Weisdorf DJ, Bloomfield CD. Acute myeloid leukemia. N Engl J Med. 2015;373:1136–52.
2. Sengsayadeth S, Savani BN, Blaise D, Malard F, Nagler A, Mohty M. Reduced intensity conditioning allogeneic hematopoietic cell transplantation for adult acute myeloid leukemia in complete remission - a review from the Acute Leukemia Working Party of the EBMT. Haematologica. 2015;100:859–69.
3. Malard F, Chevallier P, Guillaume T, Delaunay J, Rialland F, Harousseau JL, Moreau P, Mechinaud F, Milpied N, Mohty M. Continuous reduced nonrelapse mortality after allogeneic hematopoietic stem cell transplantation: a single-institution's three decade experience. Biol Blood Marrow Transplant. 2014;20:1217–23.
4. Flowers ME, Inamoto Y, Carpenter PA, Lee SJ, Kiem HP, Petersdorf EW, Pereira SE, Nash RA, Mielcarek M, Fero ML, et al. Comparative analysis of risk factors for acute graft-versus-host disease and for chronic graft-versus-host disease according to National Institutes of Health consensus criteria. Blood. 2011;117:3214–9.
5. Anasetti C, Logan BR, Lee SJ, Waller EK, Weisdorf DJ, Wingard JR, Cutler CS, Westervelt P, Woolfrey A, Couban S, et al. Peripheral-blood stem cells versus bone marrow from unrelated donors. N Engl J Med. 2012;367:1487–96.
6. Arai S, Arora M, Wang T, Spellman SR, He W, Couriel DR, Urbano-Ispizua A, Cutler CS, Bacigalupo AA, Battiwalla M, et al. Increasing incidence of chronic graft-versus-host disease in allogeneic transplantation: a report from the Center for International Blood and Marrow Transplant Research. Biol Blood Marrow Transplant. 2015;21:266–74.
7. Bacigalupo A, Lamparelli T, Bruzzi P, Guidi S, Alessandrino PE, di Bartolomeo P, Oneto R, Bruno B, Barbanti M, Sacchi N, et al. Antithymocyte globulin for graft-versus-host disease prophylaxis in transplants from unrelated donors: 2

randomized studies from Gruppo Italiano Trapianti Midollo Osseo (GITMO). Blood. 2001;98:2942–7.

8. Finke J, Bethge WA, Schmoor C, Ottinger HD, Stelljes M, Zander AR, Volin L, Ruutu T, Heim DA, Schwerdtfeger R, et al. Standard graft-versus-host disease prophylaxis with or without anti-T-cell globulin in haematopoietic cell transplantation from matched unrelated donors: a randomised, open-label, multicentre phase 3 trial. Lancet Oncol. 2009;10:855–64.

9. Walker I, Panzarella T, Couban S, Couture F, Devins G, Elemary M, Gallagher G, Kerr H, Kuruvilla J, Lee SJ, et al. Pretreatment with anti-thymocyte globulin versus no anti-thymocyte globulin in patients with haematological malignancies undergoing haemopoietic cell transplantation from unrelated donors: a randomised, controlled, open-label, phase 3, multicentre trial. Lancet Oncol. 2016;17:164–73.

10. Kroger N, Solano C, Wolschke C, Bandini G, Patriarca F, Pini M, Nagler A, Selleri C, Risitano A, Messina G, et al. Antilymphocyte globulin for prevention of chronic graft-versus-host disease. N Engl J Med. 2016;374:43–53.

11. Bacigalupo A, Lamparelli T, Barisione G, Bruzzi P, Guidi S, Alessandrino PE, di Bartolomeo P, Oneto R, Bruno B, Sacchi N, et al. Thymoglobulin prevents chronic graft-versus-host disease, chronic lung dysfunction, and late transplant-related mortality: long-term follow-up of a randomized trial in patients undergoing unrelated donor transplantation. Biol Blood Marrow Transplant. 2006;12:560–5.

12. Soiffer RJ, Kim HT, McGuirk J, Horwitz ME, Johnston L, Patnaik MM, Rybka W, Artz A, Porter DL, Shea TC, et al. Prospective, randomized, double-blind, phase iii clinical trial of anti-T-lymphocyte globulin to assess impact on chronic graft-versus-host disease-free survival in patients undergoing HLA-matched unrelated myeloablative hematopoietic cell transplantation. J Clin Oncol. 2017. https://doi.org/10.1200/JCO.2017.75.8177.

13. Mohty M, Malard F. Antithymocyte globulin for graft-versus-host disease prophylaxis after allogeneic hematopoietic stem-cell transplantation. J Clin Oncol. 2017. https://doi.org/10.1200/JCO.2017.76.0512.

14. Kottaridis PD, Milligan DW, Chopra R, Chakraverty RK, Chakrabarti S, Robinson S, Peggs K, Verfuerth S, Pettengell R, Marsh JC, et al. In vivo CAMPATH-1H prevents graft-versus-host disease following nonmyeloablative stem cell transplantation. Blood. 2000;96:2419–25.

15. Devine SM, Carter S, Soiffer RJ, Pasquini MC, Hari PN, Stein A, Lazarus HM, Linker C, Stadtmauer EA, Alyea EP 3rd, et al. Low risk of chronic graft-versus-host disease and relapse associated with T cell-depleted peripheral blood stem cell transplantation for acute myelogenous leukemia in first remission: results of the blood and marrow transplant clinical trials network protocol 0303. Biol Blood Marrow Transplant. 2011;17:1343–51.

16. Papadopoulos EB, Carabasi MH, Castro-Malaspina H, Childs BH, Mackinnon S, Boulad F, Gillio AP, Kernan NA, Small TN, Szabolcs P, et al. T-cell-depleted allogeneic bone marrow transplantation as postremission therapy for acute myelogenous leukemia: freedom from relapse in the absence of graft-versus-host disease. Blood. 1998;91:1083–90.

17. Jakubowski AA, Small TN, Kernan NA, Castro-Malaspina H, Collins N, Koehne G, Hsu KC, Perales MA, Papanicolaou G, van den Brink MR, et al. T cell-depleted unrelated donor stem cell transplantation provides favorable disease-free survival for adults with hematologic malignancies. Biol Blood Marrow Transplant. 2011;17:1335–42.

18. Jakubowski AA, Petrlik E, Maloy M, Hilden P, Papadopoulos E, Young JW, Boulad F, Castro-Malaspina H, Tamari R, Dahi PB, et al. T cell depletion as an alternative approach for patients 55 years or older undergoing allogeneic stem cell transplantation as curative therapy for hematologic malignancies. Biol Blood Marrow Transplant. 2017;23:1685–94.

19. Pasquini MC, Devine S, Mendizabal A, Baden LR, Wingard JR, Lazarus HM, Appelbaum FR, Keever-Taylor CA, Horowitz MM, Carter S, et al. Comparative outcomes of donor graft CD34+ selection and immune suppressive therapy as graft-versus-host disease prophylaxis for patients with acute myeloid leukemia in complete remission undergoing HLA-matched sibling allogeneic hematopoietic cell transplantation. J Clin Oncol. 2012;30:3194–201.

20. Jakubowski AA, Small TN, Young JW, Kernan NA, Castro-Malaspina H, Hsu KC, Perales MA, Collins N, Cisek C, Chiu M, et al. T cell depleted stem-cell transplantation for adults with hematologic malignancies: sustained engraftment of HLA-matched related donor grafts without the use of antithymocyte globulin. Blood. 2007;110:4552–9.

21. Bayraktar UD, de Lima M, Saliba RM, Maloy M, Castro-Malaspina HR, Chen J, Rondon G, Chiattone A, Jakubowski AA, Boulad F, et al. Ex vivo T cell-depleted versus unmodified allografts in patients with acute myeloid leukemia in first complete remission. Biol Blood Marrow Transplant. 2013;19:898–903.

22. Keever-Taylor CA, Devine SM, Soiffer RJ, Mendizabal A, Carter S, Pasquini MC, Hari PN, Stein A, Lazarus HM, Linker C, et al. Characteristics of CliniMACS(R) system CD34-enriched T cell-depleted grafts in a multicenter trial for acute

myeloid leukemia-Blood and Marrow Transplant Clinical Trials Network (BMT CTN) protocol 0303. Biol Blood Marrow Transplant. 2012;18:690–7.

23. Dohner H, Estey EH, Amadori S, Appelbaum FR, Buchner T, Burnett AK, Dombret H, Fenaux P, Grimwade D, Larson RA, et al. Diagnosis and management of acute myeloid leukemia in adults: recommendations from an international expert panel, on behalf of the European LeukemiaNet. Blood. 2010;115:453–74.

24. Peric Z, Cahu X, Chevallier P, Brissot E, Malard F, Guillaume T, Delaunay J, Ayari S, Dubruille V, Le Gouill S, et al. Features of Epstein-Barr virus (EBV) reactivation after reduced intensity conditioning allogeneic hematopoietic stem cell transplantation. Leukemia. 2011;25:932–8.

25. Ruggeri A, Labopin M, Ciceri F, Mohty M, Nagler A. Definition of GvHD-free, relapse-free survival for registry-based studies: an ALWP-EBMT analysis on patients with AML in remission. Bone Marrow Transplant. 2016;51:610–1.

26. Przepiorka D, Weisdorf D, Martin P, Klingemann HG, Beatty P, Hows J, Thomas ED. 1994 Consensus Conference on Acute GVHD Grading. Bone Marrow Transplant. 1995;15:825–8.

27. Filipovich AH, Weisdorf D, Pavletic S, Socie G, Wingard JR, Lee SJ, Martin P, Chien J, Przepiorka D, Couriel D, et al. National Institutes of Health consensus development project on criteria for clinical trials in chronic graft-versus-host disease: I. Diagnosis and staging working group report. Biol Blood Marrow Transplant. 2005;11:945–56.

28. Shulman HM, Sullivan KM, Weiden PL, McDonald GB, Striker GE, Sale GE, Hackman R, Tsoi MS, Storb R, Thomas ED. Chronic graft-versus-host syndrome in man. A long-term clinicopathologic study of 20 Seattle patients. Am J Med. 1980;69:204–17.

29. Wagner JE, Thompson JS, Carter SL, Kernan NA, Unrelated Donor Marrow Transplantation Trial. Effect of graft-versus-host disease prophylaxis on 3-year disease-free survival in recipients of unrelated donor bone marrow (T-cell Depletion Trial): a multi-centre, randomised phase II-III trial. Lancet. 2005;366:733–41.

30. Goldberg JD, Zheng J, Ratan R, Small TN, Lai KC, Boulad F, Castro-Malaspina H, Giralt SA, Jakubowski AA, Kernan NA, et al. Early recovery of T-cell function predicts improved survival after T-cell depleted allogeneic transplant. Leuk Lymphoma. 2017;58:1859–71.

31. Kosuri S, Adrianzen Herrera D, Scordo M, Shah GL, Cho C, Devlin SM, Maloy MA, Nieves J, Borrill T, Carlow DC, et al. The impact of toxicities on first-year outcomes after ex vivo CD34(+)-selected allogeneic hematopoietic cell transplantation in adults with hematologic malignancies. Biol Blood Marrow Transplant. 2017;23:2004–11.

32. Scordo M, Shah GL, Kosuri S, Herrera DA, Cho C, Devlin SM, Maloy MA, Nieves J, Borrill T, Avecilla ST, et al. Effects of late toxicities on outcomes in long-term survivors of ex-vivo CD34(+)-selected allogeneic hematopoietic cell transplantation. Biol Blood Marrow Transplant. 2018;24:133–41.

33. Shah GL, Scordo M, Kosuri S, Herrera DA, Cho C, Devlin SM, Borrill T, Carlow DC, Avecilla ST, Meagher RC, et al. Impact of toxicity on survival for older adult patients after CD34(+) selected allogeneic hematopoietic stem cell transplantation. Biol Blood Marrow Transplant. 2018;24:142–9.

34. Cho C, Hsu M, Barba P, Maloy MA, Avecilla ST, Barker JN, Castro-Malaspina H, Giralt SA, Jakubowski AA, Koehne G, et al. Long-term prognosis for 1-year relapse-free survivors of CD34+ cell-selected allogeneic hematopoietic stem cell transplantation: a landmark analysis. Bone Marrow Transplant. 2017;52:1629–36.

35. Huang YT, Kim SJ, Lee YJ, Burack D, Nichols P, Maloy M, Perales MA, Giralt SA, Jakubowski AA, Papanicolaou GA. Co-infections by double-stranded DNA viruses after ex vivo T cell-depleted, CD34(+) selected hematopoietic cell transplantation. Biol Blood Marrow Transplant. 2017;23:1759–66.

36. Huang YT, Neofytos D, Foldi J, Kim SJ, Maloy M, Chung D, Castro-Malaspina H, Giralt SA, Papadopoulos E, Perales MA, et al. Cytomegalovirus infection after CD34(+)-selected hematopoietic cell transplantation. Biol Blood Marrow Transplant. 2016;22:1480–6.

37. Storek J, Mohty M, Boelens JJ. Rabbit anti-T cell globulin in allogeneic hematopoietic cell transplantation. Biol Blood Marrow Transplant. 2015;21:959–70.

38. Barba P, Martino R, Zhou Q, Cho C, Castro-Malaspina H, Devlin S, Esquirol A, Giralt S, Jakubowski AA, Caballero D, et al. cd34+ selection vs. reduced-intensity conditioning and unmodified graft for allogeneic hematopoietic cell transplantation in patients with AML and MDS > 50 years. Biol Blood Marrow Transplant. 2018;24:964–72.

39. Ayuk F, Diyachenko G, Zabelina T, Wolschke C, Fehse B, Bacher U, Erttmann R, Kroger N, Zander AR. Comparison of two doses of antithymocyte globulin in patients undergoing matched unrelated donor allogeneic stem cell transplantation. Biol Blood Marrow Transplant. 2008;14:913–9.

40. Locatelli F, Bernardo ME, Bertaina A, Rognoni C, Comoli P, Rovelli A, Pession A, Fagioli F, Favre C, Lanino E, et al. Efficacy of two different doses of rabbit anti-T-lymphocyte globulin to prevent graft-versus-host disease in children with haematological malignancies transplanted from an unrelated donor: a multicentre, randomised, open-label, phase 3 trial. Lancet Oncol. 2017;18:1126–36.

41. Admiraal R, Nierkens S, de Witte MA, Petersen EJ, Fleurke GJ, Verrest L, Belitser SV, Bredius RGM, Raymakers RAP, Knibbe CAJ, et al. Association between anti-thymocyte globulin exposure and survival outcomes in adult unrelated haemopoietic cell transplantation: a multicentre, retrospective, pharmacodynamic cohort analysis. Lancet Haematol. 2017;4:e183–91.

13

Evaluation of an alternative ruxolitinib dosing regimen in patients with myelofibrosis

Moshe Talpaz[1], Susan Erickson-Viitanen[2], Kevin Hou[2], Solomon Hamburg[3] and Maria R. Baer[4*]

Abstract

Background: Ruxolitinib improves splenomegaly and symptoms in patients with intermediate-2 or high-risk myelofibrosis; however, nearly half develop grade 3/4 anemia and/or thrombocytopenia, necessitating dose reductions and/or transfusions. We report findings from an open-label phase 2 study exploring a dose-escalation strategy aimed at preserving clinical benefit while reducing hematological adverse events early in ruxolitinib treatment.

Methods: Patients with myelofibrosis received ruxolitinib 10 mg twice daily (BID), with incremental increases of 5 mg BID at weeks 12 and 18 for lack of efficacy (maximum, 20 mg BID). Symptom severity was measured using the Myelofibrosis Symptom Assessment Form Total Symptom Score (MFSAF TSS).

Results: Forty-five patients were enrolled, 68.9% of whom had a Dynamic International Prognostic Scoring System score of 1 to 2 (i.e., intermediate-1 disease risk). Median percentage change in spleen volume from baseline to week 24 was − 17.3% (≥ 10% reduction achieved by 26 patients [57.8%]), with a clear dose response. Median percentage change in MFSAF TSS from baseline at week 24 was − 45.6%, also with a dose response. The most frequent treatment-emergent adverse events were anemia (26.7%), fatigue (22.2%), and arthralgias (20.0%). Grade 3/4 anemia (20.0%) and dose decreases due to anemia (11.1%) or thrombocytopenia (6.7%) were infrequent.

Conclusions: A dose-escalation approach may mitigate worsening anemia during early ruxolitinib therapy in some patients with myelofibrosis.

Keywords: Anemia, Janus kinase, Myelofibrosis, Ruxolitinib, Thrombocytopenia, Transfusion

Background

Ruxolitinib, an orally bioavailable potent inhibitor of Janus kinase (JAK)1/JAK2 signaling, is approved for use in a twice-daily (BID) dosage regimen to treat intermediate- or high-risk myelofibrosis (MF) [1]. Dysregulation of the JAK signaling pathway is thought to play a central role in the pathobiology of MF, and 50 to 60% of patients with MF harbor a *JAK2* V617F gain-of-function mutation [2–4]. Ruxolitinib has been shown to inhibit proliferation of hematopoietic progenitor cells, improve splenomegaly, and prolong overall survival in preclinical models of

disease [5], as well as in patients with MF [6–8]. In the phase 3 Controlled Myelofibrosis Study with Oral JAK Inhibitor Treatment (COMFORT)-I and COMFORT-II studies, administration of ruxolitinib reduced splenomegaly, as measured by magnetic resonance imaging [7, 8], and improved symptoms, as measured by the Myelofibrosis Symptom Assessment Form Total Symptom Score (MFSAF TSS) in COMFORT-I [7, 9] and the European Organization for Research and Treatment of Cancer Quality of Life questionnaire core model for global health status in COMFORT-II [8]. Although baseline hemoglobin levels were grade 0/1 for most patients [7, 8], grade 3/4 anemia was reported as an adverse event (AE) for 45.2 and 42% of patients receiving ruxolitinib, compared with 19.2 and 31% of those receiving placebo in COMFORT-I and best

* Correspondence: mbaer@umm.edu
[4]University of Maryland, Greenebaum Comprehensive Cancer Center, 22 S. Greene St, Baltimore, MD 21201, USA
Full list of author information is available at the end of the article

available therapy in COMFORT-II, respectively [7, 8]. Additionally, overall rates of thrombocytopenia were increased in patients receiving ruxolitinib compared with placebo in COMFORT-I (any grade, 70 vs 31%, respectively; grade 3/4, 13 vs 1%) [7] and with best available therapy in COMFORT-II (any grade, 68 vs 27%; grade 3/4, 8 vs 7%) [8]. High rates of anemia and thrombocytopenia within the initial weeks of ruxolitinib therapy may lead to discontinuation in clinical practice, and therefore subsequent risk of disease rebound.

Criteria for dose adjustments in the COMFORT studies focused on managing decreases in platelet and neutrophil counts and did not provide specific dose modification criteria for new-onset or continuing anemia. In COMFORT-I, approximately one half of all grade 3/4 anemia and grade 3/4 thrombocytopenia observed in patients receiving ruxolitinib occurred during the first 8 weeks of therapy [7, 10]. In both studies, mean hemoglobin reached a nadir after 8 to 12 weeks of ruxolitinib treatment, then recovered to new steady-state levels by week 24 [7, 8, 10]. Similarly, platelet counts primarily decreased in the first 8 to 12 weeks of ruxolitinib treatment before stabilizing over the longer term [10]. The dose adjustment approach used in the COMFORT studies resulted in low rates of discontinuation due to anemia or thrombocytopenia [7, 8, 10], but the proportion of patients receiving transfusions peaked between weeks 8 and 12 [7, 11].

Similar dose-escalation strategies to those described in the current study are being pursued in patients with MF with baseline/screening platelet counts of $50–100 \times 10^9$/L in an ongoing phase 2 study in which ruxolitinib was administered at a starting dose of 5 mg BID [12], and an ongoing phase 1b study in which ruxolitinib was initiated at 5 mg BID, 5 mg AM/10 mg PM, 10 mg BID, 10 mg AM/15 mg PM, or 15 mg BID [13]. The present study explored whether a ruxolitinib dose-escalation strategy could provide clinically meaningful reductions in splenomegaly and symptoms while abating the early hematologic toxicities observed during the first 8 to 12 weeks of ruxolitinib therapy in patients with baseline platelet counts $\geq 100 \times 10^9$/L. A regimen using a lower starting dose followed by incremental dose increases might decrease the frequency and severity of new-onset or worsening anemia or thrombocytopenia.

The current study evaluated an alternative dosing regimen (ruxolitinib 10 mg BID starting dose) in patients with primary MF (PMF), post-polycythemia vera MF (PPV-MF), or post-essential thrombocythemia MF (PET-MF). The effects of starting ruxolitinib at 10 mg BID on spleen volume, palpable spleen length, symptom burden, and safety and tolerability of ruxolitinib, including evaluation of new-onset transfusion dependence and grade ≥ 3 anemia, were assessed.

Methods
Study design
INCB 18424-261 (NCT01445769) was an open-label, multicenter, single-arm, phase 2 study evaluating an alternative dose regimen of ruxolitinib in adults with PMF, PET-MF, or PPV-MF. The study consisted of four phases: screening (up to 21 days), baseline (7 days), treatment (24 weeks), and follow-up (30–37 days after the last on-study ruxolitinib dose).

Inclusion/exclusion criteria
All patients were men or women (age ≥ 18 years) diagnosed with PMF, PPV-MF, or PET-MF; platelet counts $\geq 100 \times 10^9$/L; and hemoglobin levels ≥ 6.5 g/dL; all were willing to receive blood transfusions. At screening, all patients had a palpable spleen, life expectancy > 6 months, and an Eastern Cooperative Oncology Group (ECOG) performance status of 0 to 3. At screening and baseline, all patients had < 5% peripheral blasts. Prior MF therapies were permitted, but patients were required to discontinue all drugs used to treat underlying MF disease no later than day −1 of treatment initiation.

Patients were excluded if they had MF disease that was well controlled with current therapy per investigator assessment or had inadequate bone marrow reserves, demonstrated by absolute neutrophil count (ANC) < 1 × 10^9/L or platelet count < 100×10^9/L. Patients also were excluded if they had inadequate liver or renal function (direct bilirubin $\geq 2\times$ the upper limit of normal [ULN], alanine aminotransferase > 2.5× ULN, or glomerular filtration rate < 30 mL/min), an invasive malignancy within the previous 5 years, recent severe or unstable cardiac disease, or an unknown transfusion history during the 12 weeks before screening.

Dosage and administration of study drug
Ruxolitinib was administered orally as 5-mg tablets for 24 weeks. The initial ruxolitinib dose for all patients was 10 mg BID. Doses were taken in the morning and evening, approximately 12 h apart, without regard to food intake. Doses could be adjusted at any point during the study for safety, including protocol-defined anemia, declining platelet count, or declining ANC count (Table 1).

With the exception of any safety-related dose interruptions or reductions, the 10-mg BID starting dose of ruxolitinib was maintained through week 12. At weeks 12 and 18, doses could be increased by 5 mg BID up to a maximum dose of 20 mg BID in patients with demonstrated lack of efficacy, defined as palpable spleen length below the costal margin reduced by < 40% from baseline or a change in Patient's Global Impression of Change (PGIC) score from 3 to 7 [14]. The PGIC was used to evaluate patients' overall sense of treatment effect on their MF symptoms using a 7-point scale: 1, very much improved;

Table 1 Ruxolitinib dose modifications for safety

Patient status	Maximum ruxolitinib dose or action taken
Protocol-defined anemia*	5 mg BID[†]
Platelet count 75 to < 100 × 10⁹/L (inclusive)	10 mg BID
Platelet count 25 to < 75 × 10⁹/L	5 mg BID[‡]
Platelet count < 25 × 10⁹/L or ANC < 0.5 × 10⁹/L	Interrupt administration

ANC absolute neutrophil count, BID twice daily

*For patients who were transfusion-dependent at baseline, anemia was defined as a ≥ 50% increase in transfusion frequency vs the transfusion frequency before day 1. For patients who were transfusion-independent at baseline, anemia was defined as (1) a ≥ 2 g/dL decline in hemoglobin to < 8 g/dL, unless not confirmed by repeat laboratory assessment within 7 days without an intervening change in dose, use of an erythropoiesis stimulant, or receipt of a transfusion; or (2) receipt of any transfusions (2 units minimum) in the previous 6-week period

[†]If protocol-defined anemia occurred at a dose of 5 mg BID (after, for example, a dose reduction for declining platelet counts), the dose could continue at 5 mg BID

[‡]Patients already receiving 5 mg BID could continue at 5 mg BID with further declines in platelets to < 75 × 10⁹/L and ≥ 25 × 10⁹/L, but dosing was interrupted if platelet count was < 25 × 10⁹/L

2, much improved; 3, minimally improved; 4, no change; 5, minimally worse; 6, much worse; 7, very much worse. Additional criteria for dose increases at weeks 12 and 18 included protocol-defined minimum platelet count (week 12: ≥ 100 × 10⁹/L at study visit and ≥ 75 × 10⁹/L during the previous 6 weeks; week 18: ≥ 150 × 10⁹/L at study visit and ≥ 100 × 10⁹/L during the previous 6 weeks) and lack of any safety-related dose interruptions or reductions (Table 1). No dose increases were permitted beyond week 18. Patients benefiting from treatment were able to participate in an extension phase of the study.

The primary study endpoint was the mean percentage change from baseline in spleen volume at week 24 measured by independent central review of magnetic resonance imaging (MRI) or computed tomography scans in patients who were not candidates for MRI or if MRI was not readily available. Secondary endpoints included spleen measurements; MF symptoms, as measured by the modified Myelofibrosis Symptom Assessment Form v2.0 diary total symptom score (MFSAF TSS; sum of seven symptoms, including night sweats, itching, abdominal discomfort, pain under left ribs, early satiety, muscle/bone pain, and inactivity); transfusion status; and safety and tolerability. Spleen length was assessed by manual palpation using a soft ruler to measure from the left costal margin (typically at the midclavicular line) to the point of greatest splenic protrusion. Mean percentage change in palpable spleen length from baseline and the proportion of patients with ≥ 40% reduction in palpable spleen length were assessed. The 40% reduction represents a robust response, as a 25 to < 50% reduction in palpable spleen length in ruxolitinib-treated patients was associated with an approximate 35% reduction in spleen volume in a secondary analysis of the COMFORT-I trial [15].

Pre-specified safety assessments included evaluation of clinically notable anemia, defined as new onset of grade ≥ 3 anemia in patients who were transfusion-independent at baseline, new onset of transfusion dependence in patients who were transfusion-independent at baseline, or a 50% increase in transfusions from baseline in patients who were transfusion-dependent at baseline.

Statistical analysis

The primary endpoint was analyzed using the intent-to-treat population (1-sample t test). The mean and median change and percentage change in spleen volume from baseline (weeks 12 and 24), the percentage of patients with ≥ 35% (based on the COMFORT-I and COMFORT-II primary endpoints [7, 8]), or ≥ 10% (arbitrary cut-off to identify small but durable changes in spleen volume) reduction in spleen volume from baseline at week 24, change in palpable spleen length from baseline to every study visit, and percentage change from baseline to every study visit were each estimated with 95% confidence intervals (CIs). The proportions of patients with a ≥ 50 or ≥ 20% reduction from baseline in MFSAF TSS (week 24) and the mean and median change and percentage change from baseline in individual symptoms and MFSAF TSS (weeks 6, 12, 18, and 24) were also estimated with 95% CIs.

Clinical safety data were analyzed using summary statistics. Descriptive statistics were provided for duration of treatment, average daily dose (mg) of ruxolitinib, and total dose (mg) of ruxolitinib for safety-evaluable patients. For key laboratory parameters, value was graded based on the Common Terminology Criteria for Adverse Events v4.03 grading system, and incidence rates of newly occurring or worsening abnormalities were calculated. Transfusion dependence was defined as receipt of ≥ 2 units of packed red blood cells in a ≤ 12-week interval.

Efficacy analyses were performed for the overall study population as well as on cohorts stratified by ruxolitinib final titrated daily dose. All tables, graphs, and statistical analyses were generated using SAS® software (SAS Institute Inc., Cary, NC; version 9 or later). All CIs were two-sided 95%, unadjusted for multiplicity.

Results

Patient disposition

Forty-five patients were enrolled in the study (Table 2). Forty-two patients (93.3%) completed the 24-week treatment period; five were lost to follow-up before the end of the study. The remaining 37 patients (82.2%) completed the study through the follow-up phase.

Patient demographics and disease characteristics

The study population included 24 men and 21 women, with a median (range) age of 70 (48–85) years; 95.6%

Table 2 Patient disposition

Disposition, n (%)	Patients (N = 45)
Completed through week 24	42 (93.3)
Discontinued during the treatment phase	3 (6.7)
Consent withdrawn	2 (4.4)
Disease progression	1 (2.2)
Deaths*	1 (2.2)
Completed the study†	37 (82.2)

*The patient who withdrew because of disease progression later died
†Completed the study, including the follow-up phase, which was up to 37 days after the final ruxolitinib dose. One patient was lost to follow-up and four patients discontinued during the study for other reasons

were white. Most patients (82.2%) had an ECOG performance status of 0 to 1, 68.9% had a Dynamic International Prognostic Scoring System (DIPSS) score of 1 to 2 (intermediate-1 disease risk), and 64.4% had *JAK2* mutations (Table 3). Per protocol, all patients had platelet counts $\geq 100 \times 10^9$/L at study entry.

Efficacy

Spleen volume

The mean (standard deviation [SD]) percentage reduction from baseline in spleen volume at weeks 12 and 24 was 16.3% (12.4%) and 14.9% (21.1%), respectively. A clear dose-response relationship was observed, with week 24 mean (SD) spleen volume reductions of 20.1% (18.3%) and 32.9% (12.9%) among patients receiving average total daily doses of ruxolitinib > 20 to 30 mg and > 30 to 40 mg, respectively (Fig. 1). The median (range) change from baseline in spleen volume at week 24 was − 17.3% (− 54.2 to 58.5%; Fig. 2). Three patients had a > 20% increase in spleen volume from baseline, which influenced the mean value. At week 24, 26 patients (57.8%) had a ≥ 10% reduction in spleen volume from baseline; the week 24 total daily ruxolitinib dose distribution was as follows: > 0 to 5 mg, n = 1; > 5 to 10 mg, n = 6; > 10 to 20 mg, n = 6; > 20 to 30 mg, n = 8; > 30 to 40 mg, n = 5. At week 24, seven patients (15.6%) had ≥ 35% reduction in spleen volume (95% CI 4.97–26.14) from baseline; the week 24 total daily ruxolitinib dose distribution was as follows: > 5 to 10 mg, n = 1; > 20 to 30 mg, n = 3; > 30 to 40 mg, n = 3.

Other spleen measurements

The mean percentage reduction in palpable spleen length was approximately 40% from study week 6 to week 18. At week 24, the mean reduction in palpable spleen length from baseline was 47.6%. The proportions of patients with a ≥ 40% reduction from baseline in palpable spleen length at study weeks 6, 12, 18, and 24 were 44.4, 35.6, 31.1, and 44.4%, respectively.

Table 3 Patient demographics and baseline disease characteristics*

Characteristic	Patients (N = 45)
Median (range) age, years	70 (48–85)
45–< 65, n (%)	8 (17.8)
65–< 75, n (%)	21 (46.7)
≥ 75, n (%)	16 (35.6)
Sex, n (%)	
Male	24 (53.3)
Female	21 (46.7)
Race, n (%)	
White	43 (95.6)
Black	1 (2.2)
Other	1 (2.2)
Median (range) height, cm	168 (152–193)
Median (range) weight, kg	74 (46–114)
Type of MF, n (%)	
PMF	25 (55.6)
PPV-MF	13 (28.9)
PET-MF	7 (15.6)
Median (range) spleen volume,† cm³	1798.5 (763.2–6633.4)
Median (range) palpable spleen length below costal margin, cm	13 (0–34)
Prior hydroxyurea use, n (%)	29 (64.4)
ECOG performance status, n (%)	
0	17 (37.8)
1	20 (44.4)
2	7 (15.6)
3	1 (2.2)
DIPSS score, n (%)	
High risk (5–6)	6 (13.3)
Intermediate-2 (3–4)	7 (15.6)
Intermediate-1 (1–2)	31 (68.9)
Low (0)	1 (2.2)
Transfusion status, n (%)	
Independent	30 (66.7)
Dependent	15 (33.3)
JAK2 mutation status, n‡ (%)	
Present	29 (64.4)
Absent	15 (33.3)
Median (range) V617F at baseline for patients with *JAK2* mutation, %§	77 (1–96)

DIPSS Dynamic International Prognostic Scoring System, *ECOG* Eastern Cooperative Oncology Group, *JAK* Janus kinase, *MF* myelofibrosis, *PET-MF* post-essential thrombocythemia myelofibrosis, *PMF* primary myelofibrosis, *PPV-MF* post-polycythemia vera myelofibrosis
*Intent-to-treat population
†n = 42
‡One patient had a missing baseline value for JAK mutation status
§n = 29

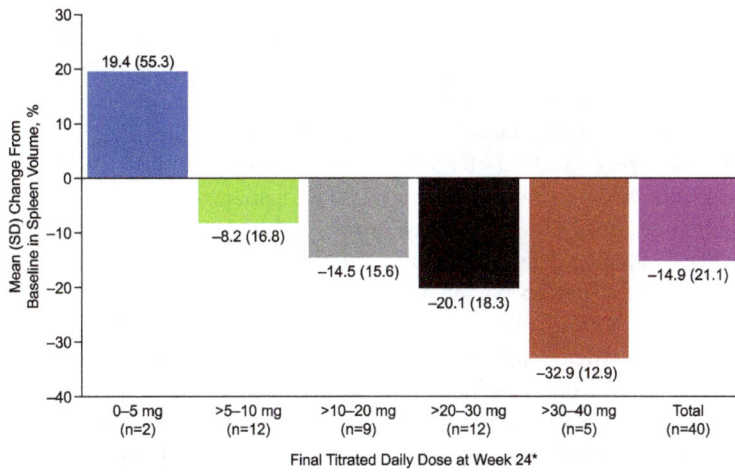

Fig. 1 Mean percentage change in spleen volume from baseline to week 24. Includes patients from the intent-to-treat population with data at week 24. *The average daily dose during the 28 days before the spleen volume assessment (inclusive) at week 24

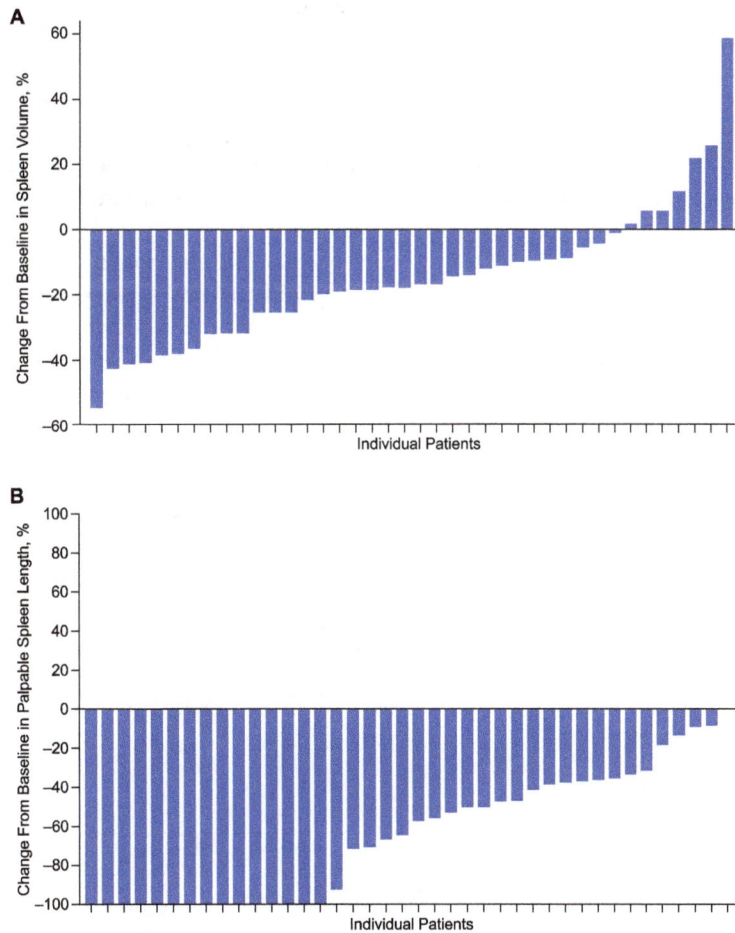

Fig. 2 Maximum change in **a** spleen volume and **b** palpable spleen length from baseline to week 24. Includes patients from the intent-to-treat population (n = 40). Each bar represents an individual patient

MF symptoms

The mean (SD) MFSAF TSS at baseline and study weeks 6, 12, 18, and 24 were 16.6 (10.1), 10.5 (7.2), 10.0 (7.6), 8.4 (6.4), and 9.3 (8.0), respectively. The median (range) percentage changes in MFSAF TSS from baseline at study weeks 6, 12, 18, and 24 were – 31.3% (– 89.3 to 265.7%), – 39.3% (– 96.8 to 380.0%), – 49.3% (– 98.0 to 223.8%), and – 45.6% (– 100.0 to 261.9%), respectively. At week 24, patients receiving an average daily ruxolitinib dose > 30 to 40 mg had the greatest median percentage reduction from baseline in MFSAF TSS (Fig. 3).

At study weeks 12 and 24, 30 patients (66.7%) had a ≥ 20% reduction in MFSAF TSS from baseline. At week 24, MFSAF TSS reductions ≥ 20% were observed in 56.3% of patients who received ruxolitinib ≤ 10 mg daily and 72.4% of patients who received > 10 mg daily.

At weeks 12 and 24, 17 patients (37.8%) and 18 patients (40.0%), respectively, achieved a ≥ 50% improvement in MFSAF TSS from baseline. At week 24, ≥ 50% MFSAF TSS reductions were observed in 12.5% of patients who received an average daily ruxolitinib dose ≤ 10 mg and in 55.2% of patients who received an average daily ruxolitinib dose > 10 mg.

At week 24, ≥ 30% of patients had a ≥ 50% reduction of all individual components of the MFSAF TSS from baseline. At weeks 12 and 24, 19 patients (42.2%) and 20 patients (44.4%), respectively, had a ≥ 50% reduction in the abdominal symptom score (composite score for abdominal discomfort, pain under ribs on left side, and early satiety) from baseline.

Safety
Exposure

All 45 patients received ≥ 1 dose of ruxolitinib. The median (range) duration of ruxolitinib treatment was 169 (31–257)

days. The mean and median total daily doses of ruxolitinib were 19.7 and 20 mg, respectively, corresponding to approximately 10 mg BID.

Adverse events

Overall, 42 patients (93.3%) had a treatment-emergent AE (TEAE); anemia (26.7%) was the most frequently reported, followed by fatigue (22.2%) and arthralgia (20.0%). TEAEs occurring in ≥ 10% of patients and all grade 3/4 TEAEs are summarized in Table 4. Seventeen patients (37.8%) had a TEAE of grade 3 or higher, and 24 patients (53.3%) had treatment-related AEs. One TEAE (myelodysplastic syndrome [MDS]) led to discontinuation of ruxolitinib and study withdrawal for one patient. Serious AEs were reported in two patients (4.4%; cholelithiasis and dehydration occurring in one patient each), and the patient with MDS died of MDS during the study.

Nine patients (20.0%) had TEAEs leading to dose reduction. The most frequently reported TEAEs leading to dose decrease were anemia (n = 5, 11.1%) and thrombocytopenia (n = 3, 6.7%).

Hematologic parameters

Figure 4 depicts median hemoglobin, platelets, and ANC through study week 24. After a small decrease at week 4, median hemoglobin returned to baseline levels at week 10 and remained similar to baseline through week 24. Twenty patients (44.4%) had a grade 3 decrease in hemoglobin level on study; no patients had a grade 4 decrease.

Median platelet count declined from baseline (277 × 10^9/L) in the first 4 weeks of treatment to 176 × 10^9/L, then increased and remained in a range of 193.5 × 10^9/L to 230.0 × 10^9/L from week 6 to week 20 (median 172 × 10^9/L at week 24). One patient each had a grade 3 and

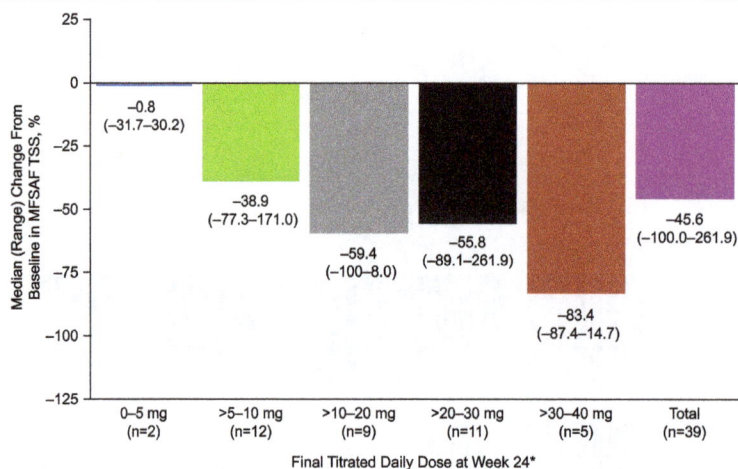

Fig. 3 Median percentage change in MFSAF TSS from baseline to week 24. Includes patients from the intent-to-treat population with data at week 24. MFSAF TSS, Myelofibrosis Symptom Assessment Form Total Symptom Score. *The average daily dose during the 28 days before the spleen volume assessment (inclusive) at week 24

Table 4 TEAEs occurring in ≥ 10% of patients and any grade 3/4 TEAEs*

Preferred term, n (%)	Ruxolitinib (N = 45)	
	TEAEs	Grade 3/4 TEAEs
Any	42 (93.3)	17 (37.8)
Anemia	12 (26.7)	9 (20.0)
Fatigue	10 (22.2)	0
Arthralgia	9 (20.0)	0
Nausea	8 (17.8)	0
Thrombocytopenia	8 (17.8)	1 (2.2)
Dizziness	7 (15.6)	1 (2.2)
Abdominal pain	6 (13.3)	0
Cough	6 (13.3)	0
Diarrhea	6 (13.3)	0
Edema peripheral	6 (13.3)	0
Muscle spasms	6 (13.3)	0
Pain in extremity	6 (13.3)	0
Back pain	5 (11.1)	0
Contusion	5 (11.1)	0
Umbilical hernia	0	1 (2.2)
Cholelithiasis	0	1 (2.2)
Dehydration	0	1 (2.2)
Blood creatine phosphokinase increased	0	1 (2.2)
Blood triglycerides increased	0	1 (2.2)
Lipase increased	0	1 (2.2)
Hyperkalemia	0	1 (2.2)
Hypermagnesemia	0	1 (2.2)
Myelodysplastic syndrome[†]	0	1 (2.2)

TEAE treatment-emergent adverse event
*Safety-evaluable population
[†]Myelodysplastic syndrome was the only grade 4 TEAE

grade 4 thrombocytopenia on study. In general, median ANC counts remained stable through week 24.

Transfusions

Of the 30 patients who were red blood cell transfusion-independent at baseline, 21 (70.0%) maintained transfusion independence throughout the treatment phase of the study. Of the 15 patients who were red blood cell transfusion-dependent at baseline, a shift to transfusion independence occurred in one patient (6.7%) from day 1 to week 12 and in three patients each (20.0%) during weeks 6 to 18 and weeks 12 to 24.

Discussion

This 24-week, open-label study examined whether initiating ruxolitinib therapy at a lower dose affected the initial drop in hemoglobin that was observed during the first 8 to 12 weeks of therapy in COMFORT-I [7]

and COMFORT-II [8], while retaining efficacy. This study protocol allowed clinicians the opportunity to titrate doses based on safety and efficacy and resulted in lower rates of grade 3/4 anemia compared with COMFORT-I and COMFORT-II (grade 3: 20.0% vs 34% and 34%, respectively; grade 4: 0% vs 11% and 8%) [1, 8]. Furthermore, the majority of patients who were transfusion-independent at baseline remained so during the study. Although the patient population for this study was small, with 37 patients (82% of initial enrollment) completing through the follow-up phase, these findings suggest that a dose-escalation approach may be advantageous in patients for whom anemia is, or is likely to become, a problem while receiving ruxolitinib therapy (i.e., patients with low baseline hemoglobin levels).

Eligibility criteria and patient populations in this study and in COMFORT-I [7] and COMFORT-II [8] were similar. However, unlike the COMFORT-I and COMFORT-II studies, in which nearly all patients (> 99%) treated with ruxolitinib were intermediate-2 or high-risk as assessed by the International Prognostic Scoring System [7, 8], more than two thirds (68.9%) of patients in the current study were intermediate-1 risk status at baseline, and 28.9% had DIPSS scores indicating intermediate-2 or high-risk. Current National Comprehensive Cancer Network (NCCN) clinical practice guidelines recommend treatment with ruxolitinib for patients with intermediate-1, intermediate-2, and high-risk MF, depending on their symptom status (intermediate-1 MF) or their transplant eligibility and platelet status (intermediate-2 or high-risk MF) [16]. Per these NCCN guidelines and based on the presence of symptomatic splenomegaly and/or constitutional symptoms, intermediate-1 risk patients enrolled in this study had indications for ruxolitinib treatment similar to those of intermediate-2 risk and high-risk patients.

In the present study, reduction in spleen volume from baseline showed a clear dose response. Mean week 24 reductions in spleen volume in COMFORT-I and COMFORT-II were 31.6 and 29.2%, respectively, among patients taking initial ruxolitinib doses of 15 or 20 mg BID (decreased to 10–15 mg BID during the first 8–12 weeks in some cases) [7, 8, 10]. Interestingly, compared with the COMFORT studies [8, 10], spleen volume decreased less at week 24 across all dose levels in the present study. It should also be noted that 58.7 and 32% of patients originally randomized to ruxolitinib in COMFORT-I and COMFORT-II, respectively, achieved a ≥ 35% reduction in spleen volume during study follow-up, most by week 12, as compared with 15.6% in the present study. The correlation between reductions in palpable spleen length and spleen volume was also higher in COMFORT-I than in the present study [8, 17].

Compared with changes in spleen volume, changes in MFSAF TSS depended less on ruxolitinib dose. The median

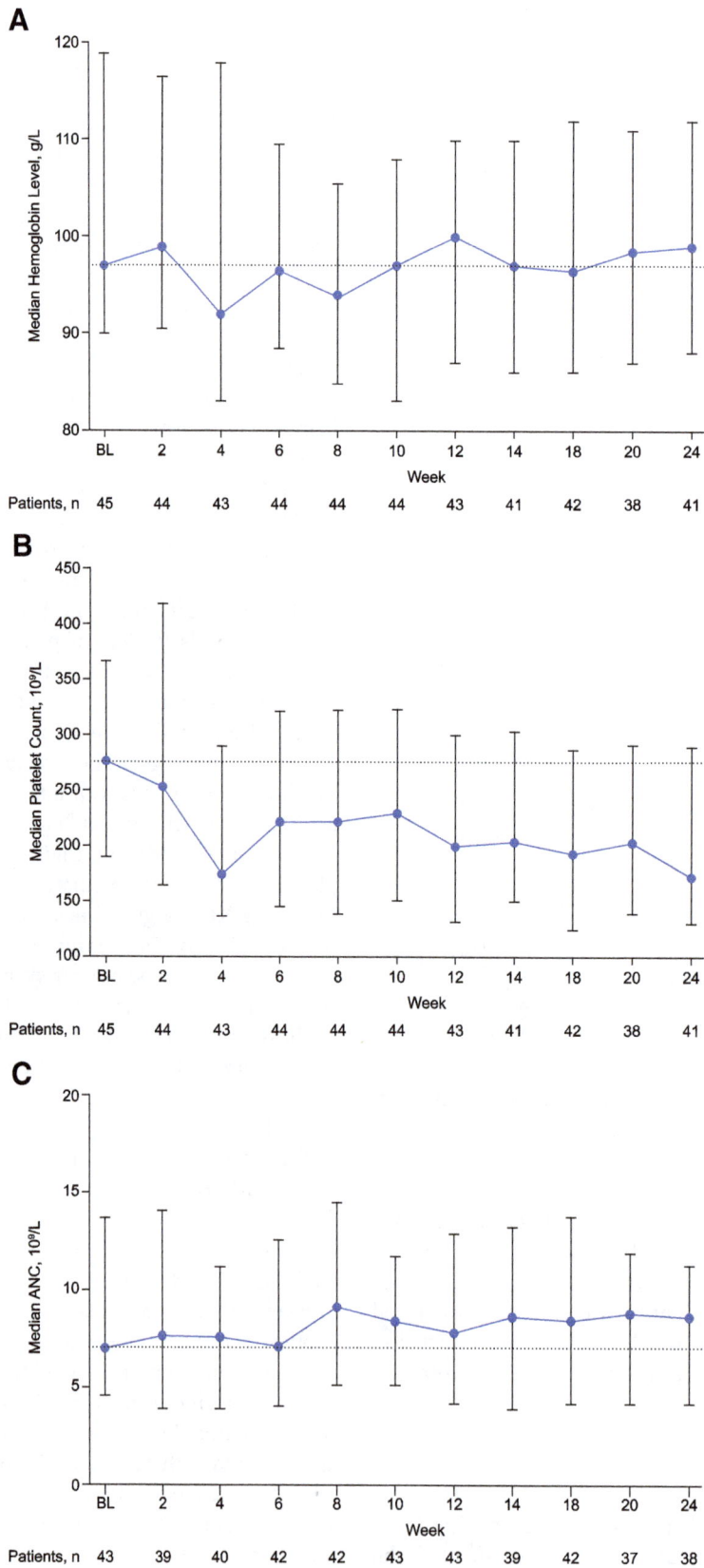

Fig. 4 (See legend on next page.)

percentage reduction (improvement) in MFSAF TSS was 45.6% at 24 weeks. This finding was similar to 24-week data from COMFORT-I, in which median reduction in MFSAF TSS was 56.2% [7]. Notably, in COMFORT-I, the majority of patients with a ≥ 50% reduction in MFSAF TSS characterized their disease as "improved" or "very much improved" per PGIC [18].

The alternative dosing scheme explored in this study (ruxolitinib 10 mg BID) provided benefit with regard to symptoms and reduced palpable spleen length in most patients; however, improvements in efficacy outcomes observed here with the 10-mg BID dose were smaller compared with those observed in COMFORT-I, in which the mean doses at the end of 24 weeks were ~ 10 mg (for a starting dose of 15 mg BID) and 15 to 20 mg BID (for a starting dose of 20 mg BID) [10]. In COMFORT-II, starting doses were 15 mg BID in 38% of patients and 20 mg BID in 62% of patients (median [range] dose intensity of ruxolitinib, 30 [10–49] mg/day). The difference may have occurred because of the protocol's mandate to increase the dose of study drug only for patients who had a reduction in palpable spleen length < 40% (or a PGIC of minimally improved or worse), preventing patients from attaining greater reductions in spleen volume with higher doses.

Current guidelines for the use of ruxolitinib to manage symptoms consider dose-response relationships and dose adjustments in the development of specific recommendations for the clinical management of MF. The European LeukemiaNet and the Italian Society of Hematology have strongly recommended ruxolitinib for improving symptomatic or severe splenomegaly (> 15 cm below the costal margin) in patients with intermediate-2 or high-risk disease, as well as for improving systemic symptoms in patients with a score of ≥ 44 on the MPN10 (a validated tool used to assess the severity of 10 symptoms related to myeloproliferative neoplasms), refractory severe itching, unintended weight loss not attributable to other causes, or unexplained fever [19]. However, the panel provided no specific recommendations regarding the tapering of drug doses, the use of combination therapies, or the method and timing of response assessment.

Conclusions

Concerns of progressive cytopenias in patients with MF treated with ruxolitinib are well established. Results from this open-label, multicenter, single-arm, phase 2 study suggest that initiating therapy at lower doses can be performed safely and may provide clinical benefit, including improvements in splenomegaly and symptoms, in patients with MF for whom anemia is, or is likely to become, a concern while receiving treatment with ruxolitinib. Current recommendations, including those detailed in the NCCN Clinical Practice Guidelines in Oncology: Myeloproliferative Neoplasms [16], continue to adhere to ruxolitinib dosing as described in the product label [1], in which the initial ruxolitinib dose is based on baseline platelet count. However, the NCCN does recognize that there are specific clinical situations that may support the initiation of ruxolitinib at a lower dose, followed by dose increases [16]. Alternative strategies should be considered for patients who have anemia or are likely to become anemic.

Abbreviations
AE: Adverse event; ANC: Absolute neutrophil count; BID: Twice daily; CI: Confidence interval; COMFORT: Controlled Myelofibrosis Study with Oral JAK Inhibitor Treatment; DIPSS: Dynamic International Prognostic Scoring System; ECOG: Eastern Cooperative Oncology Group; GCP: Good Clinical Practice; JAK: Janus kinase; MDS: Myelodysplastic syndrome; MF: Myelofibrosis; MFSAF TSS: Myelofibrosis Symptom Assessment Form Total Symptom Score; NCCN: National Comprehensive Cancer Network; PET-MF: Post-essential thrombocythemia myelofibrosis; PGIC: Patient's Global Impression of Change; PMF: Primary myelofibrosis; PPV-MF: Post-polycythemia vera myelofibrosis; SD: Standard deviation; TEAE: Treatment-emergent adverse event; ULN: Upper limit of normal

Acknowledgements
We gratefully acknowledge the assistance of Ramon Tiu, MD, as the coordinating principal investigator for this study. Medical writing assistance was provided by Tania R. Iqbal, PhD, of Complete Healthcare Communications, LLC (West Chester, PA), a CHC Group company, and was funded by Incyte Corporation (Wilmington, DE).

Funding
The study and writing support were funded by Incyte Corporation. The study design and collection, analysis, and interpretation of data were conducted by the authors, some of whom are employees of Incyte Corporation.

Authors' contributions
MT, SE-V, KH, SH, and MRB wrote the manuscript. MT, SE-V, and MRB designed the research. MT, SE-V, SH, and MRB performed the research. MT, SE-V, KH, SH, and MRB analyzed the data. All authors read and approved the final manuscript.

Consent for publication
Not applicable

Competing interests

MT has participated as an investigator in clinical trials funded by Incyte Corporation, NS Pharma, CTI BioPharma, and Gilead. SE-V and KH are employees and stockholders of Incyte Corporation. SH is a member of the speaker's bureau for Incyte Corporation. MRB has participated as an investigator in clinical trials funded by Incyte Corporation.

Author details

[1]University of Michigan, Ann Arbor, MI, USA. [2]Incyte Corporation, Wilmington, DE, USA. [3]Tower Hematology Oncology Medical Group, Beverly Hills, CA, USA. [4]University of Maryland, Greenebaum Comprehensive Cancer Center, 22 S. Greene St, Baltimore, MD 21201, USA.

References

1.   JAKAFI® (ruxolitinib). Full prescribing information. Wilmington: Incyte Corporation; 2017.
2.   Agarwal A, Morrone K, Bartenstein M, Zhao ZJ, Verma A, Goel S. Bone marrow fibrosis in primary myelofibrosis: pathogenic mechanisms and the role of TGF-beta. Stem Cell Investig. 2016;3:5.
3.   Baxter EJ, Scott LM, Campbell PJ, East C, Fourouclas N, Swanton S, et al. Acquired mutation of the tyrosine kinase JAK2 in human myeloproliferative disorders. Lancet. 2005;365:1054–61.
4.   Kralovics R, Passamonti F, Buser AS, Teo SS, Tiedt R, Passweg JR, et al. A gain-of-function mutation of JAK2 in myeloproliferative disorders. N Engl J Med. 2005;352:1779–90.
5.   Quintás-Cardama A, Vaddi K, Liu P, Manshouri T, Li J, Scherle PA, et al. Preclinical characterization of the selective JAK1/2 inhibitor INCB018424: therapeutic implications for the treatment of myeloproliferative neoplasms. Blood. 2010;115:3109–17.
6.   Verstovsek S, Kantarjian H, Mesa RA, Pardanani AD, Cortes-Franco J, Thomas DA, et al. Safety and efficacy of INCB018424, a JAK1 and JAK2 inhibitor, in myelofibrosis. N Engl J Med. 2010;363:1117–27.
7.   Verstovsek S, Mesa RA, Gotlib J, Levy RS, Gupta V, DiPersio JF, et al. A double-blind, placebo-controlled trial of ruxolitinib for myelofibrosis. N Engl J Med. 2012;366:799–807.
8.   Harrison C, Kiladjian JJ, Al-Ali HK, Gisslinger H, Waltzman R, Stalbovskaya V, et al. JAK inhibition with ruxolitinib versus best available therapy for myelofibrosis. N Engl J Med. 2012;366:787–98.
9.   Mesa RA, Schwager S, Radia D, Cheville A, Hussein K, Niblack J, et al. The Myelofibrosis Symptom Assessment Form (MFSAF): an evidence-based brief inventory to measure quality of life and symptomatic response to treatment in myelofibrosis. Leuk Res. 2009;33:1199–203.
10. Verstovsek S, Mesa RA, Gotlib J, Levy RS, Gupta V, DiPersio JF, et al. Efficacy, safety and survival with ruxolitinib in patients with myelofibrosis: results of a median 2-year follow-up of COMFORT-I. Haematologica. 2013;98:1865–71.
11. Cervantes F, Vannucchi AM, Kiladjian JJ, Al-Ali HK, Sirulnik A, Stalbovskaya V, et al. Three-year efficacy, safety, and survival findings from COMFORT-II, a phase 3 study comparing ruxolitinib with best available therapy for myelofibrosis. Blood. 2013;122:4047–53.
12. Talpaz M, Paquette R, Afrin L, Hamburg SI, Prchal JT, Jamieson K, et al. Interim analysis of safety and efficacy of ruxolitinib in patients with myelofibrosis and low platelet counts. J Hematol Oncol. 2013;6:81.
13. Vannucchi AM, Gisslinger H, Harrison CN, Al-Ali HK, Pungolino E, Kiladjian JJ, et al. EXPAND: a phase 1b, open-label, dose-finding study of ruxolitinib in patients with myelofibrosis (MF) and low platelet counts (50×10^9/L to 99×10^9/L) at baseline. Blood. 2015;126:2817.
14. Hurst H, Bolton J. Assessing the clinical significance of change scores recorded on subjective outcome measures. J Manip Physiol Ther. 2004;27:26–35.
15. Miller CB, Komrokji RS, Mesa RA, Sun W, Montgomery M, Verstovsek S. Practical measures of clinical benefit with ruxolitinib therapy: an exploratory analysis of COMFORT-I. Clin Lymphoma Myeloma Leuk. 2017;17:479–87.
16. National Comprehensive Cancer Network. NCCN clinical practice guidelines in oncology. Myeloproliferative neoplasms. Version 2.2018. Available at: https://www.nccn.org/professionals/physician_gls/pdf/mpn.pdf. Accessed 14 February 2018.
17. Verstovsek S, Mesa RA, Gotlib J, Levy RS, Gupta V, DiPersio JF, et al. Efficacy, safety, and survival with ruxolitinib in patients with myelofibrosis: results of a median 3-year follow-up of COMFORT-I. Haematologica. 2015;100:479–88.
18. Mesa RA, Gotlib J, Gupta V, Catalano JV, Deininger MW, Shields AL, et al. Effect of ruxolitinib therapy on myelofibrosis-related symptoms and other patient-reported outcomes in COMFORT-I: a randomized, double-blind, placebo-controlled trial. J Clin Oncol. 2013;31:1285–92.
19. Marchetti M, Barosi G, Cervantes F, Birgegard G, Griesshammer M, Harrison C, et al. Which patients with myelofibrosis should receive ruxolitinib therapy? ELN-SIE evidence-based recommendations. Leukemia. 2017;31:882–8.

14

Long non-coding RNA-SNHG7 acts as a target of miR-34a to increase GALNT7 level and regulate PI3K/Akt/mTOR pathway in colorectal cancer progression

Yang Li[1†], Changqian Zeng[2†], Jialei Hu[1], Yue Pan[1], Yujia Shan[1], Bing Liu[1] and Li Jia[1*] ⓘ

Abstract

Background: Colorectal cancer (CRC) arises in a multistep molecular network process, which is from either discrete genetic perturbation or epigenetic dysregulation. The long non-coding RNAs (lncRNAs), emerging as key molecules in human malignancy, has become one of the hot topics in RNA biology. Aberrant *O*-glycosylation is a well-described hallmark of many cancers. GALNT7 acts as a glycosyltransferase in protein *O*-glycosylation, involving in the occurrence and development of CRC.

Methods: The microarrays were used to survey the lncRNA and mRNA expression profiles of primary CRC cell line SW480 and metastatic CRC cell line SW620. Cell proliferation, migration, invasion, and apoptosis were assayed. Xenograft mouse models were used to determine the role of lncRNA-SNHG7 in CRC in vivo. In addition, CNC analysis and competing endogenous analysis were used to detect differential SNHG7 and relational miRNAs expression in CRC cell lines.

Results: SNHG7 expression showed a high fold (SW620/SW480) in CRC microarrays. The CRC patients with high expression of SNHG7 had a significantly poor prognosis. Furthermore, SNHG7 promoted CRC cell proliferation, metastasis, mediated cell cycle, and inhibited apoptosis. SNHG7 and GALNT7 were observed for co-expression by CNC analysis, and a negative correlation of SNHG7 and miR-34a were found by competing endogenous RNA (ceRNA) analysis. Further results indicated that SNHG7 facilitated the proliferation and metastasis as a competing endogenous RNA to regulate GALNT7 expression by sponging miR-34a in CRC cell lines. SNHG7 also played the oncogenic role in regulating PI3K/Akt/mTOR pathway by competing endogenous miR-34a and GALNT7.

Conclusion: The CRC-related SNHG7 and miR-34a might be implicated in CRC progression via GALNT7, suggesting the potential usage of SNHG7/miR-34a/GALNT7 axis in CRC treatment.

Keywords: lncRNA-SNHG7, miR-34a, GALNT7, Progression

* Correspondence: jiali0386@sina.com
†Yang Li and Changqian Zeng contributed equally to this work.
[1]College of Laboratory Medicine, Dalian Medical University, Dalian 116044, Liaoning Province, China
Full list of author information is available at the end of the article

Background

Colorectal cancer (CRC), a high-risk digestive tract tumor, is one of the most frequent malignant tumors worldwide [1]. The pathogenesis of CRC involves multiple factors, including environmental and genetic variables, while detailed molecular mechanisms remain unclear [2]. Hence, a better understanding of the mechanisms and finding predictive biomarkers are urgently needed to detect CRC.

Long non-coding RNAs (lncRNAs) are over 200 nucleotides in length without protein-coding capacity. Mounting evidence demonstrates that lncRNAs may be emerged as essential regulators in many biological processes [3]. MicroRNAs (miRNAs, 20–25 nt) bind to the 3′-untranslated region (3′-UTR) of mRNA, catalyzed by the RNA-induced silencing complex (RISC), which subsequently cause degradation of the target mRNA or inhibition of its translation [4]. Recent literature has documented that lncRNAs enrich in the cytoplasm typically participate in post-transcriptional regulation by interacting with miRNAs or mRNAs [5], and play an active role in regulating miRNA availability within the cell and form regulatory networks [6].

SNHG7 (small nucleolar RNA host gene 7) is one of the recognized lncRNAs, which is located on chromosome 9q34.3, with a length of 2176 bp [7]. SNHG7 promotes the proliferation, migration, and invasion and inhibits apoptosis in many cancers, such as malignant pleural mesothelioma [8], breast cancer [9], chromophobe renal cell carcinoma [10], and lung cancer [11]. However, the clinical significance and biological mechanisms of SNHG7 in the progression of CRC remain largely to be elucidated.

Glycosylation is a common and highly diverse form of protein modification [12] and plays a pivotal role in malignancy. As a member of the acetylgalactosaminyltransferase family, GALNT7 materializes a certain biological effect by regulating the interaction between tumor cells and the extracellular environment. GALNT7 expression is a well-described hallmark of many cancers such as cervical cancer, pancreatic cancer, and laryngocarcinoma [13–15]. Recently, promising evidence has shown that the mRNA encoded by competing endogenous RNA (ceRNA) genes could be involved in distinct biological processes. Exploration of the function and involvement of lncRNA-miRNA-mRNA crosstalk may become a key development in exploring the molecular mechanisms of cancer.

In the present study, differences between the lncRNA and mRNA expression profiles of CRC cell lines were assessed in lncRNA microarray. High level of lncRNA-SNHG7 was correlated with tumor size, lymphatic metastasis, distant metastasis, and tumor stage. In addition, we investigated whether SNHG7 directly bound to miR-34a to de-repress the target gene of GALNT7 and participated in the regulation of CRC progression via PI3K/Akt/mTOR pathway. Our findings provided further evidence that SNHG7 regulated GALNT7 by sponging miR-34a and contributed to CRC progression, which might provide novel insights into the function of lncRNA-driven in CRC.

Methods

Clinical samples, cell lines, and culture condition

Two independent cohorts were enrolled. Cohort 1: Fresh CRC and adjacent tissues were collected from 53 patients between March 2015 and January 2018. Cohort 2: Liquid nitrogen storage tissues from 70 CRC patients who initially underwent tumor between January 2011 and May 2012. Tumor tissues and adjacent tissues (5 cm from the tumor edge) were obtained at the First Affiliated Hospital of Dalian Medical University (Dalian, China). None of the patients received any chemotherapy or radiation treatment prior to the surgery. The study and its informed consent have been examined and certified by the Ethics Committee.

CRC cell lines caco2, SW480, SW620, Hct116, and LoVo, and human normal colon epithelial cell line (FHC) were purchased from KeyGEN Company (Nanjing, China). The primary CRC cell line was established from a primary carcinoma of the CRC. Cells were cultured in 90% DMEM (Gibco) supplemented with 10% heat-inactivated fetal bovine serum (Gibco) and 1% penicillin–streptomycin (HyClone, Logan, UT, USA) at 37 °C with 5% CO_2.

RNA labeling and array hybridization

Labeled sample and array hybridization were analyzed according to the Agilent One-Color Microarray-Based Gene Expression Analysis protocol (Agilent Technology). The rRNA was removed, and mRNA was purified from total RNA (mRNA-ONLY™ Eukaryotic mRNA Isolation Kit, Epicentre). Then, each specimen was amplified and transcribed into fluorescent cRNA (Arraystar Flash RNA Labeling Kit, Arraystar). The labeled cRNAs were purified using RNeasy Mini Kit (Qiagen). The concentration and specific activity of the labeled cRNAs (pmol Cy3/μg cRNA) were determined by NanoDrop ND-1000. Each labeled cRNA (1 μg) was fragmented by adding 5 μl 10 × Blocking Agent and 1 μl of 25 × Fragmentation Buffer. The mixture was heated at 60 °C for 30 min, and 25 μl 2 × GE Hybridization buffer was added. Hybridization solution (50 μl) was applied and assembled to the lncRNA expression microarray slide. The slides were treated for 17 h at 65 °C in an Agilent Hybridization Oven. The hybridized arrays were scanned by the Agilent DNA Microarray Scanner (part number G2505C).

Microarray and computational analysis

LncRNA expression profiles of SW480 and SW620 ($n = 3$/group) were used to synthesize double-stranded cDNA and hybridized to the 8x60K. RNA quantity and quality were measured by NanoDrop ND-1000. RNA integrity was assessed by standard denaturing agarose gel electrophoresis or Agilent 2100 Bioanalyzer. Arraystar Human LncRNA Microarray V4.0 was designed for the global profiling of human lncRNAs and protein-coding transcripts.

Agilent Feature Extraction software (version 11.0.1.1) was used to analyze acquired array images. Quantile normalization and subsequent data processing were performed with GeneSpring GX v12.1 software package (Agilent Technologies). Differentially expressed lncRNAs and mRNAs were identified through fold change/p value/FDR filtering (fold change ≥ 2.0, a P value ≤ 0.05, and FDR ≤ 0.05). Hierarchical clustering was performed based on differentially expressed mRNAs and lncRNAs using Cluster_Treeview software. The microarray analysis was performed by KangChen Bio-tech, Shanghai, China.

Gene ontological and pathway analysis

The Gene Ontology (GO) project provided a controlled vocabulary to describe gene and gene product attributed in any organism (http://www.geneontology.org). The ontology covers three domains: biological process, cellular component, and molecular function. Fisher's exact test was used to determine whether the overlap between the differentially expressed list and the GO annotation list was greater than that expected by chance. The lower the P value was the more significant in the GO term enrichment among differentially expressed genes (P value ≤ 0.05 was recommended).

Pathway analysis was a functional analysis that mapped genes to KEGG (Kyoto Encyclopedia of Genes and Genomes) pathways (http://www.genome.jp/kegg/). The P value (EASE-score, Fisher P value, or hypergeometric P value) denoted the significance of the pathway correlated to the condition. The GO and KEGG pathways were analyzed by KangChen Bio-tech, Shanghai, China.

CNC analyses and ceRNA analyses

A coding/non-coding gene co-expression network using 21 mRNAs and the differentially expressed lncRNAs were constructed. The CNC analysis was based on calculating the Pearson correlation coefficient between the expression of coding and noncoding genes. Two correlated genes were screened based on the Pearson correlation using the selection parameters PCC ≥ 0.99 and FDR < 0.05. The co-expression network was illustrated using Cytoscape (v3.4.0). Analyses were performed by KangChen Bio-tech, Shanghai, China.

The potential miRNA response elements were searched on the sequences of lncRNAs and mRNAs. The miRNA binding sites were predicted by miRcode (http://www.mircode.org/), and the miRNA-mRNA interaction was predicted by Targetscan (http://www.targetscan.org/).

RNA isolation and qRT-PCR analyses

RNA isolation and qRT-PCR analyses were performed. The primers to amplify SNHG7: forward, 5′-TTGC TGGCGTCTCGGTTAAT-3′; reverse, 5′-GGAAGTC CATCACAGGCGAA-3′; GALNT7: forward, 5-GGTA CCAT GGCCTCATGTTG-3; reverse, 5-GCCACCACA CTGCCATATCT-3′; miR-34a: forward, 5′-CACG GACTC GGGGCATTTGGAGATTTT-3′; reverse, 5′-CTGTCTAGATCGCTTATCTTCCC CTTGG3′. U6: forward 5′-CTCGCTTCGGCAGCACA-3′; reverse 5′-A ACGCTT CACGAATTTGCGT-3′; GAPDH: forward 5′-AACGTGTCAGTGGTGGACCTG-3′; reverse, 5′-A GTGGGTGTCGCTGTTGAAGT-3′; miR-34a was normalized to U6, lncRNA-SNHG7 and mRNA expression data were normalized to GAPDH. The relative expression was calculated using the 2-$\Delta\Delta$CT method.

Plasmids, oligonucleotides, siRNA, transfection, and dual luciferase assay

SNHG7 pcDNA3.1 vector (SNHG7), GALNT7 pcDNA3.1 vector (GALNT7), and empty vector (vector) were subcloned into the expression vector pcDNA3.1 (Invitrogen, USA). MiR-34a mimic, negative control oligonucleotides (miR-NC), miR-34a inhibitor, negative control oligonucleotide (NC inhibitor), small interfering RNA of SNHG7 or GALNT7 (siSNHG7, siGALNT7), and scramble siRNA of SNHG7 or GALNT7 (siSCR) were purchased from RiboBio (Guangzhou, China). The cells were seeded into six-well plates, and transfection was performed using Lipofectamine 2000 (Invitrogen, Carlsbad, CA, USA) according to the manufacturer's instruction. ShSCR and shSNHG7 were purchased from RiboBio (Guangzhou, China) and constructed into CRC cell lines for further in vivo experiments. The transfection efficiency was evaluated by fluorescence microscopy by calculating the percentage of fluorescein-labeled cells.

Cells were cultured overnight until 70–80% confluence. Next, cells were co-transfected with pcDNA3.1 SNHG7-wt, pcDNA3.1 SNHG7-mut, pcDNA3.1 GALNT7-wt or pcDNA3.1 GALNT7-mut was transfected into HEK-293T cells together with miR-34a mimic or the control, respectively. Lipofectamine 2000 (Invitrogen Co., Carlsbad, CA, USA) was used according to the manufacturer's instructions. After 48 h, cells were harvested for luciferase detection using the dual-luciferase reporter gene assay system (Promega, Madison, WI, USA). All values were obtained from at least three independent repetitions of the transfection.

RNA immunoprecipitation (RIP) assay

RIP assay was performed using the Magna RIP™ RNA Binding Protein Immunoprecipitation Kit (Millipore, Bedford, MA, USA). Cells were collected and lysed in complete RIPA buffer containing a protease inhibitor cocktail and RNase inhibitor. Next, the cell extracts were incubated with RIP buffer containing magnetic bead conjugated with human anti-Ago2 antibody (Millipore) or mouse immunoglobulin G (IgG) control. The protein was digested with proteinase K, and subsequently, the immunoprecipitated RNA was obtained. The purified RNA was finally subjected to a qRT-PCR analysis to demonstrate the presence of the binding targets.

Ethynyldeoxyuridine (Edu) analysis

Edu detection kit (KeyGENBioTECH, Nanjing, China) was used to assess cell proliferation. Cells were cultured in 96-well plates at 4×10^4 cells/well. Twenty-micromolar Edu labeling media was added to the 96-well plates, and they were then incubated for 2 h at 37 °C under 5% CO_2. After treatment with 4% paraformaldehyde and 0.5% Triton X-100, the cells were stained with the anti-Edu working solution.

Viability assay, colony formation assay, and tumorigenicity assays in nude mice

The cell viability was monitored using the Cell Counting Kit-8 (CCK8) according to the manufacturer's protocol. Measured the OD (optical density) value by microplate computer software (Bio-Rad Laboratories, Hercules, CA). Absorbance at 450 nM (A450) was read on a microplate reader (168–1000 Model 680, Bio-Rad).

Colony formation assay was performed to measure the capacity of cell proliferation. Briefly, 1×10^3 cells were plated in six-well plates. After incubated for 12 days, cells were fixed, stained, photographed, and analyzed.

Tumorigenicity assays in nude mice were performed. Briefly, the mice in groups were inoculated subcutaneously with 1×10^7 cells in the right flank with SNHG7, shSNHG7, or control. Tumor volumes were calculated by using the equation volume $(mm^3) = A \times B^2/2$, where A is the largest diameter, and B is the perpendicular diameter.

Cell cycle analysis and apoptosis analysis

Cell cycle and apoptosis analysis were cultured as previously described [16].

Wound healing, transwell migration, transwell invasion, and endothelial tube formation assay

Wound healing assay was performed to measure the capacity of cell migration. Detailed description of wound healing assay was cultured as previously describe [16]. The results were photographed using an inverted microscope (Olympus, Japan) and analyzed by software IPP Image-Pro Plus 6.0.

Transwell assay was performed using Boyden chambers containing a transwell membrane filter (Corning, New York, USA). Transwell assay analysis was cultured as previously described [16]. Evaluation of invasive capacity was performed by counting invading cells under a microscope (40×10). Five random fields of view were analyzed for each chamber.

Detailed description of angiogenesis assay was cultured as previously described [16] and analyzed by ImageJ software (National Institutes of Health, Bethesda, MD).

Western blot analysis

Western blot analysis was cultured as previously described [16]. GALNT7 monoclonal antibody (1:1000, Abcam, Cambridge, UK), PI3K, p-PI3K Tyr458, Akt, p-Akt Ser473, mTOR, p-mTOR Ser2248 antibody (1:1000 Proteintech, Chicago, USA). Immunoreactive bands were visualized using ECL Western blotting kit (Amersham Biosciences, Buckinghamshire, UK) and were normalized to GAPDH.

Statistical procedures

The data were presented as the mean ± SD. Comparison between two groups was assessed using an unpaired two-tailed t test. A one-way analysis of variance, the chi-square test, and the Fisher's exact test were performed. The survival curves were calculated using the Kaplan-Meier method, and the differences were assessed by a log-rank test. The Cox proportional hazards model was used to determine the independent factors. p value < 0.05 was considered to be statistically significant. All results were reproduced across triplicate experiments. Statistical analyses were carried out using GraphPad Prism (GraphPad Software, Inc., USA).

Results

Expressional profiles of lncRNAs and mRNAs in CRC cell lines

Microarray analysis revealed lncRNAs and mRNAs expression in CRC cells. After screening (fold change ≥ 2.0, *p value < 0.05), 2130 lncRNAs (1175 were upregulated, and 955 were downregulated) notably changed in metastatic cell SW620 relative to primary cell SW480 (Fig. 1a). A total of 3442 mRNAs (1771 were upregulated, and 1671 were downregulated) significantly changed (Fig. 1b). The top 10 upregulated and downregulated lncRNA/

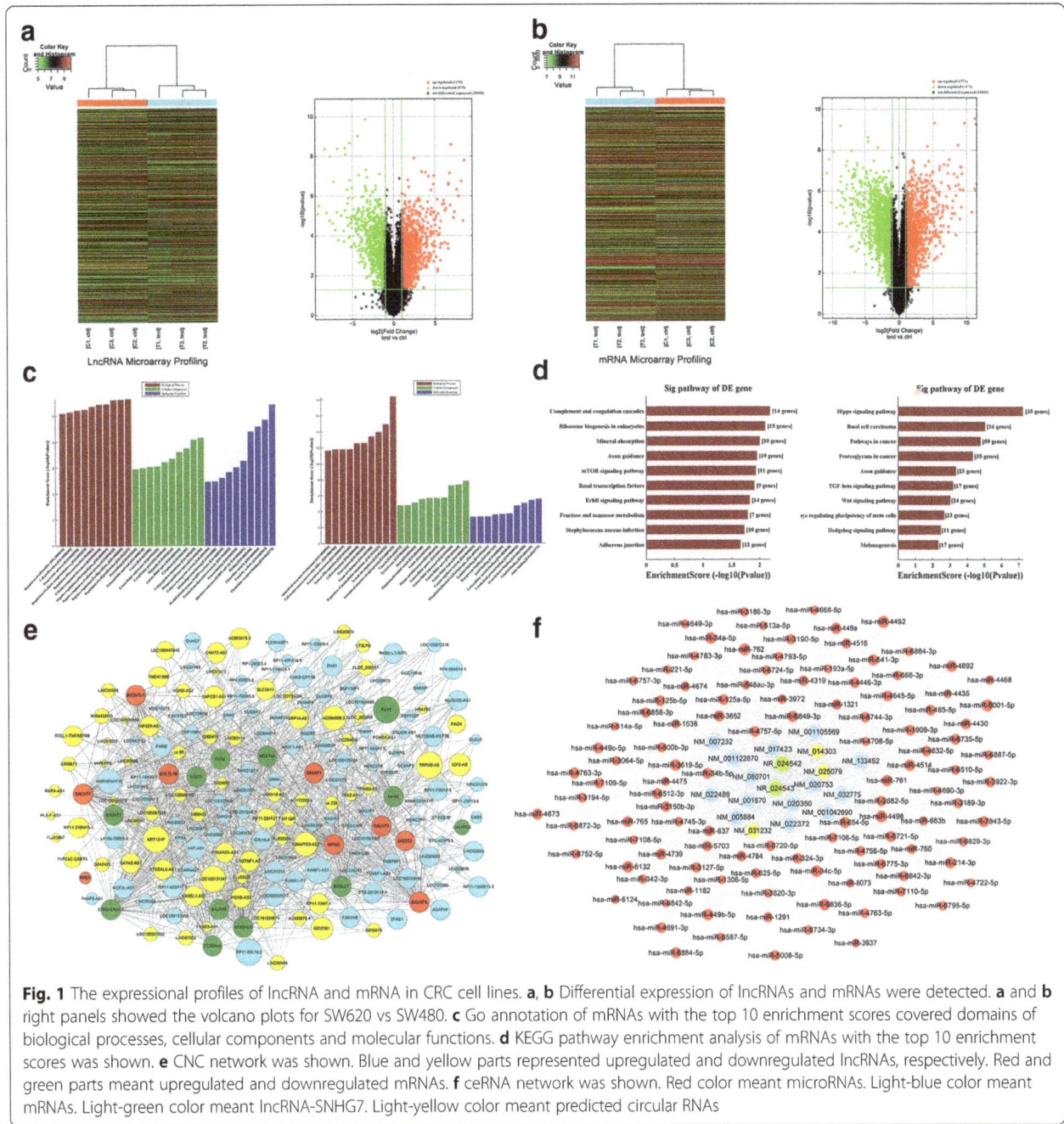

Fig. 1 The expressional profiles of lncRNA and mRNA in CRC cell lines. **a, b** Differential expression of lncRNAs and mRNAs were detected. **a** and **b** right panels showed the volcano plots for SW620 vs SW480. **c** Go annotation of mRNAs with the top 10 enrichment scores covered domains of biological processes, cellular components and molecular functions. **d** KEGG pathway enrichment analysis of mRNAs with the top 10 enrichment scores was shown. **e** CNC network was shown. Blue and yellow parts represented upregulated and downregulated lncRNAs, respectively. Red and green parts meant upregulated and downregulated mRNAs. **f** ceRNA network was shown. Red color meant microRNAs. Light-blue color meant mRNAs. Light-green color meant lncRNA-SNHG7. Light-yellow color meant predicted circular RNAs

mRNAs were listed in Table 1, respectively. Function of upregulated lncRNAs would be discussed.

GO analysis showed that the aberrant mRNA mainly took part in following biological processes in CRC. The upregulated transcripts involved in regulation of cell proliferation, plasma membrane region, and chemokine receptor binding (Fig. 1c). KEGG pathway enrichment analysis for significantly dysregulated mRNAs was useful to reveal related pathways and molecular interaction. These results demonstrated that the upregulated and downregulated mRNAs were associated with 10 pathways

(Fig. 1d). MTOR pathway was one of the most upregulated pathways.

Gene co-expression network was constructed to study the relationship between the lncRNAs and mRNAs. One hundred ninety-one lncRNAs (116 were upregulated and 76 were downregulated) and 21 mRNAs (9 were upregulated and 12 were downregulated) were involved in the co-expression network (Fig. 1e). The CNC networks indicated that mRNA was correlated with lncRNAs. CeRNA hypothesis showed RNA transcripts could crosstalk by competing for miRNAs. The ceRNA network of

Table 1 The top 10 upregulated and downregulated lncRNAs

Upregulated lncRNAs			Downregulated lncRNAs		
Sequence name	Gene symbol	Fold change	Sequence name	Gene symbol	Fold change
NR_024543	SNHG7	19.3	NR_033203	HOXB-AS3	32.1
NR_038108	SNHG16	18.5	T105469	G024903	25.4
T117110	G027615	17.2	NR_033877	LINC00548	19.8
T117111	G027616	15.8	T377350	G089269	14.8
ENST00000606186	RP4-680D5.8	9.1	NR_039989	MIR4458HG	11.0
ENST00000430859	AC005083.1	9.0	NR_110078	UBXN10-AS1	10.7
NR_109758	LOC644919	8.3	NR_110845	LOC101928674	10.7
TCONS_00019861	XLOC_009079	7.2	NR_120685	LINC01503	10.5
ENST00000602939	RP11-395P17.11	7.1	T232938	G053602	10.1
NR_034119	LINC00460	6.9	NR_034121	CKMT2-AS1	9.2
Upregulated mRNAs			Downregulated mRNAs		
Gene symbol	Fold change		Gene symbol		Fold change
LCP1	90.2		IGFBP3		59.3
S100P	60.6		GLI3		56.5
CNN3	50.8		PTGR1		46.2
TPM2	46.6		ISM2		44.3
GALNT7	43.7		ZAP70		37.7
GALNT1	40.6		RGCC		33.1
CA9	39.9		ARL4C		33.1
GYLTL1B	34.4		CADM1		32.9
GPX2	32.0		TBC1D4		30.8
MFNG	31.9		KRT85		27.8

lncRNA-SNHG7 was first built by integrating expression profiles and regulatory relationships of mRNAs, miRNAs, and SNHG7 (Fig. 1f).

LncRNA SNHG7 is upregulated in CRC tissues and cell lines and correlated with poor progression

The microarray results showed that SNHG7 level was significantly higher in SW620 than in SW480 cells. To further explore SNHG7 expression, CRC cell lines were validated. SNHG7 expression was significantly higher in SW620 cells than in SW480 cells (Fig. 2a). In parallel, SNHG7 level was also higher in CRC tissues than that in adjacent tissues (Fig. 2b, c).

In order to examine the correlation between SNHG7 level and clinical pathological features, we stratified 53 tumor tissue samples (cohort 1) into high and low expression groups (Table 2) and found that SNHG7 expression was significantly correlated with tumor size (< 5 vs. ≥ 5 cm, $P = 0.025$), lymphatic metastasis (absent vs. present, $P = 0.002$), distant metastasis (absent vs. present, $P = 0.004$), and tumor stage (I/II vs. III/IV $P = 0.002$, Fig. 2d–g). Multivariate analysis indicated that SNHG7 expression (95% CI 1.035–5.268; $P = 0.030$), lymphatic metastasis (95% CI 0.869–4.012; $P = 0.045$), distant metastasis (95%

CI 1.586–5.275; $P = 0.011$), and tumor stage (95% CI 1.301–6.684; $P = 0.002$) were independent predictors of the prognosis of CRC (Table 3).

To understand the prognostic value of SNHG7, the overall survival (OS) and disease-free survival (DFS) rates were analyzed. High expression of SNHG7 had poorer prognosis than low expression of SNHG7 ($P = 0.0105$, OS, and $P = 0.0043$, DFS, Fig. 2h, i) by Kaplan-Meier and log-rank test analyses. These results implied that SNHG7 overexpression might be useful for the novel prognostic markers in CRC.

SNHG7 mediates CRC cell proliferation, cell cycle progression, and apoptosis in vitro

To investigate the biological significance of SNHG7 in CRC progression, the cell proliferation was analyzed. Following SNHG7 overexpression, the proliferative capability of CRC cell lines was increased using CCK8 assay (Fig. 3a), clone formation (Fig. 3b), and Edu staining (Fig. 3c). Knockdown of SNHG7 attenuated the proliferative ability. In addition, the cell cycle was analyzed following SNHG7 overexpression or silencing by fluorescence-activated cell sorting (FACS). G1/S phase was driven in SW480 cell transfected with SNHG7,

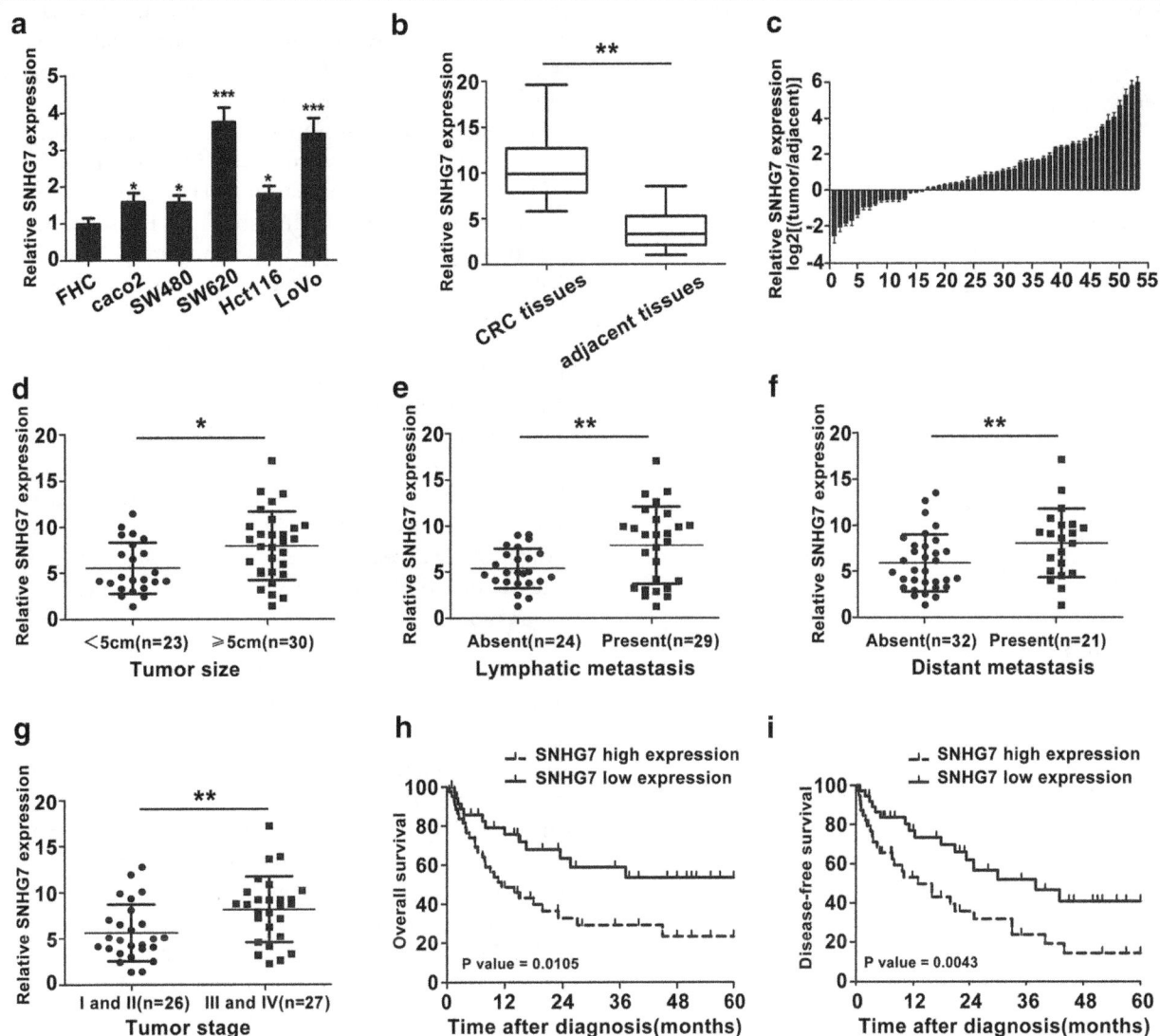

Fig. 2 Expression of SNHG7 in CRC tissues, CRC cell lines, and its clinical significance. **a** Expression of SNHG7 in CRC cells was analyzed by qRT-PCR. **b** SNHG7 expression in CRC tissues were determined (cohort 2, $n = 70$). **c** Relative expression of SNHG7 in CRC tissues in comparison with non-tumor tissues was analyzed (cohort 1, $n = 53$). **d–g** The correlation between SNHG7 expression and clinical pathological features was shown. SNHG7 upregulation was correlated with larger tumor size, lymphatic metastasis, distant metastasis, and advanced pathological stage in CRC. **h**, **i** Kaplan–Meier OS and DFS rates of 53 patients were shown. The error bars in graphs represented SD. Each experiment was repeated thrice. $*P < 0.05$, $**P < 0.01$, $***P < 0.001$

whereas stalled G1/S was observed in SW620 cell transfected with siSNHG7 in Fig. 3d. The apoptosis cells were decreased in transfected with SNHG7 group, while in transfected with siSNHG7, SW620 cells had a significantly higher percentage of Annexin V-positive cells by FACS analysis (Fig. 3e). Furthermore, upregulation of SNHG7 led to reduced levels of cleaved caspase 3 and cleaved PARP in SW480 cells, and opposite trend was found in SW620 cells transfected with siSNHG7 compared with siSCR (Fig. 3f). These data indicated that

SNGH7 promoted cell proliferation, facilitated cell cycle progression, and inhibited apoptosis in vitro.

SNHG7 promotes CRC cell migration, invasion, vasculogenic mimicry in vitro, and proliferation in vivo

To measure the migratory and invasive ability of CRC cells, wound healing and transwell assays were utilized. The results showed that the ability of migration and invasion were increased in SW480 cell transfected with SNHG7, while the migratory and invasive ability were

Table 2 Relationship between SNHG7 expression and clinicopathologic parameters of 53 colorectal cancer patients (cohort 1)

Characteristics	Number of case	SNHG7 expression		P value
		High (n = 30) %	Low (n = 23) %	
	53			
Age (years)				0.477
< 60	27	14	13	
> 60	26	16	10	
Gender				0.337
Male	33	17	16	
Female	20	13	7	
Tumor size				0.025*
< 5 cm	23	9	14	
≥ 5 cm	30	21	9	
Tumor location				0.745
Colon	29	17	12	
Rectum	24	13	11	
Depth of invasion				0.194
T1,T2	34	17	17	
T3,T4	19	13	6	
Histologic grade				0.206
Well/moderately	27	13	14	
Poorly/others	26	17	9	
Lymphatic metastasis				0.002**
Absent	24	8	16	
Present	29	22	7	
Venous invasion				0.132
Absent	27	18	9	
Present	26	12	14	
Nervous invasion				0.414
Absent	31	19	12	
Present	22	11	11	
Distant metastasis				0.004**
Absent	32	13	19	
Present	21	17	4	
Tumor stage*				0.002**
I and II	26	9	17	
III and IV	27	21	6	

*Tumor stage was obtained according to the TNM criteria
**P<0.05

decreased in SW620 cell transfected with siSNHG7 (Fig. 4a–c).

It is well known that new blood vessel is essential in tumor development. The endothelial tube formation assay was used to assess the ability of SNHG7 in CRC cell progression. The results showed that neovascularization rate was increased after transfecting with SNHG7 or decreased after transfecting with siSNHG7 compared with their negative controls (Fig. 4d).

To confirm whether SNHG7 affect CRC tumorigenesis, SW480 cells (transfected with SNHG7 or NC) and SW620 cells (transfected with shSNHG7 or shSCR) were inoculated into nude mice. As shown in Fig. 4e, f, tumor growth in SNHG7 group was significantly faster than that in NC group, while tumor growth was slower in shSNHG7 group than that in shSCR group. Furthermore, the average tumor weight was obviously changed than their corresponding control group. In order to further validate the growth ability mediated by SNHG7 in vivo, the tumor tissues were for IHC staining with ki67 antibody. These results were consistent with our above data that SNHG7 overexpression enhanced the growth and downregulation of SNHG7 decreased the tumor growth of CRC cell lines (Fig. 4g, h). Collectively, these data demonstrated that SNHG7 promoted CRC cell progression.

SNHG7 is a direct target of miR-34a and regulates GALNT7 expression in CRC cell lines

Recently, accumulating evidence has suggested that lncRNA has an inhibitory effect on miRNA expression and activity [17]. CeRNA analysis and bioinformatics software (Starbase v2.0) were used to predict the potential miRNA binding sites in SNHG7. We found that miR-34a was among the numerous possible targets of SNHG7 (Fig. 5a). MiR-34a level was much lower in CRC tissues than that in adjacent tissues (Fig. 5b). Pearson correlation coefficient analysis showed a significant negative correlation between SNHG7 and miR-34a in CRC tissues (Fig. 5c). The luciferase activity of wt-SNHG7 was significantly reduced by miR-34a mimic (Fig. 5d). In contrast, the luciferase activity of mut-SNHG7 experienced no statistical changes. These findings indicated that there were interaction between miR-34a and the binding sites of SNHG7.

The previous study indicated that lncRNAs might act as the sponge of miRNAs and function through binding the miRNAs and Argonaute 2 (Ago2) [18, 19]. According to the bioinformatics software, the sites of SNHG7/miR-34a could also bind the protein Ago2 protein. So, RIP assay was performed in SW480 and SW620 cell extracts utilizing the antibody against Ago2. SNHG7 and miR-34a expression were detected by qRT-PCR. The results illustrated that both SNHG7 and miR-34a were enriched in the Ago2 pellet relative to control IgG immunoprecipitate (Fig. 5e), suggesting that SNHG7 was present in Ago-contained miRNPs, likely through an association with miR-34a.

Table 3 Univariate and multivariate Cox regression analyses of clinicopathological features association with prognosis of 53 CRC patients (cohort 1)

Variables	Subset	Univariate analysis		Multivariate analysis	
		HR (95% CI)	P value	HR (95% CI)	P value
Age (years)	< 60 vs. ≥ 60	1.379(0.525–2.484)	0.495	–	–
Gender	Male vs. female	1.514(0.701–2.916)	0.410	–	–
Tumor size	< 5 cm vs. ≥ 5 cm	2.438(1.003–5.105)	0.062	–	–
Tumor location	Colon vs. rectum	1.028(0.712–1.582)	0.875	–	–
Histologic grade	Well/moderately vs. poorly/others	1.847(0.571–2.896)	0.289	–	–
Depth of invasion	T1,T2 vs. T3,T4	2.561(0.911–4.616)	0.124	–	–
Lymphatic metastasis	Absent vs. Present	3.054(1.008–5.531)	0.028*	2.313(0.869–4.012)	0.045*
Venous invasion	Absent vs. Present	1.478(0.491–3.292)	0.353	–	–
Distant metastasis	Absent vs. Present	3.681(1.308–5.928)	0.004*	3.163(1.586–5.275)	0.011*
Tumor stage	I-II vs. III-IV	4.422(1.849–8.241)	< 0.001*	3.549(1.301–6.684)	0.002*
SNHG7 expression	Low vs. high	3.317(1.331–5.609)	0.008*	2.924(1.035–5.268)	0.030*

HR hazard ratio, *CI* confidence interval
*$P < 0.05$

Gene co-expression networks indicated that SNHG7 was correlated with nine mRNAs (B3GLCT, FUT2, MFNG, MGAT4A, GALNT1, GALNT5, GALNT7, ST3GAL5, ST6GALNAC2). GALNT7 was the highest correlation among these mRNAs in Pearson analysis. GALNT7 level was identified in CRC tissues and metastasis cell lines (Fig. 5f, g), and a positive relationship between the levels of SNHG7 and GALNT7 mRNA was found (Fig. 5h). The expression of GALNT7 mRNA and protein were significantly increased in SW480 cells overexpressing SNHG7 (Fig. 5i). In contrast, GALNT7 level was downregulated in SW620 cells with silencing SNHG7 (Fig. 5j). These results showed that SNHG7 indeed regulated GALNT7 level.

GALNT7 is a target gene of miR-34a in CRC cell lines

Lately, ceRNA hypothesis was proposed to describe the crosstalk of RNA transcripts with each other by using MREs. LncRNAs participate in ceRNA networks and mRNA-miRNA-lncRNA crosstalk [20]. We initially identified GALNT7 as potential target of miR-34a using public prediction algorithms (Target-Scan, miroRNA.org and Starbase v2.0) (Fig. 6a). Then, Pearson analysis showed a negative correlation with miR-34a and GALNT7 in CRC samples (Fig. 6b). Next, the dual luciferase reporter assay revealed that GALNT7 was the direct target of miR-34a (Fig. 6c).

To verify the phenomenon of mRNA and lncRNA competed for the binding of miRNA, GALNT7 expression was analyzed. The GALNT7 level was higher in SW480 cell transfected with Wt-SNHG7 than that transfected with Mut-SNHG7 (Fig. 6d). The influence of Wt-SNHG7 could be reversed by transfecting miR-34a mimic in SW480 cells, which identified that SNHG7 regulated

GALNT7 by sponging for miR-34a. SNHG7 knockdown led to a decreased GALNT7 expression, while GALNT7 level could be reversed by co-transfecting siSNHG7 and miR-34a inhibitor in SW620 cells (Fig. 6e).

SNHG7 or GALNT7 and miR-34a mimic were co-transfected into SW480 cells; the ability of proliferation, migration, invasion, and vasculogenic mimicry were recovered (Fig. 6f). By contrary, knockdown of SNHG7 or GALNT7 expression weakened the proliferation and metastasis in SW620 cells. Suppression of miR-34a relieved the reduced level of SNHG7 or GALNT7 (Fig. 6g). All of the outcomes above explained that SNHG7 functioned as a ceRNA to regulate GALNT7 expression by sponging miR-34a in CRC progression.

SNHG7 activates the PI3K/AKT/mTOR pathway

KEGG pathway enrichment analysis identified that mTOR pathway was one of the most enriched pathways, involved in the development of CRC. In order to figure out the molecular mechanism induced by SNHG7, miR-34a, and GALNT7, the activity of PI3K/AKT/mTOR pathway was detected in the SW480 and SW620 cells. The results showed that high levels of p-PI3K, p-Akt, and p-mTOR were observed in SW480 cells transfected with SNHG7 or GALNT7 than control groups, respectively. The degree of PI3K/Akt/mTOR pathway was decreased in SW480 cell transfected with miR-34a mimic (Fig. 7a, c). Correspondingly, the expression of PI3K/Akt/mTOR pathway proteins was decreased in SW620 cell transfected with siSNHG7 or siGALNT7 (Fig. 7b, d). SW620 cells treated with LY294002 or siSNHG7 exhibited apparently decreased levels of the main signal molecules of PI3K/Akt/mTOR pathway (Additional file 1: Figure S1a). The inhibition of PI3K/Akt/mTOR pathway resulted in decreased

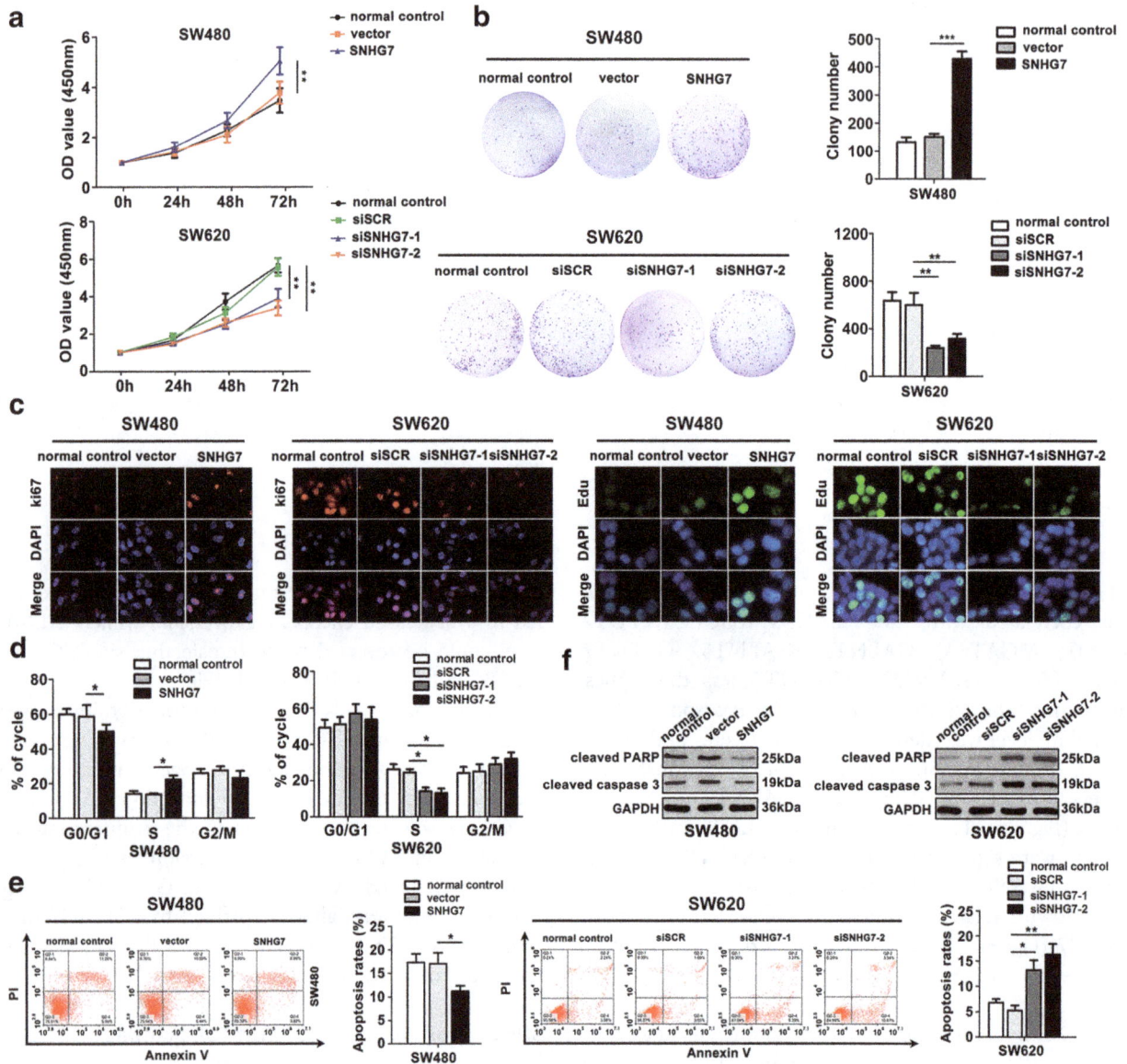

Fig. 3 SNHG7 mediates cell proliferation, cell cycle, and apoptosis of CRC cells in vitro. **a–c** Cell proliferation was analyzed by CCK-8 assay, colony formation assay, and immunofluorescence analysis with ki67 and Edu. **d** The influence of CRC cell lines in S phase transfected with SNHG7 or siSNHG7 was investigated by FACS analysis. **e** Apoptosis rates of CRC cells transfected with SNHG7 or siSNHG7 was detected by FACS analysis. **f** Relative cleaved PARP and cleaved caspase-3 expression following transfected or silencing SNHG7 in CRC cells were analyzed by Western blot. The error bars in graphs represented SD, and each experiment was repeated thrice. *$P < 0.05$, **$P < 0.01$, ***$P < 0.001$

proliferation and invasion of SW620 cells (Additional file 1: Figure S1b). These data suggested that the SNHG7, miR-34a, and GALNT7 played an important role in CRC progression via PI3K/AKT/mTOR pathway.

Discussion

Early diagnosis, especially biomarkers, is an effective means to reduce the mortality of CRC patients. In this study, we explored the possible mechanism of lncRNA-SNHG7, as

competing endogenous RNA, modulating GALNT7 by sponging miR-34a in human CRC cell lines.

LncRNAs exerted more complex effects on cell proliferation, differentiation, and epigenetic processes [21, 22]. LncRNA-ATB as a biomarker involved in the progression of CRC [23]. LncRNA-CCAT1-L regulated MYC locus in CRC progression [24]. In this study, we used lncRNA microarray to analyze the composition profiling of lncRNAs in CRC cells. The differences in lncRNA expression, especially SNHG7 were found. SNHG7 was

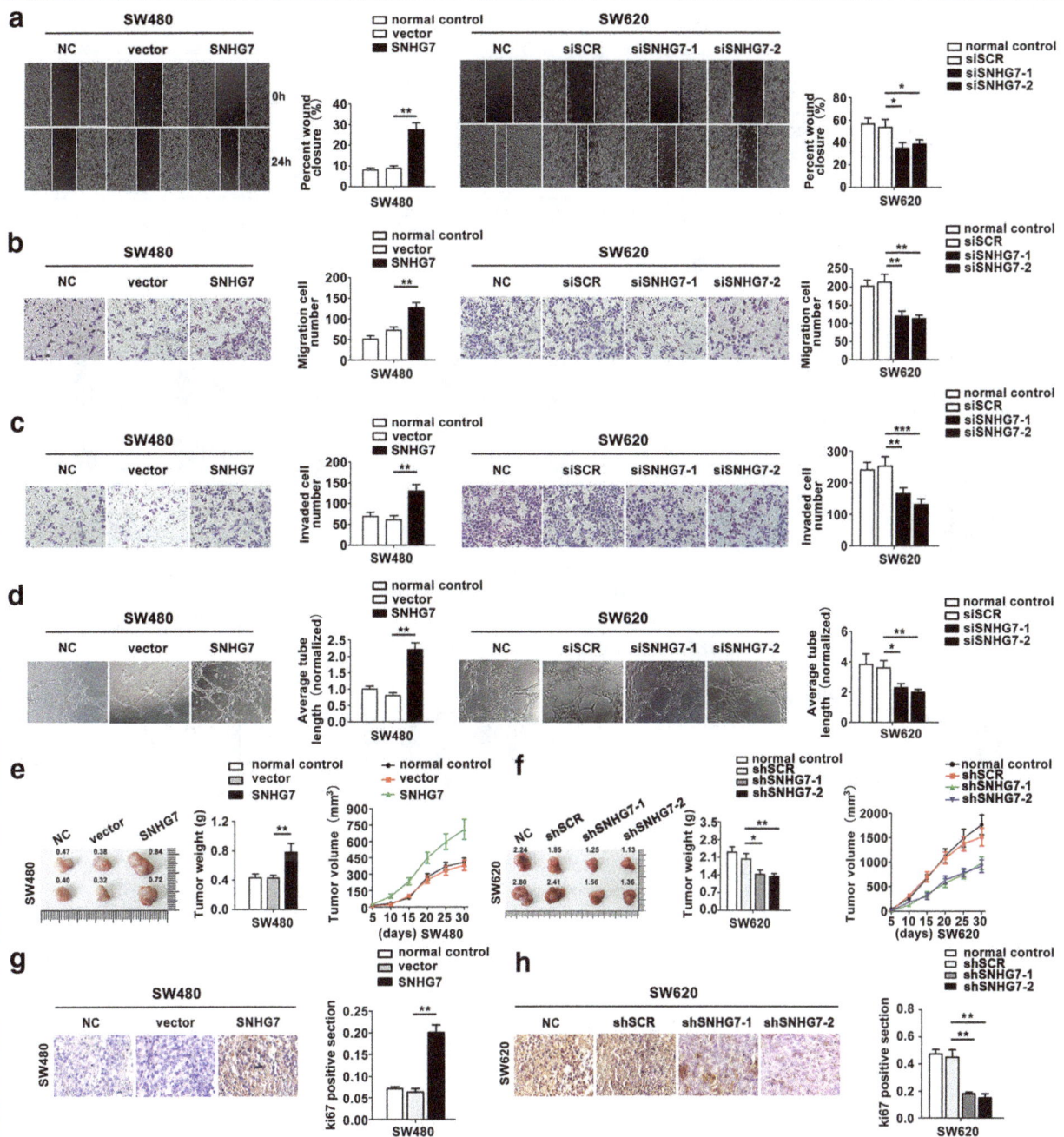

Fig. 4 SNHG7 promotes cell migration, invasion, vasculogenic mimicry of CRC cells in vitro, and proliferation in vivo. **a, b** The cell migration rates were determined by performing wound healing and transwell assay. **c** Transwell invasion assays were performed. **d** The abilities of neovascularization were determined by endothelial tube formation assay. **e** Effects of SNHG7 overexpression on tumor growth in vivo. Left: images of tumors in nude mice injected with SNHG7-overexpressed SW480 cells. Middle: tumor weights. Right: tumor growth curves. **f** Effects of SNHG7 knockdown on tumor growth in vivo. Left: images of tumors in nude mice injected with shSNHG7 SW620 cells. Middle: tumor weights. Right: tumor growth curves. **g, h** Ki67 was detected by IHC assay. The error bars in all graphs represented SD, and each experiment was repeated thrice. *$P < 0.05$, **$P < 0.01$, ***$P < 0.001$

upregulated in CRC tissues and metastatic cell lines. Furthermore, SNHG7 upregulation was correlated with tumor size, lymphatic metastasis, distant metastasis, and tumor stage of clinicopathologic parameters. The OS

and DFS of CRC patients with low expression of SNHG7 were longer than that with high expression of SNHG7. Moreover, SNHG7 promoted CRC cell progression both in vitro and in vivo. Recent studies showed that SNHG7

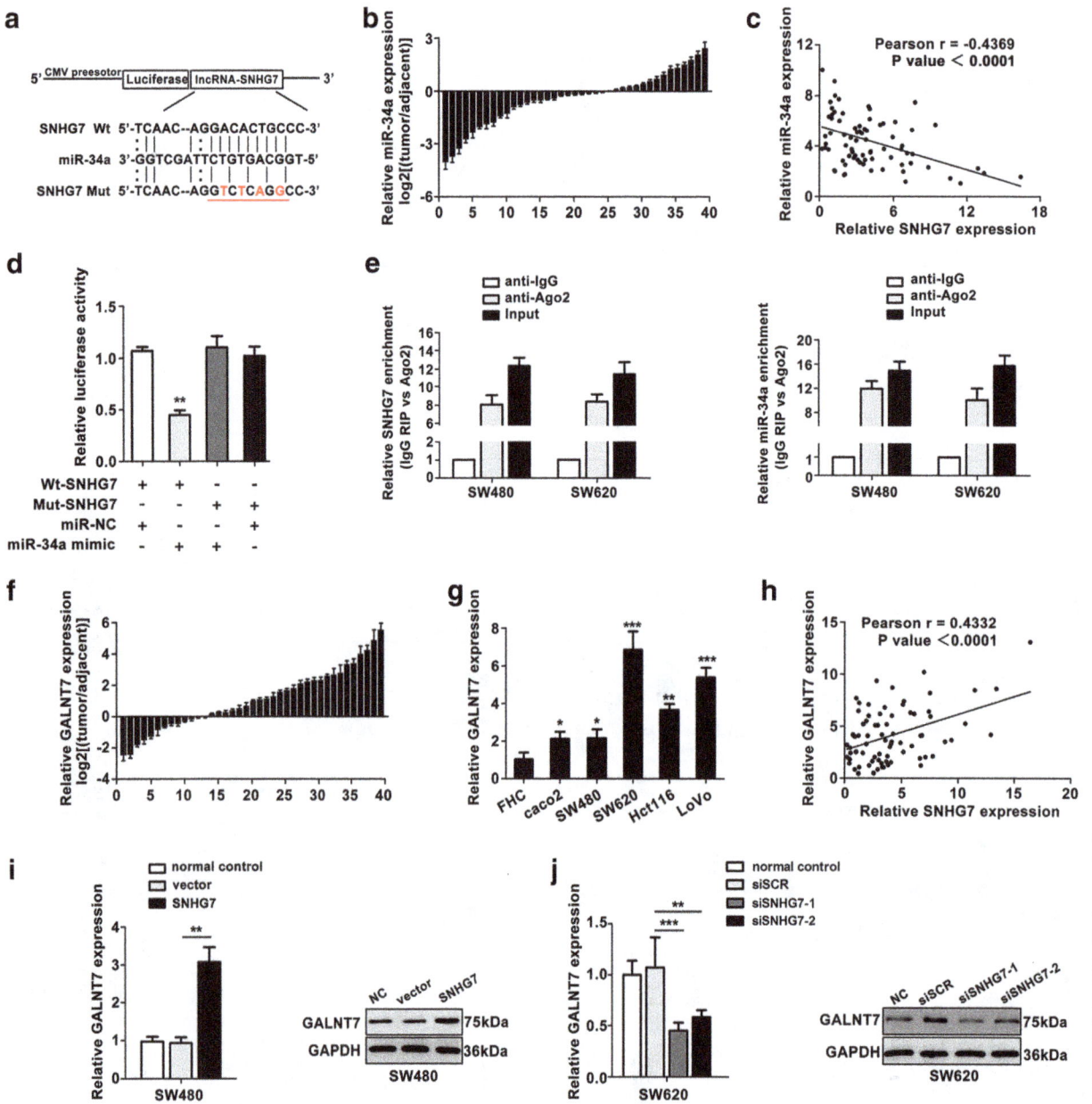

Fig. 5 SNHG7 is a direct target of miR-34a and regulates GALNT7 expression in CRC cells. **a** Sequence alignment of miR-34a with the binding sites in the wild-type and mutant-type regions of SNHG7 was shown. **b** miR-34a expression in CRC tissues were determined. **c** The negative relevance between SNHG7 and miR-34a was revealed by Pearson's correlation curve. **d** The relative luciferase activity of 293T cells was tested after co-transfection with SNHG7 wide-type and miR-34a mimic. **e** RIP assay was performed, and the co-precipitated RNA was subjected to qRT-PCR. RNA levels were presented as fold enrichment in Ago2 relative to IgG immunoprecipitates. **f, g** Relative GALNT7 expression of CRC tissues and CRC cells were analyzed. **h** The positive relevance between SNHG7 and GALNT7 expression was revealed by Pearson's correlation curve. **i** GALNT7 level in SW480 cells transfected with SNHG7 was shown. **j** GALNT7 level in SW620 cells transfected with siSNHG7 was shown. The error bars in graphs represented SD, and each experiment was repeated thrice. *$P < 0.05$, **$P < 0.01$, ***$P < 0.001$

was correlated with breast cancer [9], chromophobe renal cell carcinoma [10], and lung cancer [11]. These data suggested that SNHG7 was CRC progression-related. Further investigation was needed to elucidate the role of SNHG7 in CRC.

CeRNA hypothesis emerged as an alternative function for lncRNAs [25]. The novel regulatory mechanism has been identified in crosstalk between lncRNAs and mRNAs. LncRNA HULC promoted tumorigenesis via the miR-200a-3p/ZEB1 pathway in hepatocellular carcinoma

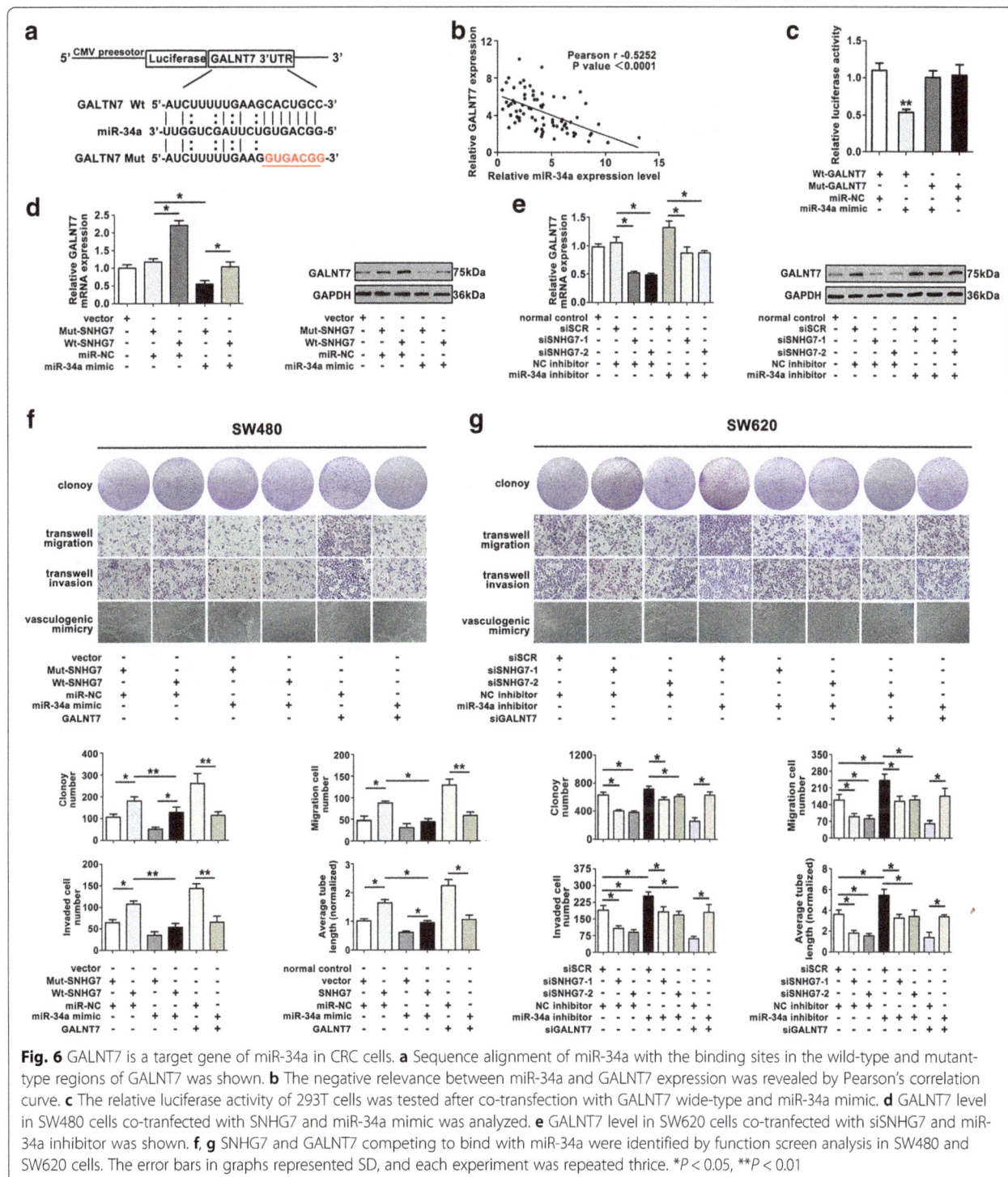

Fig. 6 GALNT7 is a target gene of miR-34a in CRC cells. **a** Sequence alignment of miR-34a with the binding sites in the wild-type and mutant-type regions of GALNT7 was shown. **b** The negative relevance between miR-34a and GALNT7 expression was revealed by Pearson's correlation curve. **c** The relative luciferase activity of 293T cells was tested after co-transfection with GALNT7 wide-type and miR-34a mimic. **d** GALNT7 level in SW480 cells co-tranfected with SNHG7 and miR-34a mimic was analyzed. **e** GALNT7 level in SW620 cells co-tranfected with siSNHG7 and miR-34a inhibitor was shown. **f, g** SNHG7 and GALNT7 competing to bind with miR-34a were identified by function screen analysis in SW480 and SW620 cells. The error bars in graphs represented SD, and each experiment was repeated thrice. *$P < 0.05$, **$P < 0.01$

[26]. LncRNA RSU1P2, acting as a ceRNA against let-7a, promoted tumorigenesis in cervical cancer [27]. Our current research observed an inverse correlation between SNHG7 and miR-34a. MiR-34a could bind the SNHG7 by conducting the dual luciferase assay. Also, we found an endogenous interaction between SNHG7 and miR-34a by utilizing RIP assays with the Ago2 antibody in CRC cells.

SNHG7 regulated CRC cell progression partially mediated by miR-34a, which was highly correlated with CRC malignancy [28].

Aberrant *O*-glycosylation is a hallmark of metabolic disorders and many cancers. Altered cell-surface *O*-glycoproteins are often implicated in proliferation, invasion, and metastasis [29]. GALNTs were illustrated as the importance in cancer

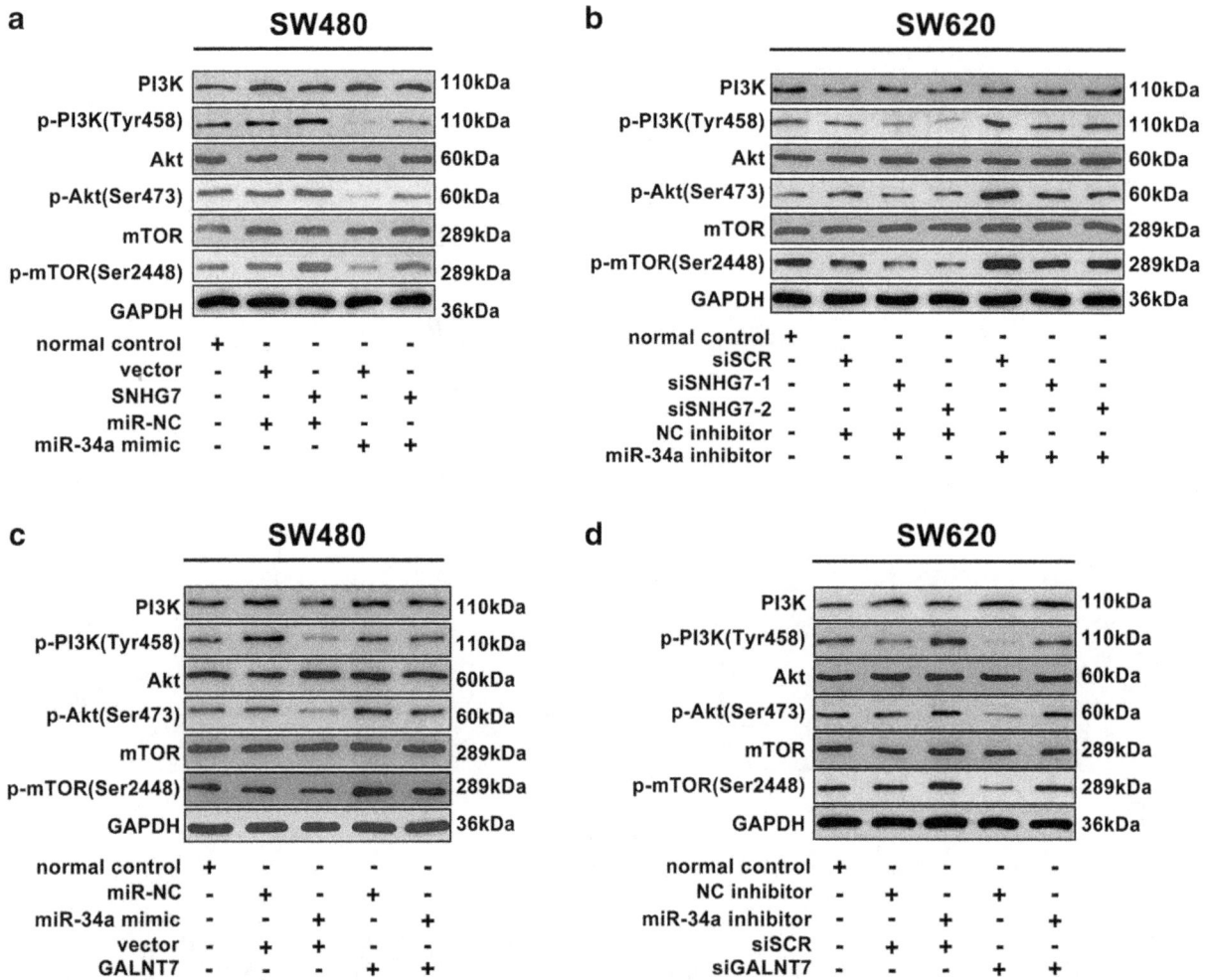

Fig. 7 SNHG7 and GALNT7 compete for the binding of miR-34a to activate the PI3K/Akt/mTOR pathway. **a, c** The levels of main molecules of PI3K/Akt/mTOR pathway in SW480 cell co-transfected SNHG7, GALNT7 or vector with miR-34a mimic or miR-NC were analyzed. **b, d** The levels of main molecules of PI3K/Akt/mTOR pathway in SW620 cells co-transfected siSNHG7, siGALNT7 or siSCR with miR-34a inhibitor or NC inhibitor were shown. The error bars in graphs represented SD, and each experiment was repeated thrice

pathogenesis. The GALNT levels vary with cell type, differentiation, and malignant transformation [30, 31]. GALNT12 mutation inactivated the normal function of the GALNT enzyme in initiating mucin type O-linked protein glycosylation in colon cancers [32]. MiRNA cluster controlled glycosylation by targeting GALNTs, responsible for initiating mucin-type O-linked glycosylation [33]. Aberrant glycosylation resulting from GALNT1 involved in melanoma [34], ovarian [35], and bladder cancers [36]. Overexpression of GALNT2 inhibited IGF-l-stimulated growth, migration, and invasion of neuroblastoma cells [37]. GALNT3 was predicted as an independent prognostic factor in renal cell carcinomas [38], and GALNT6 was found to function in pancreatic cancer [39]. Upregulation of GALNT5 played a major role in hepatoblastoma progression [40]. GALNT7, as a downstream target of miR-34a, encoded GalNAc-transferase 7 to participate

in laryngeal squamous cell carcinoma [13]. Several studies have reported the function of GALNT7 in the regulation of hepatocellular carcinoma [41] and cervical cancer [14]. These findings suggested that genetic defects in the O-glycosylation in part underlied aberrant glycosylation in CRC. In our study, GALNT7 expression was increased in metastatic CRC cells and tumor tissues. Therefore, GALNT7 implicated as a prognostic marker and therapeutic target for CRC.

In recent years, miRNAs could serve functionally as oncogenes or tumor suppressors in cancers. MiR-30e regulated GALNT7 transcripts in cervical cancer [42]. MiR-34a was downregulated in colon cancer specimens compared to normal colonic mucosa [43]. MiR-30a-5p regulated GALNT7 transcripts in renal cell carcinoma [44]. In this study, miR-34a also regulated endogenous GALNT7 expression in CRC cell lines and directly

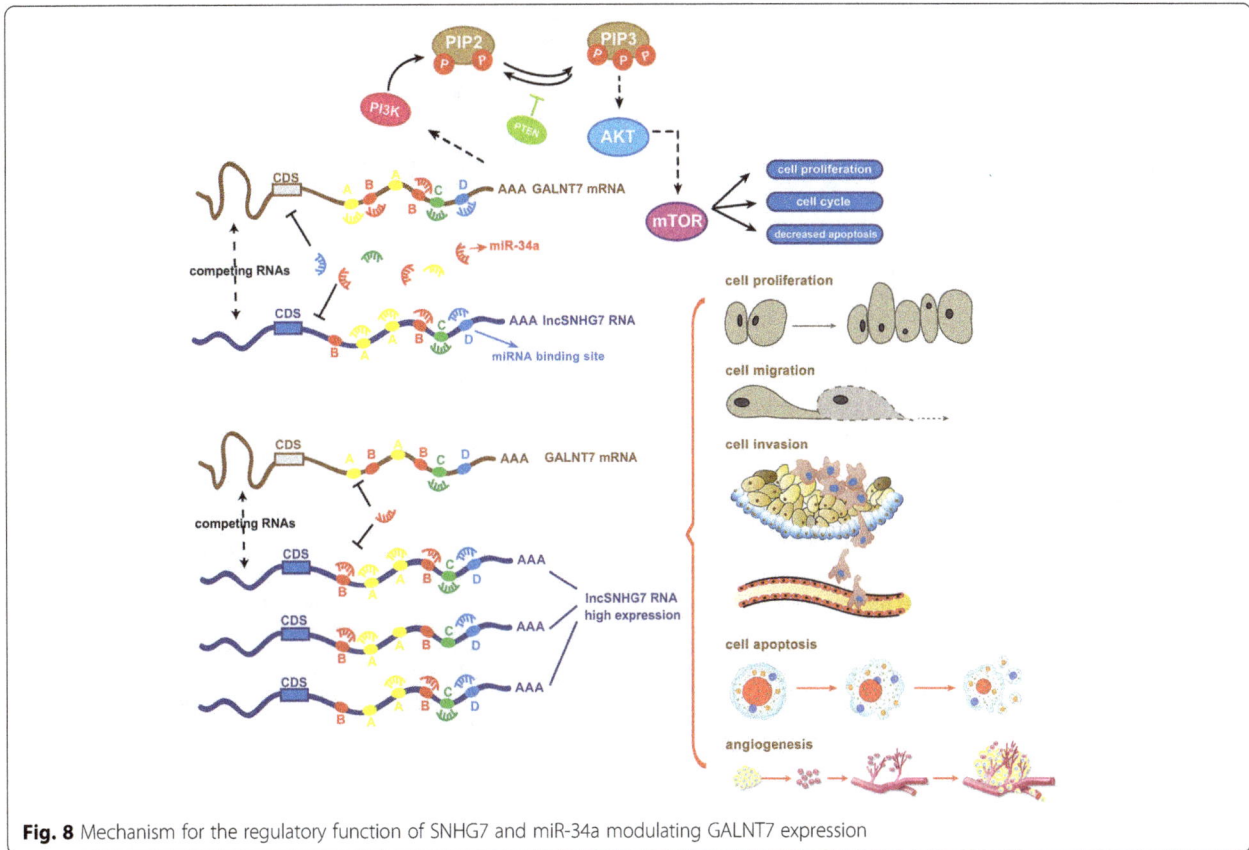

Fig. 8 Mechanism for the regulatory function of SNHG7 and miR-34a modulating GALNT7 expression

targeted GALNT7. LncRNAs played a part in ceRNA networks and lncRNA-miRNA-mRNA crosstalk. SNHG7 and GALNT7 were constructed in gene co-expression networks, and SNHG7 could regulate GALNT7 level. MiR-34a directly targeted SNHG7-3′UTR. Altered levels of SNHG7, miR-34a, and GALNT7 were associated with progression of CRC cells. Taken together, these data indicated that SNHG7 participated in ceRNA networks and SNHG7-miR-34a-GALNT7 crosstalk played a vital role in CRC progression.

PI3K/Akt/mTOR pathway is known to control the progression of cancer [45]. SNHG7 has potential to influence ribosome biogenesis, which could regulate mTOR transcription [46]. MiR-34a could regulate diffuse malignant peritoneal mesothelioma progression by modulating Akt [47]. CRC cell lines SW480 and SW620 with differently metastatic potential were used in this study. SNHG7, miR-34a, and GALNT7 expression altered between SW480 and SW620 cells. SNHG7 acted as ceRNA to regulate miR-34a availability for the target gene GALNT7, which modulated the PI3K/Akt/mTOR pathway. LY294002 represented the first generation inhibitors with highly potent PI3K-inhibitory property [48]. The inhibition of PI3K/Akt/mTOR pathway by LY294002 or siSNHG7 altered proliferative and invasive abilities of SW620 cells. Therefore, targeting the SNHG7/miR34a/GALNT7 interaction might represent a novel therapeutic application, thus contributing to the metastatic mechanism in CRC patients.

Our study defined a mechanism for the regulatory function of SNHG7 and miR-34a modulating GALNT7 expression in Fig. 8. The identification of these ceRNAs will undoubtedly enhance our knowledge to clarify the mechanism of SNHG7-miR-34a-GALNT7 axis involving in CRC progression.

Conclusion

In summary, our study showed that SNHG7 as a ceRNA to regulated GALNT7 by sponging miR-34a in CRC and played the oncogenic role in regulating PI3K/Akt/mTOR pathway. Targeting the SNHG7/miR34a/GALNT7 interaction may represent a novel therapeutic application, thus contributing to better knowledge of the metastatic mechanism in CRC patients.

Additional file

Additional file 1: Figure S1. PI3K/Akt/mTOR pathway inhibition modulates the proliferation and invasion of SW620 cells. (a) SW620 cells were treated LY294002 or siSNHG7. The main molecular expression of

PI3K/Akt/mTOR pathway was detected by western blot. (b) LY294002 or siSNHG7 treatment also alleviated proliferation and invsion of SW620 cells. (TIF 2009 kb)

Abbreviations
3'UTR: 3'-Untranslated region; AGO2: Argonaute 2; ceRNA: Competing endogenous RNA; CNC networks: Coding-non-coding gene co-expression network; CRC: Colorectal cancer; DFS: Disease-free survival; FACS: Fluorescence-activated cell sorting; GALNT7: UDP-*N*-acetyl-α-D-galactosamine: polypeptide-*N*-acetylgalactosaminyltransferase 7; LncRNAs: Long non-coding RNAs; miRNAs: MicroRNAs; MREs: MicroRNA response elements; OS: Overall survival; RIP: RNA immunoprecipitation; SNHG7: Small nucleolar RNA host gene 7; VM: Vasculogenic mimicry

Acknowledgements
We thank Nana Li, Yuan Miao, Tianming Qiu, and Yining Zhang for the technical assistance. We also thank Huimin Zhou for the comments and advice.

Funding
This work was supported by grants from the National Natural Science Foundation of China (81772277).

Authors' contributions
YL and CZ were responsible for doing experiments, acquisition of data, and analysis and drafted the manuscript. JH and YP provided technical and material support. YS and BL provided and collected the clinical data. LJ was responsible for designing the experiments and study supervision. All authors read and approved the final manuscript.

Consent for publication
Not applicable.

Competing interests
The authors declare that they have no competing interests.

Author details
[1]College of Laboratory Medicine, Dalian Medical University, Dalian 116044, Liaoning Province, China. [2]Medical College, Dalian University, Dalian 116622, Liaoning Province, China.

References
1. Siegel RL, Miller KD, Fedewa SA, Ahnen DJ, Meester RG, Barzi A, et al. Colorectal cancer statistics, 2017. CA Cancer J Clin. 2017;67(3):177-93.
2. O'Brien JM. Environmental and heritable factors in the causation of cancer: analyses of cohorts of twins from Sweden, Denmark, and Finland, by P. Lichtenstein, N.V. Holm, P.K. Verkasalo, A. Iliadou, J. Kaprio, M. Koskenvuo, E. Pukkala, A. Skytthe, and K. Hemminki. N Engl J Med 343:78–84, 2000. Survey of ophthalmology. 2000;45:167–8.
3. Zhang H, Chen Z, Wang X, Huang Z, He Z, Chen Y. Long non-coding RNA: a new player in cancer. J Hematol Oncol. 2013;6:37.
4. Hayes J, Peruzzi PP, Lawler S. MicroRNAs in cancer: biomarkers, functions and therapy. Trends Mol Med. 2014;20:460–9.
5. Salmena L, Poliseno L, Tay Y, Kats L, Pandolfi PP. A ceRNA hypothesis: the Rosetta Stone of a hidden RNA language? Cell. 2011;146:353–8.
6. Topalian SL, Taube JM, Anders RA, Pardoll DM. Mechanism-driven biomarkers to guide immune checkpoint blockade in cancer therapy. Nat Rev Cancer. 2016;16:275–87.
7. Ota T, Suzuki Y, Nishikawa T, Otsuki T, Sugiyama T, Irie R, et al. Complete sequencing and characterization of 21,243 full-length human cDNAs. Nat Genet. 2004;36:40–5.
8. Quinn L, Finn SP, Cuffe S, Gray SG. Non-coding RNA repertoires in malignant pleural mesothelioma. Lung cancer (Amsterdam, Netherlands). 2015;90:417–26.
9. Zhou M, Zhong L, Xu W, Sun Y, Zhang Z, Zhao H, et al. Discovery of potential prognostic long non-coding RNA biomarkers for predicting the risk of tumor recurrence of breast cancer patients. Sci Rep. 2016;6:31038.
10. He HT, Xu M, Kuang Y, Han XY, Wang MQ, Yang Q. Biomarker and competing endogenous RNA potential of tumor-specific long noncoding RNA in chromophobe renal cell carcinoma. Onco Targets Therapy. 2016;9: 6399–406.
11. She K, Huang J, Zhou H, Huang T, Chen G, He J. lncRNA-SNHG7 promotes the proliferation, migration and invasion and inhibits apoptosis of lung cancer cells by enhancing the FAIM2 expression. Oncol Rep. 2016;36:2673–80.
12. Khoury GA, Baliban RC, Floudas CA. Proteome-wide post-translational modification statistics: frequency analysis and curation of the swiss-prot database. Sci Rep. 2011;1:90.
13. Li W, Ma H, Sun J. MicroRNA34a/c function as tumor suppressors in Hep2 laryngeal carcinoma cells and may reduce GALNT7 expression. Mol Med Rep. 2014;9:1293–8.
14. Peng RQ, Wan HY, Li HF, Liu M, Li X, Tang H. MicroRNA-214 suppresses growth and invasiveness of cervical cancer cells by targeting UDP-N-acetyl-alpha-D-galactosamine:polypeptide N-acetylgalactosaminyltransferase 7. J Biol Chem. 2012;287:14301–9.
15. Taniuchi K, Cerny RL, Tanouchi A, Kohno K, Kotani N, Honke K, et al. Overexpression of GalNAc-transferase GalNAc-T3 promotes pancreatic cancer cell growth. Oncogene. 2011;30:4843–54.
16. Shan Y, Liu Y, Zhao L, Liu B, Li Y, Jia L. MicroRNA-33a and let-7e inhibit human colorectal cancer progression by targeting ST8SIA1. Int J Biochem Cell Biol. 2017;90:48–58.
17. Jalali S, Bhartiya D, Lalwani MK, Sivasubbu S, Scaria V. Systematic transcriptome wide analysis of lncRNA-miRNA interactions. PLoS One. 2013;8:e53823.
18. Prensner JR, Chinnaiyan AM. The emergence of lncRNAs in cancer biology. Cancer Discov. 2011;1:391–407.
19. Thomas M, Lieberman J, Lal A. Desperately seeking microRNA targets. Nat Struct Mol Biol. 2010;17:1169–74.
20. Qu J, Li M, Zhong W, Hu C. Competing endogenous RNA in cancer: a new pattern of gene expression regulation. Int J Clin Exp Med. 2015;8:17110–6.
21. Hauptman N, Glavac D. Long non-coding RNA in cancer. Int J Mol Sci. 2013; 14:4655–69.
22. Maass PG, Luft FC, Bahring S. Long non-coding RNA in health and disease. J Mol Med (Berlin, Germany). 2014;92:337–46.
23. Iguchi T, Uchi R, Nambara S, Saito T, Komatsu H, Hirata H, et al. A long noncoding RNA, lncRNA-ATB, is involved in the progression and prognosis of colorectal cancer. Anticancer Res. 2015;35:1385–8.
24. Xiang JF, Yin QF, Chen T, Zhang Y, Zhang XO, Wu Z, et al. Human colorectal cancer-specific CCAT1-L lncRNA regulates long-range chromatin interactions at the MYC locus. Cell Res. 2014;24:513–31.
25. Tay Y, Rinn J, Pandolfi PP. The multilayered complexity of ceRNA crosstalk and competition. Nature. 2014;505:344–52.
26. Li SP, Xu HX, Yu Y, He JD, Wang Z, Xu YJ, et al. LncRNA HULC enhances epithelial-mesenchymal transition to promote tumorigenesis and metastasis of hepatocellular carcinoma via the miR-200a-3p/ZEB1 signaling pathway. Oncotarget. 2016;7:42431–46.
27. Liu Q, Guo X, Que S, Yang X, Fan H, Liu M, et al. LncRNA RSU1P2 contributes to tumorigenesis by acting as a ceRNA against let-7a in cervical cancer cells. Oncotarget. 2016;8(27):43768-81.
28. Tazawa H, Tsuchiya N, Izumiya M, Nakagama H. Tumor-suppressive miR-34a induces senescence-like growth arrest through modulation of the E2F pathway in human colon cancer cells. Proc Natl Acad Sci U S A. 2007; 104:15472–7.
29. Hollingsworth MA, Swanson BJ. Mucins in cancer: protection and control of the cell surface. Nat Rev Cancer. 2004;4:45–60.

30. Bennett EP, Mandel U, Clausen H, Gerken TA, Fritz TA, Tabak LA. Control of mucin-type O-glycosylation: a classification of the polypeptide GalNAc-transferase gene family. Glycobiology. 2012;22:736–56.

31. Schjoldager KT, Clausen H. Site-specific protein O-glycosylation modulates proprotein processing—deciphering specific functions of the large polypeptide GalNAc-transferase gene family. Biochim Biophys Acta. 2012; 1820:2079–94.

32. Guda K, Moinova H, He J, Jamison O, Ravi L, Natale L, et al. Inactivating germ-line and somatic mutations in polypeptide N-acetylgalactosaminyltransferase 12 in human colon cancers. Proc Natl Acad Sci U S A. 2009;106:12921–5.

33. Gaziel-Sovran A, Hernando E. miRNA-mediated GALNT modulation of invasion and immune suppression: a sweet deal for metastatic cells. Oncoimmunology. 2012;1:746–8.

34. Cheng SL, Huang Liu R, Sheu JN, Chen ST, Sinchaikul S, Tsay GJ. Toxicogenomics of kojic acid on gene expression profiling of a375 human malignant melanoma cells. Biol Pharm Bull. 2006;29:655–69.

35. Phelan CM, Tsai YY, Goode EL, Vierkant RA, Fridley BL, Beesley J, et al. Polymorphism in the GALNT1 gene and epithelial ovarian cancer in non-Hispanic white women: the Ovarian Cancer Association Consortium. Cancer Epidemiol Biomark Prev. 2010;19:600–4.

36. Ding MX, Wang HF, Wang JS, Zhan H, Zuo YG, Yang DL, et al. ppGalNAc T1 as a potential novel marker for human bladder cancer. Asian Pac J Cancer Prev: APJCP. 2012;13:5653–7.

37. Ho WL, Chou CH, Jeng YM, Lu MY, Yang YL, Jou ST, et al. GALNT2 suppresses malignant phenotypes through IGF-1 receptor and predicts favorable prognosis in neuroblastoma. Oncotarget. 2014;5:12247–59.

38. Kitada S, Yamada S, Kuma A, Ouchi S, Tasaki T, Nabeshima A, et al. Polypeptide N-acetylgalactosaminyl transferase 3 independently predicts high-grade tumours and poor prognosis in patients with renal cell carcinomas. Br J Cancer. 2013;109:472–81.

39. Li Z, Yamada S, Inenaga S, Imamura T, Wu Y, Wang KY, et al. Polypeptide N-acetylgalactosaminyltransferase 6 expression in pancreatic cancer is an independent prognostic factor indicating better overall survival. Br J Cancer. 2011;104:1882–9.

40. Rodrigues TC, Fidalgo F, da Costa CM, Ferreira EN, da Cunha IW, Carraro DM, et al. Upregulated genes at 2q24 gains as candidate oncogenes in hepatoblastomas. Future Oncol (London, England). 2014;10:2449–57.

41. Shan SW, Fang L, Shatseva T, Rutnam ZJ, Yang X, Du W, et al. Mature miR-17-5p and passenger miR-17-3p induce hepatocellular carcinoma by targeting PTEN, GalNT7 and vimentin in different signal pathways. J Cell Sci. 2013;126:1517–30.

42. Roy S, Levi E, Majumdar AP, Sarkar FH. Expression of miR-34 is lost in colon cancer which can be re-expressed by a novel agent CDF. J Hematol Oncol. 2012;5:58.

43. Wu H, Chen J, Li D, Liu X, Li L, Wang K. MicroRNA-30e functions as a tumor suppressor in cervical carcinoma cells through targeting GALNT7. Transl Oncol. 2017;10:876–85.

44. Li Y, Li Y, Chen D, Jin L, Su Z, Liu J, et al. miR30a5p in the tumorigenesis of renal cell carcinoma: a tumor suppressive microRNA. Mol Med Rep. 2016;13:4085–94.

45. Engelman JA. Targeting PI3K signalling in cancer: opportunities, challenges and limitations. Nat Rev Cancer. 2009;9:550–62.

46. Zhang R, Lahens NF, Ballance HI, Hughes ME, Hogenesch JB. A circadian gene expression atlas in mammals: implications for biology and medicine. Proc Natl Acad Sci U S A. 2014;111:16219–24.

47. El Bezawy R, De Cesare M, Pennati M, Deraco M, Gandellini P, Zuco V, et al. Antitumor activity of miR-34a in peritoneal mesothelioma relies on c-MET and AXL inhibition: persistent activation of ERK and AKT signaling as a possible cytoprotective mechanism. J Hematol Oncol. 2017;10(1):19.

48. Akinleye A, Avvaru P, Furqan M, Song Y, Liu D. Phosphatidylinositol 3-kinase (PI3K) inhibitors as cancer therapeutics. J Hematol Oncol. 2013;6:88.

15

Mouse avatar models of esophageal squamous cell carcinoma proved the potential for EGFR-TKI afatinib and uncovered Src family kinases involved in acquired resistance

Zhentao Liu[1†], Zuhua Chen[1†], Jingyuan Wang[1], Mengqi Zhang[1], Zhongwu Li[2], Shubin Wang[3], Bin Dong[2], Cheng Zhang[1], Jing Gao[1,3*] and Lin Shen[1,3*]

Abstract

Background: No approved targeted agents are available for esophageal squamous cell carcinoma (ESCC). Informative genomic analysis and mouse patient-derived xenografts (PDX) also called mouse avatar can greatly expedite drug discovery.

Methods: Six ESCC cell lines and 7 out of 25 PDX models derived from 188 biopsies with clear molecular features were employed to evaluate the sensitivity of several EGFR blockers in vitro and in vivo, as well as the underlying antitumor mechanisms of the most promising EGFR-TKI afatinib. Mechanisms involved in acquired resistance of afatinib were explored based on established resistant cell lines and PDX models followed by an attempt to reverse resistance.

Results: Compared with other EGFR blockers, the second-generation EGFR-TKI afatinib exerted superior antitumor effects in ESCC, and *EGFR* copy number gain (CNG) or overexpression was proposed to be predictive biomarkers. Afatinib played its antitumor effects by inhibiting EGFR downstream pathways, as well as inducing apoptosis and cell cycle arrest at G1. It was increased phosphorylation of Src family kinases (SFKs), rather than MET upregulation, that conferred to acquired resistance of afatinib. Dual blockade of EGFR and SFKs could overcome afatinib resistance and warrants validation in clinical practice.

Conclusion: Both ESCC cell lines and PDXs with *EGFR* CNG or overexpression are potential candidates for afatinib, and concomitant EGFR/SFKs inhibition could reverse afatinib-acquired resistance caused by SFKs activation in ESCC.

Keywords: ESCC, Mouse avatar, Afatinib, Src family kinases, Acquired resistance

Background

Different from western countries, esophageal squamous cell carcinoma (ESCC) is the predominant histopathological type in China, which poses great threats to people's health [1]. A large portion of patients with ESCC are diagnosed with advanced-stage disease and lose the

opportunity for radical therapy, resulting in a very poor overall survival [2]. Current treatments for patients with unresectable advanced disease focus on chemotherapy and chemoradiotherapy, but the efficacy is quite limited [2, 3]. Although targeted therapies play an increasingly important role in the treatment of many cancers, no targeted agents are available in ESCC [4]. Consequently, developing new targeted agents based on potential targets is an urgent need in ESCC.

Currently, several large-scale genomics studies on ESCC have highlighted the roles of multiple recurrently dysregulated pathways and genes in ESCC, including

* Correspondence: gaojing_pumc@163.com; shenlin@bjmu.edu.cn
†Zhentao Liu and Zuhua Chen contributed equally to this work.
[1]Key laboratory of Carcinogenesis and Translational Research (Ministry of Education/Beijing), Department of Gastrointestinal Oncology, Peking University Cancer Hospital and Institute, 52 Fucheng Road, Haidian District, Beijing 100142, China
Full list of author information is available at the end of the article

receptor tyrosine kinase (RTK), cell cycle, Wnt/Notch, and Hippo pathways [5–7]. Among these altered pathways and genes, epidermal growth factor receptor (EGFR) is very promising, and attempts to target EGFR are never given up in ESCC even if no targeted agents are approved till now. Although *EGFR* mutation is rare in ESCC, frequency of *EGFR* amplification or copy number variation (CNV) ranges from 6 to 24.3% [5–9], suggesting a potential for EGFR-targeted therapy in ESCC.

EGFR blockers contain monoclonal antibodies (mAbs) and small-molecule tyrosine kinase inhibitors (TKI) and have been updated a few generations [10]. Despite the failure of some EGFR blockers in ESCC such as EGFR monoclonal antibodies (mAbs) cetuximab and tyrosine kinase inhibitors (TKIs) gefitinib as confirmed by several clinical trials [11–14], subsequent stratified analysis of these trials suggested that patients with squamous histopathological type, *EGFR* copy number gain (CNG), or overexpression might benefit from EGFR-targeted therapy [15–17], which motivated us greatly to initiate the deeper exploration. Previously, we have established many patient-derived xenografts (PDX) of advanced ESCC using gastroscopic biopsies [18], which faithfully resembled the original patients' tumors and had been regarded as the optimal preclinical mouse avatar [19]. Here in this study, we utilized ESCC PDXs and cell lines to systematically identify the most promising EGFR blocker and provide a more accurate evidence for clinical trials, followed by its further investigations of underlying mechanisms, predictive biomarkers, and acquired resistant mechanisms together with reversing strategies.

Methods

Drugs and antibodies

Afatinib dimaleate was provided by Boehringer Ingelheim International GmbH (Germany). Gefitinib (#S1025), osimertinib (#S7297), dasatinib hydrochloride (#HY-10181A), and crizotinib hydrochloride (#HY-50878A) were purchased from Selleck Chemicals or MedChem Express. Cetuximab (#205923-56-4) and nimotuzumab (#828933-51-3) were separately obtained from Merck (Germany) and Biotech Pharma Co., Ltd. (China). Afatinib was dissolved in water, and the other drugs were dissolved in dimethyl sulfoxide (DMSO, #0231, Amresco) for in vitro studies. Antibodies are listed in Additional file 1: Materials and Methods.

Cell lines and cell culture

Human ESCC cell lines EC109, KYSE450, KYSE140, KYSE510, TE-1, and TE-10 were purchased from the cell bank of Peking Union Medical College (Beijing, China). Cells were cultured in RPMI 1640 medium (Gibco) supplemented with 10% FBS (Gibco) in a humidified incubator with 5% CO_2 at 37 °C. All cell lines were confirmed by short-tandem repeat (STR) analysis and no mycoplasma

contamination certified by using a Mycoplasma Detection Kit (#FM311–01, TransGen Biotech, China).

Cell proliferation assay

A total of 3000–5000 cells per well were seeded in 96-well plates and treated with drugs. Seventy-two hours after treatment, CCK-8 (#CK04, Dojindo, Japan) was added to assess cell viability, and the absorbance at 450 nm was measured on a Microplate Absorbance Reader (Bio-Rad). The IC50 was calculated using GraphPad software. All assays were repeated at least three times.

Generation of afatinib-resistant cell lines

EC109 and KYSE450 cells were cultured with stepwise escalating concentrations of afatinib, starting at 100 nM and increasing to 2 μM (EC109) or 5 μM (KYSE450), at which cells could proliferate. Control cells were parallel treated with vehicle. Cell proliferation assays were conducted to confirm the resistance, and parental analysis was performed by STR genotyping.

Cell cycle and apoptosis analysis

Cells were treated with afatinib or vehicle for 48 h. Apoptosis was measured by PE Annexin V Apoptosis Detection Kit I (#559763, BD Pharmingen), and cell cycle distribution was performed using PI/RNase staining buffer solution (#550825, BD Pharmingen) according to manufacturer's instructions. The results were analyzed using FlowJo 7.6 software and ModFit LT 4.0 software.

Animal experiments in mouse

All animal studies were approved by the Ethics Committee of Animal Experiments of Peking University Cancer Hospital and were conducted in compliance with the Guide for the Care and Use of Laboratory Animals of the National Institutes of Health. For cell line-derived xenografts (CDX), five million cells were injected subcutaneously into one flank of 6-week-old non-obese diabetic/severe combined immunodeficiency (NOD/SCID) female mice (Beijing HFK Bioscience Co., Ltd., China). The PDX models were established and passed serially as described previously [18, 20, 21]. When xenografts reached 200–300 mm^3, mice were randomly assigned to different groups with five mice per group. Dissolution and administration methods of all drugs were described in Additional file 1: Materials and Methods. Tumor size and body weight were measured every 3 days. Tumor volume was determined using the formula volume = (length × width^2)/2, where length and width were the long and short diameters of the tumor, respectively. Tumor growth inhibition (TGI) rate was determined using the formula TGI = $(1-\Delta T/\Delta C) \times 100\%$, where ΔT is the change of tumor volume in the treatment group on the final day of the study and ΔC is the change of tumor volume in the control group.

Generating the afatinib-resistant PDX model

Afatinib-sensitive PDX03 was chosen to establish the afatinib-refractory PDX model. When tumor volumes reached 200–300 mm^3, the mice were given 15 mg/kg/day of afatinib until the fast growth of tumor after afatinib exposure for ~ 8 months containing three passages, indicating that the tumor was resistant to afatinib. Resistant PDX was named PDX03-R, and the parental PDX03-P was also generated after continuous vehicle treatment.

Western blotting

The proteins of cells or xenograft tissues were extracted and western blotting was performed as previously described [22]. The proteins were then detected by chemiluminescence using Immobilon Western Chemiluminescent HRP Substrate (#WBKLS0500, Millipore) and visualized with a chemiluminescent detection system (GE Healthcare). Protein bands were quantified by ImageJ software. All western blotting results shown are representative of at least three experiments with independent cell lysates.

Immunohistochemistry (IHC) and hematoxylin and eosin (H&E) staining

After the mice were sacrificed, tumors were dissected and formalin-fixed paraffin embedded (FFPE) tissue blocks were generated. IHC and H&E staining were performed as described previously [23] and were interpreted by two pathologists in our hospital independently. Ki-67 scoring was in accordance with a previous report [24]. Scoring for EGFR, pERK, and pS6 used the following scale: 0 = no staining, 1+ = weak or focal staining, 2+ = moderate staining, and 3+ = strong staining.

TaqMan copy number assays

Genomic DNA was extracted from cell lines or xenograft tissues using an EasyPure Genomic DNA Kit (#EE101, TransGen Biotech) following the manufacturer's instructions. DNA was then subjected to *EGFR* copy number analysis using TaqMan Copy Number Assays (*EGFR* Hs02925916_cn, #4400291, ThermoFisher) on an ABI 7500 FAST real-time PCR system (Applied Biosystems). *RNase P* (#4403326, ThermoFisher) was used as the control gene. Copy number was then calculated by Copy Caller v 2.0 software using the comparative Ct ($\Delta\Delta$Ct) method. Normal human control DNA (#4312660, ThermoFisher) was used as the reference. When the relative copy number was ≥ 3.0, the *EGFR* copy number was determined to be gained.

MET knockdown

The *MET* short-hairpin RNA (shRNA) virus was purchased from Genechem, China. Cells were seeded in a six-well plate and infected at a density of 3×10^5 per well with 10 μL virus following the manufacturer's instructions. The shRNA sequences are as follows: sh-Ctrl: TTCTCCGAACGTGTCACGT; sh-*MET*#1: TGGCTGGTGGCACTTTACTTA; sh-*MET*-#2: GAGGGACAAGGCTGACCATAT.

Next-generation panel sequencing

Next-generation panel sequencing and subsequent data analysis were performed as by Novogene, Beijing and were described in Additional file 1: Materials and Methods.

Transcriptome sequencing (RNA-seq)

Total mRNA was extracted using TRIzol reagent (#15596018, Invitrogen) according to the manufacturer's instructions. RNA-seq and subsequent data analysis were performed by Novogene Bioinformatics Institute (China) and were described in Additional file 1: Materials and Methods.

Statistical analysis

Statistical analyses were performed using SPSS 23.0 software or Graphpad software. Differences were analyzed using unpaired two-tailed t tests (two groups) or one-way ANOVA analysis (more than two groups). All data are presented as means $\pm$ SDs. P values < 0.05 were considered significant for all analyses.

Results

Afatinib demonstrates greater anti-tumor activity than other generation EGFR-TKIs or mAbs in ESCC in vitro and in vivo

We first evaluated six ESCC cell lines and two established ESCC PDXs for their in vitro and in vivo sensitivity to the first-, second-, and third-generation EGFR-TKIs (namely gefitinib, afatinib, and osimertinib, respectively) and two EGFR-mAbs (cetuximab and nimotuzumab), respectively. As shown in Additional file 2: Table S1 and Additional file 3: Figure S1A, for in vitro cells, EGFR-mAbs exhibited limited anti-proliferative activities, and EC109, KYSE450, and KYSE140 cells were more sensitive to EGFR-TKIs than the other three cells. Meanwhile, the second-generation EGFR-TKI, afatinib, exerted stronger anti-proliferative activities than gefitinib or osimertinib in EC109, KYSE450, and KYSE140 cells. For in vivo PDXs, afatinib also exhibited the greatest anti-tumor effects among the EGFR blockers, with a TGI of 100.22% for PDX03 and 82.65% for PDX06 (Additional file 3: Figure S1B).

Based on the above results, the inhibitory effects of very promising afatinib were further validated in two cell-derived xenografts and five another ESCC PDXs. Figure 1a showed that EC109, KYSE450, and KYSE140

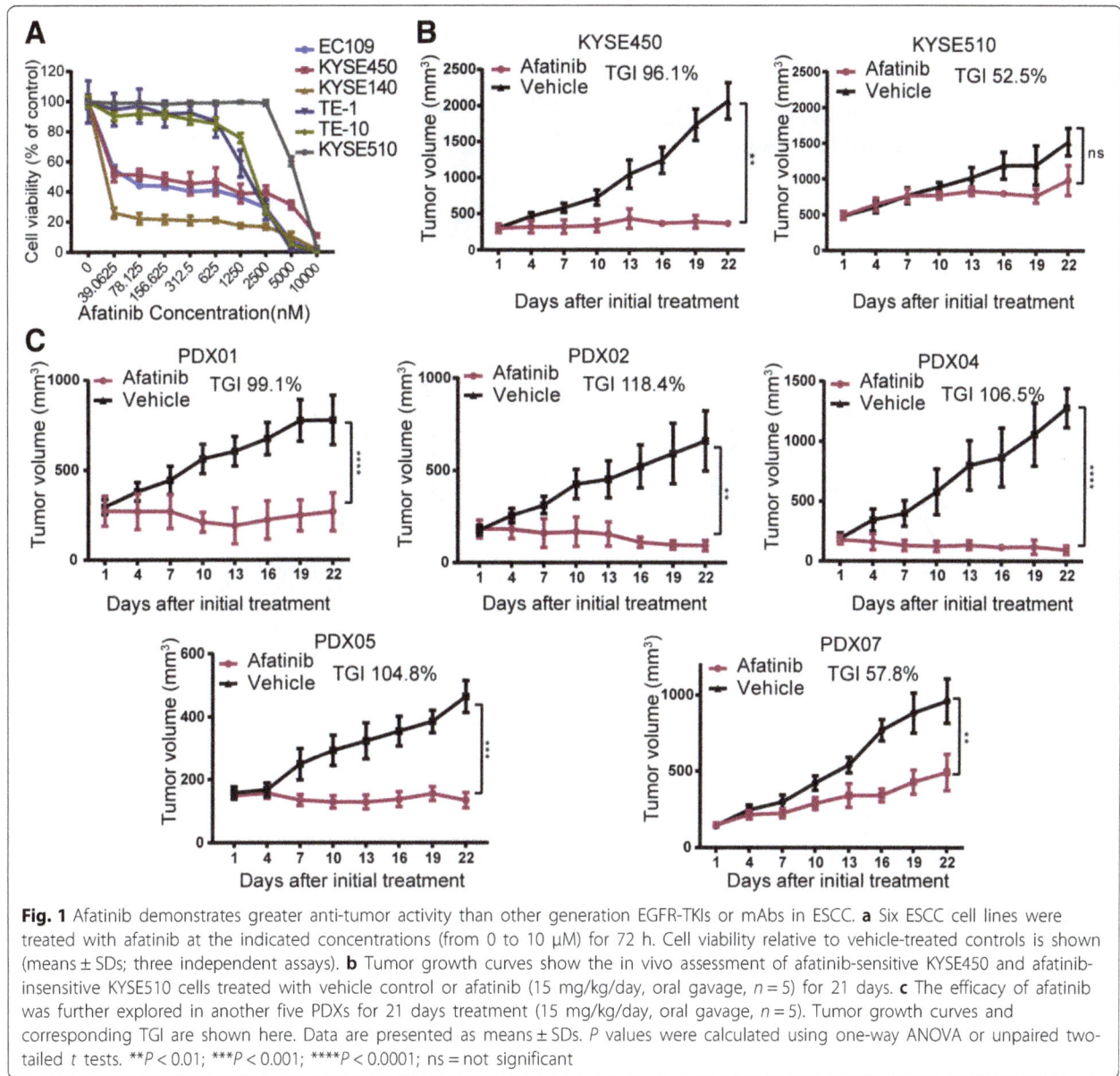

Fig. 1 Afatinib demonstrates greater anti-tumor activity than other generation EGFR-TKIs or mAbs in ESCC. **a** Six ESCC cell lines were treated with afatinib at the indicated concentrations (from 0 to 10 μM) for 72 h. Cell viability relative to vehicle-treated controls is shown (means ± SDs; three independent assays). **b** Tumor growth curves show the in vivo assessment of afatinib-sensitive KYSE450 and afatinib-insensitive KYSE510 cells treated with vehicle control or afatinib (15 mg/kg/day, oral gavage, $n = 5$) for 21 days. **c** The efficacy of afatinib was further explored in another five PDXs for 21 days treatment (15 mg/kg/day, oral gavage, $n = 5$). Tumor growth curves and corresponding TGI are shown here. Data are presented as means ± SDs. P values were calculated using one-way ANOVA or unpaired two-tailed t tests. **$P < 0.01$; ***$P < 0.001$; ****$P < 0.0001$; ns = not significant

cells were more sensitive to afatinib than KYSE510, TE-1, and TE-10 cells in vitro. Therefore, we selected KYSE450 and KYSE510 cells to evaluate the sensitivity to afatinib in vivo. Consistent with the in vitro assay, afatinib significantly inhibited the growth of KYSE450 xenografts (TGI, 96.1%) but had a limited inhibitory effect on KYSE510 xenografts (TGI, 52.5%; Fig. 1b). Moreover, four out of five PDXs showed cessation or shrinkage of tumor growth with TGIs ranging from 99.1 to 118.4% thereby illustrating a high sensitivity to afatinib (Fig. 1c). However, PDX07 showed tumor increase under afatinib treatment with a TGI of 57.8%, which illustrated a low sensitivity to afatinib.

EGFR CNG or overexpression predicts a higher sensitivity to afatinib

Since different ESCC cell lines and PDXs demonstrated a wide range of sensitivity to afatinib, the potential predictive biomarkers for EGFR-targeted therapy were investigated. Western blotting showed EGFR was the major molecule among the four pan-HER family members which expressed in the six ESCC cell lines (Fig. 2a), whereas HER2, HER3, and HER4 were hardly detected. The expression level of EGFR in EC109, KYSE450, and KYSE140 cells, which were sensitive to afatinib, was higher than that in other cells (Fig. 2). Meanwhile, these three afatinib-sensitive cell lines had an *EGFR* copy number gain, with copy numbers of

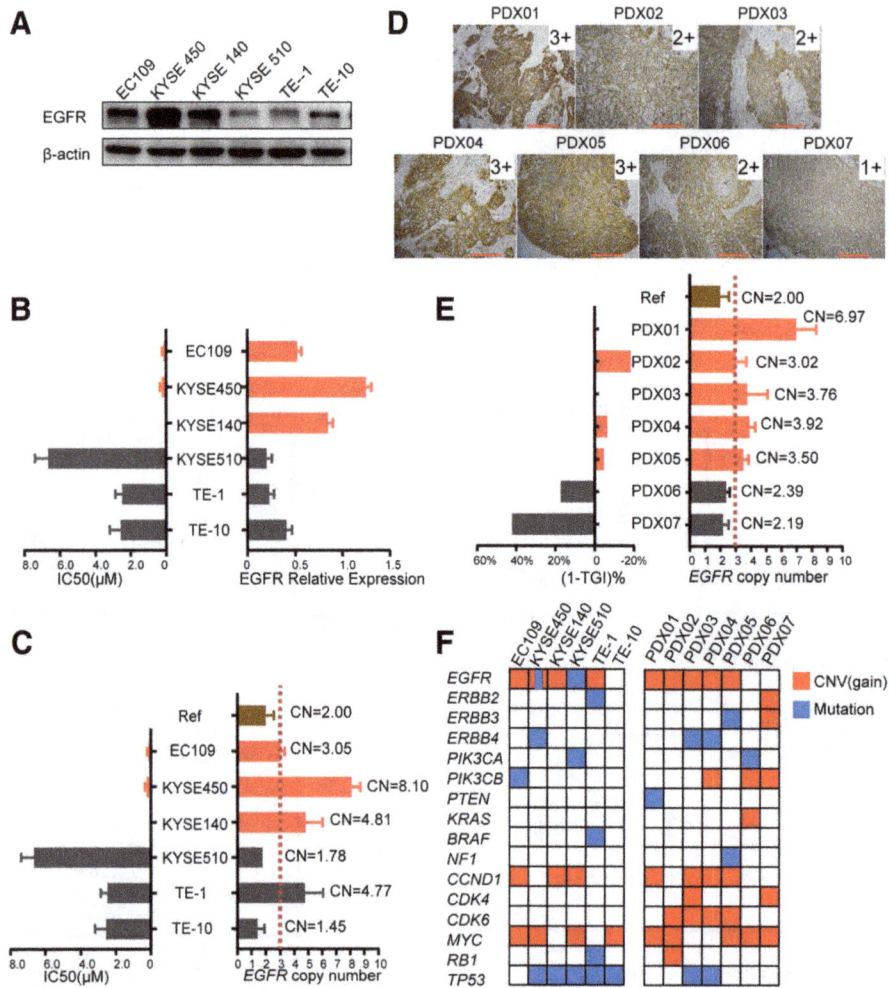

Fig. 2 *EGFR* CNG or overexpression predicts a higher sensitivity to afatinib. **a** Western blotting showed the basal protein levels of EGFR expression in six ESCC cell lines. **b** The relative EGFR expression across six ESCC cell lines was calculated according to the above western blotting after normalized to β-actin using ImageJ software. The bar chart of IC50 was drawn using the data in Additional file 2: Table S1. EC109, KYSE450, and KYSE140 are drawn in red while KYSE510, TE-1, and TE-10 are drawn in gray according to their sensitivity to afatinib. **c** The *EGFR* copy number of the six ESCC cell lines was detected using copy number assays. A copy number ≥ 3 was defined as an *EGFR* copy number gain. Data are presented as means ± SDs of three independent assays. CN, copy number; Ref, normal human control DNA . **d** The expression of EGFR in seven ESCC PDXs was detected by IHC (× 200 magnification; scale bars = 100 μM). **e** This bar chart demonstrated ESCC PDXs with *EGFR* CNG were more sensitive to afatinib treatment.1-TGI% was calculated using the data in Additional file 3: Figure S1B and Fig. 1c. When 1-TGI% was close to 0 or a negative value, the xenografts showed growth cessation or shrinkage. When 1-TGI% was a positive value or far greater than 0, the xenografts exhibited tumor growth. Data are presented as means ± SDs of three independent assays. **f** The main genetic features of ESCC cell lines and PDX models were detected using next-generation panel sequencing. Only genes in EGFR-related pathways or important tumor suppressor genes are listed. Mutations containing single nucleotide variant (SNV) and InDel are depicted in blue whereas CNV (only copy number gain) is depicted in red

3.05, 8.10, and 4.81, respectively (Fig. 2c). A significant reverse correlation was found between EGFR expression or copy number and afatinib sensitivity as indicated by IC50 (Fig. 2b and c), which was further validated in PDXs. PDXs (PDX01–05) with cessation or shrinkage of tumor growth after afatinib treatment showed a high EGFR expression (IHC score of 3+ or 2+, Fig. 2d) and a copy number > 3 (Fig. 2e). Also, a very good correlation was presented between *EGFR* copy number and inhibitory effects of afatinib in PDXs (Fig. 2e). We further explored whether other

genomic alterations could affect the response of these models to afatinib. Panel sequencing of these cell lines and PDXs showed that KYSE450 harbored an activating *EGFR* mutation (S7681), TE-1 harbored an activating *BRAF* mutation at codon 326 (I326V), and KYSE510 and PDX06 harbored an activating *PIK3CA* mutation (E545K and H1047L, respectively), which partially provided rationale for the sensitivity and resistance of these models to afatinib (Fig. 2f). Importantly, there was high consistency in *EGFR* CNV between next-generation sequencing and copy number assays.

Together, these results provided a convictive evidence for using *EGFR* CNG or overexpression as a predictive biomarker in future clinical trial design.

Afatinib plays inhibitory effects by blocking EGFR phosphorylation and downstream signaling pathways as well as inducing cell cycle arrest and apoptosis

We next evaluated the biochemical effects of afatinib in these ESCC cell lines and PDXs. EGFR phosphorylation was effectively blocked by 10 nM afatinib in all cell lines (Fig. 3a). S6 and ERK phosphorylation (pS6 and pERK) were significantly inhibited by 100 nM afatinib in the afatinib-sensitive lines EC109, KYSE450, and KYSE140, but 100 nM afatinib did not inhibit pS6 in KYSE510 or pERK in TE-1 cells possibly due to the abovementioned PIK3CA and BRAF mutations, respectively (Fig. 3a). Phosphorylated AKT (S473) was either inhibited or activated among different cell lines (Fig. 3a), which was possibly due to the feedback bypass activation [25] and need to be further investigated. Similarly, afatinib effectively inhibited pS6 and pERK in PDXs tissue as detected by IHC (Fig. 3b). Moreover, afatinib significantly decreased the expression level of Ki-67 and further verified its anti-proliferative activities (Fig. 3b). In addition, afatinib could induce obvious G1 phase arrest and apoptosis in a dose-dependent manner in afatinib-sensitive KYSE450, KYSE140, and EC109 cells, but not in afatinib-insensitive KYSE510 cells (Fig. 3c, d, f, and g; Additional file 4: Figure S2A, S2B, S2D, and S2E). Consistent with G1 phase arrest evaluated by flow cytometry, levels of P21 and P27, two negative regulators of the cell cycle, were increased, whereas CDK4, CDK6, and CCND1 were decreased in KYSE450, KYSE140, and EC109 cells other than KYSE510 cells after afatinib treatment (Fig. 3e and Additional file 4: Figure S2C). Also, along with cell apoptosis, cleaved form of caspase-8 and PARP were increased, and the anti-apoptotic protein BCL2 was decreased in KYSE450, KYSE140, and EC109 cells other than KYSE510 cells under afatinib treatment (Fig. 3h and Additional file 4: Figure S2F).

Distinct differences are presented in afatinib-refractory ESCC models compared with its parental sensitive models

Undergoing a long-term exposure to afatinib (Fig. 4a), two afatinib acquired resistant cell lines and one afatinib-acquired resistant PDX model were established and named as KYSE450-R, EC109-R, and PDX03-R, respectively. Compared with their parental cells or PDX named as KYSE450-P, EC109-P, and PDX03-P, refractory models demonstrated obvious resistance to afatinib (Fig. 4b) indicated as significantly increased IC50 (about 20 folds) in cells and decreased TGI (decreased by 58.72%) in PDX. Besides, no obvious morphological changes were obtained between afatinib-acquired resistant models and their parental sensitive models (Fig. 4c). In afatinib-refractory cells or PDX, phosphorylated S6

and ERK could no longer be inhibited by afatinib in contrast with their sensitive counterparts (Fig. 4d), which also verified the success of afatinib-acquired resistant models. Transcriptome sequencing results indicated that compared with their parental sensitive cells or PDX, afatinib-resistant models showed distinct differential gene profiles (Fig. 4e) which involved in many signaling pathways (Additional file 5: Figure S3A-C). In addition, variant analysis did not reveal any new mutations within the EGFR kinase domain or mutations in the downstream effectors like *PIK3CA, KRAS*, or *BRAF* after afatinib-acquired resistance (data not shown). However, the transcriptome sequencing data failed to help us find a specific gene or pathway to rationally explain the mechanisms of acquired resistance here.

The common emergence of MET upregulation does not confer afatinib-acquired resistance in ESCC

Previous studies suggested that the epithelial to mesenchymal transition (EMT) lead to acquired resistance to EGFR TKIs in lung cancer and ESCC [8, 10]. However, the EMT process was proved not to play an important role in this study (Fig. 5a). To elucidate whether a bypass signaling pathway participated in the acquisition of resistance, the expression of some RTKs was examined, and MET upregulation was observed in all three resistant models (Fig. 5b), which suggested the possible role of MET in afatinib-acquired resistance. Crizotinib, a MET inhibitor, was added to afatinib-resistant KYSE450-R and EC109-R cells, but no any difference was found compared with afatinib monotherapy (Fig. 5c). An alternative strategy was employed by *MET* knockdown, and results also confirmed that MET downregulation could not re-sensitize the resistant cells to afatinib (Fig. 5d). Deep-going analysis demonstrated that neither combining crizotinib with afatinib nor *MET* knockdown had effects on phosphorylated S6 and ERK (Fig. 5e and f), which provided a solid evidence that targeting MET was not a strategy for overcoming acquired resistance to afatinib in ESCC.

Increased phosphorylation of Src family kinases leads to acquired afatinib resistance in ESCC

We then turned to Src family kinases (SFKs), as SFKs are well-known upstream regulators of PI3K and MAPK pathways [26]. Western blotting showed increased SFKs phosphorylation at Tyr-416 in the KYSE450-R and PDX03-R models but not in EC109-R (Fig. 6a). However, no obvious upregulation in total SFKs levels was observed. Therefore, we explored whether increased pSFKs levels lead to the acquired resistance. The SFKs inhibitor, dasatinib, could re-sensitize KYSE450-R and EC109-R cells to afatinib treatment (Fig. 6b), which was validated by results that dasatinib combined with afatinib could significantly inhibit phosphorylated S6 and ERK (Fig. 6c),

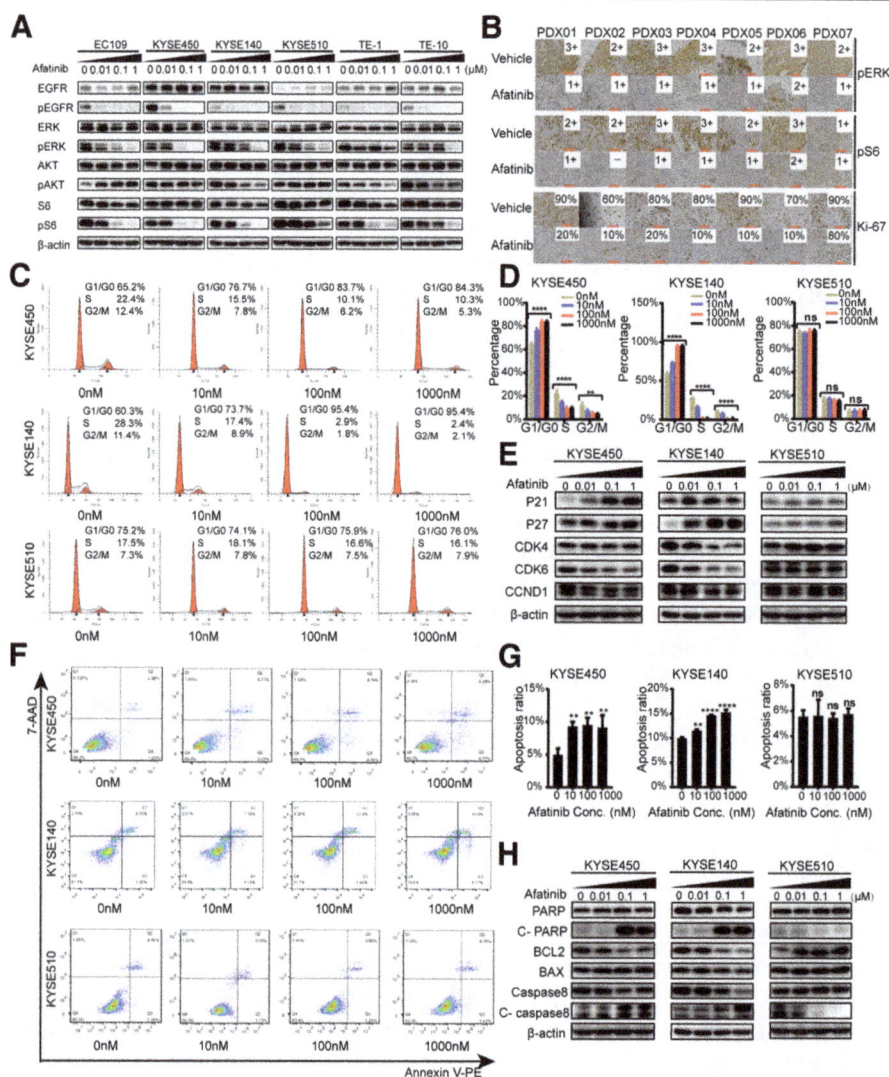

Fig. 3 The anti-tumor mechanisms of afatinib in ESCC cell lines and PDXs. **a** Six ESCC cell lines were treated with 0, 10 nM, 100 nM, and 1 μM afatinib and harvested after 48 h. Immunoblots show the response of EGFR downstream signaling molecules to afatinib. **b** IHC staining for pERK, pS6, and Ki-67 in seven PDXs tumors after 21 days treatment. Representative images and interpretation (by two independent pathologists) are shown (× 200 magnification; scale bars = 100 μM). **c–h** KYSE450, KYSE140, and KYSE510 cells were treated with 0, 10 nM, 100 nM, and 1 μM afatinib after serum-starvation for 12 h. After 48 h of treatment, the cells were harvested and assayed as described below. The effects of afatinib on cell cycle distribution were assessed using flow cytometry after PI/RNase staining (**c**). The distribution of cells in the cell cycle is depicted (**d**). G1 phase-associated proteins (P21, P27, CDK4, CDK6, and CCND1) were assessed using western blotting (**e**). Flow cytometry showed the apoptosis induced by afatinib treatment using PE-annexin V and 7-AAD staining (**f**). The percentage of cells in early apoptosis (Q3) and late apoptosis (Q2) was calculated as the total apoptosis ratio (**g**). Apoptosis-related proteins (c-PARP, c-caspase8, BCL2, and BAX) were measured by western blotting after afatinib treatment (**h**). Data are presented as means ± SDs of three independent assays. P values were calculated using one-way ANOVA or unpaired two-tailed t tests.*$P < 0.05$; **$P < 0.01$; ***$P < 0.001$; ****$P < 0.0001$; ns = not significant

although no obvious increase of pSFKs was observed in EC109-R. These data were further confirmed in vivo xenografts. As shown in Fig. 6d and e, compared with any single drug or afatinib combined with crizotinib, a combination of afatinib with dasatinib could greatly inhibit the growth of xenografts derived from KYSE450-R and PDX03-R, with TGIs of 96.47% and 102.10%, respectively. Further analysis also verified the in vivo results indicated as the inactivation of phosphorylated S6 and

ERK after afatinib combined with dasatinib treatment (Fig. 6f and g). Based on our results, the molecular mechanisms that afatinib works or not followed by the subsequential strategies are depicted schematically in Fig. 6h.

Discussion

The present study demonstrated that afatinib exerted greater anti-tumor effects on ESCC cell lines and PDXs than other-generation EGFR-TKIs or mAbs in vitro and

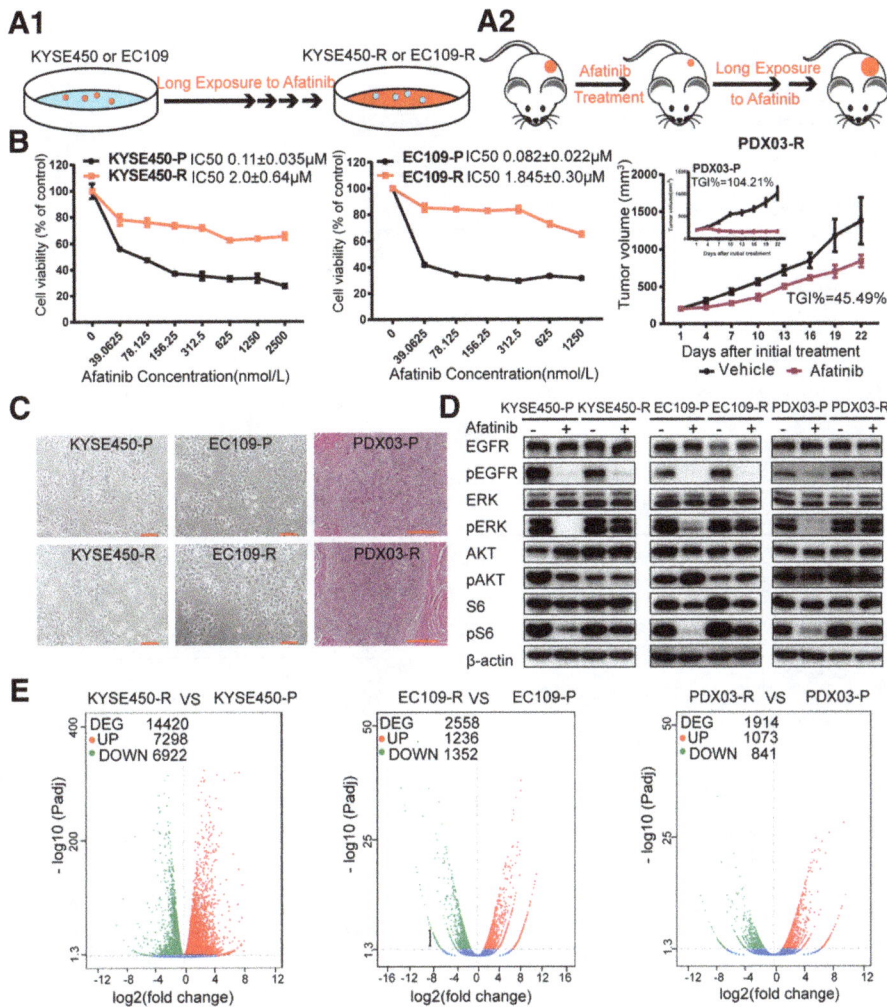

Fig. 4 Distinct differences are presented in afatinib-refractory ESCC models compared with its parental sensitive models. **a** The cartoon depicts the process of generating two afatinib-resistant ESCC cell lines in vitro (**a1**) and one afatinib-resistant ESCC PDX in vivo (**a2**). **b** Dose-response curves were generated to confirm the resistant phenotype of KYSE450-R and EC109-R after 72 h of afatinib treatment. Data are presented as means ± SDs of three independent assays. In vivo xenograft experiments were conducted to confirm the resistant phenotype of PDX03-R. PDX03-P and PDX03-R were treated with afatinib for 21 days by oral gavage at a dose of 15 mg/kg/day (n = 5). Data are presented as means ± SDs. **c** Representative images of resistant and parental cells or PDX (× 100 magnification for cells; × 200 magnification for PDX; scale bars = 100 μM). The morphology of the resistant PDX model was detected by H&E staining. **d** Responses of the EGFR downstream signaling to afatinib treatment in parental and resistant cells or PDX. Cells were harvested after 200 nM afatinib treatment for 48 h. Tissue lysates were extracted from PDX03-R and PDX03-P xenografts after 21 days of afatinib treatment. All experiments were repeated three times independently. **e** Volcano plots showed the distinct differential gene profiles after the acquisition of a resistant phenotype, as detected by RNA-seq. Red dots represented upregulated genes and green dots indicated downregulated genes in resistant models compared with their counterparts. DEG, differential genes; UP, upregulated genes; DOWN, downregulated genes

in vivo. Previous in vitro kinase assays revealed that afatinib had a higher affinity for wild-type EGFR than gefitinib or osimertinib [27, 28], which were consistent with the current findings that afatinib exhibited better efficacy than other EGFR blockers in ESCC because of its higher potency for wild-type EGFR and broader irreversible ErbB blockade compared with inhibitors that block EGFR alone. Two clinical trials uncovered that afatinib achieved better clinical improvements than erlotinib in lung squamous

cell carcinoma (LUSC) [29] or methotrexate in head and neck squamous cell carcinoma (HNSCC) [30], illustrating afatinib's outstanding clinical efficacy in tumors with wild-type EGFR. Given the similar genomic landscape among ESCC, HNSCC, and LUSC [5], we speculate that afatinib will have promising performance in select ESCC patients. The current study provided encouraging evidence for evaluating afatinib in the clinical trials for ESCC patients.

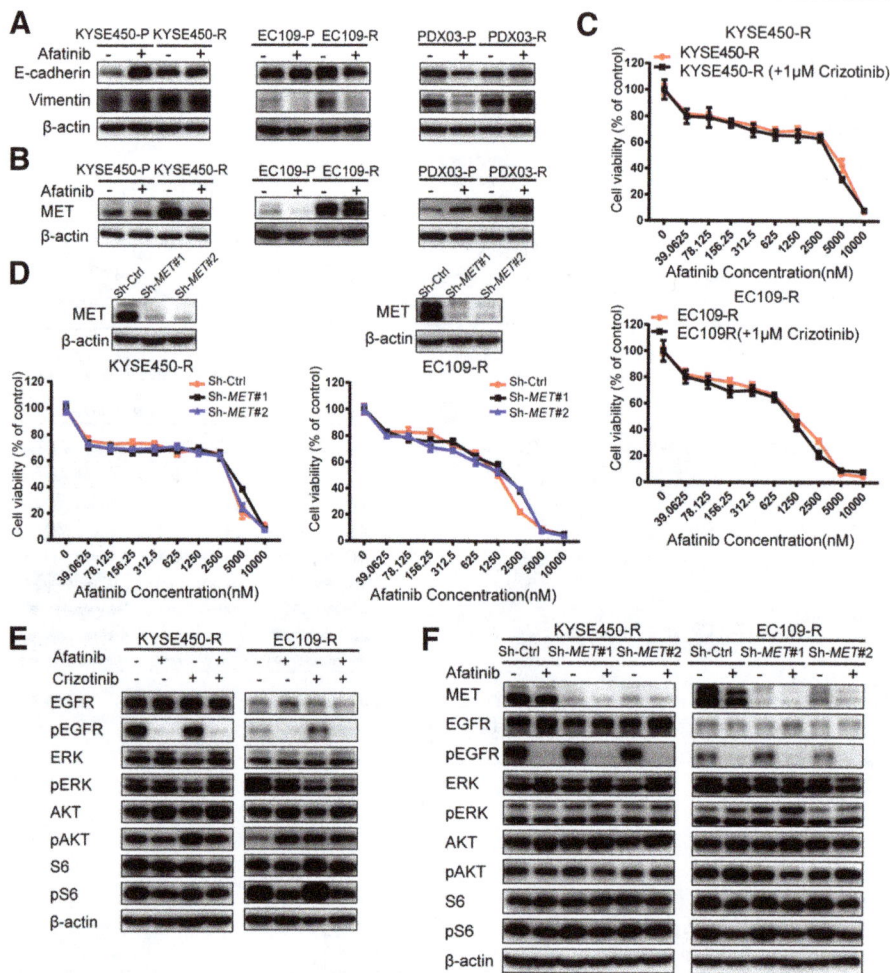

Fig. 5 The common emergence of MET upregulation does not confer afatinib-acquired resistance in ESCC. **a** The levels of the EMT markers (E-cadherin and vimentin) between resistant and parental models. **b** MET expression was upregulated in all three afatinib-resistant models. Cells were harvested after treatment with 200 nM afatinib for 48 h. The PDX lysates used were the same as those described in Fig. 4d. All assays were repeated three times independently. **c** KYSE450-R and EC109-R cells were treated with increasing concentrations of afatinib in the presence or absence of 1 μM crizotinib for 72 h, and CCK-8 assays were performed to assess cell viability. Data are presented as the means ± SDs of three independent assays. **d** After *MET* was knocked down in KYSE450-R and EC109-R cells, cells were treated with increasing concentrations of afatinib for 72 h, and then CCK-8 assays were performed to assess cell viability. Data are presented as the means ± SDs of three independent assays. **e** Resistant cells were treated with 200 nM afatinib alone or in combination with 1 μM crizotinib for 48 h. **f** Resistant cells after *MET* knockdown were treated with 200 nM afatinib for 48 h. All experiments were repeated three times independently

Previous clinical trials of gefitinib (the COG study) [14, 15] and icotinib (first-generation EGFR-TKIs) [31] demonstrated that EGFR-TKIs exhibited favorable efficacy in ESCC patients with *EGFR* amplification as detected by fluorescence in situ hybridization (FISH) method. Despite with different detection methods for *EGFR* copy number, we showed that *EGFR* CNG, as detected by copy number assays, was proved to be the predictor for afatinib efficacy, which further verified the role of EGFR as a potential target in ESCC and was consistent with what we have found in gastric cancer [21]. However, TE-1 cells with *EGFR* CNG were not sensitive to afatinib. Further genomic analysis showed that in addition to *EGFR* CNG, TE-1 harbored a *BRAF* mutation at codon 326

(I326V), which had been reported to result in primary resistance to panitumumab [32]. Besides, KYSE510 harbored a non-activating *EGFR* mutation (A702D) in the juxtamembrane region and showed no correlations with sensitivity to EGFR-TKIs according to previous studies [33]; KYSE450 harbored an activating *EGFR* mutation (S768I) in tyrosine kinase domain, and this mutation was reported to be sensitive to afatinib [34]. Since afatinib is a pan-HER inhibitor, we also examined the expression levels and genetic alterations of HER2, HER3, and HER4 in these ESCC cell lines and PDX models, but all these three molecules were hardly detected by western blotting or IHC, and no genetic alterations were found to be correlated with the afatinib sensitivity (data

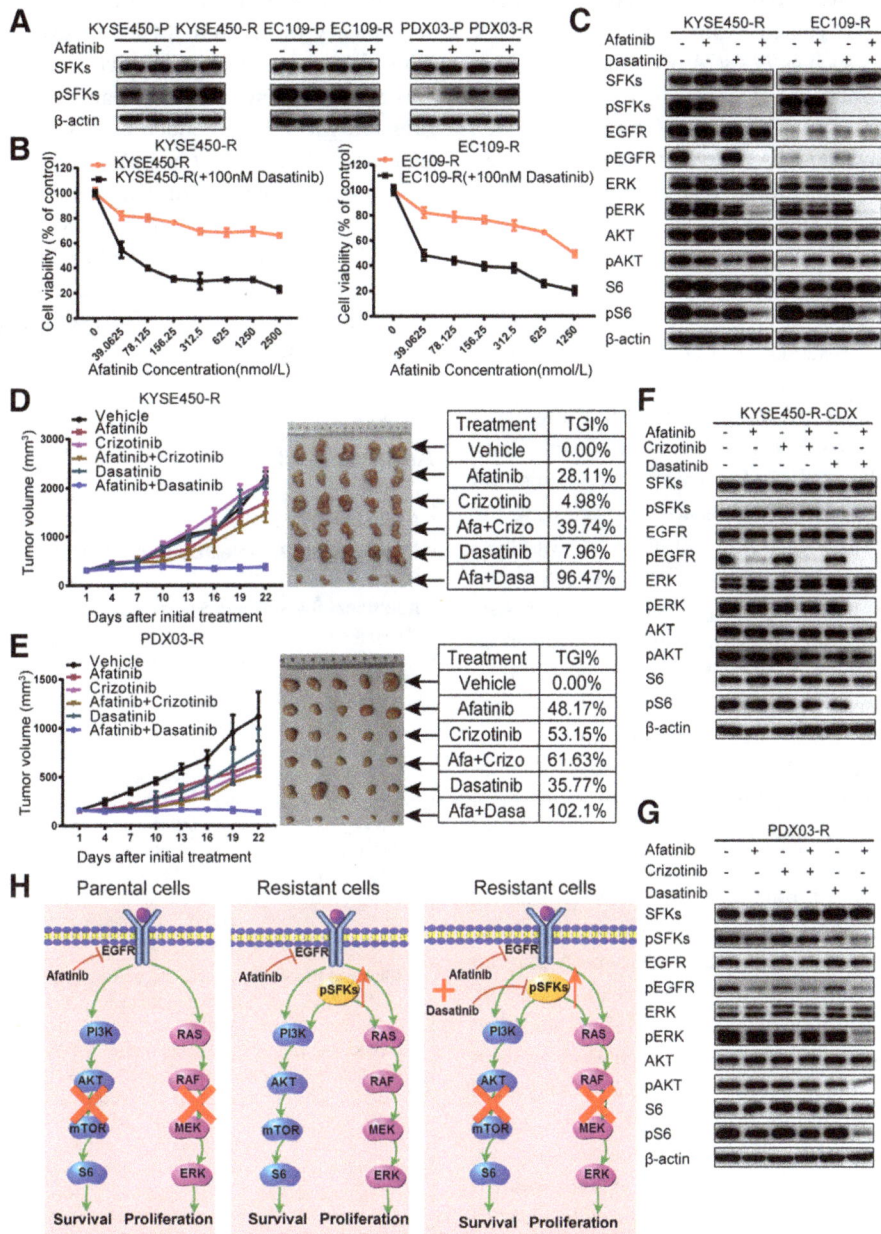

Fig. 6 Increased phosphorylation of Src family kinases leads to acquired afatinib resistance in ESCC. **a** Increased pSFKs levels were observed in KYSE450-R and PDX03-R resistant models, but total SFKs levels were unchanged. Cells were harvested after treatment with 200 nM afatinib for 48 h. The PDX lysates used were the same as those described in Fig. 4d. All assays were repeated three times independently. **b** Resistant cells were treated with the indicated concentrations of afatinib in the presence or absence of 100 nM dasatinib for 72 h, and CCK-8 assays were performed to assess cell viability. Data are presented as the means ± SDs of three independent assays. **c** KYSE450-R and EC109-R cells were treated with 200 nM afatinib alone or in combination with 100 nM dasatinib for 48 h. **d, e** Curves showing the xenografts growth of KYSE450-R (**d**) and PDX03-R (**e**) treated with vehicle control, afatinib (15 mg/kg), crizotinib (25 mg/kg), afatinib (15 mg/kg) plus crizotinib (25 mg/kg), dasatinib (15 mg/kg), or afatinib (15 mg/kg) plus dasatinib (15 mg/kg). Data are presented as means ± SDs; $n = 5$. Mice were sacrificed after 21 days of treatment, and xenografts were isolated. Pictures of the xenografts are shown with the corresponding TGI listed in the tables. **f, g** Lysates were extracted from KYSE450-R (**f**) and PDX03-R (**g**) xenografts after 21 days of treatment with the corresponding inhibitors and analyzed by western blotting to explore the downstream signaling responses. The lysates were then probed with the indicated antibodies. All experiments were repeated three times independently. **h** A schematic of the molecular mechanisms of acquired resistance revealed in this study

not shown). Above all, *EGFR* CNG or amplification may be a promising predictive biomarker for EGFR-targeted therapy in ESCC patients, but patients with mutations in EGFR downstream effectors such as *PIK3CA* or *BRAF* may exhibit de novo resistance to afatinib.

Despite the initial response of most targeted agents, resistance inevitably emerges. Previous studies revealed several mechanisms of acquired resistance to EGFR inhibitors in lung cancer such as *EGFR* T790 M mutation, *MET* amplification, IGF-1R upregulation, AXL upregulation, or histologic changes like transformation to small-cell lung cancer or EMT [35].However, the mechanisms of acquired resistance to EGFR-targeted therapy in an ESCC setting, where *EGFR* is wild-type, are poorly understood. Zhou et al. [8] showed that EMT mediated the acquired resistance to erlotinib in ESCC cell lines. However, EMT did not play a key role in the acquisition of resistance in our resistant models. After excluding the emergence of mutations in *EGFR* and downstream effectors such as *PIK3CA*, *KRAS*, and *BRAF*, we speculated that bypass signaling pathways might result in the resistance. We first focused on MET for its upregulation in all three resistant models, but it was finally proved to be irrelevant to the resistance in vitro and in vivo. Others [36] also found that MET upregulation without amplification was not associated with acquired resistance to EGFR-TKIs in lung cancer, but instead only enhanced migratory and invasive abilities, which was consistent with the current findings.

SFKs are a group of non-receptor tyrosine kinases containing nine members and are well-known upstream regulators of PI3K and MAPK pathways, which play an important role in cell proliferation, survival, adhesion, and invasion during tumor development [37]. Takeshi et al. [38] and Eiki et al. [25] revealed that SFKs activation could mediate resistance to EGFR-TKIs and suggested that concomitant inhibition of SFKs and EGFR could overcome this resistance in lung cancer. Here, we showed that SFKs phosphorylation at Tyr-416 was increased in the afatinib-refractory ESCC models without upregulation of total SFKs levels. Dual EGFR and SFKs blockade could abolish the downstream phosphorylation of S6 and ERK and therefore overcome the resistance. In Eiki's study, they found that increased pSFKs levels were caused by amplification of *YES1*, one member of the SFKs, and further led to EGFR-TKIs resistance [25]. However, since the total protein levels of SFKs or the transcriptional levels of the nine SFKs members as indicated by RNA-seq (data not shown) were unchanged, we did not further explore which member of the nine SFKs lead to such resistance. Future studies need to elucidate the reasons for the increased pSFKs levels in our resistant models, and explore whether dual EGFR/SFKs blockade could delay the emergence of resistance.

Conclusions

In conclusion, our work is the first attempt to compare the efficacy of different EGFR blockers using ESCC preclinical models in vitro and in vivo. We found that afatinib was a better choice for ESCC, and *EGFR* CNG or overexpression was recommended as a predictive biomarker for EGFR-targeted therapy in ESCC patients. Afatinib can inhibit EGFR downstream pathways as well as inducing apoptosis and G1 phase arrest in ESCC preclinical models. In addition, activated SFKs could mediate acquired resistance to afatinib and dual EGFR/SFKs blockade can overcome this resistance in an ESCC setting, which need to be further validated in clinical practice.

Additional files

Additional file 1: Materials and Methods. (DOCX 22 kb)

Additional file 2: Table S1. Efficacy of different EGFR blockers on ESCC cell lines. (DOCX 17 kb)

Additional file 3: Figure S1. Efficacy of different EGFR blockers on ESCC cell lines and PDX models. (A) Six ESCC cell lines were treated with different EGFR blockers (gefitinib, afatinib, osimertinib, cetuximab, and nimotuzumab) at the indicated concentrations (from 0 to 10 μM for TKIs and 0–1000 μg/mL for mAbs). After treatment for 72 h, cell growth inhibition was detected using CCK-8 assays. Cell viability at different doses relative to vehicle-treated controls is shown (means ± SD; three independent assays). (B) Curves plots the growth of PDX03 and PDX06 treated with vehicle control, gefitinib (50 mg/kg/day, oral gavage), afatinib (15 mg/kg/day, oral gavage), osimertinib (15 mg/kg/day, oral gavage), cetuximab (0.5 mg per mouse, twice a week, i.p.), or nimotuzumab (0.5 mg per mouse, twice a week, i.p.). Mice were sacrificed after 21 days of treatment and xenografts were isolated. Pictures of the xenografts are shown and the corresponding TGI is listed in the tables. Data are presented as means ± SDs; $n = 5$. (DOCX 1320 kb)

Additional file 4: Figure S2. Effects of afatinib on cell cycle and apoptosis in EC109 cells. EC109 cells were treated with 0, 10 nM, 100 nM, and 1 μM afatinib after serum-starvation for 12 h. After 48 h treatment, the cells were harvested and assayed as described below. The effects of afatinib on cell cycle distribution were assessed using flow cytometry after PI/RNase staining (A). The distribution of cells in the cell cycle is depicted (B). G1 phase-associated proteins (P21, P27, CDK4, CDK6, and CCND1) were assessed using western blotting (C).Flow cytometry showed the apoptosis induced by afatinib treatment using PE-annexin V and 7-AAD staining (D). The percentage of cells in early apoptosis (Q3) and late apoptosis (Q2) was calculated as the total apoptosis ratio (E). Apoptosis-related proteins (c-PARP, c-caspase8, BCL2, and BAX) were measured by western blotting after afatinib treatment (F). Data are presented as means ± SDs of three independent assays. P values were calculated using one-way ANOVA or unpaired two-tailed t-tests.*$P < 0.05$; **$P < 0.01$; ***$P < 0.001$; ****$P < 0.0001$; ns = not significant. (DOCX 570 kb)

Additional file 5: Figure S3. Pathway enrichment by RNA-Seq. Dot plots showing the enrichment results of KEGG pathway analysis for KYSE450-R versus KYSE450-P (A), EC109-R versus EC109-P (B), and PDX03-R versus PDX03-P (C), as detected by RNA-seq. The size of the dots indicates the number of genes enriched in the corresponding pathways. The color of the dots indicates the significance level of the enriched pathways, as represented by the value of *Padj*. (DOCX 549 kb)

Abbreviations
CDX: Cell line-derived xenografts; CNG: Copy number gain; CNV: Copy number variation; DMSO: Dimethyl sulfoxide; EGFR: Epidermal growth factor

receptor; EMT: Epithelial to mesenchymal transition; ESCC: Esophageal squamous cell carcinoma; FISH: Fluorescence in situ hybridization; H&E: Hematoxylin and eosin; HNSCC: Head and neck squamous cell carcinoma; IHC: Immunohistochemistry; LUSC: Lung squamous cell carcinoma; mAbs: Monoclonal antibodies; NOD/SCID: Non-obese diabetic/severe combined immunodeficiency; PCR: Polymerase chain reaction; PDXs: Patient-derived xenografts; RNA-seq: Transcriptome sequencing; RTK: Receptor tyrosine kinase; SFKs: Src family kinases; shRNA: Short-hairpin RNA; STR: Short-tandem repeat; TGI: Tumor growth inhibition; TKI: Tyrosine kinase inhibitors

Acknowledgments

We would like to thank LetPub (http://www.letpub.com) for providing linguistic assistance during the preparation of this manuscript.

Funding

This work was supported by the National Key Research and Development Program of China (no. 2017YFC1308900, 2017YFC0908400) and Boehringer Ingelheim International GmbH.

Authors' contributions

This study was conceived and designed by LS and JG. ZL and ZC performed the experiments. ZL, ZL, SW, and BD analyzed the data. JW, MZ, and CZ contributed the reagents, materials, and analysis tools. ZL wrote the manuscript. All of the authors have read and approved the final manuscript.

Consent for publication

This is not applicable for this study.

Competing interests

The authors declare that they have no competing interests.

Author details

[1]Key laboratory of Carcinogenesis and Translational Research (Ministry of Education/Beijing), Department of Gastrointestinal Oncology, Peking University Cancer Hospital and Institute, 52 Fucheng Road, Haidian District, Beijing 100142, China. [2]Key Laboratory of Carcinogenesis and Translational Research (Ministry of Education/Beijing), Department of Pathology, Peking University Cancer Hospital and Institute, 52 Fucheng Road, Haidian District, Beijing 100142, China. [3]Department of Oncology, Peking University Shenzhen Hospital, 1120 Lianhua Road, Shenzhen 518036, Guangdong, China.

References

1. Zeng H, Zheng R, Zhang S, Zuo T, Xia C, Zou X, et al. Esophageal cancer statistics in China, 2011: estimates based on 177 cancer registries. Thorac Cancer. 2016;7(2):232–7.
2. Rustgi AK, El-Serag HB. Esophageal carcinoma. N Engl J Med. 2014;371(26): 2499–509.
3. Pennathur A, Gibson MK, Jobe BA, Luketich JD. Oesophageal carcinoma. Lancet. 2013;381(9864):400–12.
4. Domper Arnal MJ, Ferrandez Arenas A, Lanas Arbeloa A. Esophageal cancer: risk factors, screening and endoscopic treatment in western and eastern countries. World J Gastroenterol. 2015;21(26):7933–43.
5. Song Y, Li L, Ou Y, Gao Z, Li E, Li X, et al. Identification of genomic alterations in oesophageal squamous cell cancer. Nature. 2014;509(7498):91–5.
6. Lin DC, Hao JJ, Nagata Y, Xu L, Shang L, Meng X, et al. Genomic and molecular characterization of esophageal squamous cell carcinoma. Nat Genet. 2014;46(5):467–73.
7. Gao YB, Chen ZL, Li JG, Hu XD, Shi XJ, Sun ZM, et al. Genetic landscape of esophageal squamous cell carcinoma. Nat Genet. 2014;46(10):1097–102.

8. Zhou J, Wu Z, Wong G, Pectasides E, Nagaraja A, Stachler M, et al. CDK4/6 or MAPK blockade enhances efficacy of EGFR inhibition in oesophageal squamous cell carcinoma. Nat Commun. 2017;8:13897.
9. Wang X, Niu H, Fan Q, Lu P, Ma C, Liu W, et al. Predictive value of EGFR overexpression and gene amplification on icotinib efficacy in patients with advanced esophageal squamous cell carcinoma. Oncotarget. 2016;7(17): 24744–51.
10. Rotow J, Bivona TG. Understanding and targeting resistance mechanisms in NSCLC. Nat Rev Cancer. 2017;17(11):637–58.
11. Crosby T, Hurt CN, Falk S, Gollins S, Mukherjee S, Staffurth J, et al. Chemoradiotherapy with or without cetuximab in patients with oesophageal cancer (SCOPE1): a multicentre, phase 2/3 randomised trial. Lancet Oncol. 2013;14(7):627–37.
12. Suntharalingam M, Winter K, Ilson D, Dicker AP, Kachnic L, Konski A, et al. Effect of the addition of cetuximab to paclitaxel, cisplatin, and radiation therapy for patients with esophageal cancer: the NRG oncology RTOG 0436 phase 3 randomized clinical trial. JAMA Oncol. 2017;3(11):1520–8.
13. Lorenzen S, Schuster T, Porschen R, Al-Batran SE, Hofheinz R, Thuss-Patience P, et al. Cetuximab plus cisplatin-5-fluorouracil versus cisplatin-5-fluorouracil alone in first-line metastatic squamous cell carcinoma of the esophagus: a randomized phase II study of the Arbeitsgemeinschaft Internistische Onkologie. Ann Oncol. 2009;20(10):1667–73.
14. Dutton SJ, Ferry DR, Blazeby JM, Abbas H, Dahle-Smith A, Mansoor W, et al. Gefitinib for oesophageal cancer progressing after chemotherapy (COG): a phase 3, multicentre, double-blind, placebo-controlled randomised trial. Lancet Oncol. 2014;15(8):894–904.
15. Petty RD, Dahle-Smith A, Stevenson DAJ, Osborne A, Massie D, Clark C, et al. Gefitinib and EGFR gene copy number aberrations in esophageal Cancer. J Clin Oncol. 2017;35(20):2279–87.
16. Janmaat ML, Gallegos-Ruiz MI, Rodriguez JA, Meijer GA, Vervenne WL, Richel DJ, et al. Predictive factors for outcome in a phase II study of gefitinib in second-line treatment of advanced esophageal cancer patients. J Clin Oncol. 2006;24(10):1612–9.
17. Ilson DH, Kelsen D, Shah M, Schwartz G, Levine DA, Boyd J, et al. A phase 2 trial of erlotinib in patients with previously treated squamous cell and adenocarcinoma of the esophagus. Cancer. 2011;117(7):1409–14.
18. Zou J, Liu Y, Wang J, Liu Z, Lu Z, Chen Z, et al. Establishment and genomic characterizations of patient-derived esophageal squamous cell carcinoma xenograft models using biopsies for treatment optimization. J Transl Med. 2018;16(1):15.
19. Lai Y, Wei X, Lin S, Qin L, Cheng L, Li P. Current status and perspectives of patient-derived xenograft models in cancer research. J Hematol Oncol. 2017;10(1):106.
20. Zhu Y, Tian T, Li Z, Tang Z, Wang L, Wu J, et al. Establishment and characterization of patient-derived tumor xenograft using gastroscopic biopsies in gastric cancer. Sci Rep. 2015;5:8542.
21. Chen Z, Huang W, Tian T, Zang W, Wang J, Liu Z, et al. Characterization and validation of potential therapeutic targets based on the molecular signature of patient-derived xenografts in gastric cancer. J Hematol Oncol. 2018;11(1):20.
22. Chen Z, Liu Z, Huang W, Li Z, Zou J, Wang J, et al. Gimatecan exerts potent antitumor activity against gastric cancer in vitro and in vivo via AKT and MAPK signaling pathways. J Transl Med. 2017;15(1):253.
23. Wang J, Liu Z, Wang Z, Wang S, Chen Z, Li Z, et al. Targeting c-Myc: JQ1 as a promising option for c-Myc-amplified esophageal squamous cell carcinoma. Cancer Lett. 2018;419:64–74.
24. Vorreuther R, Hake R, Borchmann P, Lukowsky S, Thiele J, Engelmann U. Expression of immunohistochemical markers (PCNA, Ki-67, 486p and p53) on paraffin sections and their relation to the recurrence rate of superficial bladder tumors. Urol Int. 1997;59(2):88–94.
25. Ichihara E, Westover D, Meador CB, Yan Y, Bauer JA, Lu P, et al. SFK/FAK signaling attenuates osimertinib efficacy in both drug-sensitive and drug-resistant models of EGFR-mutant lung cancer. Cancer Res. 2017; 77(11):2990–3000.
26. Zhang S, Yu D. Targeting Src family kinases in anti-cancer therapies: turning promise into triumph. Trends Pharmacol Sci. 2012;33(3):122–8.
27. Li D, Ambrogio L, Shimamura T, Kubo S, Takahashi M, Chirieac LR, et al. BIBW2992, an irreversible EGFR/HER2 inhibitor highly effective in preclinical lung cancer models. Oncogene. 2008;27(34):4702–11.

28. Cross DA, Ashton SE, Ghiorghiu S, Eberlein C, Nebhan CA, Spitzler PJ, et al. AZD9291, an irreversible EGFR TKI, overcomes T790M-mediated resistance to EGFR inhibitors in lung cancer. Cancer Discov. 2014;4(9):1046–61.

29. Soria J-C, Felip E, Cobo M, Lu S, Syrigos K, Lee KH, et al. Afatinib versus erlotinib as second-line treatment of patients with advanced squamous cell carcinoma of the lung (LUX-Lung 8): an open-label randomised controlled phase 3 trial. Lancet Oncol. 2015;16(8):897–907.

30. Machiels J-PH, Haddad RI, Fayette J, Licitra LF, Tahara M, Vermorken JB, et al. Afatinib versus methotrexate as second-line treatment in patients with recurrent or metastatic squamous-cell carcinoma of the head and neck progressing on or after platinum-based therapy (LUX-Head & Neck 1): an open-label, randomised phase 3 trial. Lancet Oncol. 2015;16(5):583–94.

31. Huang J, Fan Q, Lu P, Ying J, Ma C, Liu W, et al. Icotinib in patients with pretreated advanced esophageal squamous cell carcinoma with EGFR overexpression or EGFR gene amplification: a single-arm, multicenter phase 2 study. J Thoracic Oncol. 2016;11(6):910–7.

32. Tajima Y, Shimada Y, Yagi R, Okamura T, Nakano M, Kameyama H, et al. A systematic analysis of oncogene and tumor suppressor genes for panitumumab-resistant rectal cancer with wild RAS gene - a case report. Gan To Kagaku Ryoho Cancer Chemother. 2016;43(12):2280–2.

33. Reckamp KL, Krysan K, Morrow JD, Milne GL, Newman RA, Tucker C, et al. A phase I trial to determine the optimal biological dose of celecoxib when combined with erlotinib in advanced non-small cell lung cancer. Clin Cancer Res. 2006;12(11 Pt 1):3381–8.

34. Banno E, Togashi Y, Nakamura Y, Chiba M, Kobayashi Y, Hayashi H, et al. Sensitivities to various epidermal growth factor receptor-tyrosine kinase inhibitors of uncommon epidermal growth factor receptor mutations L861Q and S768I: what is the optimal epidermal growth factor receptor-tyrosine kinase inhibitor? Cancer Sci. 2016;107(8):1134–40.

35. Sequist LV, Waltman BA, Dias-Santagata D, Digumarthy S, Turke AB, Fidias P, et al. Genotypic and histological evolution of lung cancers acquiring resistance to EGFR inhibitors. Sci Transl Med. 2011;3(75):75ra26.

36. Rho JK, Choi YJ, Lee JK, Ryoo BY, Na II, Yang SH, et al. The role of MET activation in determining the sensitivity to epidermal growth factor receptor tyrosine kinase inhibitors. Mol Cancer Res. 2009;7(10):1736–43.

37. Kim LC, Song L, Haura EB. Src kinases as therapeutic targets for cancer. Nat Rev Clin Oncol. 2009;6(10):587–95.

38. Yoshida T, Zhang G, Smith MA, Lopez AS, Bai Y, Li J, et al. Tyrosine phosphoproteomics identifies both codrivers and cotargeting strategies for T790M-related EGFR-TKI resistance in non-small cell lung cancer. Clin Cancer Res. 2014;20(15):4059–74.

16

Control of triple-negative breast cancer using ex vivo self-enriched, costimulated NKG2D CAR T cells

Yali Han[1,2], Wei Xie[1,3], De-Gang Song[1,5*] and Daniel J. Powell Jr[1,4*]

Abstract

Background: Triple-negative breast cancer (TNBC) is an aggressive disease that currently lacks effective targeted therapy. NKG2D ligands (NKG2DLs) are expressed on various tumor types and immunosuppressive cells within tumor microenvironments, providing suitable targets for cancer therapy.

Methods: We applied a chimeric antigen receptor (CAR) approach for the targeting of NKG2DLs expressed on human TNBCs. Lentiviral vectors were used to express the extracellular domain of human NKG2D that binds various NKG2DLs, fused to signaling domains derived from T cell receptor CD3 zeta alone or with CD27 or 4-1BB (CD137) costimulatory domain.

Results: Interleukin-2 (IL-2) promoted the expansion and self-enrichment of NKG2D-redirected CAR T cells in vitro. High CD25 expression on first-generation NKG2D CAR T cells was essential for the self-enrichment effect in the presence of IL-2, but not for CARs containing CD27 or 4-1BB domains. Importantly, self-enriched NKG2D CAR T cells effectively recognized and eliminated TNBC cell lines in vitro, and adoptive transfer of T cells expressing NKG2D CARs with CD27 or 4-1BB specifically enhanced NKG2D CAR surface expression, T cell persistence, and the regression of established MDA-MB-231 TNBC in vivo. NKG2D-z CAR T cells lacking costimulatory domains were less effective, highlighting the need for costimulatory signals.

Conclusions: These results demonstrate that CD27 or 4-1BB costimulated, self-enriched NKG2D CAR-redirected T cells mediate anti-tumor activity against TNBC tumor, which represent a promising immunotherapeutic approach to TNBC treatment.

Keywords: Chimeric antigen receptor, T cells, NKG2D ligands, Immunotherapy, Triple-negative breast cancer

Background

Triple-negative breast cancers (TNBC), an aggressive form of breast cancer that lacks significant expression of the human epidermal growth factor receptor 2 (HER2), estrogen receptor (ER), and progesterone receptor (PR), accounts for approximately 15~20% of invasive breast cancers. In the absence of obvious targets, patients with TNBC do not benefit from endocrine therapy or other available targeted agents [1]. To date, the standard treatment still depends on surgery and adjuvant chemotherapy and radiotherapy. Patients with TNBC have a worse outcome after chemotherapy, compared to breast cancers patients with other subtypes [2], a finding that reflects the intrinsically adverse prognosis associated with the disease. Thus, effective therapeutic strategies are urgently needed for TNBC patients.

Cancer cells including TNBC cells frequently upregulate "stress" induced ligands recognized by the NK cell activating receptors NKG2D (natural-killer group 2, member D) and DNAM-1(CD226) [3, 4]. Therefore, the adoptive transfer of NK cells may represent a promising treatment strategy for these cancers. Large numbers of autologous NK cells can be infused to patients but often do not mediate tumor regression [5]. The feasibility of targeting NKG2D ligands (NKG2DLs) utilizing chimeric antigen receptor (CAR) engineered T cell approach was

* Correspondence: degangsong@gmail.com; poda@pennmedicine.upenn.edu
[1]Ovarian Cancer Research Center, Department of Obstetrics and Gynecology, Perelman School of Medicine, University of Pennsylvania, 3400 Civic Center Blvd, Smilow CTR, Philadelphia, PA 19104, USA
Full list of author information is available at the end of the article

demonstrated by Sentman and colleagues [6] in 2005, and early clinical trial results now show the significant promise of this approach [7]. This CAR construct contained the full-length NKG2D fused to the cytoplasmic domain of CD3z with costimulation provided endogenously by Dap10. We and others [8, 9] have utilized 4-1BB or CD28 signaling platform-based NKG2D CAR T cells, in which the NKG2D extracellular domain (ECD) was connected to a transmembrane portion of the platform in a reverse orientation that maintained the ligand binding specificity and function. In these CARs, the human NKG2D ECD recognize several distinct ligands, including the MIC (MHC class I-related chain) family and six members of the ULBP/RAET (UL16-binding protein, or retinoic acid early transcript) family [10], which are generally absent or expressed at low levels by healthy tissues but widely expressed on cancer cells. In the present study, we identify for the first time NKG2DL-expressing TNBCs as being sensitive to NKG2D CAR T cell attack, offering a new strategy for effective therapy. Further, we identify an unexpected role for IL-2 in the self-enrichment of first-generation NKG2D CAR T cells as well as the impact of 4-1BB and CD27 costimulatory signaling domains in NKG2D CARs in generating more potent T cells against TNBCs in vitro and in vivo.

Methods
Cell lines
Human cell lines used in immune-based assays include the established human breast cancer cell line MCF7 and TNBC cell lines MDA-MB-231, MDA-MB-436, MDA-MB-468, MDA-MB-453, and BT549. The mouse malignant mesothelioma cell line, AE17 (kindly provided by Steven Albelda, University of Pennsylvania), was used as antigen negative control. For bioluminescence assays, the cancer cell lines were transfected to express firefly luciferase (fluc). Lentivirus packaging was executed using the immortalized normal fetal renal 293T cell line purchased from ATCC. All cell lines were maintained in complete medium: RPMI-1640 supplemented with 10% heat inactivated FBS, 100 U/ml penicillin, and 100 mg/ml streptomycin sulfate.

CAR construction and lentivirus production
The NKG2D CAR constructs are comprised of the extracellular portion of human NKG2D (aa 82–216) linked to a CD8a hinge and transmembrane region, followed by a CD3z signaling moiety alone (NKG2D-z) or in tandem with the 4-1BB or CD27 intracellular signaling motif, which was previously described [11, 12]. CAR sequences were preceded in frame by a green fluorescent protein (GFP) sequence followed by the 2A ribosomal skipping sequence.

High-titer replication-defective lentivirus were produced and concentrated as previously described [13]. Briefly, 293T cells were seeded in 150-cm^2 flask and transfected using TurboFect (Life Technologies) according to the manufacturer's instructions. NKG2D CAR transgene plasmid (15 μg) was co-transfected with 18 μg pRSV.REV (Rev expression plasmid), 18 μg pMDLg/p.RRE (Gag/Pol expression plasmid), and 7 μg pVSV-G (VSV glycoprotein expression plasmid) with 174-ul transfection reagent Express In (1 μg/ul) per flask. Supernatants were collected at 24 and 48 h after transfection, concentrated tenfold by ultracentrifugation for 2 h at 28,000 rpm with a Beckman SW32Ti rotor (Beckman Coulter). The viruses were aliquoted and stored at − 80 °C until ready to use for titering or experiments. All lentiviruses used in the experiments were from concentrated stocks.

Human T cells and transfection
Primary human T cells, purchased from the Human Immunology Core at University of Pennsylvania, were isolated from healthy, normal donors following leukapheresis by negative selection. All T cell samples were collected under a protocol approved by a University Institutional Review Board, and written informed consent was obtained from each healthy, normal donor. T cells were cultured in R10 medium and stimulated with anti-CD3 and anti-CD28 monoclonal antibodies (mAb)-coated beads (Invitrogen). Approximately 18 to 24 h after activation, human T cells were transduced. Briefly, 0.5×10^6 T cells were infected with a multiplicity of infection (MOI) 2 of the NKG2D receptor lentiviral vector and expanded for 2 weeks. Human recombinant interleukin-2 (IL-2; Novartis) was added every 2–3 days to a 50-IU/ml final concentration, and a cell density of 0.5×10^6 to 1×10^6 cells/ml was maintained. Engineered CAR T cells were rested in cytokine-free medium for 24 h and were then used for functional analysis.

Flow cytometric analysis
The following fluorochrome-conjugated monoclonal antibodies, purchased from BD Biosciences, were used for T cell phenotypic analysis: APC-Cy7 anti-human CD3, FITC anti-human CD4, APC anti-human CD8, PE anti-human CD45, and APC anti-human NKG2D. PE anti-human CD137, APC anti-human PD-1, and Pacific Blue anti-human TIM-3 were purchased from Biolegend. 7-Aminoactinomycin D (7-AAD) was used for viability staining. Expression of NKG2D CAR was detected by GFP and surface NKG2D expression using anti-NKG2D Ab. For the in vivo experiments, peripheral blood was obtained via retro-orbital bleeding and stained for the presence of human CD45, CD4, and CD8 T cells. Gating specifically on the human CD45+ population, the CD4+

and CD8+ subsets were quantified using TruCount tubes (BD Biosciences) with known numbers of fluorescent beads as described in the manufacturer's instructions.

NKG2DLs were analyzed using PE anti-MICA/B (clone 6D4, BD Pharmingen), PE anti-ULBP1 (clone 170818, R&D System), PE anti-ULBP2/5/6 (clone 165903, R&D System), anti-ULBP3 (clone 2F9, Santa Cruz), and polyclonal Per-CP-anti-human ULBP4 (R&D System). Recombinant human NKG2D Fc chimera and a control recombinant human folate receptor-alpha (FRA) Fc chimera were purchased from R&D System. Matched secondary and isotype antibodies were used in all analyses. Flow cytometry was performed on BD FACSCanto II flow cytometer, and flow cytometric data were analyzed using FlowJo Version 7.2.5 software.

Cytokine release assays

Cytokine release assays were performed by co-culturing 1×10^5 T cells with 1×10^5 target cells in triplicate in a 96-well flat bottom plate in a total volume of 200-ul R10 media. After 20~24 h, cells free co-culture supernatants were collected and ELISA (Biolegend, San Diego) was performed, according to manufacturer's instructions, to measure the secretion of IFN-γ. The values shown represent the mean of triplicate wells.

Cytotoxicity assays

For cell-based bioluminescence assays, 5×10^4 firefly luciferase (fLuc)-expressing tumor cells were cultured with R10 media in the presence of different T cell ratios in a 96-well microplate (BD Biosciences). After incubation for ~ 20 h at 37 °C, each well was filled with 50 ul of D-luciferin (0.015 g/ml) resuspended with PBS and imaged with the Xenogen IVIS Spectrum. Tumor cell viability percentage was calculated as the mean luminescence of the experimental sample minus background divided by the mean luminescence of the input number of target cells used in the assay minus background times 100. All data are represented as a mean of triplicate wells.

Additional cytotoxicity of NKG2D CAR-T cells was measured in real time using an xCELLigence (ACEA Bioscience) label-free, impedance-based cell sensing device. AE17, MDA-MB-436, MDA-MB-468, or BT549 cells (2×10^4/well) were left to adhere for 24 h to xCELLigence E-plates. Cell proliferation was measured as a change in relative impedance, termed cell index (CI). After 24 h, the effector cells were added at the ratio of the effector to target cell ($E:T = 2:1$, 1:1, and 1:2) in a total volume of 200 μl. The cytotoxicity was then monitored by measuring changes in impedance as CI values recorded by the xCELLigence RTCA SP device.

Xenograft model of TNBC

NOD/SCID/γ-chain-/- (NSG) mice were bred, treated, and maintained under pathogen-free conditions in-house under the University of Pennsylvania IACUC-approved protocols. All animals were obtained from the Stem Cell and Xenograft Core (SCXC) of the Abramson Cancer Center, University of Pennsylvania. To establish a TNBC model, 6~10-week-old female NSG mice were inoculated subcutaneously (s.c.) on the flank with 3×10^6 MDA-MB-231 fluc(+) cells on day 0. After the tumors become palpable at about 3 weeks, primary human T cells were activated and transduced. After the primary human T cells were expanded for 2 weeks and the mouse tumor burden was about 200~300 mm³, the mice were treated with the T cells. To investigate the roles of CD27 and 4-1BB costimulated NKG2D CAR in vivo, NKG2D CAR T cells were adjusted from 90 to ~ 30% by adding UNT T cells. The route, dose, and timing of T cell injections are indicated in the individual figure legends. Tumor dimensions were measured with the calipers, and tumor volumes calculated using the formula $V = 1/2(\text{length} \times \text{width}^2)$, where length is the greatest longitudinal diameter and width is the greatest transverse diameter. Animals were imaged prior to T cell transfer and 3 weeks thereafter to evaluate tumor growth. Photon emission from fluc+ cells was quantified using the "Living Image" software (Xenogen) for all in vivo experiments. Approximately 50 days after the first T cell injection, the mice were euthanized and the tumors were resected immediately.

Bioluminescence imaging

Tumor growth was also monitored using bioluminescent imaging (BLI). BLI was conducted using Xenogen IVIS imaging system. The photons emitted from fLuc-expressing cells within the animal body were quantified using Living Image software (Xenogen). Briefly, mice bearing MDA-MB-231fLuc tumors were injected intraperitoneally (i.p.) with D-luciferin (150 mg/kg stock, 100 μL of D-luciferin per 10 g of mouse body weight) suspended in PBS and imaged under isoflurane anesthesia after 5~10 min. A pseudocolor image representing light intensity (blue, least intense; red, most intense) was generated using Living Image. BLI findings were confirmed at necropsy.

Statistical analysis

The data are reported as means and standard deviations (SD). Statistical analysis was performed using two-way repeated-measures analysis of variance (ANOVA) for the tumor burden (tumor volume, photon counts). The Student t test was used to evaluate differences in absolute numbers of transferred T cells, cytokine secretion, and specific cytolysis. GraphPad Prism 5.0 (GraphPad

Software) was used for the statistical calculations, where a *P* value of $P < 0.05$ was considered significant.

Results

Expression of NKG2D ligands on TNBC cell lines

To investigate NKG2DL expression in human TNBC, we screened five TNBC cell lines for the NKG2DL expression via flow cytometry using a recombinant NKG2D receptor–human IgG1-Fc fusion protein that recognizes all ligands for this receptor. The majority of lines bound the NKG2D-Fc protein and expressed a high to moderate level of NKG2DLs, except for BT549; a lower level of NKG2D-Fc protein binding was detected on MDA-MB-453 cells (Fig. 1). AE17, a mouse malignant mesothelioma cell line [8], served as a negative control and did not express detectable human NKG2DLs (Additional file 1: Figure S1a). We next examined the expression distribution of the individual NKG2DL family members in TNBC cell lines by flow cytometry, using antibodies specific for MICA/B, or ULBP-1, ULBP-2/5/6, ULBP-3, or ULBP-4 (Fig. 1). Although varied in level of expression, all TNBC cell lines tested expressed one or more cell surface NKG2DLs. BT549 nearly exclusively

expressed surface MICA/B and at high level, while a low level of MICA/B was detected on MDA-MB-436 cells. All other TNBC lines were MICA/B negative. The expression of the ULBPs on TNBC cell lines varied: ULBP1 was only expressed on MDA-MB-468 at low levels, while ULBP-2/5/6 were more often strongly expressed in all TNBC cell lines except for BT549; ULBP-3 and 4 were only found on the MDA-453 and MDA-MB-231, respectively. The breast cancer cell line MCF-7 that expressed various NKG2DLs which was previously characterized [14, 15] was used as a positive control. Together, NKG2DLs appear to be broadly expressed by TNBC cell lines, although some cell lines display a relatively low level of ligand expression.

NKG2D CAR design and surface expression on T cells

The build upon the earlier clinical efficacy of NKG2D CAR therapy in acute myeloid leukemia [7], NKG2D CARs were developed consisting of the extracellular portion of the human NKG2D receptor linked to a CD8a hinge and transmembrane region, followed by a CD3z signaling moiety alone (GFP-NKG2D-z) or in tandem with the 4-1BB (GFP-NKG2D-BBz) or CD27

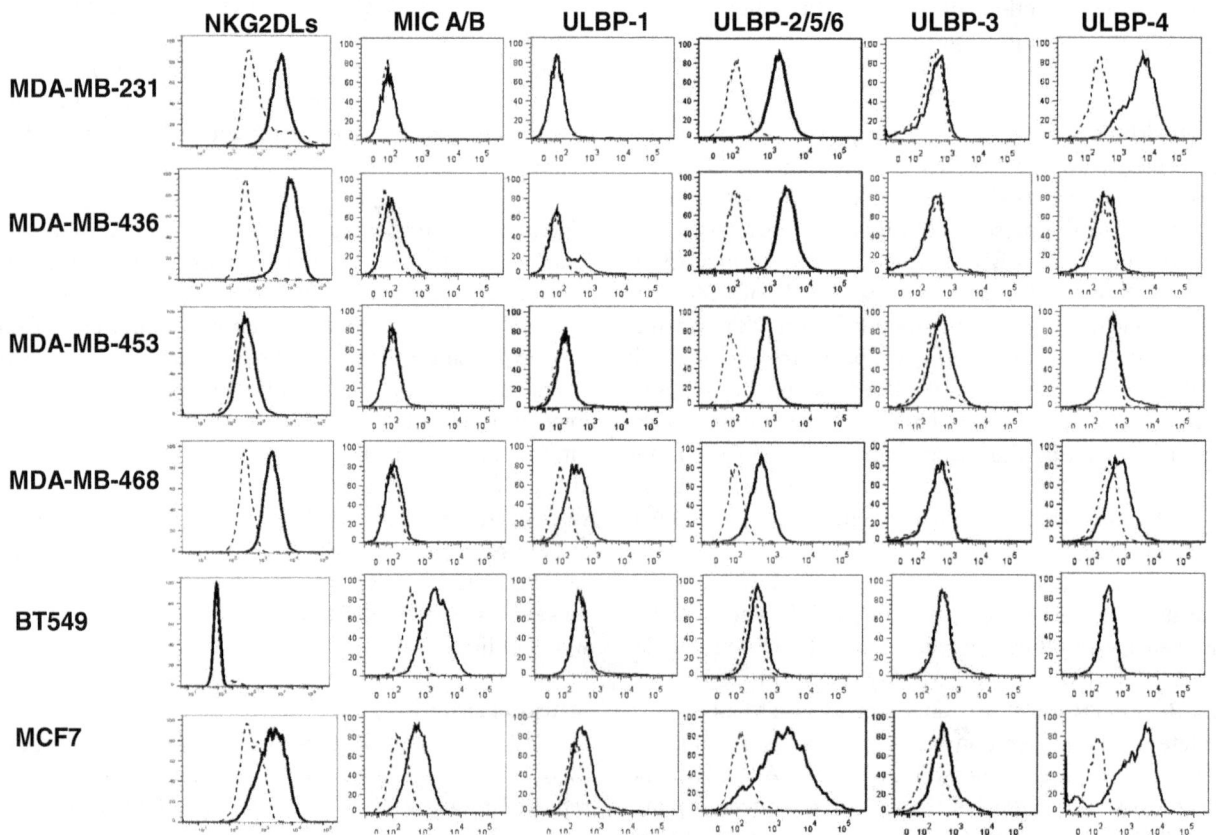

Fig. 1 Surface expression of NKG2D ligands on TNBC cell lines. A panel of human TNBC cell lines were stained with recombinant NKG2D-Fc or specific antibodies that recognize MICA/B; ULBP-1, ULBP-2/5/6, ULBP-3, or ULBP-4 (solid line histogram); matched isotype or irrelevant recombinant protein-Fc controls (dashed line histogram) and analyzed by flow cytometry. A breast cancer cell line, MCF7, was used as a positive control

(GFP-NKG2D-27z) intracellular signaling motif (Fig. 2a). Bicistronic expression vectors incorporating a 2A peptide sequence permitted dual expression analysis of GFP and the NKG2D CAR (Fig. 2b). We previously showed NKG2DLs expressed on activated T cells enrich for 4-1BB costimulated NKG2D CAR T cells [8]. Similarly, cultures of GFP-NKG2D-z, GFP-NKG2D-z-27z, and GFP-NKG2D-z-BBz CAR T cells were highly enriched for CAR+ GFP+ T cells (~ 90%) at the end of 2-week expansion in the presence of IL-2 (50 IU/ml) (Fig. 2b). Based on these results, we used GFP as a surrogate marker for detection of engineered NKG2D CAR T cells in the following experiments.

NKG2D CAR T cells effectively recognize and eliminate TNBC cell lines in vitro

To evaluate the anti-tumor function of NKG2D CAR-T cells in vitro, primary human T cells and TNBC cells were co-cultured and CAR T cell reactivity measured by proinflammatory cytokine secretion. NKG2D CAR-T cells recognized TNBC cell lines MDA-MB-231 and MDA-MB-468 and secreted high levels of IFN-γ, but not when stimulated with the NKG2DL (−) cell line AE17 (Fig. 3a), illustrating the requirement for antigen

specificity for CAR-T cell activity. Invariably, increased quantities of secreted IFN-γ were detected when NKG2D-27z and NKG2D-BBz CAR-T cells where stimulated with the NKG2DL (+) target cells, relative to the first-generation NKG2D-z CAR T cells (Fig. 3a).

We next evaluated the cytotoxicity of NKG2D CAR T cells against the NKG2DL (+) TNBC cell line, MDA-MB-231fluc, using an overnight luminescence-based assay. Compared to the control untransduced T cells, NKG2D CARs T cells demonstrated significant cytotoxicity against firefly luciferase (fLuc) expressing MDA-MB-231 cells. When the $E:T$ ratio was as low as 1:2, the cytotoxicity was more than 60% and increased as the $E:T$ ratio increased (Fig. 3b). The NKG2DL (−) cell line AE17 fLuc was not lysed by NKG2D CAR T cells. Similar to cytokine production results, costimulated NKG2D-BBz or NKG2D-27z CAR-T cells demonstrated enhanced cytotoxicity compared to their first-generation counterparts (Fig. 3b).

Similarly, xCELLigence cytotoxic data showed that 4-1BB or CD27 costimulated NKG2D CAR-T cells were cytotoxic toward NKG2DL (+) MDA-MB-468, MDA-MB-436 cells in a time- and $E:T$ ratio-dependent manner, while untransduced T cells did not inhibit the growth of these cells (Fig. 3c). As expected, NKG2D-z

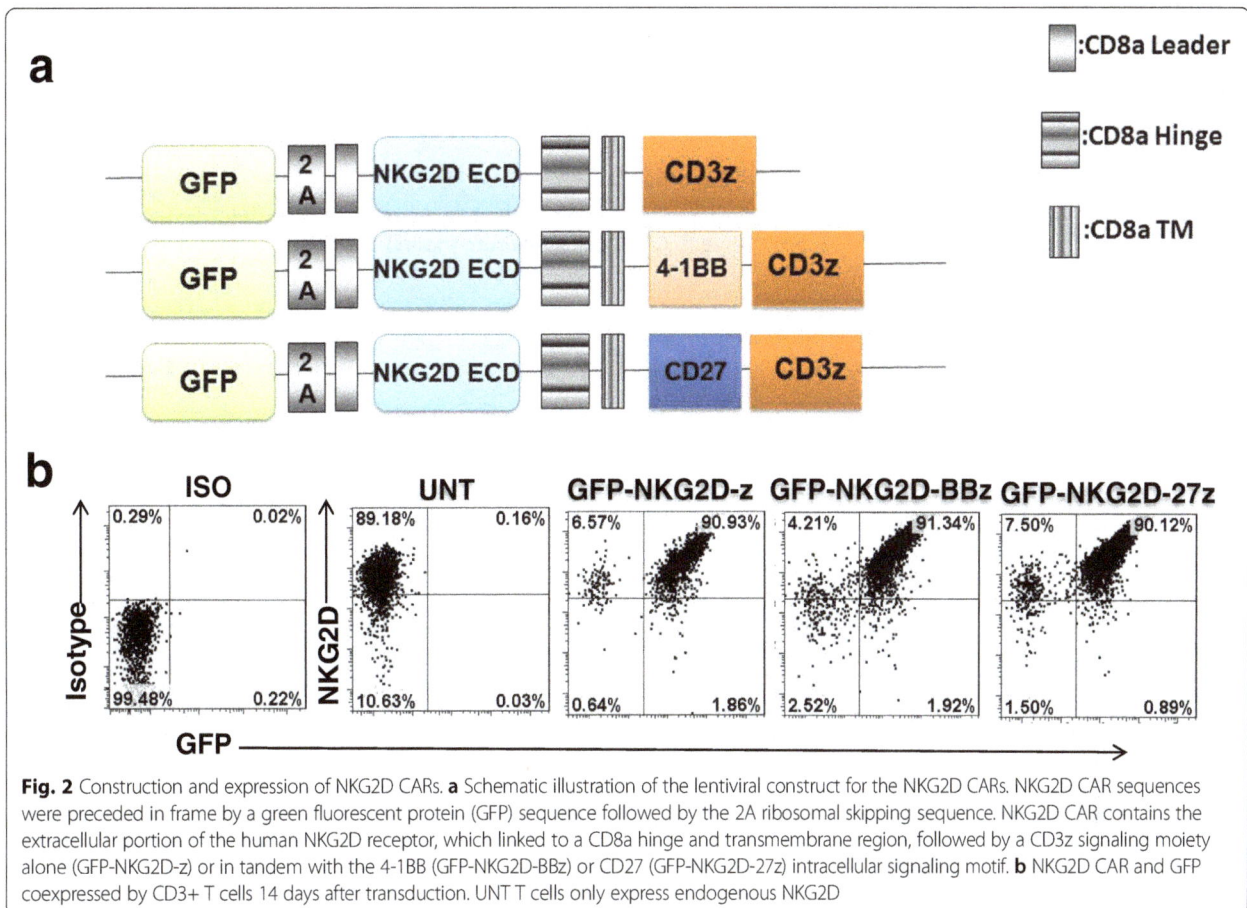

Fig. 2 Construction and expression of NKG2D CARs. **a** Schematic illustration of the lentiviral construct for the NKG2D CARs. NKG2D CAR sequences were preceded in frame by a green fluorescent protein (GFP) sequence followed by the 2A ribosomal skipping sequence. NKG2D CAR contains the extracellular portion of the human NKG2D receptor, which linked to a CD8a hinge and transmembrane region, followed by a CD3z signaling moiety alone (GFP-NKG2D-z) or in tandem with the 4-1BB (GFP-NKG2D-BBz) or CD27 (GFP-NKG2D-27z) intracellular signaling motif. **b** NKG2D CAR and GFP coexpressed by CD3+ T cells 14 days after transduction. UNT T cells only express endogenous NKG2D

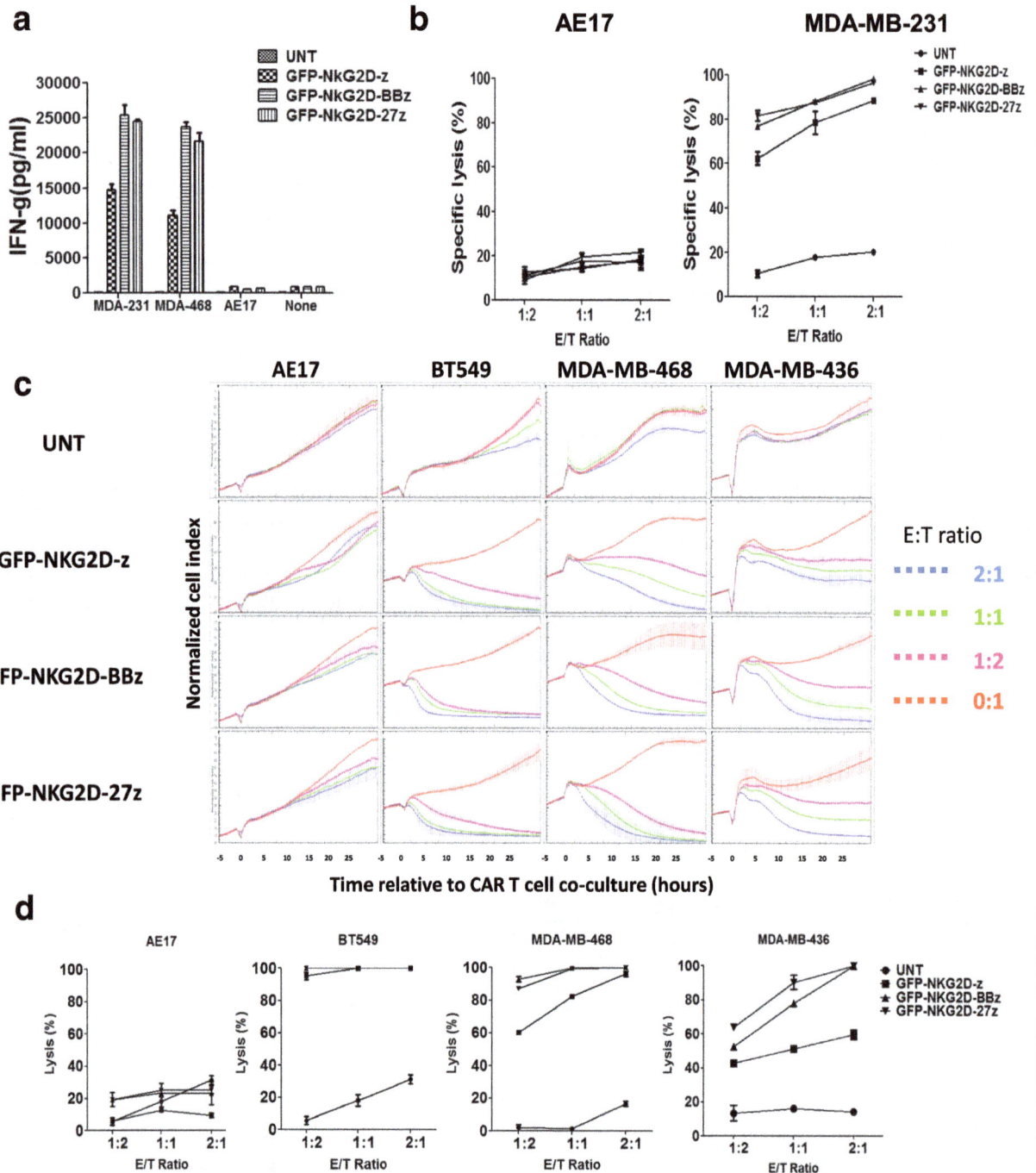

Fig. 3 Recognition of human TNBC cells by NKG2D CAR T cells in vitro. **a** NKG2D CAR-modified T cells secrete IFN-γ during overnight co-culture with NKG2DL-expressing TNBC cells, but not NKG2DL-negative AE17 mesothelioma cells. Mean IFN-γ concentration ± SD (pg/ml) from triplicate cultures is shown. **b** Lysis of NKG2DL-expressing TNBC cells (MDA-MB-231 fluc) by NKG2D CAR T cells in an 18-h bioluminescence assay at the indicated effector-to-target (*E/T*) ratios. Untransduced (UNT) CD3+ human T cells and AE17 mesothelioma cells served as negative effector and target cell controls, respectively. **c** Normalized cell index(CI) plot for target cells (AE17, BT549, MDA-MB-436, and MDA-MB-468) incubated with UNT or NKG2D CAR T cells at different *E:T* ratios for 24 h. When seeded alone, target cells adhere to the plate and proliferate, increasing the CI readout (red lines). When T cells added to target cells, NKG2CD CAR T cells cause cell cytolysis and subsequent progressive decrease in CI. *Y*-axis is the normalized CI generated by the RTCA software and displayed in real time. *X*-axis is the time of cell culture and treatment time in hour. Mean values of the CI were plotted ± standard deviation. **d** The cell index plot is converted to a % Lysis plot by the xCELLigence Immunotherapy Software

CAR T cells were less efficient in killing NKG2DL (+) target cells and required higher E/T ratios to achieve efficient response (Fig. 3c, d). Interestingly, after 24 h of co-culture, addition of any iteration of NKG2D CART cells caused BT549 cells to detach from the culture plate, consequently reducing cell index value, suggested BT459 cells were lysed efficiently even at low 1:1 E/T ratio (Fig. 3c, d), although these cells only express MIC A/B but no detectable expression of NKG2DLs measured by NKG2D-Fc (Fig. 1). This further suggests that BT549 cells may be more sensitive than MDA-MB-436 and MDA-MB-438 cells to cytolysis by CAR T cells. Similar to the luciferase release-based cytotoxicity assays, the NKG2DL (–) cell line AE17 was not lysed by NKG2D CAR T cells (Fig. 3c, d).

IL-2 promotes expansion and enrichment of NKG2D-redirected CAR T cells

During the culture of NKG2D CAR T cells in the presence of IL-2, we consistently observed the temporal enrichment of both the first and second generation of NKG2D CARs, with the frequencies of CAR+ T cells increasing temporally. To investigate the influence of IL-2 on this NKG2D CAR enrichment phenomenon, CAR T cells were washed free of IL-2 using PBS on day 5 after activation and transduction, and then cultured in complete medium in the presence or absence of exogenous IL-2 (50 IU/ml). CAR T cell count and expression level were monitored for additional 2 weeks (Additional file 1: Figure S1b). Consistently, in this assay from three different donors whose untransduced T cells express NKG2DLs when activated by anti-CD3/28 beads (Additional file 1: Figure S1c), GFP-expressing NKG2D-z, NKG2D-BBz, and NKG2D-27z CAR T cells expanded more than 300-fold (Additional file 1: Figure S1d) and were highly enriched for CAR+ cells during prolonged culture in the presence of IL-2 (Fig. 4a). Only ~ 30% of T cells were positive for GFP expression on day 5, but were preferentially enriched to more than 95% GFP+ after an additional 2 weeks of culture (Fig. 4a). In stark contrast, in the absence of IL-2, NKG2D CAR T cells did not expand well (Additional file 1: Figure S1d) and only T cells that expressed the costimulated GFP-NKG2D-BBz and GFP-NKG2D-27z CARs were still highly enriched for CAR+ cells. In contrast, the frequency of GFP-NKG2D-z CAR T cells remained stable

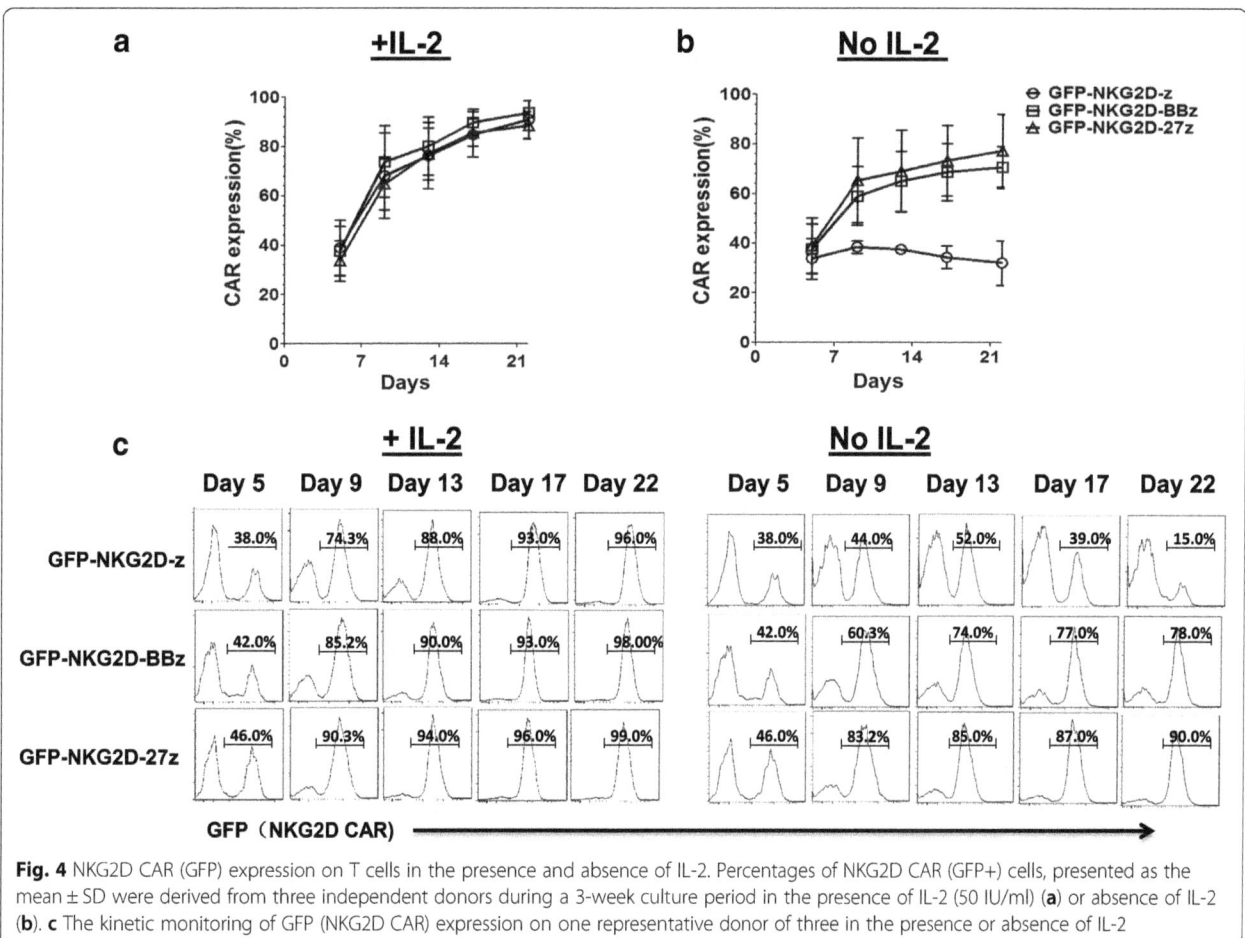

Fig. 4 NKG2D CAR (GFP) expression on T cells in the presence and absence of IL-2. Percentages of NKG2D CAR (GFP+) cells, presented as the mean ± SD were derived from three independent donors during a 3-week culture period in the presence of IL-2 (50 IU/ml) (**a**) or absence of IL-2 (**b**). **c** The kinetic monitoring of GFP (NKG2D CAR) expression on one representative donor of three in the presence or absence of IL-2

at ~ 30% over this entire time, suggesting that a costimulatory signal may be required for CAR enrichment in the absence of IL-2. The kinetic monitoring of surface CAR expression on one representative donor in the presence or absence of IL-2 is shown in Fig. 4c.

CD25 high expression on first-generation NKG2D CAR T cells is essential for CAR enrichment in the presence of IL-2

We previously showed that the enrichment of CAR may due to the "T cell fratricide" of the 4-BB costimulated NKG2D CAR T cells interacting with NKG2DLs expressed on activated T cells [8]. However, in the presence of IL-2, the first-generation NKG2D-z CAR was also highly enriched for CAR (+) cells during culture in vitro. This result suggested that IL-2 stimulation may promote the CAR T cell expansion and upregulate NKG2DLs to enrich NKG2D CAR T cells even without costimulation. To test our hypothesis, we sought to investigate whether CD25 (IL-2 receptor-alpha chain) expression is associated with NKG2D CAR enrichment.

On day 5 after activation, 4 days post transduction, nearly all of NKG2D CAR+ T cell population expressed a high level of CD25 (Fig. 5a, *left*). All NKG2D-z, NKG2D-BBz, and NKG2D-27z CAR T cells that expressed high levels of CD25 were preferentially enriched to ~ 80% after an additional 14 days of culture (Fig. 5b, *left*).). We then separated out the CD25^{low} NKG2D-z, NKG2D-BBz, and NKG2D-27z CAR T cells by depleting human CD25+ cells by magnetic separation 4 days post transduction (Fig. 5a, *right*). NKG2D-BBz and NKG2D-27z CAR T cells that were CD25^{low} were still ~ 80% enriched after additional 14 days culture in the presence of IL-2 (Fig. 5b, *right*). Alternatively, NKG2D-z CAR T cell expression frequency in the CD25^{low} population ranged between 30 and 40%, which was substantially lower than costimulated NKG2D CAR expression, suggesting that high CD25 expression is essential for IL-2-driven NKG2D CAR enrichment in the absence of costimulatory signal domains and that the CAR costimulatory domains are sufficient to drive

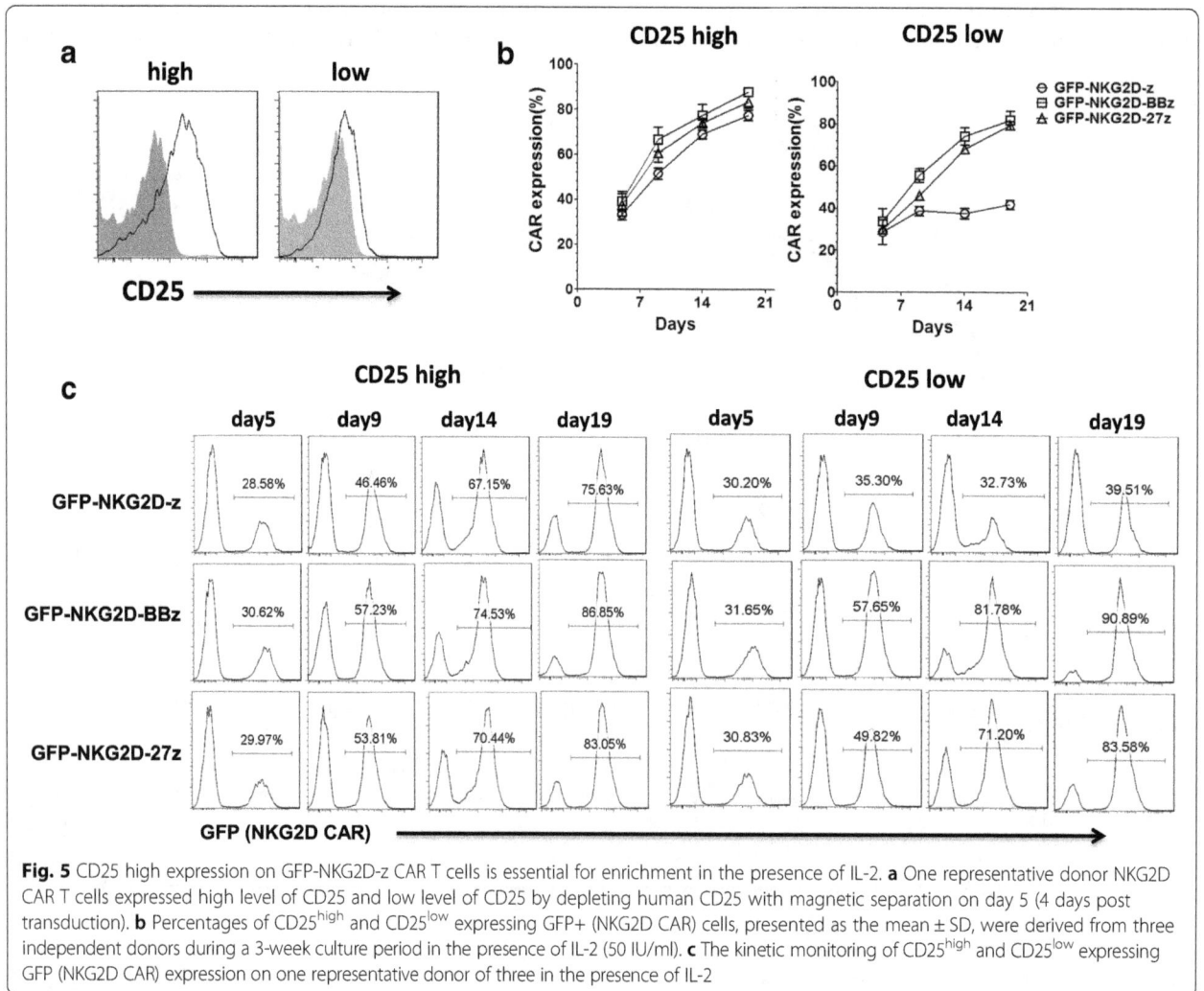

Fig. 5 CD25 high expression on GFP-NKG2D-z CAR T cells is essential for enrichment in the presence of IL-2. **a** One representative donor NKG2D CAR T cells expressed high level of CD25 and low level of CD25 by depleting human CD25 with magnetic separation on day 5 (4 days post transduction). **b** Percentages of CD25^{high} and CD25^{low} expressing GFP+ (NKG2D CAR) cells, presented as the mean ± SD, were derived from three independent donors during a 3-week culture period in the presence of IL-2 (50 IU/ml). **c** The kinetic monitoring of CD25^{high} and CD25^{low} expressing GFP (NKG2D CAR) expression on one representative donor of three in the presence of IL-2

NKG2D CAR enrichment even when surface CD25 expression levels are low. The kinetics of CAR expression in T cells with CD25^{high} or CD25^{low} expression in the presence of IL-2 is shown for one representative donor (Fig. 5c).

CAR T cells may become exhausted due to the persistent antigen exposure or tonic signaling of the CAR [16]. To ascertain whether T cell exhaustion develops during NKG2D CAR T cell expansion, we measured the expression of the two more abundantly expressed inhibitory receptors on T cells, TIM3 and PD-1. Similar to the untransduced T cells, NKG2D CAR T cells expressed low levels of the PD1 and TIM3 (Additional file 2: Figure S2a). Although these CAR T cells were highly enriched by "T cell fratricide" in the presence of IL-2, they did not become exhausted. Interestingly, first-generation NKG2D-z CAR T cells expressed relatively higher levels of PD-1 and TIM-3 compared to costimulated NKG2D-BBz or NKG2D-CD27z CAR T cells, and even untransduced T cells. High levels of PD-1 and TIM3 were however expressed on activated T cells stimulated by anti-CD3/CD28 beads (Additional file 2: Figure S2a). We also measured 4-1BB and PD-1 expression on NKG2D CAR T cells because the presence of the target antigen on T cells may sustain high tonic signaling which leads to increased activation marker and exhaustion [16]. Similar to untransduced T cells, CAR T cells lacked 4-1BB expression (Additional file 2: Figure S2b) indicating a lack of tonic signaling and suggesting insufficient stimulation by NKG2DLs, possibly due to the transient nature of expression of NKG2DLs in activated T cells. Alternatively, the small subsets of 4-1BB expressing CAR T cells might preferentially express NKG2DLs and accordingly be killed by other NKG2D CAR T cells leading to a "CAR T cells-fratricide and auto-stimulation/enrichment" cycle. Incubation of NKG2D CAR T cells with the MDA-MB-231 cell line resulted in robust activation-induced upregulation of 4-1BB restricted to CAR+ T cells and a significant upregulation of PD-1 on CAR+ cells after 24 h of incubation (Additional file 2: Figure S2b). Similar to the above experiments, first-generation NKG2D-z CAR T cells expressed relatively higher levels of PD-1 compared to costimulated NKG2D-BBz or NKG2D-CD27z CAR T cells during culture or when stimulated with MDA-MB-231 cells (Additional file 2: Figure S2b). Together, these data suggested that NKG2D CAR T cells do not become exhausted during ex vivo expansion and that 4-1BB or CD27 costimulation may enable T cells to resist immune exhaustion, consistent with a prior report focused on 4-1BB [16].

Control of TNBC by costimulated NKG2D CAR T cells in vivo

We next evaluated the therapeutic efficacy of these NKG2D CAR T cells against human TNBC in vivo. We first generated a xenograft model of TNBC by injecting

3×10^6 luciferase-labeled NKG2DL-expressing MDA-MB-231 cells (Fig. 6a) subcutaneously in NSG mice. When tumors reached a mean volume of ~ 300 mm^3, mice were assigned to the following treatment groups: administration of PBS, untransduced T cells, or NKG2D CAR (+) T cells on day 40 and day 45 after tumor implantation by tail-vein injection. MDA-MB-231 tumors in the control mice group treated with PBS or untransduced T cells grew progressively beyond the time of T cell transfer as measured by caliper-based sizing and bioluminescent imaging (BLI) (Fig. 6b, c). These mice had to be euthanized due to high tumor burden by day 90. Tumor growth was modestly delayed in mice receiving GFP-NKG2D-z T cells, compared with control groups at the latest evaluated time point. In contrast, mice receiving GFP-NKG2D-BBz or GFP-NKG2D-27z CAR T cells were protected from rapid progression (Fig. 6b, c), which was significantly better than NKG2D-z T cells ($P < 0.001$).

Peripheral blood was collected from tumor-bearing mice and quantified for persistence of infused human T cells. Ten days after the first injection of T cells, human CD4+ T cell counts were higher compared to CD8+ T cell counts in the circulation and both CD4+ and CD8+ T cells in GFP-NKG2D-z, GFP-NKG2D-BBz, and GFP-NKG2D-27z CAR cohorts were present in lower numbers in comparison to untransduced T cells, suggesting early NKG2DL-specific CAR T cell migration to specific tumor sites (Fig. 6d). NKG2D CAR expressing T cells were detectable in the peripheral blood. The level of CAR expression by NKG2D-BBz and NKG2D-27z T cells was high compared to the expression detected on NKG2D-z CAR T cells, which poorly expressed on the surface of transduced (GFP+) T cells, suggesting CAR downregulation (Fig. 6e). Twenty days after first T cell injection, significant CD4+ and CD8+ T cell expansion was now detected in the peripheral blood of mice receiving GFP-NKG2D-BBz or GFP-NKG2D-27z CAR T cells compared to untransduced and GFP-NKG2D-z treatment groups, indicating roles for 4-1BB and CD27 in T cell survival in vivo (Fig. 6f). For the costimulated CAR groups tested, the CD8 T cell counts were higher than the CD4 T cell counts. Analysis of the CD8 data in these two groups revealed statistically similar cell counts in the GFP-NKG2D-BBz CAR T cell-treated group compared to GFP-NKG2D-27z group ($P > 0.05$) (Fig. 6f). These results indicate that both 4-1BB and CD27 costimulation augment CD8 T cell persistence but also suggest 4-1BB may be slightly superior for CD8+ T cells. Similar to what we observed in vitro, 4-1BB or CD27 costimulated NKG2D CAR T cells maintained a high level of surface CAR expression in vivo without the need for additional exogenous IL-2 support; this was not the case for the NKG2D-z CAR (Fig. 6g). These data suggest

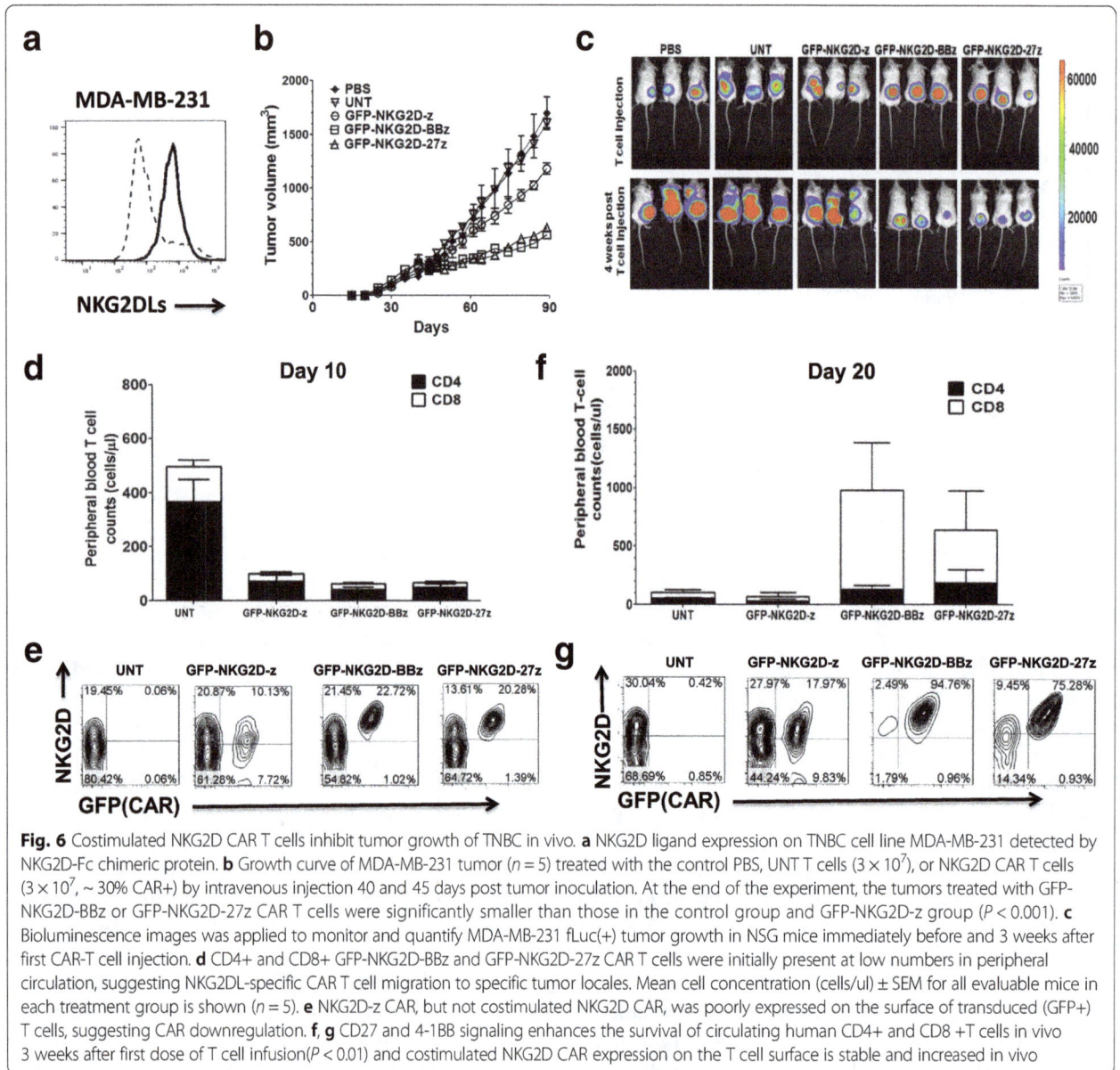

Fig. 6 Costimulated NKG2D CAR T cells inhibit tumor growth of TNBC in vivo. **a** NKG2D ligand expression on TNBC cell line MDA-MB-231 detected by NKG2D-Fc chimeric protein. **b** Growth curve of MDA-MB-231 tumor ($n = 5$) treated with the control PBS, UNT T cells (3×10^7), or NKG2D CAR T cells (3×10^7, ~ 30% CAR+) by intravenous injection 40 and 45 days post tumor inoculation. At the end of the experiment, the tumors treated with GFP-NKG2D-BBz or GFP-NKG2D-27z CAR T cells were significantly smaller than those in the control group and GFP-NKG2D-z group ($P < 0.001$). **c** Bioluminescence images was applied to monitor and quantify MDA-MB-231 fLuc(+) tumor growth in NSG mice immediately before and 3 weeks after first CAR-T cell injection. **d** CD4+ and CD8+ GFP-NKG2D-BBz and GFP-NKG2D-27z CAR T cells were initially present at low numbers in peripheral circulation, suggesting NKG2DL-specific CAR T cell migration to specific tumor locales. Mean cell concentration (cells/ul) ± SEM for all evaluable mice in each treatment group is shown ($n = 5$). **e** NKG2D-z CAR, but not costimulated NKG2D CAR, was poorly expressed on the surface of transduced (GFP+) T cells, suggesting CAR downregulation. **f, g** CD27 and 4-1BB signaling enhances the survival of circulating human CD4+ and CD8 +T cells in vivo 3 weeks after first dose of T cell infusion($P < 0.01$) and costimulated NKG2D CAR expression on the T cell surface is stable and increased in vivo

that costimulated NKG2D CAR expression on the T cell surface is stable and increased in vivo, even after antigen recognition and the proliferation of the CAR T cells. Together, these results support the use of costimulated NKG2D-BBz or NKG2D-27z CAR T cells as a cellular modality for enhanced treatment of TNBC in vivo.

Discussion

The expression of NKG2DLs on many primary tumor cells and immunosuppressive cells (e.g., T regulatory cells and myeloid-derived suppressor cells) within the tumor microenvironment makes them attractive targets for the development of novel therapeutics [17]. Targeting NKG2DLs with NKG2D CAR T cells has been shown to induce tumor elimination and long-term tumor-free

survival in various tumor models [18–20]. NKG2DLs are frequently expressed in breast cancer [21], and we found positive surface expression of NKG2DLs on all (5/5) human TNBC cell lines tested by flow cytometry. Based on these results, we rationalized the extension of our NKG2D CAR T cell-based immunotherapy approach to TNBCs.

NKG2D CAR T cells secreted IFN-γ upon stimulation with NKG2DL (+) tumor cells and displayed potent cytolytic capacity in vitro against NKG2DLs+ TNBC cells, even at low E/T ratios. Consistently, the production of proinflammatory cytokines and cytolytic capacity by NKG2D-BBz and NKG2D-27z CAR-T cells was substantially increased after co-culture with NKG2DL (+) TNBC cell lines, compared with NKG2D-z T cells. Mechanisms accounting for increased effector function by 4-1BB and CD27 costimulated CAR-T cells in vitro appear linked in part to their ability to resist antigen-induced cell death (AICD) as we reported previously [11]. These in vitro tumor killing findings further support the notion that NKG2DLs have promise as novel immunotherapy targets for TNBCs, which currently lack effective targeted therapies. Indeed, two injections of 4-1BB or CD27 costimulated NKG2D CAR T cells exhibited in vivo anti-tumor effects in a highly invasive MDA-MB-231 xenograft model of human TNBC, compared to the first-generation NKG2D CAR T cells. Consistent with clinical observations [22], tumor regression was associated with enhanced T cell persistence in vivo. The greatest number of CAR T cells persisting in the blood 20 days after the first T cell dose was observed in those animals administered NKG2D-BBz and NKG2D-27z CAR-T cells followed by NKG2D-z and untransduced T cells, indicating that simultaneous TCR CD3 signaling and 4-1BB or CD27 costimulation triggered by CAR ligation with antigen improves upon TCR signaling alone, implicating a role for 4-1BB and CD27 costimulation in memory T cell formation in vivo. Results of comparative in vivo studies of CARs containing these various costimulatory domains demonstrated that both 4-1BB and CD27, members of the TNFR superfamily, enhances T cell anti-tumor activity and persistence.

In this study, costimulated NKG2D CAR T cells failed to completely eradicate large, established tumors. Major studies suggest that administration of exogenous IL-2 may be necessary for the anti-tumor activity for the first-generation CAR T cells that lack costimulatory domains [23, 24]. We have previously found that the administration of IL-2 has little to no anti-tumor effect on human CAR T cells activity in immunodeficient mice, if the CAR contains a costimulatory domain [25]. Therefore, the omission of exogenous IL-2 is not likely the primary factor accounting for the suboptimal anti-tumor response in this study. The efficacy of NKG2D CAR T cell treatment for TNBC may also be influenced by surface antigen expression level as suggested previously [26] in the same MDA-MB-231 tumor model. Although MDA-231 cells express various NKG2DLs, a previous study [27] suggested that NKG2D can bind to only one ligand at a time. In addition, NKG2D displays varying affinities for its ligands that ranges between 600 nM and 1.1 mM [28] and NKG2D CAR may preferentially bind to the higher affinity form of ligands. Therefore, further investigation of affinity of each ligand's binding to NKG2D receptor and selecting patients with higher NKG2DL expression may help to enhance the anti-tumor activity of NKG2D CAR T cells in clinical studies. Other antigens such as folate receptor-a [26], mesothelin [29], and TEM8 [30] were also investigated as CAR targets for TNBCs with mixed efficacy results

reported. Targeting solid tumors, like TNBC, is still challenging, as it may be greatly hampered clinically by the immunosuppressive microenvironment and the inefficient homing of CAR T cells to tumor sites [31]. Combining CAR T cells with other therapies like CTLA-4 and PD-1 inhibitor offers the potential to improve anti-tumor effects.

One intriguing finding from this study is that in the presence of exogenous IL-2, a potent cytokine stimulator of activated effector lymphocyte expansion and proliferation, NKG2D CAR T cells, undergoes substantial long-term expansion without evidence of prolonged detriment from fratricide in vitro. In addition, the NKG2D CAR (+) T cell population was enriched during prolonged culture, suggesting a possible auto-stimulatory effect through endogenous expression of induced NKG2DLs after T cell stimulation. These findings are similar to a CD28 costimulated CD5-specific CAR [32], which kills both CD5(+) autologous T cells and malignant T cell lines, yet results in limited and transient T cell fratricide. However, by incorporating 4-1BB, CD27, OX40, CD30, CD28, ICOS, or HVEM into the CD5 CAR, a more recent study suggested that only CD5 CARs costimulated with non-TNFR domains (CD28, ICOS, or non-costimulated) overcome impaired the expansion of CAR T cells and resulted in complete or partial downregulate CAR expression [33]. Unlike the CD5 CAR platform, which differs significantly in expansion and transduction methodology and antigen specificity, our NKG2D CAR T cells undergo dramatic expansion and preferentially enrich for CAR expressing T cells during culture. Here, exogenous IL-2 promoted the expansion and enrichment of NKG2D-z, NKG2D-BBz, and NKG2D-27z CAR (+) T cells, which was dependent on a high expression level of the IL-2 receptor-alpha subunit, CD25. Without IL-2 support, T cells expressing any of the NKG2D constructs did not expand well and only NKG2D CAR (+) T cells containing 4-1BB or CD27 costimulatory domains enriched for CAR-positivity, demonstrating a benefit from 4-1BB and CD27 costimulation in vitro. These results suggest that incorporation of costimulatory domains into CAR constructs promotes preferential T cell survival and resistance to AICD by upregulating anti-apoptotic proteins as suggested previously [11]. These data also support the three-signal hypothesis that optimal T cell activation and expansion involves T cell receptor (TCR) activation (signal 1) in addition to costimulatory receptor engagement (signal 2) and cytokine receptor engagement (signal 3) [34]. Although NKG2DLs can be expressed on active T lymphocytes, our NKG2D CARs do not elicit tonic signaling, as seen with other CARs reported previously [16, 35]. In one report [35], tonic signaling CAR T cells displayed sustained proliferation for up to 3 months, resulting from autocrine CAR crosslinking that is independent of cognate antigen and did not require the addition of exogenous cytokines or feeder cells after a single stimulation of the TCR and CD28. NKG2D-z, NKG2D-BBz, and NKG2D-27z CAR (+) T cells do not undergo prolonged and unfettered proliferation. Whether regulated proliferation in NKG2D CAR T cells is impacted by the selection of the 4-1BB and CD27 TNFR costimulatory domains, and not CD28, is not known. However, in the setting of tonic CAR signaling, 4-1BB costimulation reduces exhaustion induced by persistent CAR signaling and augments anti-tumor activity in vivo, while CD28 costimulation does not [16].

In light of the therapeutic potential of NKG2D CAR T cells for TNBC and because of the potential for expression of NKG2DLs on healthy tissues, the concerns about potential "on-target, off-tumor" toxicity must be considered. VanSeggelen et al. [36] described lethal toxicity in mice treated with murine NKG2D CAR T cells. This toxicity was both CAR construct and strain dependent and was exacerbated upon the use of a lymphodepleting conditioning regimen. These results suggested that predicting the toxicity of NKG2D CAR approach becomes especially problematic because of the diversity of target ligands. Moreover, both efficacy and toxicity will likely be affected by the ligand tissue distribution, density, and affinity with which NKG2D binds the respective ligand. None of these parameters are very well characterized and likely vary greatly between mice and humans [37]. However, results from a phase I clinical study [38] testing the safety of NKG2D CAR-T cells in patients with AML/MDS and multiple myeloma (ClinicalTrials.gov Identifier: NCT03018405) are promising with no reported cases of cytokine-release syndrome, CAR T cell-related neurotoxicity, autoimmunity, or patient death. It is important to have adequate safety data in multiple clinical studies using different NKG2D CAR constructs. In the current ongoing clinical trial [38], the full-length NKG2D is used in a CAR design that incorporates Dap10 signaling, which was showed the enhanced CAR expression and toxicity [36]. Notably, one recent case study reports that NKG2D-based chimeric antigen receptor therapy safely induced remission in a patient with relapsed/refractory acute myeloid leukemia [7]. Our NKG2D CAR construct contains 4-1BB and lacks DAP10, yet still possesses potent anti-tumor capacity against TNBC. Therefore, future clinical studies are warranted.

Conclusions

In conclusion, we have identified a self-enrichment phenomenon of NKG2D CAR in vitro, which does not affect T cell expansion. These NKG2D CAR T cells can effectively target NKG2DLs expressing TNBC cells

in vitro, and CD27 or 4-1BB costimulated CAR T cells can significantly reduce tumor growth in vivo. NKG2D CAR T cell therapy may provide novel treatment options for patients with TNBCs and may be amenable to combination with immune checkpoint blockade, cytokines, and other strategies to transform this approach from being "promising" to being "effective" treatments for TNBC and other solid tumors.

Additional files

Additional file 1: Figure S1. a Schematic of the monitoring NKG2D CAR expression procedure in the presence or absence of IL-2. NKG2DLs are expressed on activated CD8+ and CD8-(CD4)T cells after 4 days activation by anti-CD3/28 beads. b Results for three independent donors are shown and irrelevant folate receptor-alpha (FRA)-Fc protein was used as negative control. c T cell expansion folds in the presence of IL-2 (50 IU/ml) or absence of IL-2. (PPTX 226 kb)

Additional file 2: Figure S2. a Expression of PD-1 and TIM-3 markers of exhaustion in T cells during culture.Anti-CD3/28 beads activated NKG2D-27z CAR T cells (15 h stimulation) were used as positive control for expression of PD-1 and TIM-3. b Expression of CD137 and PD-1 in T cells during culture and when co-cultured with MDA-MD-231 cells. (PPTX 147 kb)

Abbreviations

7-AAD: 7-Aminoactinomycin D; AICD: Antigen-induced cell death; CAR: Chimeric antigen receptor; ECD: Extracellular domain; ER: Estrogen receptor; GFP: Green fluorescent protein; HER2: Human epidermal growth factor receptor 2; i.p.: Intraperitoneally; IL-2R: IL-2 receptor; MIC: MHC class I-related chain; NKG2D: Natural-killer group 2, member D; NKG2DLs: NKG2D ligands; NSG: NOD/SCID/γ-chain-/-; PR: Progesterone receptor; s.c.: Subcutaneously; TCR: T cell receptor; TNBC: Triple-negative breast cancer; ULBP/RAET: UL16-binding protein, or retinoic acid early transcript

Funding

This work was supported by grants from the Ovarian Cancer Research Foundation Alliance. Yali Han was supported by the China Scholarship Council (CSC) and grants from National Science Foundation for Young Scientists of China (Grant No. 81402195 and 81602709).

Authors' contributions

DJP and DS initiated and designed the in vitro and in vivo studies. YH, WX, and DS performed the vitro experiments and preclinical animal studies. YH, DS, WX, and DJP prepared the manuscript. All authors read and approved the final manuscript.

Consent for publication

Not applicable.

Competing interests

DJP holds patents in the area of CAR T cell therapy for oncology. The remaining authors declare that they have no competing interests.

Author details

[1]Ovarian Cancer Research Center, Department of Obstetrics and Gynecology, Perelman School of Medicine, University of Pennsylvania, 3400 Civic Center Blvd, Smilow CTR, Philadelphia, PA 19104, USA. [2]Department of Radiation Oncology, Qilu Hospital of Shandong University, Jinan 250012, China. [3]Center for Stem Cell Research and Application, Union Hospital, Tongji Medical College, Huazhong University of Science and Technology, Wuhan 430022, China. [4]Department of Pathology and Laboratory Medicine, Abramson Cancer Center, Perelman School of Medicine, University of Pennsylvania, 3400 Civic Center Blvd, Rm 8-103 Smilow CTR, Philadelphia, PA 19104, USA. [5]Present address: Janssen R&D, LLC, 1400 McKean Road, Spring House, PA 19477, USA.

References

1. Foulkes WD, Smith IE, Reis-Filho JS. Triple-negative breast cancer. N Engl J Med. 2010;363(20):1938–48.
2. Tan DS, Marchió C, Jones RL, Savage K, Smith IE, Dowsett M, Reis-Filho JS. Triple negative breast cancer: molecular profiling and prognostic impact in adjuvant anthracycline-treated patients. Breast Cancer Res Treat. 2008;111(1):27–44.
3. Morisaki T, Onishi H, Katano M. Cancer immunotherapy using NKG2D and DNAM-1 systems. Anticancer Res. 2012;32(6):2241–7.
4. Roberti MP, Mordoh J, Levy EM. Biological role of NK cells and immunotherapeutic approaches in breast cancer. Front Immunol. 2012;3:375.
5. Parkhurst MR, Riley JP, Dudley ME, Rosenberg SA. Adoptive transfer of autologous natural killer cells leads to high levels of circulating natural killer cells but does not mediate tumor regression. Clin Cancer Res. 2011;17(19):6287–97.
6. Zhang T, Lemoi BA, Sentman CL. Chimeric NK-receptor–bearing T cells mediate antitumor immunotherapy. Blood. 2005;106(5):1544–51.
7. Sallman DA, Brayer J, Sagatys EM, Lonez C, Breman E, Agaugué S, Verma B, Gilham DE, Lehmann FF, Davila ML. NKG2D-based chimeric antigen receptor therapy induced remission in a relapsed/refractory acute myeloid leukemia patient. Haematologica. 2018; https://doi.org/10.3324/haematol.2017.186742.
8. Song D-G, Ye Q, Santoro S, Fang C, Best A, Powell DJ Jr. Chimeric NKG2D CAR-expressing T cell-mediated attack of human ovarian cancer is enhanced by histone deacetylase inhibition. Hum Gene Ther. 2013;24(3):295–305.
9. Lehner M, Götz G, Proff J, Schaft N, Dörrie J, Full F, Ensser A, Muller YA, Cerwenka A, Abken H. Redirecting T cells to Ewing's sarcoma family of tumors by a chimeric NKG2D receptor expressed by lentiviral transduction or mRNA transfection. PLoS One. 2012;7(2):e31210.
10. Nausch N, Cerwenka A. NKG2D ligands in tumor immunity. Oncogene. 2008;27(45):5944–58.
11. Song D-G, Ye Q, Poussin M, Harms GM, Figini M, Powell DJ. CD27 costimulation augments the survival and antitumor activity of redirected human T cells in vivo. Blood. 2012;119(3):696–706.
12. Song D-G, Ye Q, Carpenito C, Poussin M, Wang L-P, Ji C, Figini M, June CH, Coukos G, Powell DJ. In vivo persistence, tumor localization, and antitumor activity of CAR-engineered T cells is enhanced by costimulatory signaling through CD137 (4-1BB). Cancer Res. 2011;71(13):4617–27.
13. Parry RV, Rumbley CA, Vandenberghe LH, June CH, Riley JL. CD28 and inducible costimulatory protein Src homology 2 binding domains show distinct regulation of phosphatidylinositol 3-kinase, Bcl-xL, and IL-2 expression in primary human CD4 T lymphocytes. J Immunol. 2003;171(1):166–74.
14. Zhang T, Barber A, Sentman CL. Generation of antitumor responses by genetic modification of primary human T cells with a chimeric NKG2D receptor. Cancer Res. 2006;66(11):5927–33.
15. Kim J-Y, Bae J-H, Lee S-H, Lee E-Y, Chung B-S, Kim S-H, Kang C-D. Induction of NKG2D ligands and subsequent enhancement of NK cell-mediated lysis of cancer cells by arsenic trioxide. J Immunother. 2008;31(5):475–86.
16. Long AH, Haso WM, Shern JF, Wanhainen KM, Murgai M, Ingaramo M, Smith JP, Walker AJ, Kohler ME, Venkateshwara VR. 4-1BB costimulation ameliorates T cell exhaustion induced by tonic signaling of chimeric antigen receptors. Nat Med. 2015;21(6):581–90.
17. Nausch N, Cerwenka A. NKG2D ligands in tumor immunity. Oncogene. 2008;27(45):5944.
18. Barber A, Zhang T, Sentman CL. Immunotherapy with chimeric NKG2D receptors leads to long-term tumor-free survival and development of host antitumor immunity in murine ovarian cancer. J Immunol. 2008;180(1):72–8.
19. Barber A, Zhang T, DeMars LR, Conejo-Garcia J, Roby KF, Sentman CL. Chimeric NKG2D receptor–bearing T cells as immunotherapy for ovarian cancer. Cancer Res. 2007;67(10):5003–8.
20. Barber A, Zhang T, Megli CJ, Wu J, Meehan KR, Sentman CL. Chimeric NKG2D receptor–expressing T cells as an immunotherapy for multiple myeloma. Exp Hematol. 2008;36(10):1318–28.
21. de Kruijf EM, Sajet A, van Nes JG, Putter H, Smit VT, Eagle RA, Jafferji I, Trowsdale J, Liefers GJ, van de Velde CJ. NKG2D ligand tumor expression and association with clinical outcome in early breast cancer patients: an observational study. BMC Cancer. 2012;12(1):24.
22. Kalos M, Levine BL, Porter DL, Katz S, Grupp SA, Bagg A, June CH. T cells with chimeric antigen receptors have potent antitumor effects and can establish memory in patients with advanced leukemia. Sci Transl Med. 2011;3(95):95ra73.
23. Li S, Yang J, Urban F, MacGregor J, Hughes D, Chang A, McDonagh K, Li Q. Genetically engineered T cells expressing a HER2-specific chimeric receptor mediate antigen-specific tumor regression. Cancer Gene Ther. 2008;15(6):382.
24. Zhang C, Liu J, Zhong JF, Zhang X. Engineering CAR-T cells. Biomarker Res. 2017;5(1):22.
25. Xu X-J, Song D-G, Poussin M, Ye Q, Sharma P, Rodríguez-García A, Tang Y-M, Powell DJ. Multiparameter comparative analysis reveals differential impacts of various cytokines on CART cell phenotype and function ex vivo and in vivo. Oncotarget. 2016;7(50):82354.
26. Song D-G, Ye Q, Poussin M, Chacon JA, Figini M, Powell DJ. Effective adoptive immunotherapy of triple-negative breast cancer by folate receptor-alpha redirected CAR T cells is influenced by surface antigen expression level. J Hematol Oncol. 2016;9(1):56.
27. Gupta ND. NKG2D Ligands in Cancer. University of Tennessee Health Science Center. Theses and Dissertations; 2013. p. 113.
28. Spear P, Wu M-R, Sentman M-L, Sentman CL. NKG2D ligands as therapeutic targets. Cancer Immun Arch. 2013;13(2):8.
29. Tchou J, Wang L-C, Selven B, Zhang H, Conejo-Garcia J, Borghaei H, Kalos M, Vondeheide RH, Albelda SM, June CH. Mesothelin, a novel immunotherapy target for triple negative breast cancer. Breast Cancer Res Treat. 2012;133(2):799–804.
30. Byrd TT, Fousek K, Pignata A, Szot C, Samaha H, Seaman S, Dobrolecki L, Salsman V, Oo HZ, Bielamowicz K. TEM8/ANTXR1-specific CAR T cells as a targeted therapy for triple-negative breast cancer. Cancer Res. 2018;78(2):489–500.
31. Gilham DE, Debets R, Pule M, Hawkins RE, Abken H. CAR–T cells and solid tumors: tuning T cells to challenge an inveterate foe. Trends Mol Med. 2012;18(7):377–84.
32. Mamonkin M, Rouce RH, Tashiro H, Brenner MK. A T-cell–directed chimeric antigen receptor for the selective treatment of T-cell malignancies. Blood. 2015;126(8):983–92.
33. Mamonkin M, Mukherjee M, Srinivasan M, Sharma S, Gomes-Silva D, Mo F, Krenciute G, Orange JS, Brenner MK. Reversible transgene expression reduces fratricide and permits 4-1BB costimulation of CAR T cells directed to T-cell malignancies. Cancer Immunol Res. 2018;6(1):47–58.
34. Kershaw MH, Westwood JA, Darcy PK. Gene-engineered T cells for cancer therapy. Nat Rev Cancer. 2013;13(8):525.
35. Frigault MJ, Lee J, Basil MC, Carpenito C, Motohashi S, Scholler J, Kawalekar OU, Guedan S, McGettigan SE, Posey AD. Identification of chimeric antigen receptors that mediate constitutive or inducible proliferation of T cells. Cancer Immunol Res. 2015;3(4):356–67.
36. VanSeggelen H, Hammill JA, Dvorkin-Gheva A, Tantalo DG, Kwiecien JM, Denisova GF, Rabinovich B, Wan Y, Bramson JL. T cells engineered with chimeric antigen receptors targeting NKG2D ligands display lethal toxicity in mice. Mol Ther. 2015;23(10):1600–10.
37. Lynn RC, Powell DJ. Strain-dependent lethal toxicity in NKG2D ligand-targeted CAR T-cell therapy. Mol Ther. 2015;23(10):1559–61.
38. Nikiforow S, Werner L, Murad J, Jacobs M, Johnston L, Patches S, White R, Daley H, Negre H, Reder J. Safety data from a first-in-human phase 1 trial of NKG2D chimeric antigen receptor-T cells in AML/MDS and multiple myeloma. Blood. 2016;128(22):4052.

Permissions

All chapters in this book were first published in JH&O, by BioMed Central; hereby published with permission under the Creative Commons Attribution License or equivalent. Every chapter published in this book has been scrutinized by our experts. Their significance has been extensively debated. The topics covered herein carry significant findings which will fuel the growth of the discipline. They may even be implemented as practical applications or may be referred to as a beginning point for another development.

The contributors of this book come from diverse backgrounds, making this book a truly international effort. This book will bring forth new frontiers with its revolutionizing research information and detailed analysis of the nascent developments around the world.

We would like to thank all the contributing authors for lending their expertise to make the book truly unique. They have played a crucial role in the development of this book. Without their invaluable contributions this book wouldn't have been possible. They have made vital efforts to compile up to date information on the varied aspects of this subject to make this book a valuable addition to the collection of many professionals and students.

This book was conceptualized with the vision of imparting up-to-date information and advanced data in this field. To ensure the same, a matchless editorial board was set up. Every individual on the board went through rigorous rounds of assessment to prove their worth. After which they invested a large part of their time researching and compiling the most relevant data for our readers.

The editorial board has been involved in producing this book since its inception. They have spent rigorous hours researching and exploring the diverse topics which have resulted in the successful publishing of this book. They have passed on their knowledge of decades through this book. To expedite this challenging task, the publisher supported the team at every step. A small team of assistant editors was also appointed to further simplify the editing procedure and attain best results for the readers.

Apart from the editorial board, the designing team has also invested a significant amount of their time in understanding the subject and creating the most relevant covers. They scrutinized every image to scout for the most suitable representation of the subject and create an appropriate cover for the book.

The publishing team has been an ardent support to the editorial, designing and production team. Their endless efforts to recruit the best for this project, has resulted in the accomplishment of this book. They are a veteran in the field of academics and their pool of knowledge is as vast as their experience in printing. Their expertise and guidance has proved useful at every step. Their uncompromising quality standards have made this book an exceptional effort. Their encouragement from time to time has been an inspiration for everyone.

The publisher and the editorial board hope that this book will prove to be a valuable piece of knowledge for researchers, students, practitioners and scholars across the globe.

List of Contributors

Hong Li, Ke Wang and Liang Gao
Department of Neurosurgery, Shanghai Tenth People's Hospital, Tongji University School of Medicine, Shanghai 200072, People's Republic of China

Lei Chen, Jun-jie Li and Qiang Zhou
Department of Neurosurgery, Nanfang Hospital, Southern Medical University, Guangzhou 510515, Guangdong Province, People's Republic of China

Song-tao Qi and Yun-tao Lu
Department of Neurosurgery, Nanfang Hospital, Southern Medical University, Guangzhou 510515, Guangdong Province, People's Republic of China
Nanfang Neurology Research Institution, Nanfang Hospital, Guangzhou 510515, Guangdong Province, People's Republic of China
Nanfang Glioma Center, Guangzhou 510515, Guangdong Province, People's Republic of China

Annie Huang
Brain Tumor Research Center, The Hospital for Sick Children, Toronto, Canada

Wei-wen Liu
Department of Plastic and Aesthetic Surgery, Nanfang Hospital, Southern Medical University, Guangzhou 510515, Guangdong Province, People's Republic of China

Meng Zhang
Department of Pathology, Fudan University Shanghai Cancer Center, Shanghai 200032, China
Department of Pathology, Shanghai Medical College, Fudan University, Shanghai, China
Institute of Pathology, Fudan University, Shanghai, China

Xiang Du
Department of Pathology, Fudan University Shanghai Cancer Center, Shanghai 200032, China
Department of Pathology, Shanghai Medical College, Fudan University, Shanghai, China
Institute of Pathology, Fudan University, Shanghai, China
Department of Oncology, Shanghai Medical College, Fudan University, Shanghai, China
Institutes of Biomedical Sciences, Fudan University, Shanghai, China

Weiwei Weng, Qiongyan Zhang, Shujuan Ni, Cong Tan, Midie Xu and Hui Sun
Department of Pathology, Fudan University Shanghai Cancer Center, Shanghai 200032, China
Institute of Pathology, Fudan University, Shanghai, China
Department of Oncology, Shanghai Medical College, Fudan University, Shanghai, China

Ping Wei
Department of Pathology, Fudan University Shanghai Cancer Center, Shanghai 200032, China
Institute of Pathology, Fudan University, Shanghai, China
Department of Oncology, Shanghai Medical College, Fudan University, Shanghai, China
Institutes of Biomedical Sciences, Fudan University, Shanghai, China
Cancer Institute, Fudan University Shanghai Cancer Center, Shanghai, China

Yong Wu
Institute of Pathology, Fudan University, Shanghai, China
Department of Oncology, Shanghai Medical College, Fudan University, Shanghai, China

Chenchen Liu
Department of Oncology, Shanghai Medical College, Fudan University, Shanghai, China
Cancer Institute, Fudan University Shanghai Cancer Center, Shanghai, China

Pu Fang, Jin Dai, Lauren Cole and Javier Andres Camacho
Center for Metabolic Disease Research, Lewis Kats School of Medicine, Temple University, Medical Education and Research Building, Room 1060, 3500 N. Broad Street, Philadelphia, PA 19140, USA

Xiao-Feng Yang and Hong Wang
Center for Metabolic Disease Research, Lewis Kats School of Medicine, Temple University, Medical Education and Research Building, Room 1060, 3500 N. Broad Street, Philadelphia, PA 19140, USA
Department of Pharmacology, Lewis Kats School of Medicine, Temple University, Philadelphia, PA, USA

Xinyuan Li
Department of Pathology and Laboratory Medicine,
University of Pennsylvania, Philadelphia, PA, USA

Yuling Zhang and Jingfeng Wang
Cardiovascular Medicine Department, Sun Yat-
Sen Memorial Hospital, Sun Yat-Sen University,
Guangzhou 510120, China

Yong Ji
Key Laboratory of Cardiovascular Disease and
Molecular Intervention, Nanjing Medical University,
Nanjing, China

**Peiwei Yang, Jieyi Gu, Xiaowei Chi, Chen Liu,
Ying Wang, Qingbo Sun and Shengnan Zhang**
The Engineering Research Center of Peptide Drug
Discovery and Development, China Pharmaceutical
University, Nanjing 210009, People's Republic of
China

Erhao Zhang
The Engineering Research Center of Peptide Drug
Discovery and Development, China Pharmaceutical
University, Nanjing 210009, People's Republic of
China
Basic Medical Research Center, School of Medicine,
Nantong University, Nantong 226001, People's
Republic of China

Jianpeng Xue, Weiyan Qi and Jialiang Hu
The Engineering Research Center of Peptide Drug
Discovery and Development, China Pharmaceutical
University, Nanjing 210009, People's Republic of
China
State Key Laboratory of Natural Medicines, Ministry
of Education, China Pharmaceutical University,
Nanjing 210009, People's Republic of China

Hanmei Xu
The Engineering Research Center of Peptide Drug
Discovery and Development, China Pharmaceutical
University, Nanjing 210009, People's Republic of
China
State Key Laboratory of Natural Medicines, Ministry
of Education, China Pharmaceutical University,
Nanjing 210009, People's Republic of China
Nanjing Anji Biotechnology Co., Ltd, Nanjing
210046, People's Republic of China

Heming Wu
Jiangsu Key Laboratory of Oral Diseases, Department
of Oral and Maxillofacial Surgery, Affiliated Hospital
of Stomatology, Nanjing Medical University, Nanjing
211166, People's Republic of China

**Rocco Stirparo, So ie Demeyer, Charles E. de Bock,
Olga Gielen and Jan Cools**
Center for Cancer Biology, VIB, Leuven, Belgium
Center for Human Genetics, KU Leuven, Herestraat
49, B-3000 Leuven, Belgium

Carmen Vicente
Center for Cancer Biology, VIB, Leuven, Belgium
Center for Human Genetics, KU Leuven, Herestraat
49, B-3000 Leuven, Belgium
Centro de Investigación Médica Aplicada, Av. de
Pío XII, 55, 31008 Pamplona, Spain

Mardelle Atkins and Georg Halder
Center for Cancer Biology, VIB, Leuven, Belgium
Department of Oncology, KU Leuven, Leuven,
Belgium

Jiekun Yan
Center for Human Genetics, KU Leuven, Herestraat
49, B-3000 Leuven, Belgium
Center for Brain & Disease Research, VIB, Leuven,
Belgium

Bassem A. Hassan
Center for Human Genetics, KU Leuven, Herestraat
49, B-3000 Leuven, Belgium
Center for Brain & Disease Research, VIB, Leuven,
Belgium
Institut du Cerveau et de la Moelle Epinière
(ICM) - Hôpital Pitié-Salpêtrière, UPMC, Sorbonne
Universités, Inserm, CNRS, Paris, France

Federico Rossari
Institute of Life Sciences, Scuola Superiore
Sant'Anna, Piazza Martiri della Libertà, 33, 56127
Pisa, PI, Italy
University of Pisa, Pisa, Italy

Filippo Minutolo
Department of Pharmacy, University of Pisa, Pisa,
Italy

Enrico Orciuolo
Department of Clinical and Experimental Medicine,
Section of Hematology, Azienda Ospedaliero
Universitaria Pisana, Pisa, Italy

Lixin Chen
Department of Pharmacology, Medical College,
Jinan University, Guangzhou 510632, China

Zhuoyu Gu and Meisheng Yu
Department of Pharmacology, Medical College, Jinan University, Guangzhou 510632, China
Department of Pathophysiology, Medical College, Jinan University, Guangzhou, China

Xiaoya Yang
Department of Pathophysiology, Medical College, Jinan University, Guangzhou, China
Department of Physiology, Medical College, Jinan University, Guangzhou 510632, China

Yixin Li
Department of Clinical Oncology, The First Affiliated Hospital, Zhengzhou University, Zhengzhou, China

Zhanru Chen, Chan Zhao and Liwei Wang
Department of Physiology, Medical College, Jinan University, Guangzhou 510632, China

Hui Sun and Weiqi Sheng
Department of Pathology, Fudan University Shanghai Cancer Center, Shanghai 200032, China

Mi-die Xu
Department of Pathology, Fudan University Shanghai Cancer Center, Shanghai 200032, China
Department of Pathology, Tissue bank, Fudan University Shanghai Cancer Center, Shanghai 200032, China

Zhaohui Huang
Wuxi Cancer Institute, Affiliated Hospital of Jiangnan University, Wuxi, Jiangsu, China

Guoshuang Shen, Dengfeng Ren, Ziyi Wang, Fuxing Zhao, Raees Ahmad and Jiuda Zhao
Affiliated Hospital of Qinghai University, Affiliated Cancer Hospital of Qinghai University, Xining 810000, China

Fangchao Zheng
Affiliated Hospital of Qinghai University, Affiliated Cancer Hospital of Qinghai University, Xining 810000, China
Shouguang Hospital of Traditional Chinese Medicine, Weifang 262700, China

Feng Du
Peking University Cancer Hospital and Institute, Beijing 100142, China

Andrea Ghelli Luserna Di Rorà, Enrica Imbrogno, Anna Ferrari, Valentina Robustelli, Simona Righi, Elena Sabattini, Nicoletta Testoni, Carmen Baldazzi, Cristina Papayannidis, Maria Chiara Abbenante, Giovanni Marconi, Stefania Paolini, Sarah Parisi, Chiara Sartor, Maria Chiara Fontana and Michele Cavo
Department of Experimental, Diagnostic and Specialty Medicine, Institute of Hematology "L. e A. Seràgnoli", University of Bologna, Via Massarenti 9, 40138 Bologna, Italy

Ilaria Iacobucci
Department of Experimental, Diagnostic and Specialty Medicine, Institute of Hematology "L. e A.Seràgnoli", University of Bologna, Via Massarenti 9, 40138 Bologna, Italy
Department of Pathology, St.Jude Children's Research Hospital, Memphis, TN, USA

Maria Vittoria Verga Falzacappa, Chiara Ronchini and Pier Giuseppe Pelicci
Laboratory of Clinical Genomics, European Institute of Oncology, Milan, Italy

Timothy J. Yen
Cancer Biology Program, Fox Chase Cancer Center, Philadelphia, PA, USA

Neil Beeharry
Cancer Biology Program, Fox Chase Cancer Center, Philadelphia, PA, USA
LAM Therapeutics, Guilford, CT, USA

Serena De Matteis
Biosciences Laboratory, Istituto Scientifico Romagnolo per lo Studio e la Cura dei Tumori (IRST) IRCCS, Meldola, Italy

Giovanni Martinelli
Istituto Scientifico Romagnolo per lo Studio e la Cura dei Tumori (IRST) IRCCS, Meldola, Italy

Changhong Liu, Yan Zhang, Peiyao Li, Jianbo Feng, Haijuan Fu, Chunhua Zhao and Yingnan Sun
Hunan Provincial Tumor Hospital and the Affiliated Tumor Hospital of Xiangya Medical School, Central South University, Changsha 410006, Hunan, China
Cancer Research Institute, School of Basic Medical Science, Central South University, Changsha 410078, Hunan, China

Key Laboratory of Carcinogenesis and Cancer Invasion, Ministry of Education, Changsha 410078, Hunan, China
Key Laboratory of Carcinogenesis, Ministry of Health, Changsha 410078, Hunan, China

Minghua Wu
Cancer Research Institute, School of Basic Medical Science, Central South University, Changsha 410078, Hunan, China
Key Laboratory of Carcinogenesis and Cancer Invasion, Ministry of Education, Changsha 410078, Hunan, China
Key Laboratory of Carcinogenesis, Ministry of Health, Changsha 410078, Hunan, China

Xiaoling She
Second Xiangya Hospital, Central South University, Changsha 410011, Hunan, China

Li Fan
Department of Biochemistry, University of California, Riverside, CA 92521, USA

Qing Liu
Xiangya Hospital, Central South University, Changsha 410008, Hunan, China

Qiang Liu
Third Xiangya Hospital, Central South University, Changsha 410013, Hunan, China

Myriam Labopin
Service d'Hématologie Clinique et Thérapie Cellulaire, AP-HP, Hôpital Saint-Antoine, Paris F-75012, France

Christina Cho
Adult Bone Marrow Transplantation Service, Memorial Sloan Kettering Cancer Center, New York, NY, USA
Department of Medicine, Weill Cornell Medical College, New York, NY, USA

Didier Blaise
Programme de Transplantation & Therapie Cellulaire, Centre de Recherche en Cancérologie de Marseille, Institut Paoli Calmettes, Marseille, France

Edouard Forcade
CHU Bordeaux, Hôpital Haut-leveque, Pessac, France

Corentin Orvain
Service des Maladies du Sang, CHRU, Angers, France

Moshe Talpaz
University of Michigan, Ann Arbor, MI, USA

Susan Erickson-Viitanen and Kevin Hou
Incyte Corporation, Wilmington, DE, USA

Solomon Hamburg
Tower Hematology Oncology Medical Group, Beverly Hills, CA, USA

Maria R. Baer
University of Maryland, Greenebaum Comprehensive Cancer Center, 22 S. Greene St, Baltimore, MD 21201, USA

Yang Li, Jialei Hu, Yue Pan, Yujia Shan, Bing Liu and Li Jia
College of Laboratory Medicine, Dalian Medical University, Dalian 116044, Liaoning Province, China

Changqian Zeng
Medical College, Dalian University, Dalian 116622, Liaoning Province, China

Zhentao Liu, Zuhua Chen, Jingyuan Wang, Mengqi Zhang and Cheng Zhang
Key laboratory of Carcinogenesis and Translational Research (Ministry of Education/Beijing), Department of Gastrointestinal Oncology, Peking University Cancer Hospital and Institute, 52 Fucheng Road, Haidian District, Beijing 100142, China

Jing Gao and Lin Shen
Key laboratory of Carcinogenesis and Translational Research (Ministry of Education/Beijing), Department of Gastrointestinal Oncology, Peking University Cancer Hospital and Institute, 52 Fucheng Road, Haidian District, Beijing 100142, China
Department of Oncology, Peking University Shenzhen Hospital, 1120 Lianhua Road, Shenzhen 518036, Guangdong, China

Zhongwu Li and Bin Dong
Key Laboratory of Carcinogenesis and Translational Research (Ministry of Education/Beijing), Department of Pathology, Peking University Cancer Hospital and Institute, 52 Fucheng Road, Haidian District, Beijing 100142, China

Shubin Wang
Department of Oncology, Peking University Shenzhen Hospital, 1120 Lianhua Road, Shenzhen 518036, Guangdong, China

Yali Han
Ovarian Cancer Research Center, Department of Obstetrics and Gynecology, Perelman School of Medicine, University of Pennsylvania, 3400 Civic Center Blvd, Smilow CTR, Philadelphia, PA 19104, USA
Department of Radiation Oncology, Qilu Hospital of Shandong University, Jinan 250012, China

Wei Xie
Ovarian Cancer Research Center, Department of Obstetrics and Gynecology, Perelman School of Medicine, University of Pennsylvania, 3400 Civic Center Blvd, Smilow CTR, Philadelphia, PA 19104, USA
Center for Stem Cell Research and Application, Union Hospital, Tongji Medical College, Huazhong University of Science and Technology, Wuhan 430022, China

Daniel J. Powell Jr
Ovarian Cancer Research Center, Department of Obstetrics and Gynecology, Perelman School of Medicine, University of Pennsylvania, 3400 Civic Center Blvd, Smilow CTR, Philadelphia, PA 19104, USA
Department of Pathology and Laboratory Medicine, Abramson Cancer Center, Perelman School of Medicine, University of Pennsylvania, 3400 Civic Center Blvd, Rm 8-103 Smilow CTR, Philadelphia, PA 19104, USA

De-Gang Song
Ovarian Cancer Research Center, Department of Obstetrics and Gynecology, Perelman School of Medicine, University of Pennsylvania, 3400 Civic Center Blvd, Smilow CTR, Philadelphia, PA 19104, USA
Janssen R&D, LLC, 1400 McKean Road, Spring House, PA 19477, USA

Index

www.ingramcontent.com/pod-product-compliance
Lightning Source LLC
Chambersburg PA
CBHW061257190326
41458CB00011B/3697